# Exploring
# Medical Language

*A Student-Directed Approach*

# Exploring Medical Language

## A Student-Directed Approach

MYRNA LaFLEUR BROOKS, R.N., B. Ed.

Founding President of the
National Association of Health Unit Coordinators;
Director, Health Services Management Program,
GateWay Community College, Phoenix, Arizona

with 210 illustrations

Illustrations by **May S. Cheney** and **Kimberly Battista**

THIRD EDITION

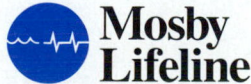

Mosby
Lifeline

St. Louis  Baltimore  Boston  Chicago  London  Madrid  Philadelphia  Sydney  Toronto

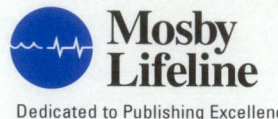

**Mosby
Lifeline**

Dedicated to Publishing Excellence

*Publisher:* David T. Culverwell
*Executive Editor:* Richard A. Weimer
*Developmental Editor:* Mary Beth Ryan Warthen
*Assistant Editor:* Julie Scardiglia
*Editorial Assistant:* Colleen E. Foley
*Project Manager:* John Rogers
*Production Editor:* Chuck Furgason
*Designer:* Julie Taugner
*Cover Designer:* GW Graphics & Publishing
*Cover Art:* Stevens Jay Carter
*Manufacturing Supervisor:* Betty Richmond

**Third Edition**

Printed in the United State of America
Composition by Clarinda Company
Printing/binding by Van Hoffman Press, Inc.

Mosby-Year Book, Inc.
11830 Westline Industrial Drive
St. Louis, Missouri 63146

**ISBN 0-8016-6984-7**

94 95 96 97 98 / 9 8 7 6 5 4 3 2 2 1

To my mother and father,
**Francis** and **Christina Weber,**
my sisters,
**Joan, Helene, Patricia,**
and my brothers,
**Jerry, Gary,** and **Richard,**
whose love through my formative years
continues to provide me with
a sense of balance and inner strength.

# Preface

## INTRODUCTION

Welcome to the third edition of *Exploring Medical Language*. The study of medical terminology continues as a requirement in health care curricula. Indeed it should. Basic knowledge of medical language facilitates the understanding of scientific and medical principles; medical language is used and understood by all members of the health care team. Many employees of law firms, insurance agencies, and other medical fields have also discovered the language used by medical professionals.

Medical knowledge continues to increase dramatically, while our fast-paced society provides less and less time for study of such knowledge. *Exploring Medical Language* is designed to assist students and others interested in learning medical terminology to master the language of medicine quickly and easily. The text can be used for formal classroom study, for independent college study, or for individual learning.

## WORD PARTS

Word parts are introduced in an orderly manner according to body systems. Many exercises are provided to help the student memorize the word parts and their meaning. At first glance the number of exercises may seem excessive and repetitive. However, after completing them, the student will have the knowledge needed to learn the medical terms built from word parts included in each chapter. Many exercises, including word building, analyzing, defining, and spelling, are provided. This approach to medical terminology allows the student to amass a large working medical vocabulary. Students will develop an appreciation for the language of medicine and a curiosity about medical terms that will linger long after the course is completed.

## MEDICAL TERMS

Medical terms not built from word parts are often omitted from programmed texts. Because the language of medicine is incomplete without them, many of these words are included in this text in separate lists and exercises. Instructors wishing to use the word part method only can easily omit these lists from the curriculum.

## ANATOMICAL TERMS

Anatomical terms for each body system are also included in each chapter. They are designed to accommodate students not versed in anatomy. These lists can also be easily omitted or used as a review if students are required to take a separate anatomy course.

## CHAPTERS

*The first chapter* in the third edition is again devoted to the introduction of word parts and rules for combining them to form meaningful medical terms. *Throughout the text more emphasis is placed on the combining form, therefore word roots will be presented in the combining form format.*

*Chapters 2 through 15* remain divided according to body structure and systems. Word lists are divided into diagnostic terms, surgical terms, diagnostic procedural terms, and additional terms. New terms reflecting advances in the medical field, such as "endoscopic surgical procedures," and terms relating to AIDS have been added. More illustrations are added to assist students to visualize the terminology and three more study tools are included throughout this new edition. Summary pages, listing the terms introduced in each chapter, can be found before the answer key sections. To aid students in their review, crossword puzzle exercises have been added. Also, new medical case studies for most chapters are written to include medical terms in a health care environment context.

*Chapter 16,* the final chapter, addresses directional terms, and anatomical planes and regions. Often this information is placed at the beginning of a text, so students can apply this information while studying the terms related to body systems. I have resisted placing this information first because it digresses from the format of the text. For those students or instructors wanting to learn directional terms, and anatomical planes and regions first, begin the course of study with Chapter 16.

## LEARNING AIDS

**Flashcards,** which were welcomed by students in the second edition, are again included. The word part as well as the meaning are recorded on the back of the card to reinforce learning. A **pronunciation audiotape** based on the text is available, and the crossword puzzles have been moved from the Instructor's Guide to the textbook. An **Instructor's Guide** and **Instructor's Resource Kit** are also available. In addition, a **computerized test-bank, computer assisted learning program,** and **computerized student self-assessment program** are available from the publisher.

If this text enables the user to acquire an appreciation and an understanding of the fascinating language of medicine, it will have met its purpose.

**Myrna LaFleur Brooks**

# Acknowledgments

Revising a textbook such as this, in which one chapter builds upon the last, requires a great deal of mental discipline. It is very easy to define a word part one way in one chapter and define the same part another way in a succeeding chapter, both correct but confusing to the learner. Therefore I am most grateful for the dedicated contributions of our reviewers who were able to assist not only with content of the chapters but also with consistency of the chapters. They are:

**Bob DeLorme, EDS, RRT, RCP**
Program Director/Instructor, Respiratory Therapy Technology
Gwinnett Technical Institute, Lawrenceville, Georgia

**David J. Fitzpatrick**
Director for Dental Center Administration
Naval Dental Center, Newport, Rhode Island

**Marty Hitchcock**
Medical Terminology Instructor
Gwinnett Technical Institute, Lawrenceville, Georgia

**Carole Howard, RRA**
Medical Record Consultant
Chabot College, Hayward, California

**Ronnie Jenkins**
Chairman, Technologies Department
Martin Community College, Williamston, North Carolina

**Trudi Kenny, RN, BSc N, CMA**
Department Chair, Allied Health
Baker College, Muskegon, Michigan

**Maryagnes Luczak, CMA**
Director of Training
Career Training Institute, Monroeville, Pennsylvania

**Kim D. Pack, MS, RRA**
Coordinator, Medical Record Technology Program
College of Dupage, Glen Ellyn, Illinois

**Trudy Parks, RT**
Instructor, Radiologic Technology
Lorain County Community College, Elyria, Ohio

**Bernice D. Stiansen, RN, B Sc N**
Medical Terminology Instructor
Grant MacEwan Community College, Edmonton, Alberta

**Pat Tate**
EMT/CPR Instructor
Mountain Empire Community College, Big Stone Gap, Virginia

Thanks to Rosemary Kesler, Director, Surgical Technology Program, GateWay Community College, Phoenix, Arizona for assisting in updating the surgical terms added to this edition.

A special thanks to Charles C. Thomas, Publisher for allowing me to use the marvelous book *The Story Behind Words* written by Harry Wain for the origin of many of the medical terms included in the text.

I wish to express thanks to the expert staff at Mosby Lifeline who gave freely of their support and expertise. Thanks to Executive Editor Rick Weimer, Developmental Editor Mary Beth Ryan Warthen, Assistant Editor Julie Scardiglia, Editorial Assistant Colleen Foley, and the rest of the Mosby staff.

And finally to the students, whose overall desire to enjoy learning and to learn as much as possible in a limited period of time and whose feedback has played a major role in revising the text to make it a better and more enjoyable product, the biggest thanks of all.

# How to Use This Text

Medical language is used by people employed in the health care field. To a newcomer, it may seem that the language is designed to be difficult and confusing. However, once you realize that many of the medical terms have a structural design and can be divided into word parts and that, once learned, the word parts can be used to define the meaning of many other words, the language of medicine becomes a fascinating subject. The following information explains how to best use this text.

## CHAPTER 1

The first chapter may well be the most important chapter in the book. It contains information, rules, and concepts used throughout the remaining chapters. In the first chapter you are introduced to the word parts—word roots, prefixes, suffixes, and combining vowels—and rules for combining them into meaningful terms. *It is important to understand the material in Chapter 1 completely before moving on to Chapter 2.* As you progress, you should refer often to Chapter 1 to refresh your memory or as a reference. Using a medical dictionary along with the textbook is helpful and will answer many questions for you.

## CHAPTERS 2 THROUGH 16
### Objectives

Each chapter begins with a list of objectives—a map describing what you can expect to learn as you progress through the chapter. Each objective is restated at the beginning of the material that relates to it. For example, the objective "Build, analyze, define, pronounce, and spell the diagnostic terms related to the digestive system" appears before the list of terms and the accompanying exercises. It tells you what you should be able to do once you complete that section of the chapter. The objective appears again at the end of the material with the instructions to place a check mark in the accompanying box when you accomplish the objective.

The objectives are repeated in this manner to help you understand where you are going and where you have been in the text. Use the objectives to help you travel this new world of knowledge.

### Anatomical Terms

The anatomical terms are the names of the body parts. Knowing them is helpful in learning the medical language. They are included in this text to assist those students not enrolled in an anatomy course. If not needed by the student, this section can be omitted or used as a review.

### Word Parts

Lists of word parts—word roots, prefixes, and suffixes—are introduced in each chapter. Learning these is important, since they are the foundation of the medical terms. Several exercises are included to assist the student in memorizing the word parts. One exercise, labeling the word roots of body parts on an anatomical diagram, is included to provide visual reinforcement. Completion of all the exercises is important for the success of the learning style used in the text. To assist you further, flash cards are included in the text.

### Medical Terms

The medical terms are divided into two lists: those that are and those that are not built from word parts. Each list has a separate objective and separate exercises. The medical terms are further divided into diagnostic terms, surgical terms, diagnostic procedural terms, and additional terms.

Once again, complete the exercises accompanying the word lists. Performing each exercise is necessary for learning this new language in a fast and easy manner. Appendix A on pages 623-637 provides a quick reference to all the word parts. Use it to assist you in completing the exercises.

## PRONUNCIATION GUIDE

The student has a readily available and simple guide to use for practicing the pronunciation of the medical terms. Since it is impractical to use all the markings of an unabridged dictionary in a medical terminology book, the pronunciations are only approximate; however, they are adequate to meet the needs of the beginning student.

In respelling for pronunciation we distorted words only minimally to indicate proper phonetic sound.

EXAMPLE:   doctor (dok-tor)
             gastric (gas-trik)

Diacritical marks are used over vowels to indicate pronunciation. The macron (ˉ) is used to indicate the long vowel sounds; the unmarked vowels indicate short vowel sounds.

EXAMPLE:   donate (dō-nāte)
             hepatoma (hep-a-tō-ma)
             ā as in ate, say
             ē as in eat, beet, see
             ī as in I, mine, sky
             ō as in oats, so
             ū as in unit, mute, loose

Vowels with no markings have the short sound.

EXAMPLE:   discuss (dis-kus)
             medical (med-i-kal)
             a as in at, lad
             e as in edge, bet
             i as in itch, wish
             o as in ox, top
             u as in sun, come

An accent mark is the stress on a certain syllable. The primary accent is indicated in this text by capital letters, and the secondary accent (which is stressed, but not as strongly as the primary accent is) is indicated by italics.

EXAMPLE:   octogenarian (*ok*-tō-jen-ĀR-ē-an)
             pancreatitis (*pan*-krē-a-TĪ-tis)

## SUMMARY PAGES

A summary at the end of each chapter contains all the words presented in the chapter. At a quick glance you can review what you need to know upon completion of the chapter. Pronunciation is included on the summary sheet. I suggest you tape record yourself pronouncing the terms and compare it with the enclosed audiotape.

After you have worked through a chapter, completing all exercises and correcting your errors, you will find that you have met the chapter objectives and feel confident and eager to move on to the next chapter and continue to build your medical vocabulary. We wish you the best as you move on to Chapter 1 and begin to discover and learn the language of medicine.

# Contents

# Color Atlas of Human Anatomy

# SKELETAL SYSTEM

**ANTERIOR VIEW OF SKELETON**
Axial skeleton is shown in blue. Appendicular system is
bone colored.

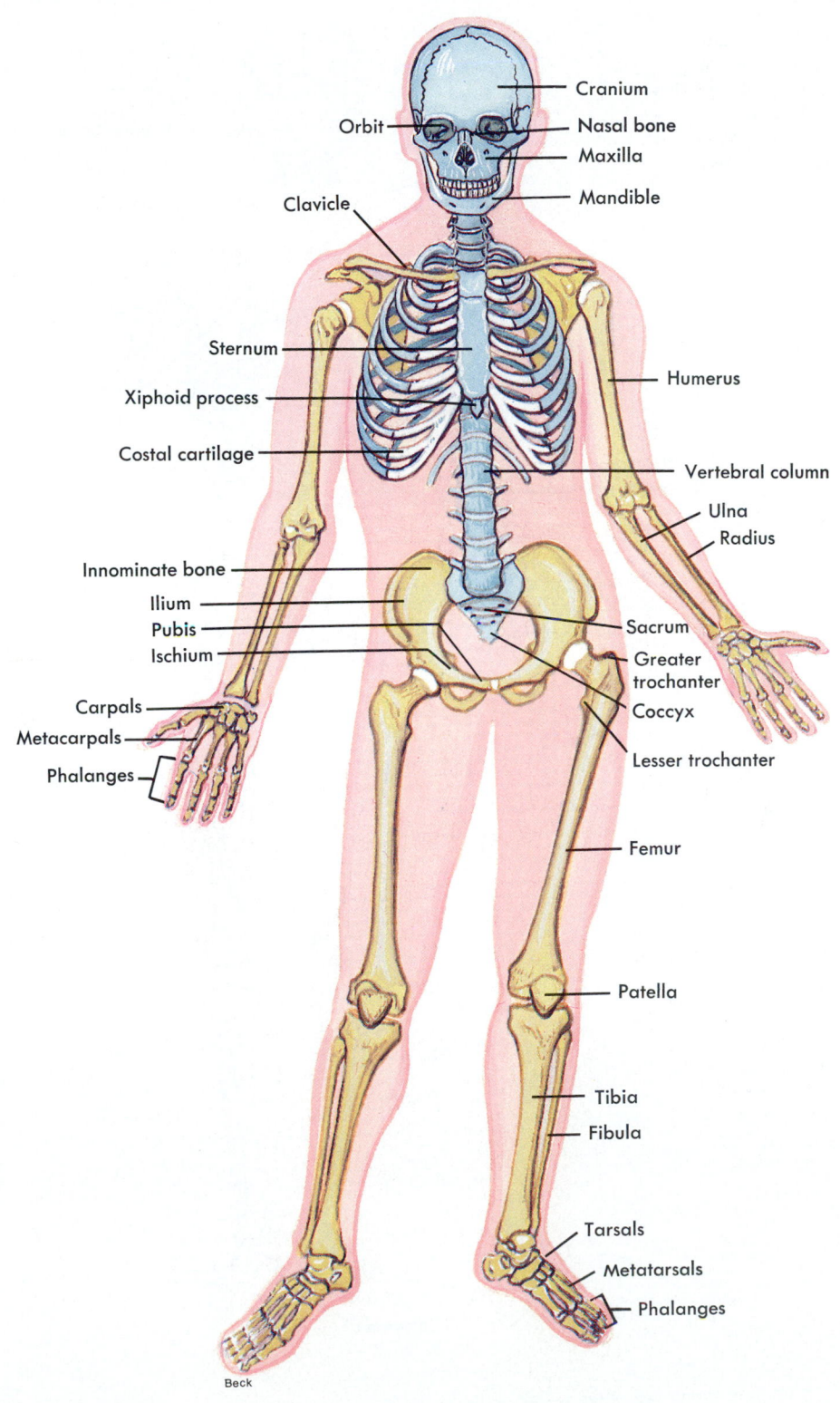

Cranium
Orbit
Nasal bone
Maxilla
Mandible
Clavicle
Sternum
Xiphoid process
Costal cartilage
Humerus
Vertebral column
Ulna
Radius
Innominate bone
Ilium
Pubis
Ischium
Sacrum
Greater trochanter
Coccyx
Lesser trochanter
Carpals
Metacarpals
Phalanges
Femur
Patella
Tibia
Fibula
Tarsals
Metatarsals
Phalanges

Beck

**A-1**

**POSTERIOR VIEW OF SKELETON**
Axial skeleton is shown in blue. Appendicular system is
bone colored.

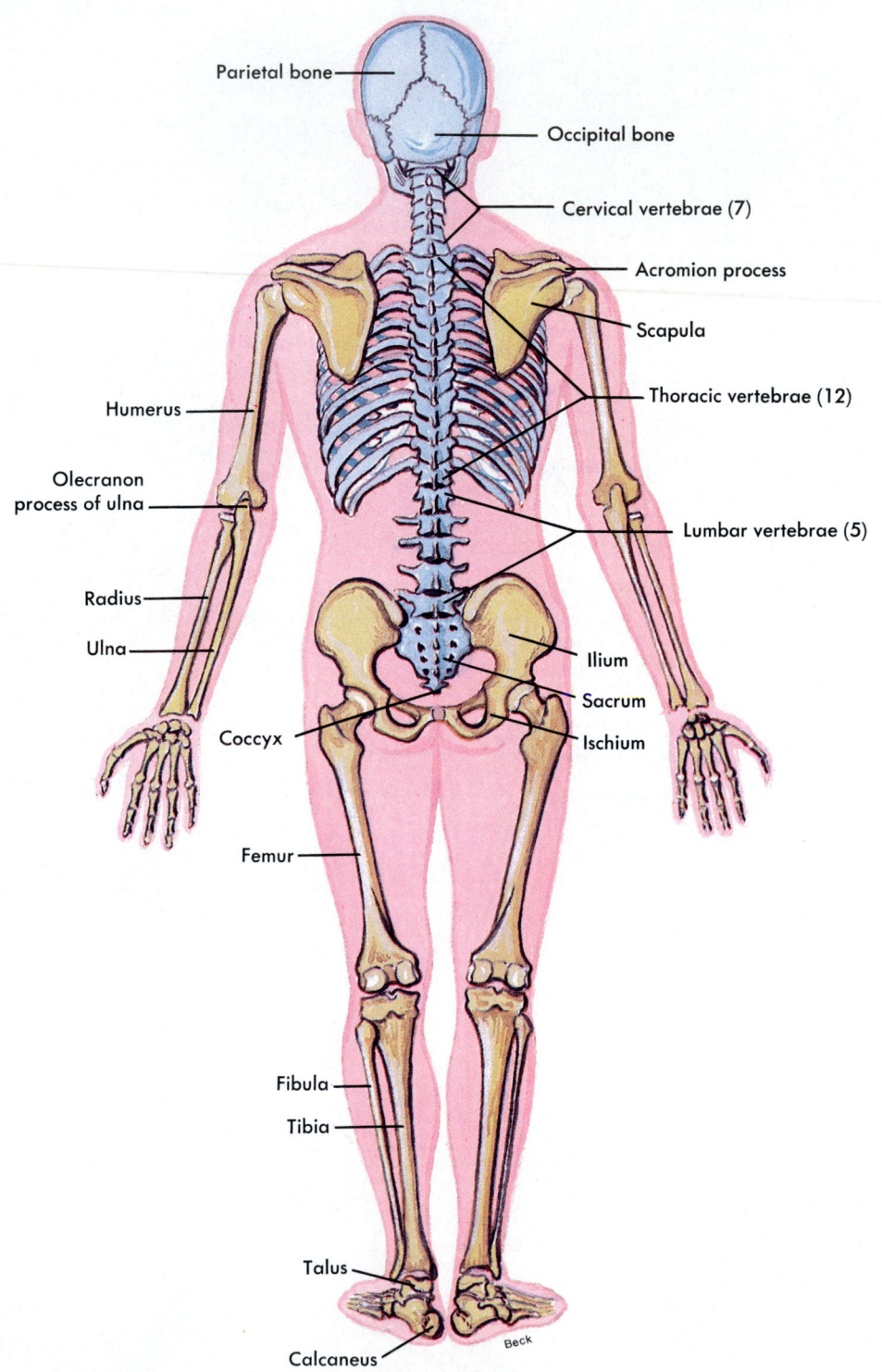

Parietal bone

Occipital bone

Cervical vertebrae (7)

Acromion process

Scapula

Thoracic vertebrae (12)

Humerus

Olecranon
process of ulna

Lumbar vertebrae (5)

Radius

Ulna

Ilium

Sacrum

Coccyx

Ischium

Femur

Fibula

Tibia

Talus

Calcaneus

Beck

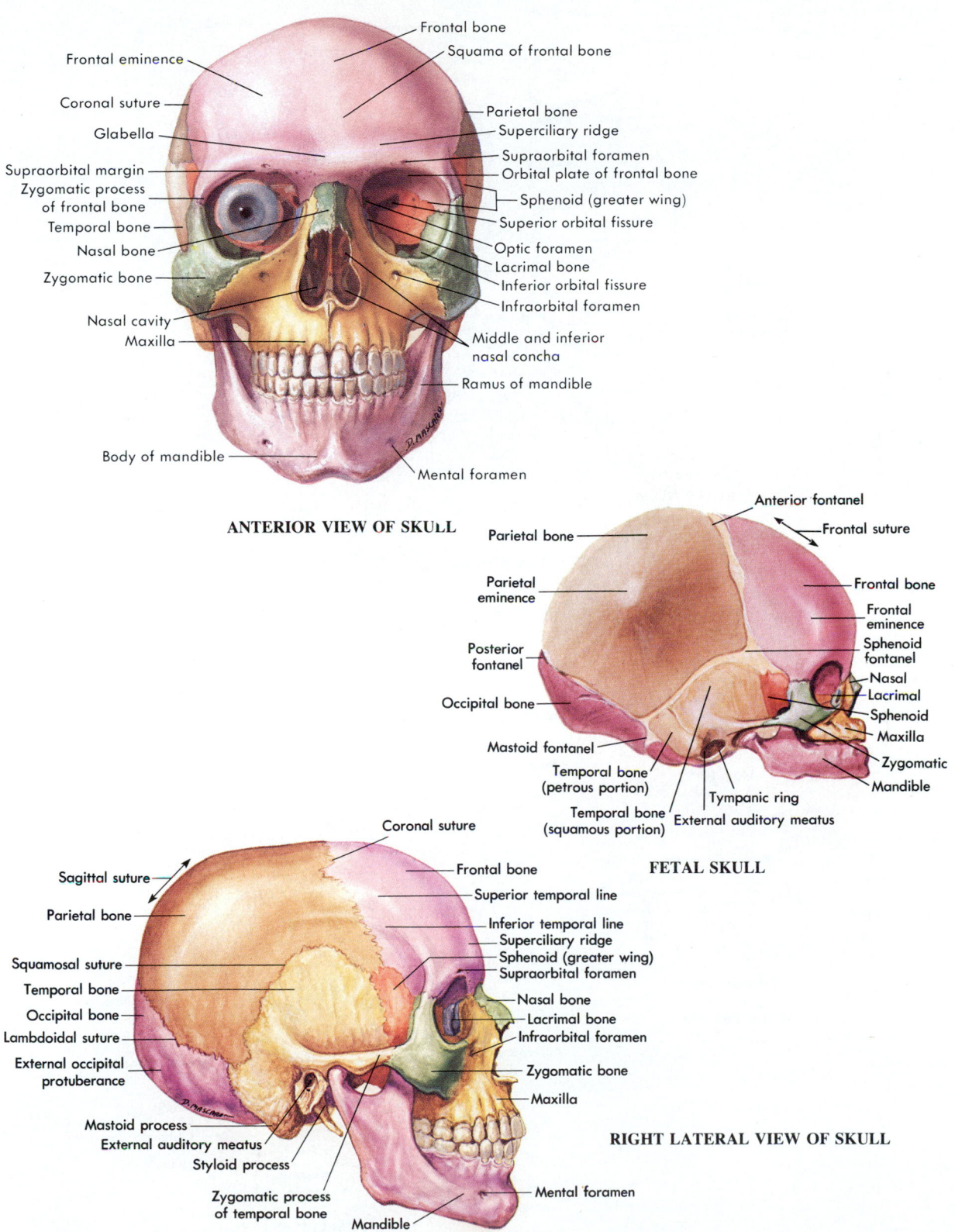

Frontal bone
Squama of frontal bone
Frontal eminence
Coronal suture
Parietal bone
Glabella
Superciliary ridge
Supraorbital foramen
Orbital plate of frontal bone
Supraorbital margin
Zygomatic process
of frontal bone
Sphenoid (greater wing)
Temporal bone
Superior orbital fissure
Nasal bone
Optic foramen
Zygomatic bone
Lacrimal bone
Inferior orbital fissure
Infraorbital foramen
Nasal cavity
Maxilla
Middle and inferior
nasal concha
Ramus of mandible
Body of mandible
Mental foramen

**ANTERIOR VIEW OF SKULL**

Anterior fontanel
Parietal bone
Frontal suture
Parietal
eminence
Frontal bone
Frontal
eminence
Sphenoid
fontanel
Posterior
fontanel
Nasal
Lacrimal
Occipital bone
Sphenoid
Maxilla
Mastoid fontanel
Zygomatic
Temporal bone
(petrous portion)
Mandible
Temporal bone
(squamous portion)
Tympanic ring
External auditory meatus

**FETAL SKULL**

Coronal suture
Sagittal suture
Frontal bone
Superior temporal line
Parietal bone
Inferior temporal line
Superciliary ridge
Squamosal suture
Sphenoid (greater wing)
Supraorbital foramen
Temporal bone
Nasal bone
Occipital bone
Lacrimal bone
Lambdoidal suture
Infraorbital foramen
External occipital
protuberance
Zygomatic bone
Maxilla
Mastoid process
External auditory meatus
Styloid process
Zygomatic process
of temporal bone
Mental foramen
Mandible

**RIGHT LATERAL VIEW OF SKULL**

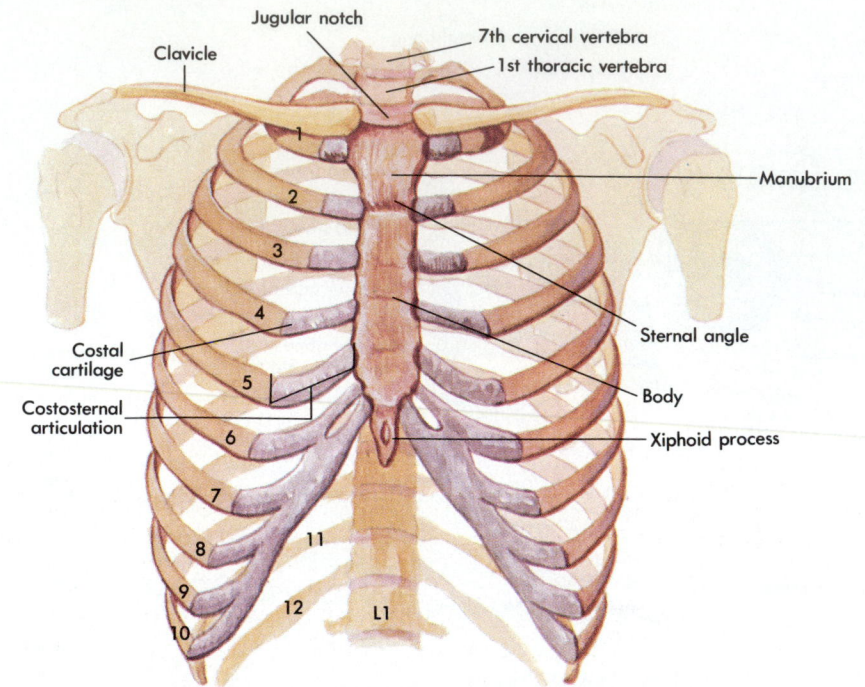

Jugular notch

Clavicle

7th cervical vertebra

1st thoracic vertebra

1

2

3

4

5

6

7

8

9

10

11

12

L1

Manubrium

Costal cartilage

Costosternal articulation

Sternal angle

Body

Xiphoid process

**THORAX AND RIBS**

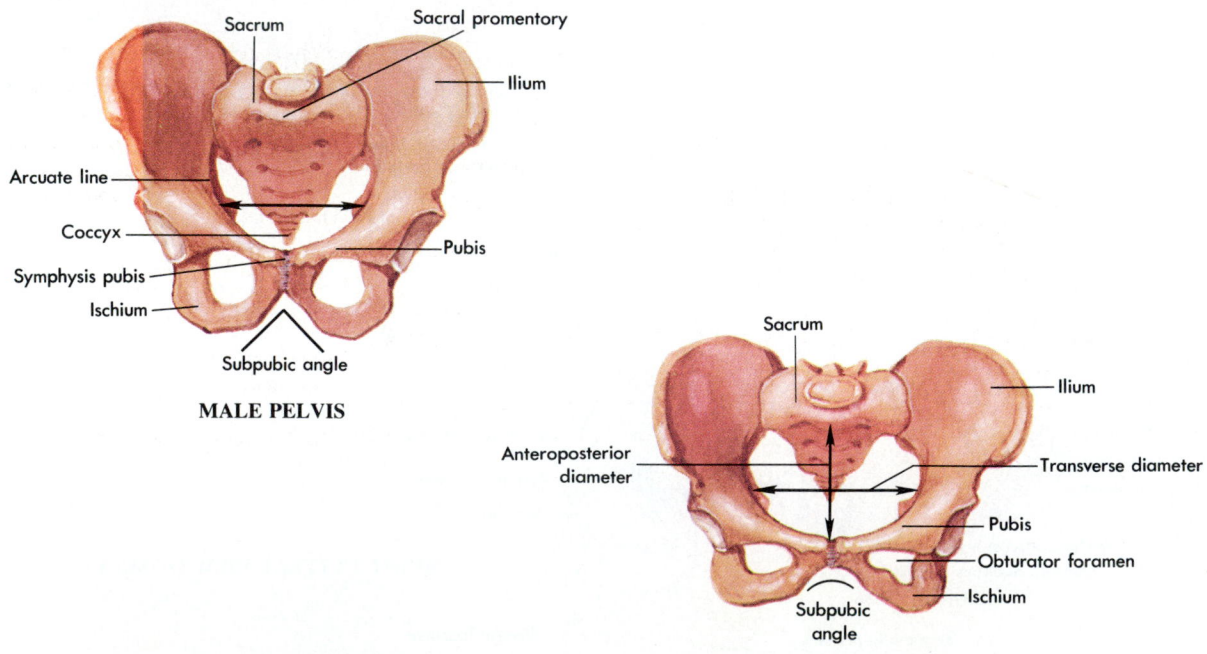

Sacrum

Sacral promentory

Ilium

Arcuate line

Coccyx

Symphysis pubis

Ischium

Subpubic angle

Pubis

**MALE PELVIS**

Sacrum

Ilium

Anteroposterior diameter

Transverse diameter

Pubis

Obturator foramen

Ischium

Subpubic angle

**FEMALE PELVIS**

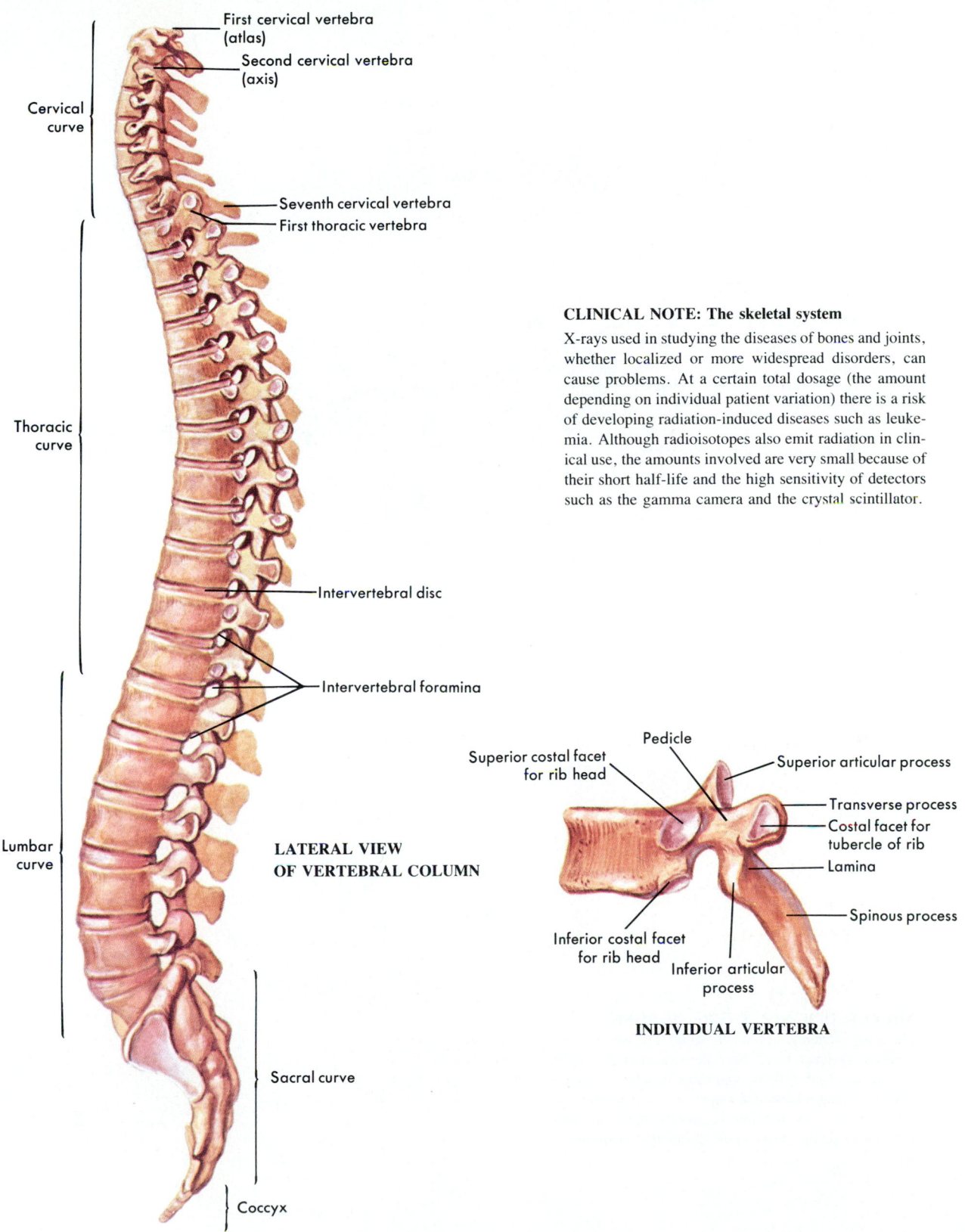

First cervical vertebra (atlas)

Second cervical vertebra (axis)

Cervical curve

Seventh cervical vertebra

First thoracic vertebra

Thoracic curve

Intervertebral disc

Intervertebral foramina

Lumbar curve

**LATERAL VIEW OF VERTEBRAL COLUMN**

Sacral curve

Coccyx

**CLINICAL NOTE: The skeletal system**

X-rays used in studying the diseases of bones and joints, whether localized or more widespread disorders, can cause problems. At a certain total dosage (the amount depending on individual patient variation) there is a risk of developing radiation-induced diseases such as leukemia. Although radioisotopes also emit radiation in clinical use, the amounts involved are very small because of their short half-life and the high sensitivity of detectors such as the gamma camera and the crystal scintillator.

Pedicle

Superior costal facet for rib head

Superior articular process

Transverse process

Costal facet for tubercle of rib

Lamina

Spinous process

Inferior costal facet for rib head

Inferior articular process

**INDIVIDUAL VERTEBRA**

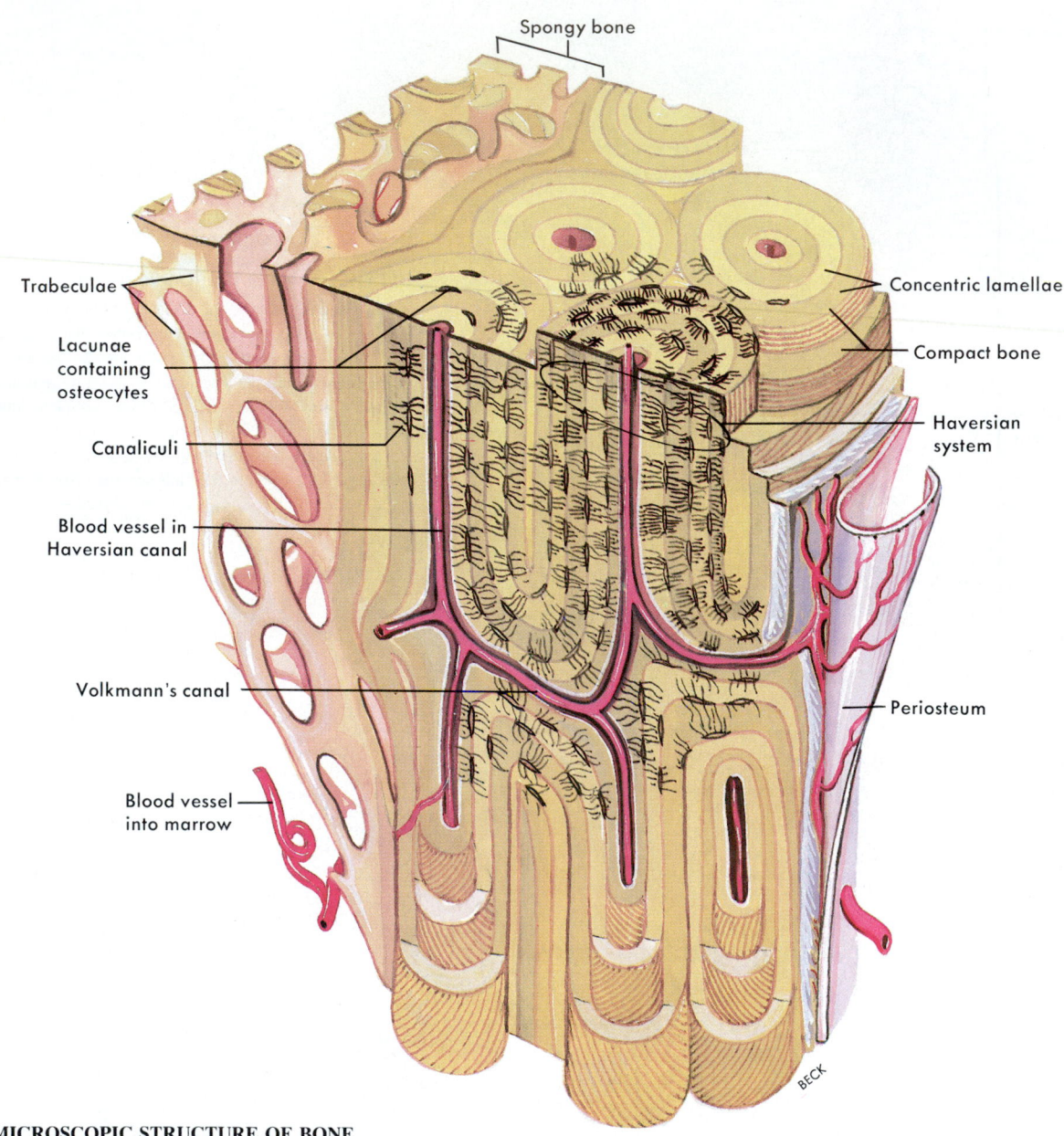

Spongy bone

Trabeculae

Lacunae
containing
osteocytes

Canaliculi

Blood vessel in
Haversian canal

Volkmann's canal

Blood vessel
into marrow

Concentric lamellae

Compact bone

Haversian
system

Periosteum

BECK

**MICROSCOPIC STRUCTURE OF BONE**
Haversian systems, several of which are shown here,
compose compact bone. Note the structures that make
up one haversian system: concentric lamellae, lacunae,
canaliculi, and a haversian canal. Shown bordering the
compact bone on the left is spongy bone, a name
descriptive of the many open spaces that characterize
it.

# MUSCULAR SYSTEM

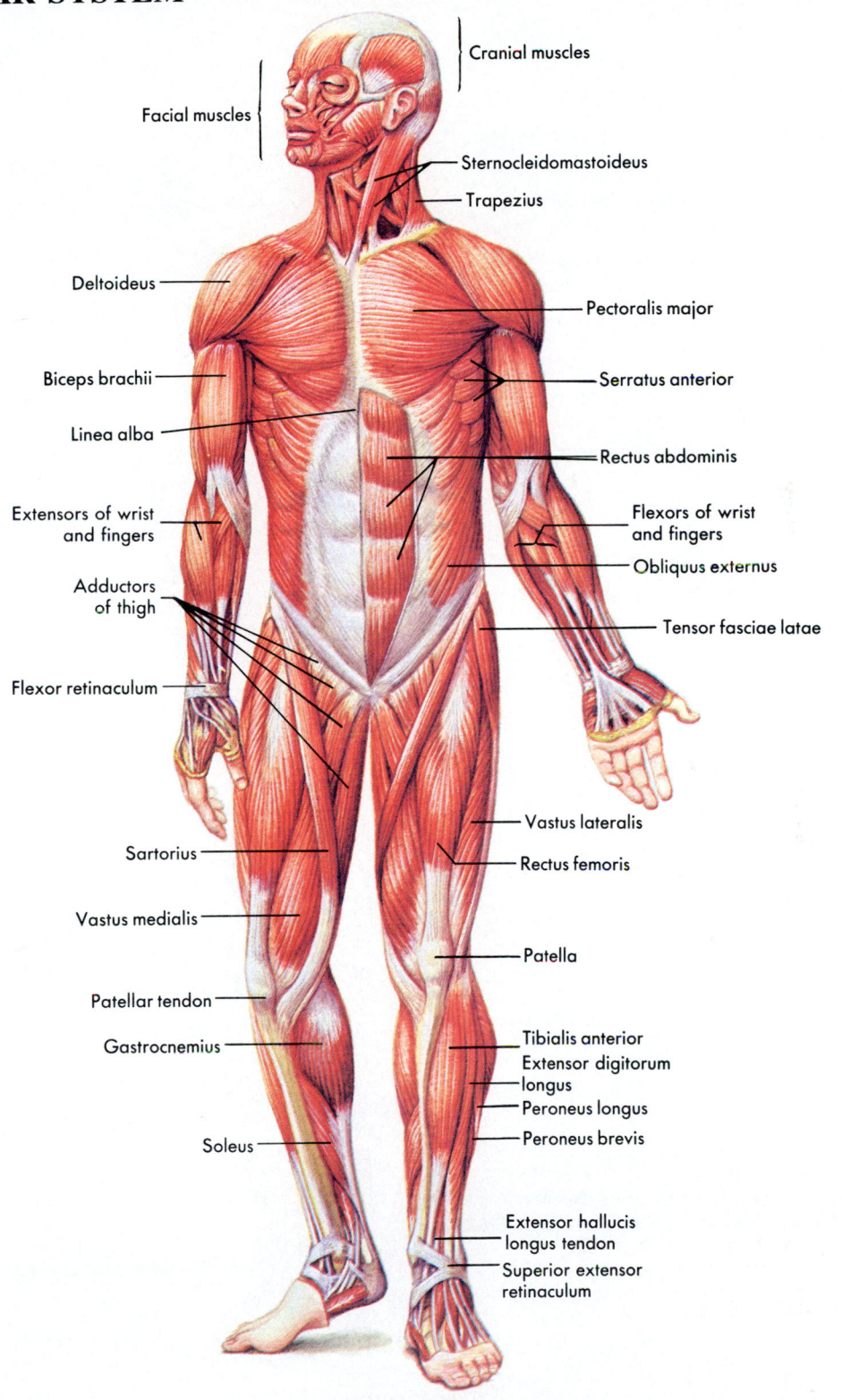

Cranial muscles

Facial muscles

Sternocleidomastoideus

Trapezius

Deltoideus

Pectoralis major

Biceps brachii

Serratus anterior

Linea alba

Rectus abdominis

Extensors of wrist
and fingers

Flexors of wrist
and fingers

Obliquus externus

Adductors
of thigh

Tensor fasciae latae

Flexor retinaculum

Vastus lateralis

Sartorius

Rectus femoris

Vastus medialis

Patella

Patellar tendon

Tibialis anterior

Gastrocnemius

Extensor digitorum
longus

Peroneus longus

Peroneus brevis

Soleus

Extensor hallucis
longus tendon

Superior extensor
retinaculum

**ANTERIOR VIEW**

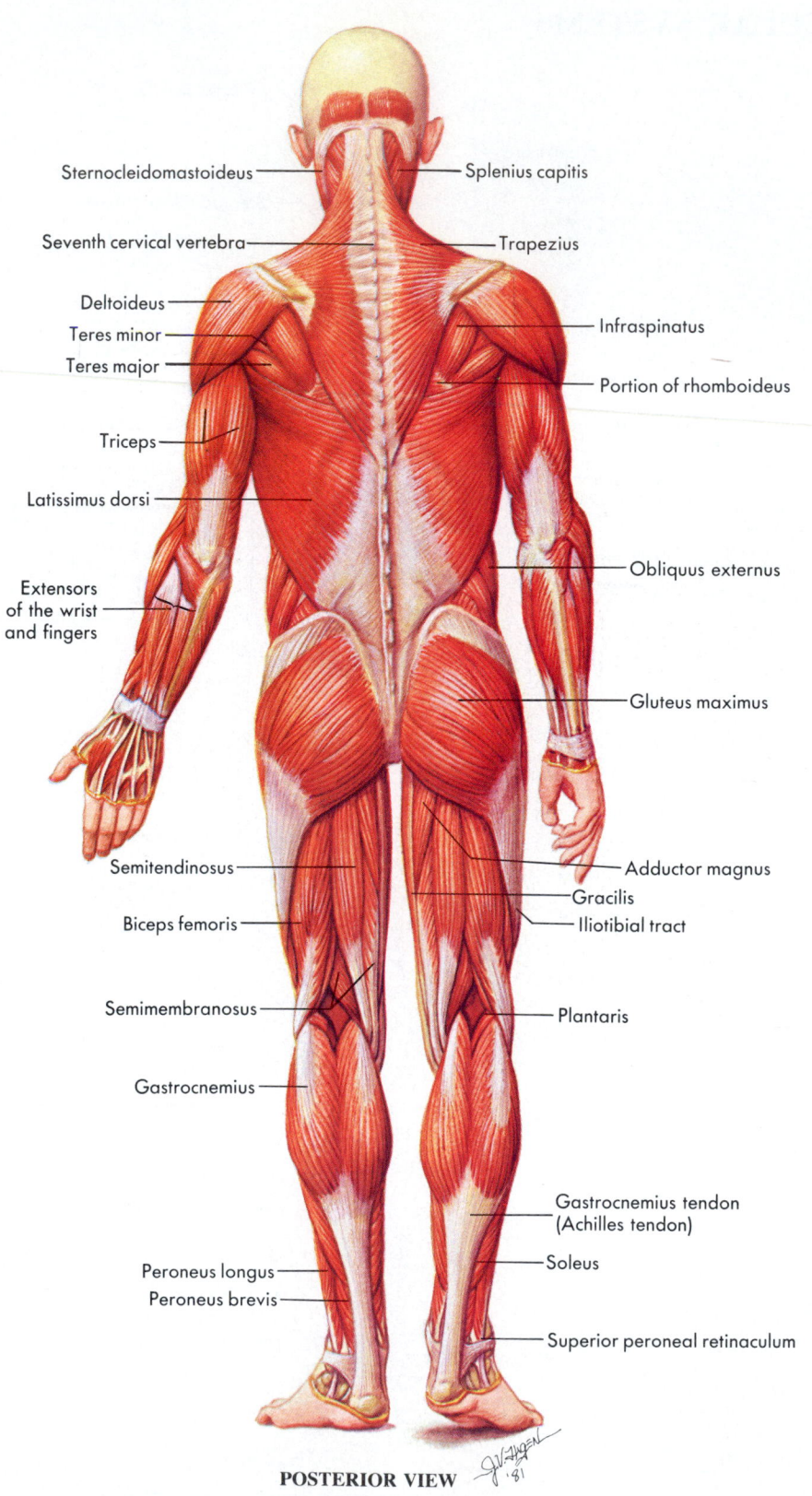

Sternocleidomastoideus — Splenius capitis

Seventh cervical vertebra — Trapezius

Deltoideus —
Teres minor — Infraspinatus
Teres major —
Portion of rhomboideus

Triceps —

Latissimus dorsi —

Obliquus externus

Extensors
of the wrist
and fingers —

Gluteus maximus

Semitendinosus — Adductor magnus
Gracilis
Biceps femoris — Iliotibial tract

Semimembranosus — Plantaris

Gastrocnemius —

Gastrocnemius tendon
(Achilles tendon)
Peroneus longus — Soleus
Peroneus brevis —
Superior peroneal retinaculum

**POSTERIOR VIEW**

# CIRCULATORY SYSTEM

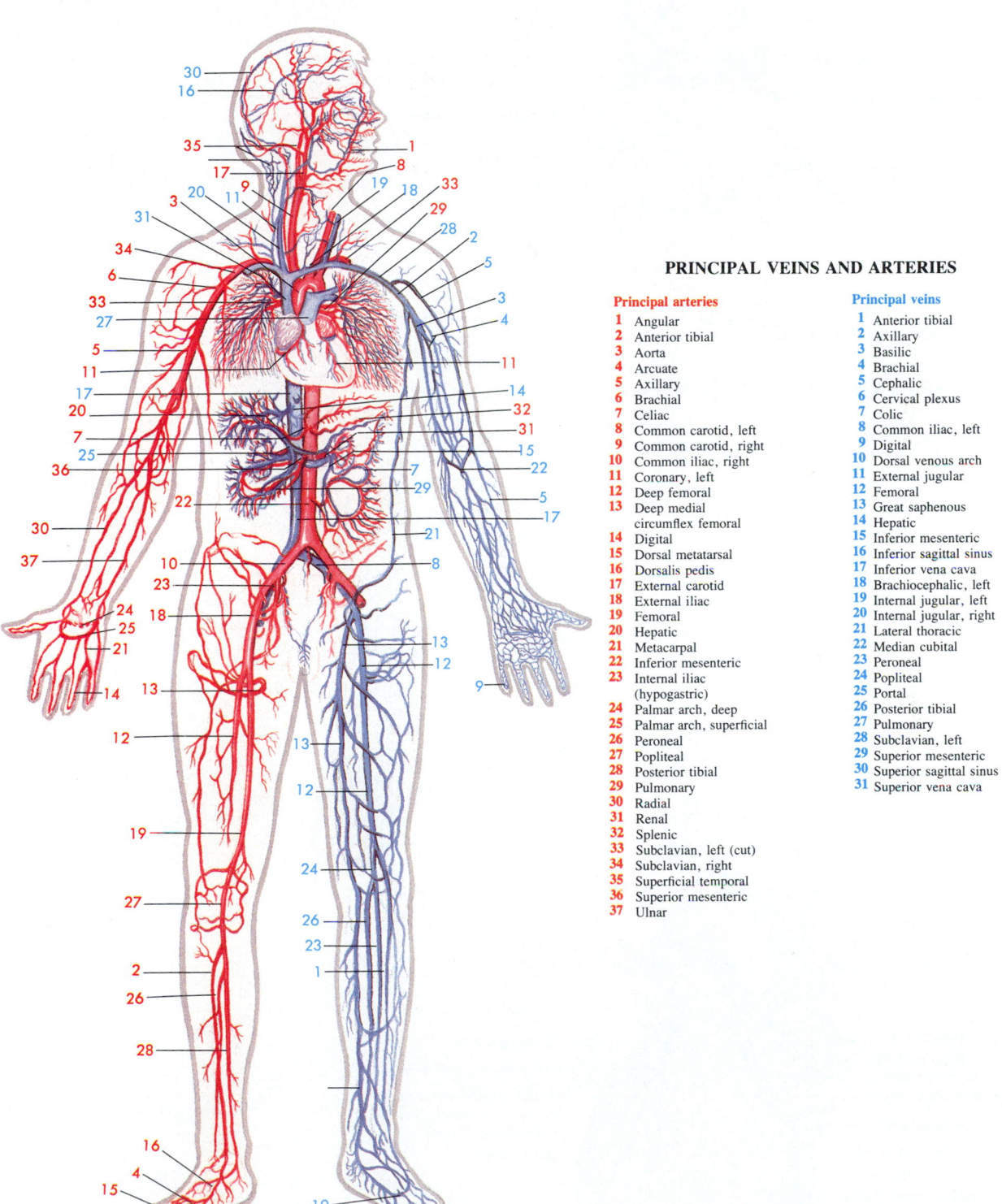

## PRINCIPAL VEINS AND ARTERIES

### Principal arteries

1 Angular
2 Anterior tibial
3 Aorta
4 Arcuate
5 Axillary
6 Brachial
7 Celiac
8 Common carotid, left
9 Common carotid, right
10 Common iliac, right
11 Coronary, left
12 Deep femoral
13 Deep medial
   circumflex femoral
14 Digital
15 Dorsal metatarsal
16 Dorsalis pedis
17 External carotid
18 External iliac
19 Femoral
20 Hepatic
21 Metacarpal
22 Inferior mesenteric
23 Internal iliac
   (hypogastric)
24 Palmar arch, deep
25 Palmar arch, superficial
26 Peroneal
27 Popliteal
28 Posterior tibial
29 Pulmonary
30 Radial
31 Renal
32 Splenic
33 Subclavian, left (cut)
34 Subclavian, right
35 Superficial temporal
36 Superior mesenteric
37 Ulnar

### Principal veins

1 Anterior tibial
2 Axillary
3 Basilic
4 Brachial
5 Cephalic
6 Cervical plexus
7 Colic
8 Common iliac, left
9 Digital
10 Dorsal venous arch
11 External jugular
12 Femoral
13 Great saphenous
14 Hepatic
15 Inferior mesenteric
16 Inferior sagittal sinus
17 Inferior vena cava
18 Brachiocephalic, left
19 Internal jugular, left
20 Internal jugular, right
21 Lateral thoracic
22 Median cubital
23 Peroneal
24 Popliteal
25 Portal
26 Posterior tibial
27 Pulmonary
28 Subclavian, left
29 Superior mesenteric
30 Superior sagittal sinus
31 Superior vena cava

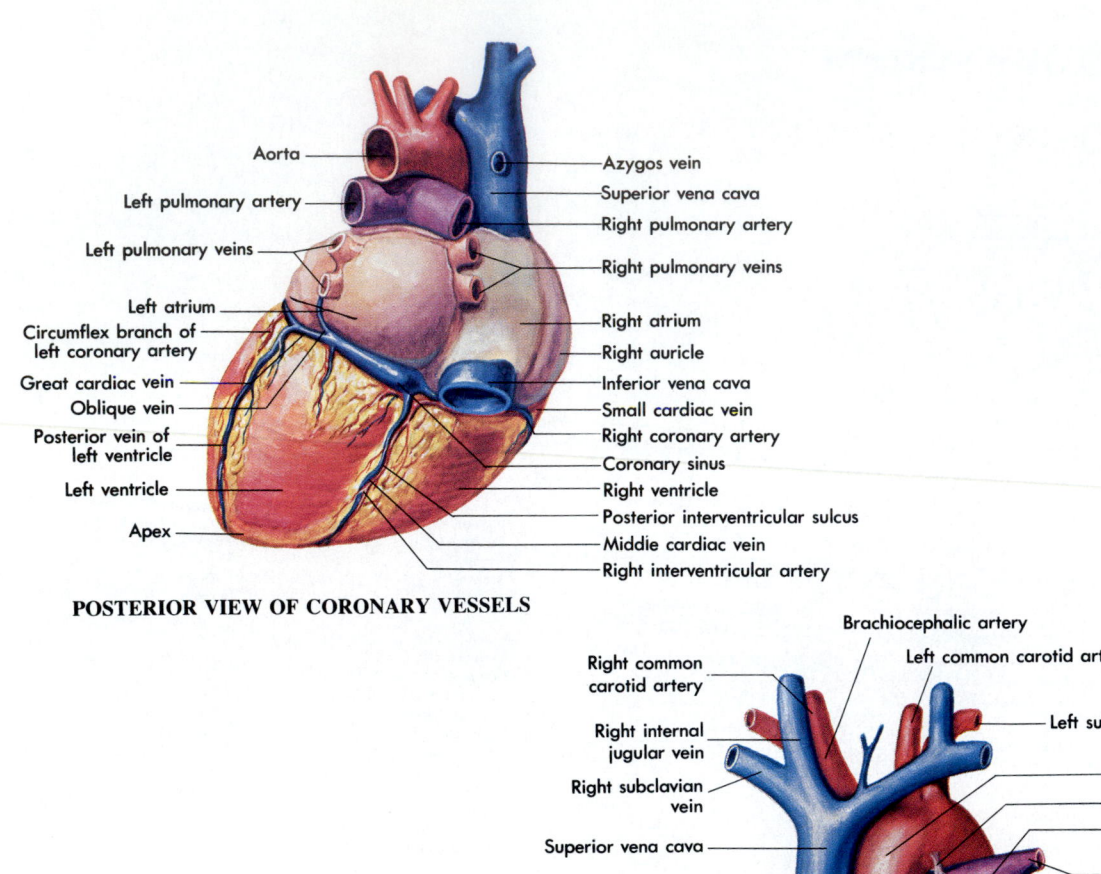

Aorta

Left pulmonary artery

Left pulmonary veins

Left atrium

Circumflex branch of
left coronary artery

Great cardiac vein

Oblique vein

Posterior vein of
left ventricle

Left ventricle

Apex

Azygos vein

Superior vena cava

Right pulmonary artery

Right pulmonary veins

Right atrium

Right auricle

Inferior vena cava

Small cardiac vein

Right coronary artery

Coronary sinus

Right ventricle

Posterior interventricular sulcus

Middle cardiac vein

Right interventricular artery

**POSTERIOR VIEW OF CORONARY VESSELS**

Brachiocephalic artery

Left common carotid artery

Right common
carotid artery

Right internal
jugular vein

Right subclavian
vein

Superior vena cava

Right pulmonary
arteries

Right pulmonary veins

Right atrium

Aortic valve (dotted lines)

Section of right
ventricle intact

Tricuspid valve

Right ventricle

Inferior vena cava

Papillary muscle

Left subclavian artery

Aortic arch

Ligamentum arteriosus

Pulmonary trunk

Left pulmonary arteries

Left pulmonary veins

Pulmonary valve leaflet

Left atrium and mitral valve

Chordae tendineae

Papillary muscle

Left ventricle

Interventricular septum

Myocardium

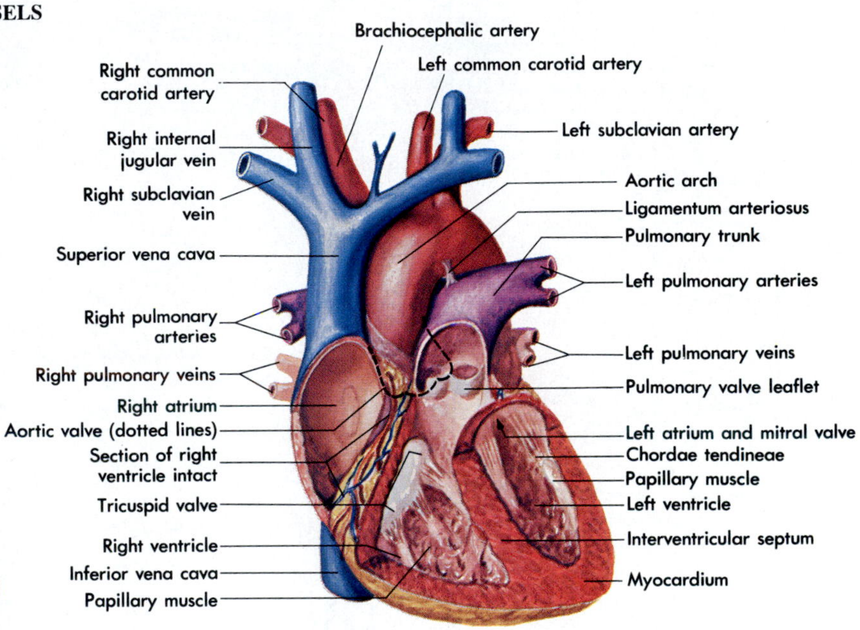

**HUMAN HEART IN FRONTAL SECTION**

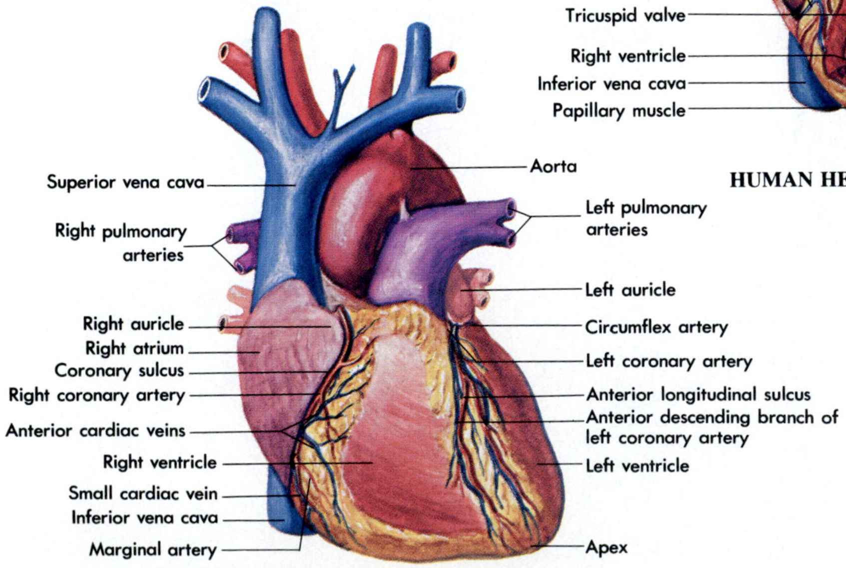

Superior vena cava

Right pulmonary
arteries

Right auricle

Right atrium

Coronary sulcus

Right coronary artery

Anterior cardiac veins

Right ventricle

Small cardiac vein

Inferior vena cava

Marginal artery

Aorta

Left pulmonary
arteries

Left auricle

Circumflex artery

Left coronary artery

Anterior longitudinal sulcus

Anterior descending branch of
left coronary artery

Left ventricle

Apex

**ANTERIOR VIEW OF CORONARY VESSELS**

**A-10**

# ENDOCRINE SYSTEM

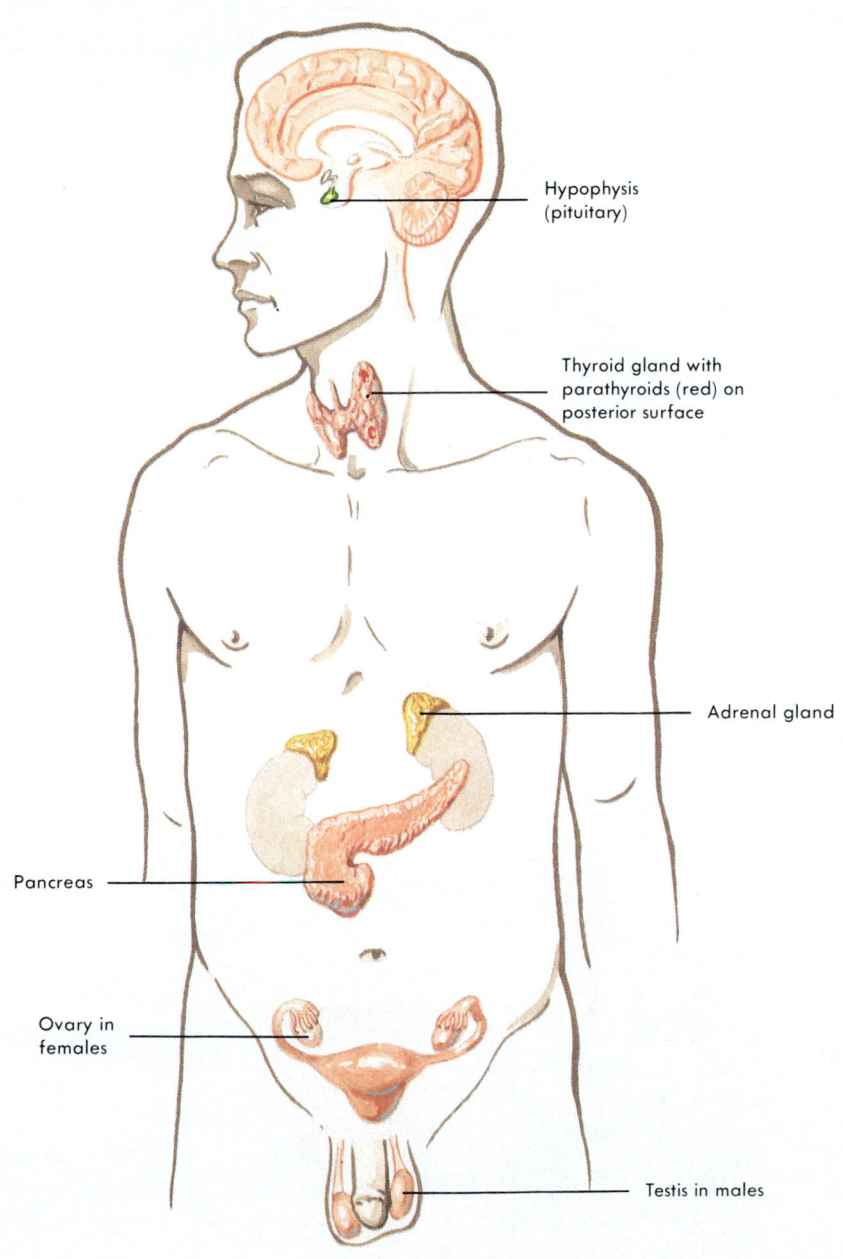

Hypophysis
(pituitary)

Thyroid gland with
parathyroids (red) on
posterior surface

Adrenal gland

Pancreas

Ovary in
females

Testis in males

**ENDOCRINE SYSTEM**

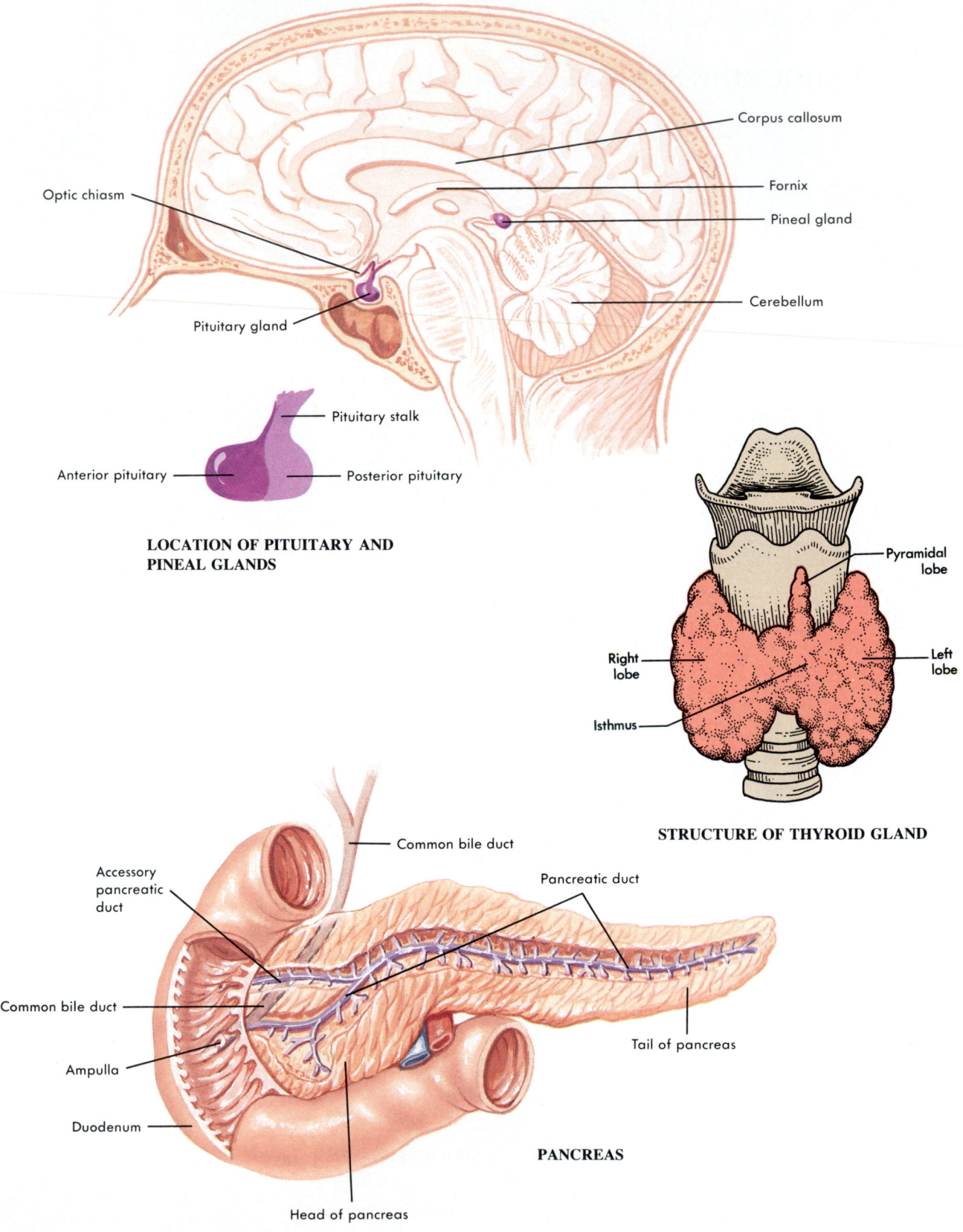

Corpus callosum

Fornix

Pineal gland

Optic chiasm

Cerebellum

Pituitary gland

Pituitary stalk

Anterior pituitary

Posterior pituitary

**LOCATION OF PITUITARY AND PINEAL GLANDS**

Pyramidal lobe

Right lobe

Left lobe

Isthmus

**STRUCTURE OF THYROID GLAND**

Common bile duct

Accessory pancreatic duct

Pancreatic duct

Common bile duct

Ampulla

Duodenum

Tail of pancreas

**PANCREAS**

Head of pancreas

# LYMPHATIC SYSTEM

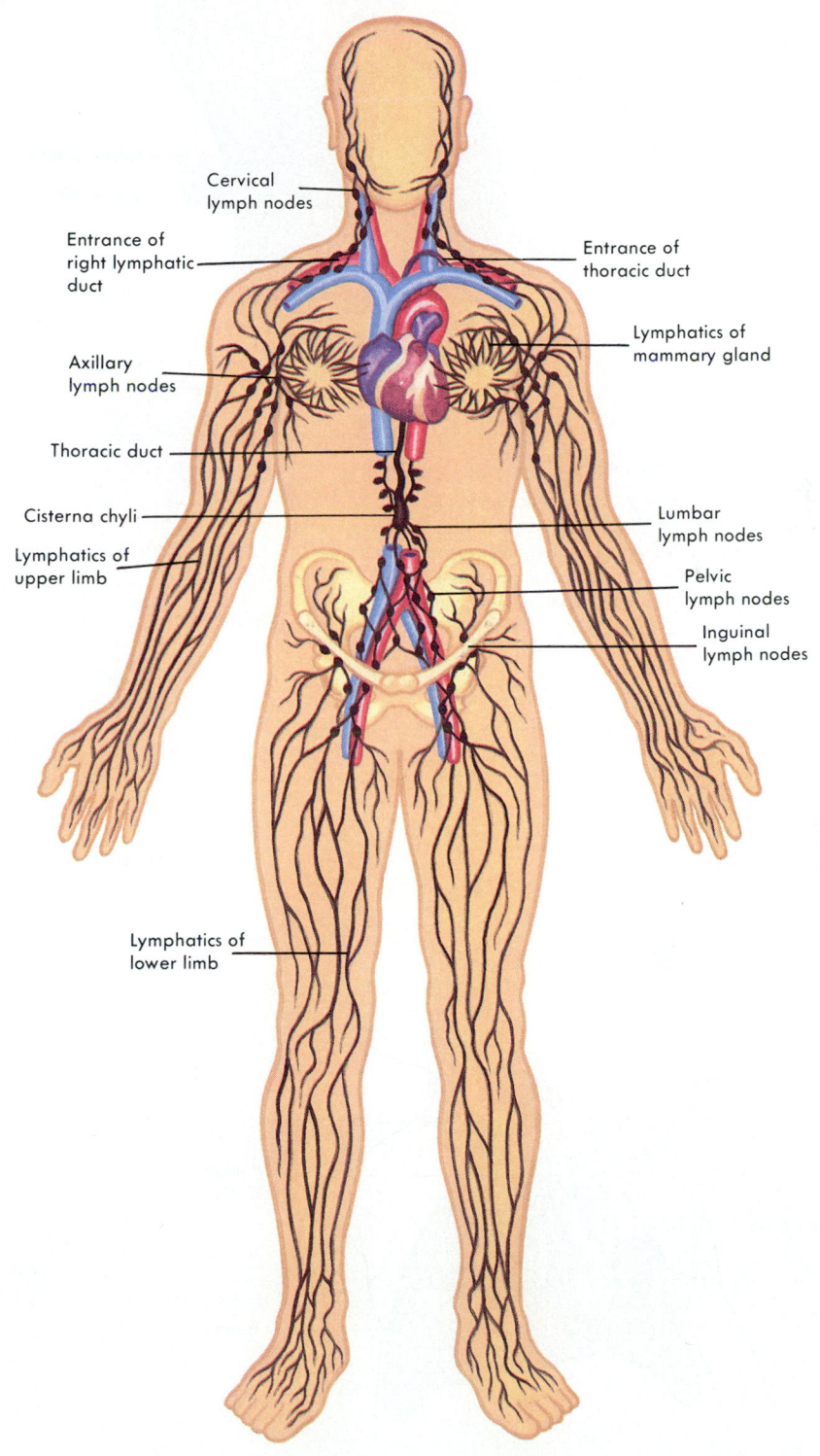

Cervical lymph nodes

Entrance of right lymphatic duct

Entrance of thoracic duct

Lymphatics of mammary gland

Axillary lymph nodes

Thoracic duct

Cisterna chyli

Lumbar lymph nodes

Lymphatics of upper limb

Pelvic lymph nodes

Inguinal lymph nodes

Lymphatics of lower limb

**LYMPHATIC SYSTEM**

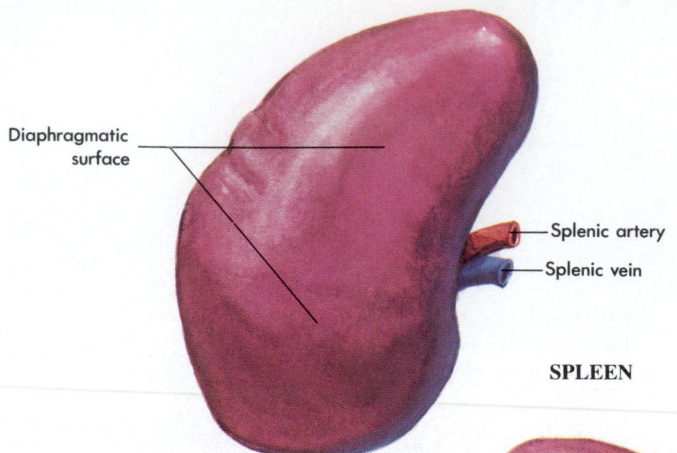

Diaphragmatic surface

Splenic artery

Splenic vein

**SPLEEN**

**CLINICAL NOTE: The spleen**

The spleen is located high in the abdomen under the left hemidiaphragm. It is involved in the creation, conservation, and destruction of various blood elements, especially erythrocytes. Arterial blood circulates through the red splenic pulp, which is rich in erythrocytes. Lymphatic tissue surrounding the smallest vessels forms a white pulp material.

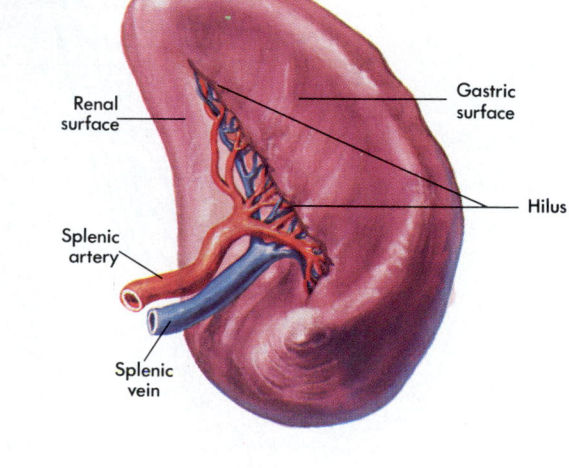

Renal surface

Gastric surface

Hilus

Splenic artery

Splenic vein

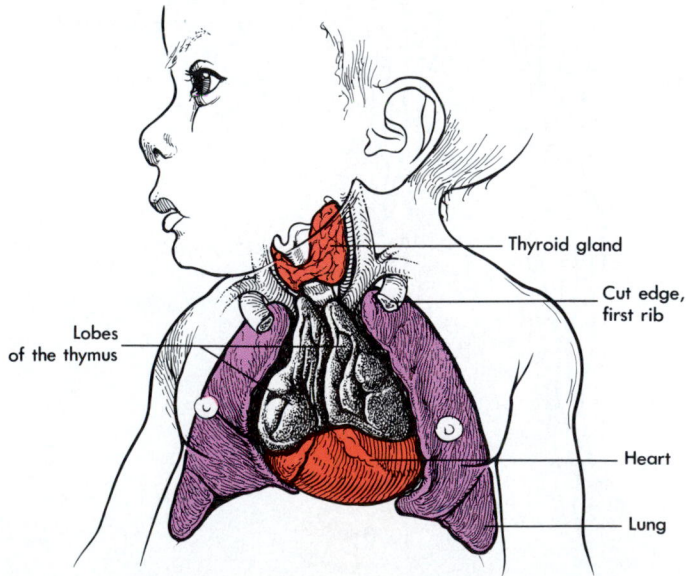

Thyroid gland

Cut edge, first rib

Lobes of the thymus

Heart

Lung

**LOCATION AND GROSS ANATOMY OF THYMUS**

# NERVOUS SYSTEM

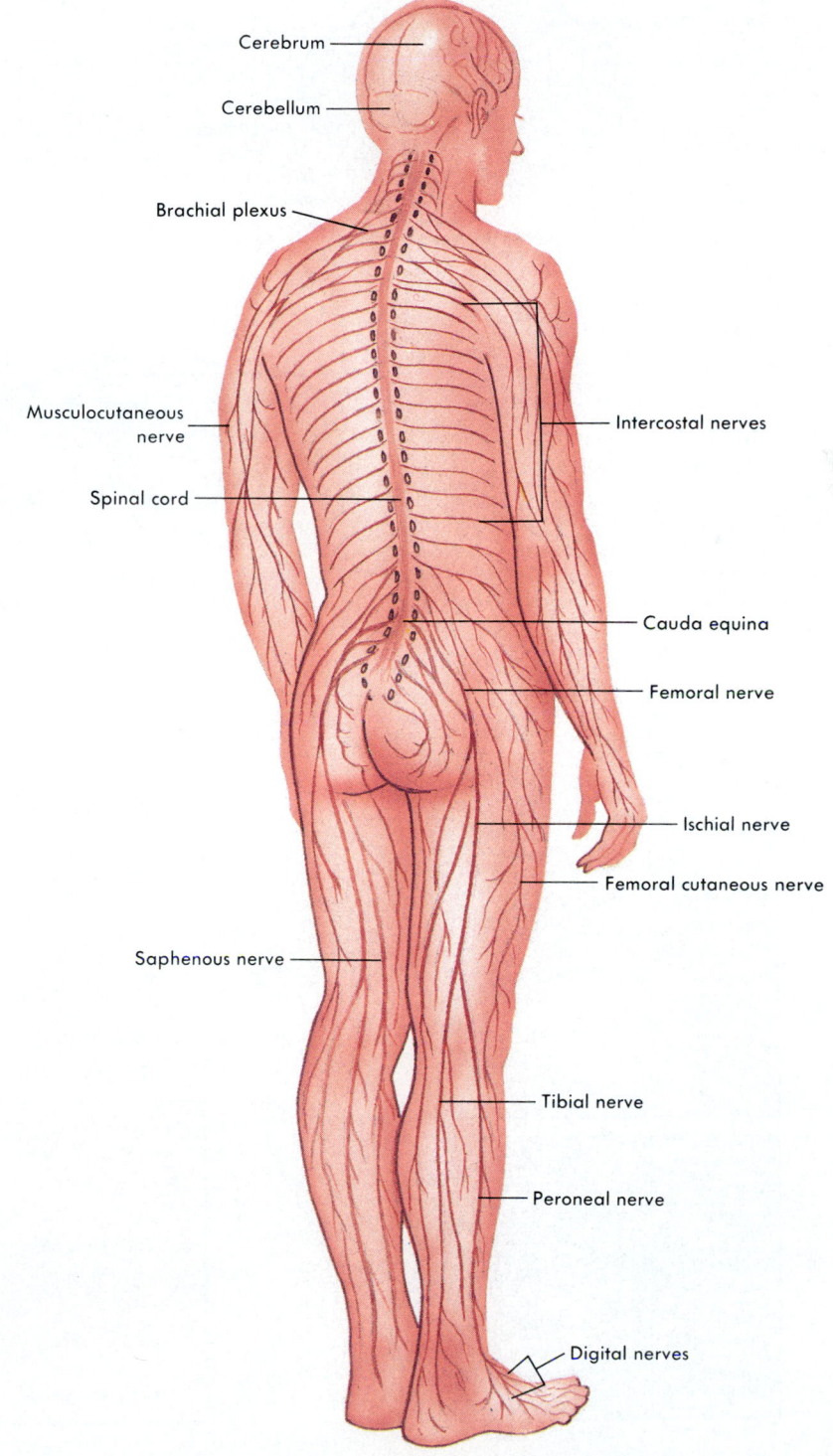

Cerebrum

Cerebellum

Brachial plexus

Musculocutaneous nerve

Spinal cord

Intercostal nerves

Cauda equina

Femoral nerve

Ischial nerve

Femoral cutaneous nerve

Saphenous nerve

Tibial nerve

Peroneal nerve

Digital nerves

**SIMPLIFIED VIEW OF NERVOUS SYSTEM**

## ANATOMY OF CEREBELLUM

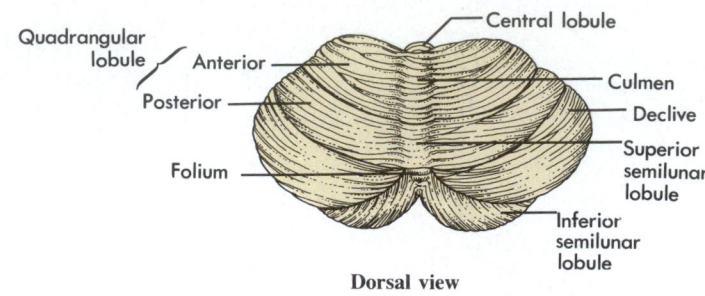

Quadrangular lobule — Anterior  
Posterior  
Folium

Central lobule  
Culmen  
Declive  
Superior semilunar lobule  
Inferior semilunar lobule

**Dorsal view**

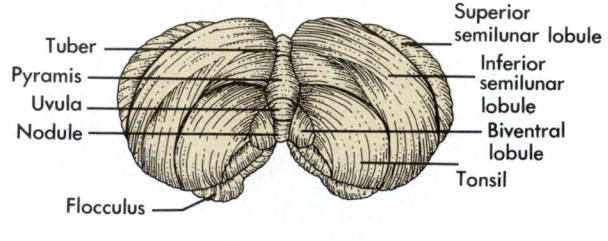

Tuber  
Pyramis  
Uvula  
Nodule  
Flocculus

Superior semilunar lobule  
Inferior semilunar lobule  
Biventral lobule  
Tonsil

**Ventral view**

| Input | Sensor | Integrator | Effector | Output |
|---|---|---|---|---|
| **External environment**<br><br>Light<br>Sound<br>Temperature<br>Barometric pressure<br>Trauma | Sight<br>Hearing<br>Taste<br>Smell<br>Touch | | Skeletal muscle<br><br>Smooth muscle | Contraction or relaxation |
| **Internal environment**<br><br>Muscular work<br>Visceral activity<br>Body chemistry<br>Trauma (pain) | Internal sensors | | Exocrine glands<br><br>Endocrine glands | Secretion |

**COMPONENTS OF NERVOUS SYSTEM**

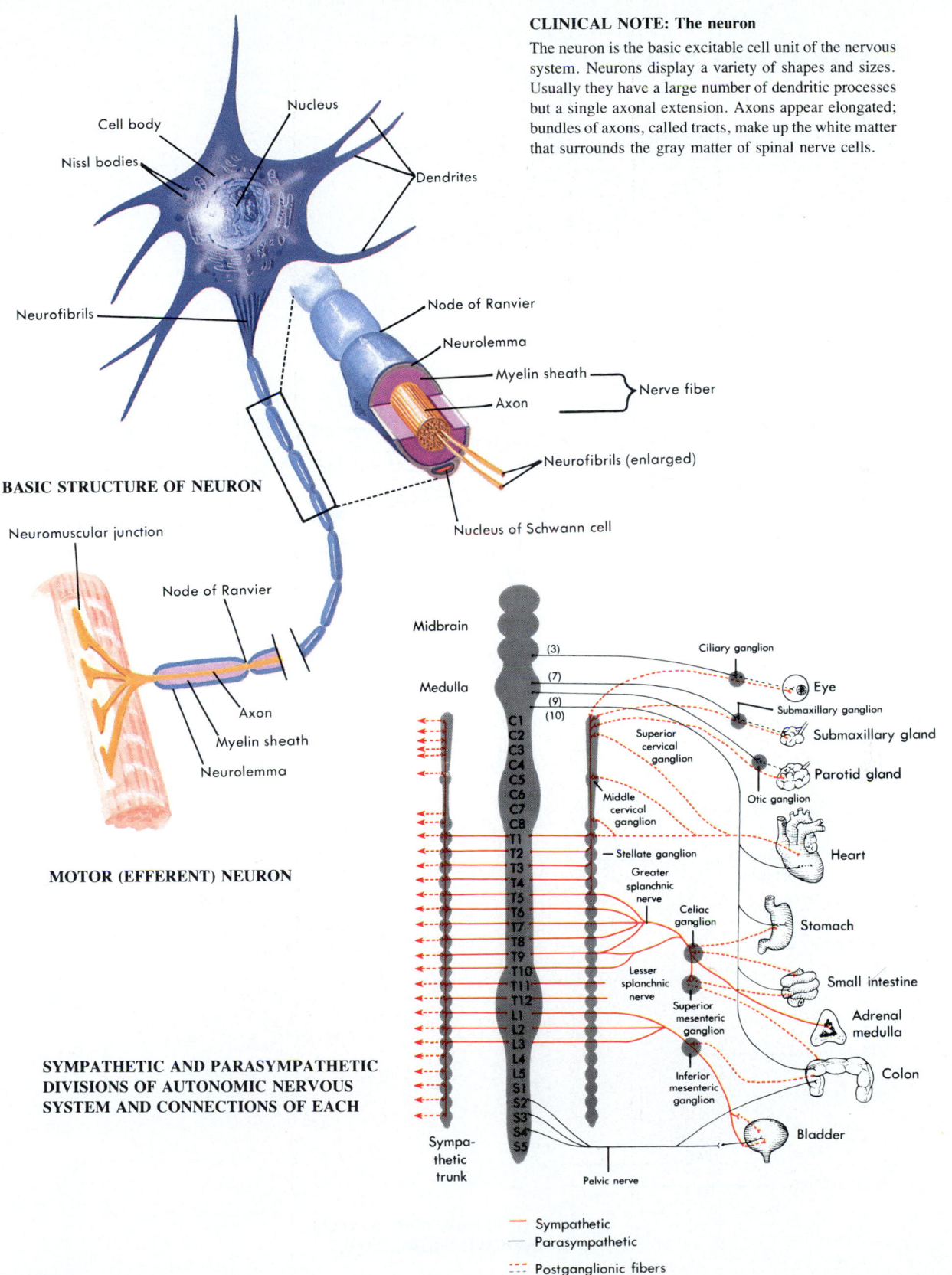

**CLINICAL NOTE: The neuron**

The neuron is the basic excitable cell unit of the nervous system. Neurons display a variety of shapes and sizes. Usually they have a large number of dendritic processes but a single axonal extension. Axons appear elongated; bundles of axons, called tracts, make up the white matter that surrounds the gray matter of spinal nerve cells.

Cell body
Nucleus
Nissl bodies
Dendrites
Neurofibrils
Node of Ranvier
Neurolemma
Myelin sheath
Axon
Nerve fiber
Neurofibrils (enlarged)
Nucleus of Schwann cell

**BASIC STRUCTURE OF NEURON**

Neuromuscular junction
Node of Ranvier
Axon
Myelin sheath
Neurolemma

**MOTOR (EFFERENT) NEURON**

Midbrain
Medulla
Ciliary ganglion
(3)
(7)
(9)
(10)
Eye
Submaxillary ganglion
Submaxillary gland
Superior cervical ganglion
Parotid gland
Otic ganglion
Middle cervical ganglion
Stellate ganglion
Heart
Greater splanchnic nerve
Celiac ganglion
Stomach
Lesser splanchnic nerve
Small intestine
Superior mesenteric ganglion
Adrenal medulla
Inferior mesenteric ganglion
Colon
Bladder
Sympathetic trunk
Pelvic nerve

C1 C2 C3 C4 C5 C6 C7 C8
T1 T2 T3 T4 T5 T6 T7 T8 T9 T10 T11 T12
L1 L2 L3 L4 L5
S1 S2 S3 S4 S5

**SYMPATHETIC AND PARASYMPATHETIC DIVISIONS OF AUTONOMIC NERVOUS SYSTEM AND CONNECTIONS OF EACH**

— Sympathetic
— Parasympathetic
--- Postganglionic fibers

# RESPIRATORY SYSTEM

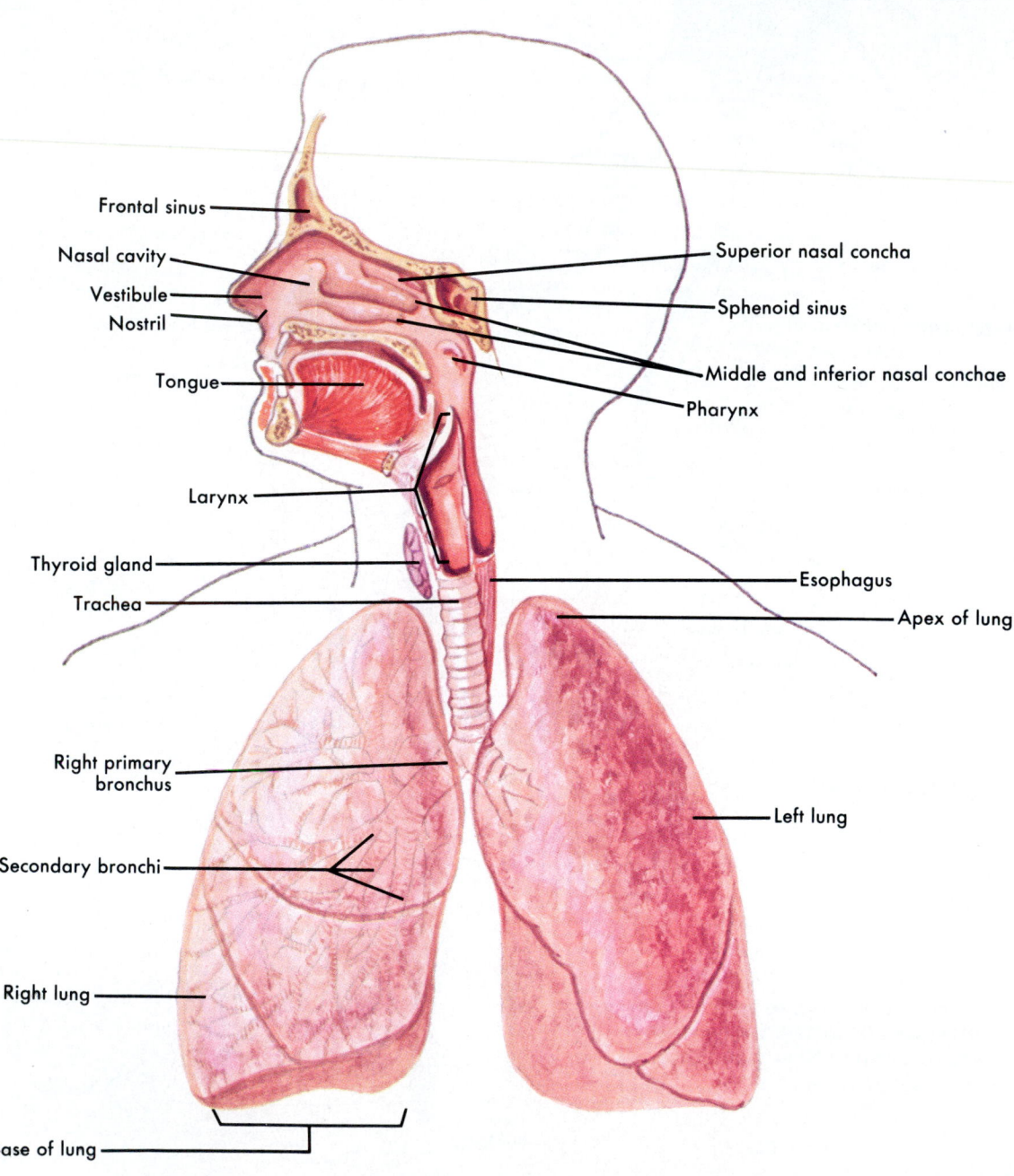

Frontal sinus

Nasal cavity

Vestibule

Nostril

Tongue

Larynx

Thyroid gland

Trachea

Right primary bronchus

Secondary bronchi

Right lung

Base of lung

Superior nasal concha

Sphenoid sinus

Middle and inferior nasal conchae

Pharynx

Esophagus

Apex of lung

Left lung

**ORGANS OF RESPIRATORY SYSTEM
AND ASSOCIATED STRUCTURES**

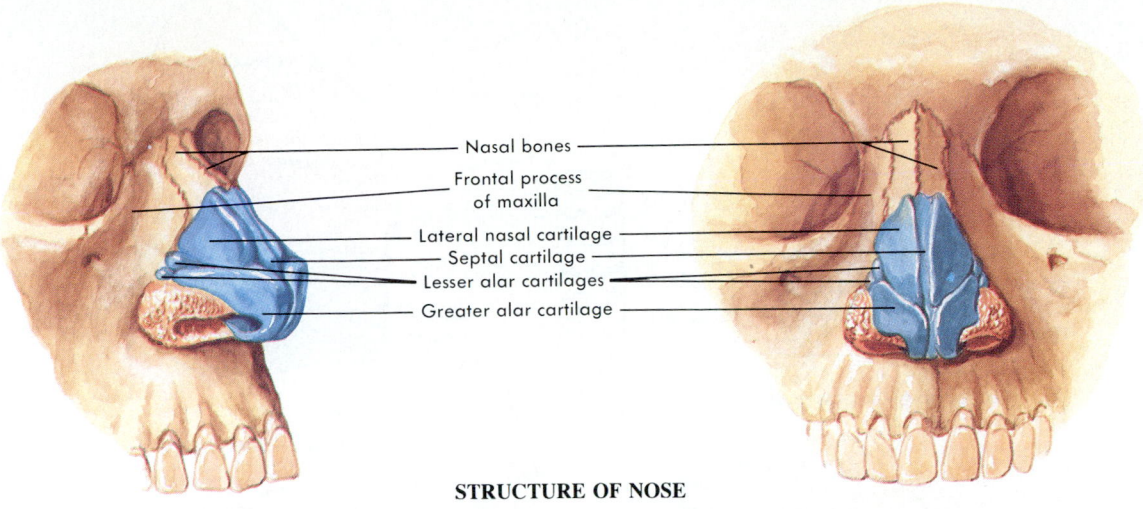

**STRUCTURE OF NOSE**

Nasal bones
Frontal process of maxilla
Lateral nasal cartilage
Septal cartilage
Lesser alar cartilages
Greater alar cartilage

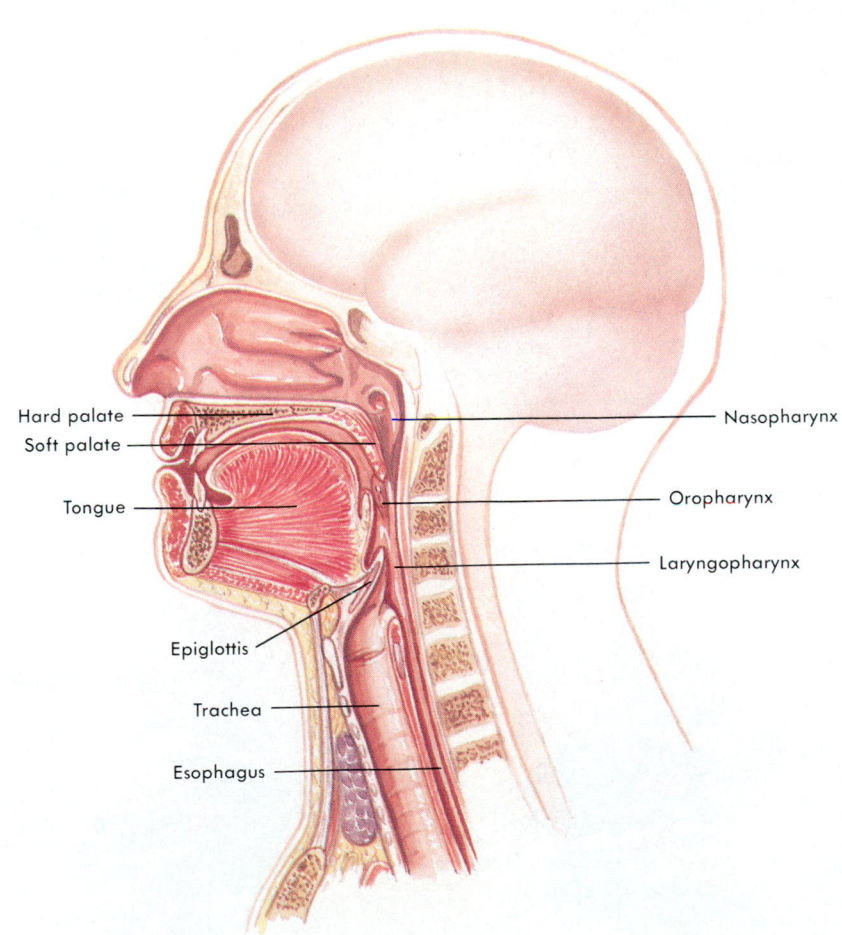

Hard palate
Soft palate
Tongue
Epiglottis
Trachea
Esophagus

Nasopharynx
Oropharynx
Laryngopharynx

**STRUCTURES OF NASAL PASSAGES AND THROAT**

**A-19**

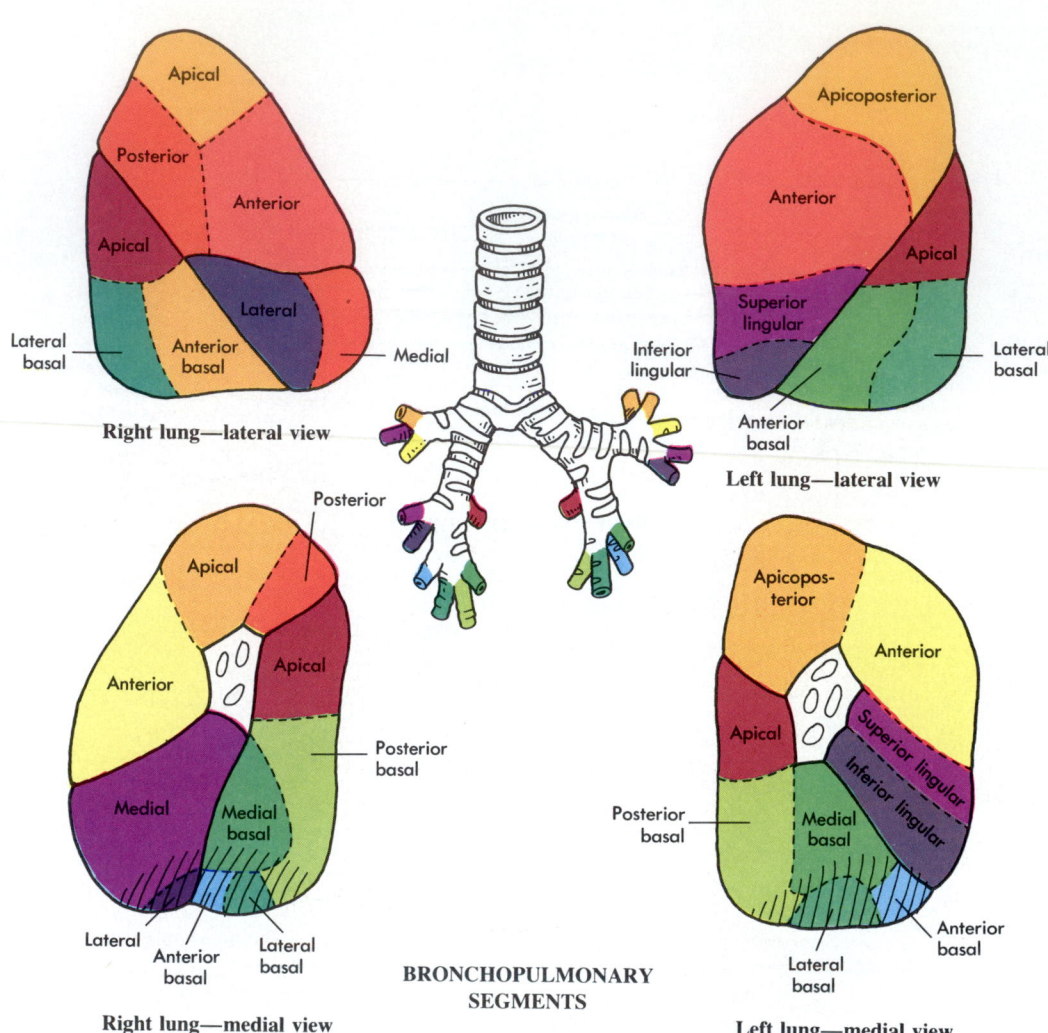

Apical

Posterior

Anterior

Apical

Lateral

Lateral basal

Anterior basal

Medial

**Right lung—lateral view**

Apicoposterior

Anterior

Apical

Superior lingular

Inferior lingular

Lateral basal

Anterior basal

**Left lung—lateral view**

Posterior

Apical

Apical

Anterior

Posterior basal

Medial

Medial basal

Lateral

Anterior basal

Lateral basal

**Right lung—medial view**

**BRONCHOPULMONARY SEGMENTS**

Apicoposterior

Anterior

Apical

Superior lingular

Inferior lingular

Posterior basal

Medial basal

Lateral basal

Anterior basal

**Left lung—medial view**

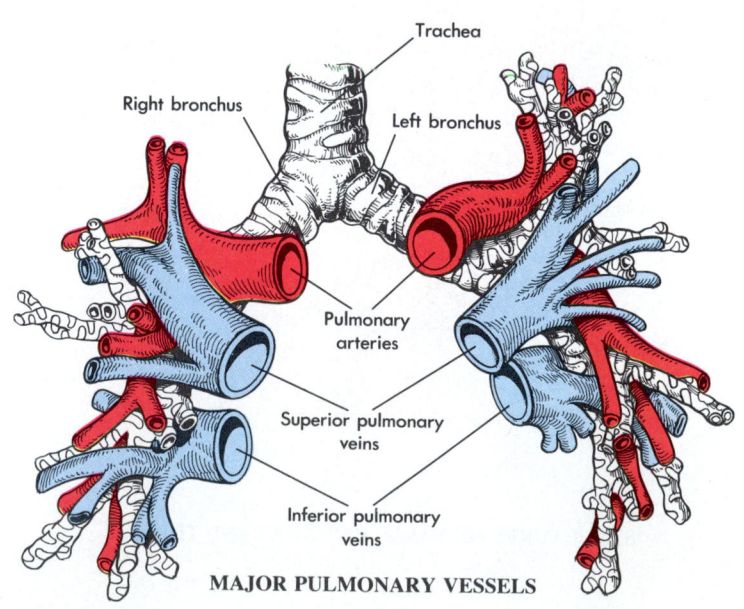

Trachea

Right bronchus

Left bronchus

Pulmonary arteries

Superior pulmonary veins

Inferior pulmonary veins

**MAJOR PULMONARY VESSELS**

# DIGESTIVE SYSTEM

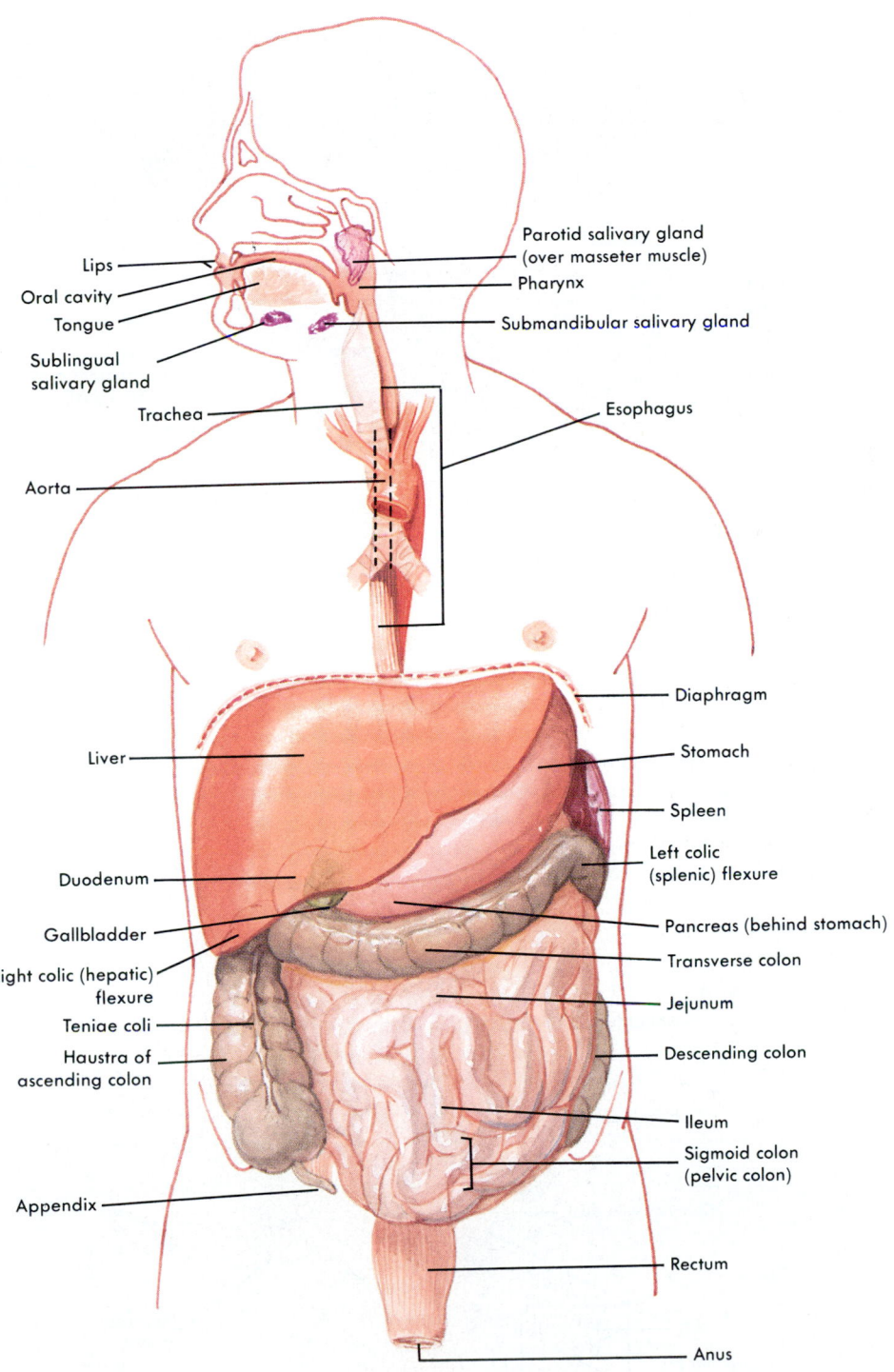

Lips

Oral cavity

Tongue

Sublingual
salivary gland

Trachea

Aorta

Parotid salivary gland
(over masseter muscle)

Pharynx

Submandibular salivary gland

Esophagus

Diaphragm

Liver

Stomach

Spleen

Left colic
(splenic) flexure

Duodenum

Pancreas (behind stomach)

Gallbladder

Transverse colon

Right colic (hepatic)
flexure

Jejunum

Teniae coli

Descending colon

Haustra of
ascending colon

Ileum

Sigmoid colon
(pelvic colon)

Appendix

Rectum

Anus

**ORGANS OF DIGESTIVE SYSTEM AND
SOME ASSOCIATED STRUCTURES**

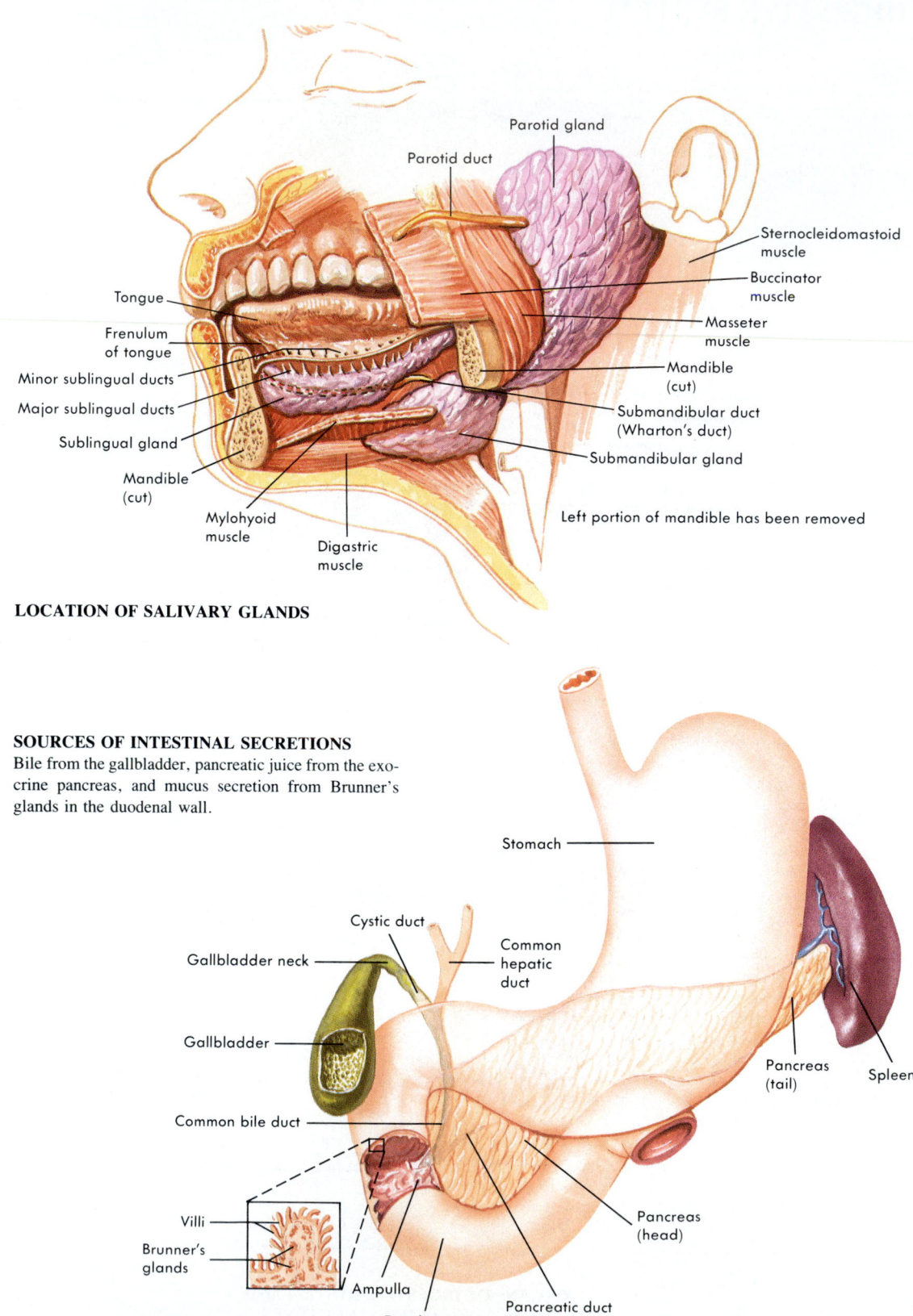

Parotid gland

Parotid duct

Sternocleidomastoid muscle

Buccinator muscle

Masseter muscle

Tongue

Frenulum of tongue

Mandible (cut)

Minor sublingual ducts

Submandibular duct (Wharton's duct)

Major sublingual ducts

Sublingual gland

Submandibular gland

Mandible (cut)

Mylohyoid muscle

Digastric muscle

Left portion of mandible has been removed

**LOCATION OF SALIVARY GLANDS**

**SOURCES OF INTESTINAL SECRETIONS**

Bile from the gallbladder, pancreatic juice from the exocrine pancreas, and mucus secretion from Brunner's glands in the duodenal wall.

Stomach

Cystic duct

Common hepatic duct

Gallbladder neck

Gallbladder

Pancreas (tail)

Spleen

Common bile duct

Villi

Brunner's glands

Pancreas (head)

Ampulla

Pancreatic duct

Duodenum

**A-22**

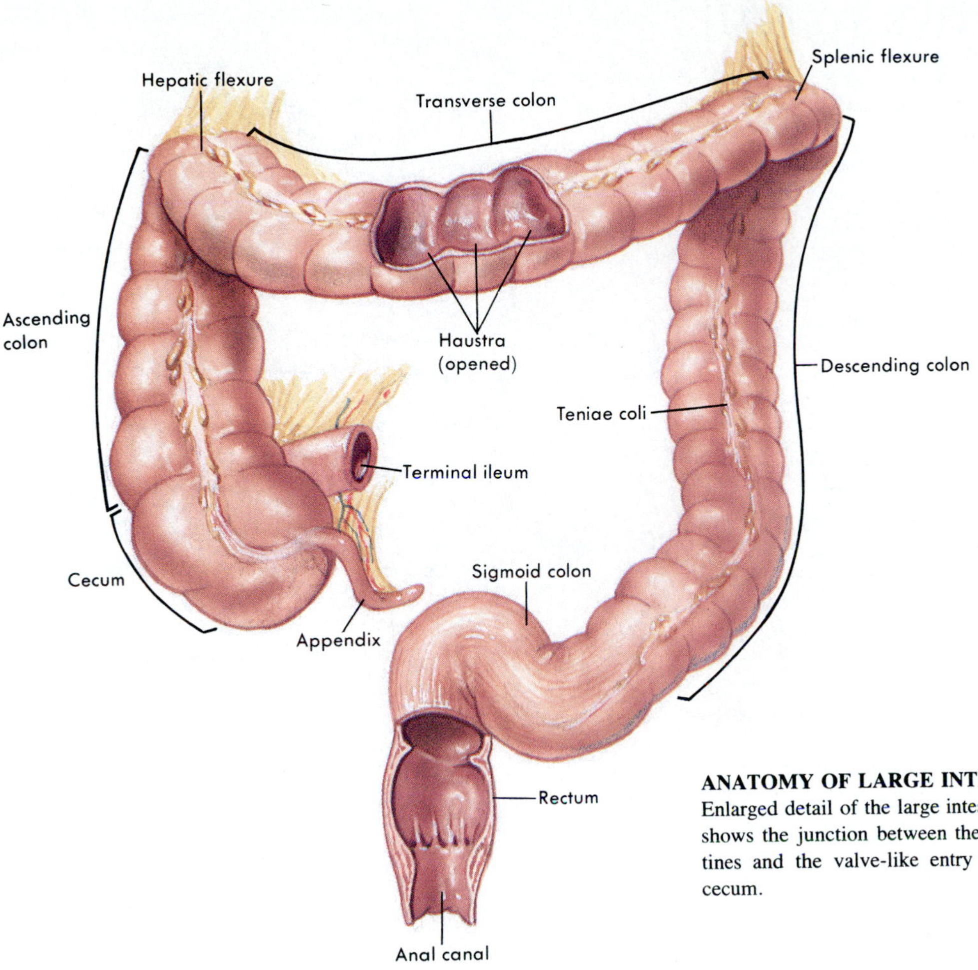

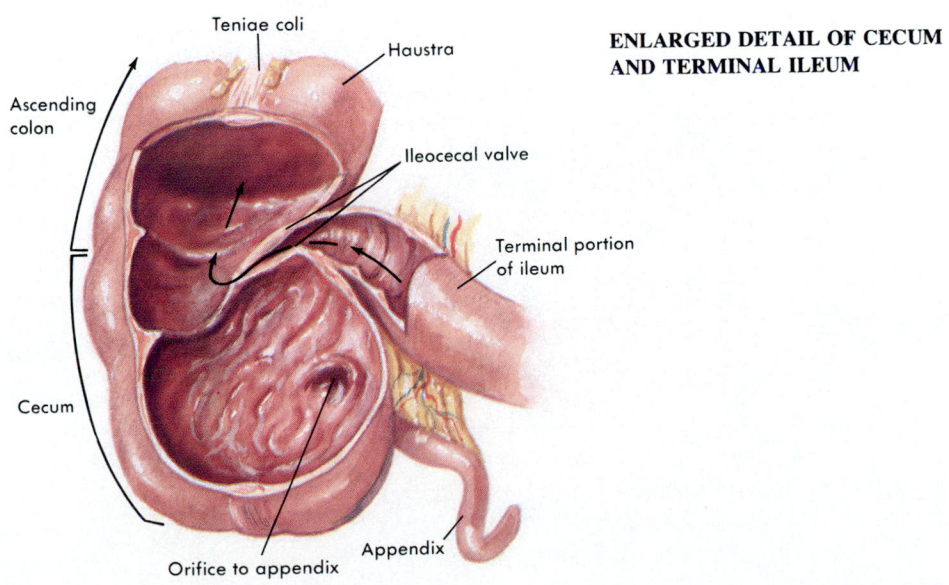

Hepatic flexure

Transverse colon

Splenic flexure

Ascending colon

Haustra (opened)

Descending colon

Teniae coli

Terminal ileum

Cecum

Sigmoid colon

Appendix

Rectum

**ANATOMY OF LARGE INTESTINE**
Enlarged detail of the large intestine, rectum, and anus shows the junction between the large and small intestines and the valve-like entry of the ileum into the cecum.

Anal canal

**ENLARGED DETAIL OF CECUM AND TERMINAL ILEUM**

Teniae coli

Haustra

Ascending colon

Ileocecal valve

Terminal portion of ileum

Cecum

Orifice to appendix

Appendix

# REPRODUCTIVE SYSTEM

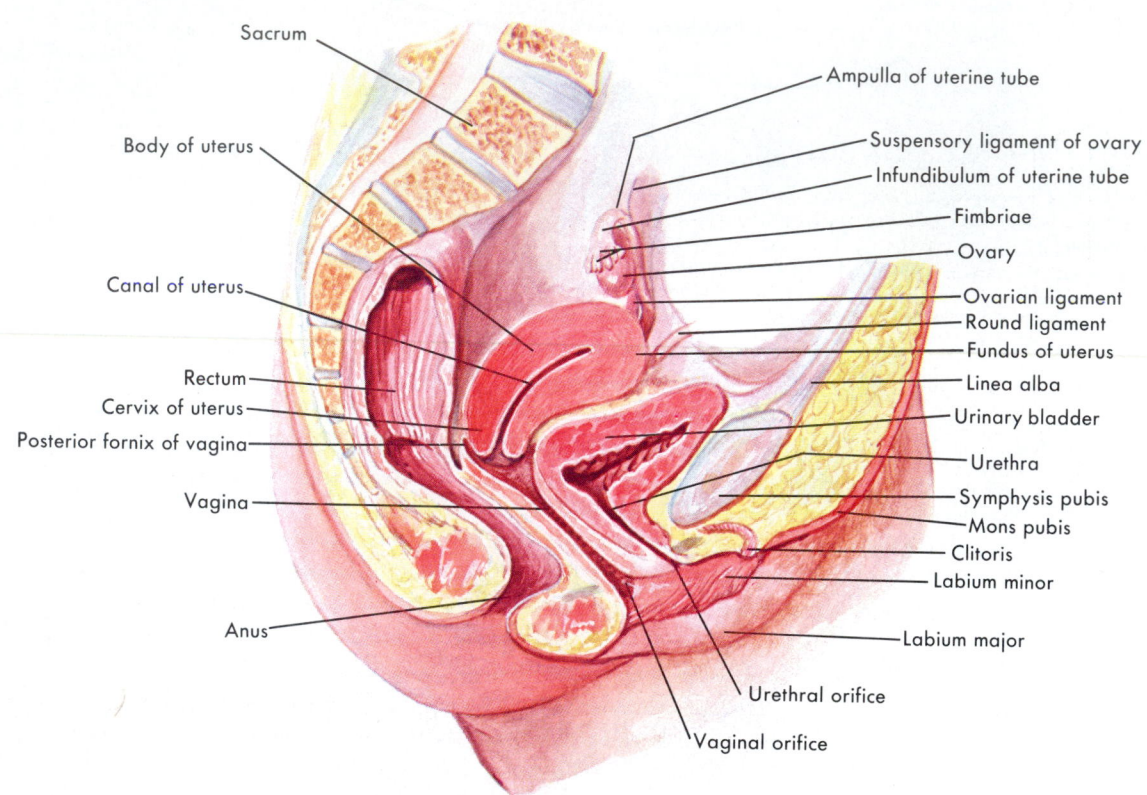

Sacrum

Body of uterus

Canal of uterus

Rectum

Cervix of uterus

Posterior fornix of vagina

Vagina

Anus

Ampulla of uterine tube

Suspensory ligament of ovary

Infundibulum of uterine tube

Fimbriae

Ovary

Ovarian ligament

Round ligament

Fundus of uterus

Linea alba

Urinary bladder

Urethra

Symphysis pubis

Mons pubis

Clitoris

Labium minor

Labium major

Urethral orifice

Vaginal orifice

**FEMALE REPRODUCTIVE ORGANS AND
ASSOCIATED STRUCTURES**

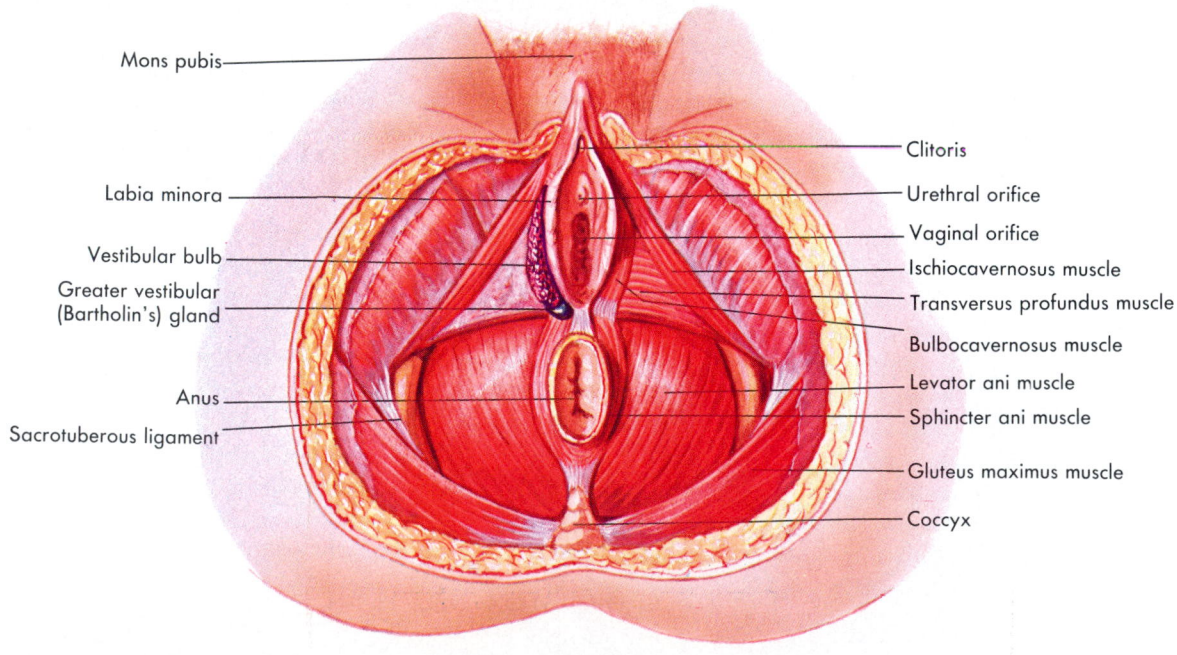

Mons pubis

Labia minora

Vestibular bulb

Greater vestibular
(Bartholin's) gland

Anus

Sacrotuberous ligament

Clitoris

Urethral orifice

Vaginal orifice

Ischiocavernosus muscle

Transversus profundus muscle

Bulbocavernosus muscle

Levator ani muscle

Sphincter ani muscle

Gluteus maximus muscle

Coccyx

**FEMALE PERINEUM**

A-24

**CLINICAL NOTE: Female reproductive system**

Immense structural changes occur within the uterus during pregnancy. However, if fertilization does not take place, then the endometrial lining is shed cyclically under hormonal control in the phenomenon of menstruation.

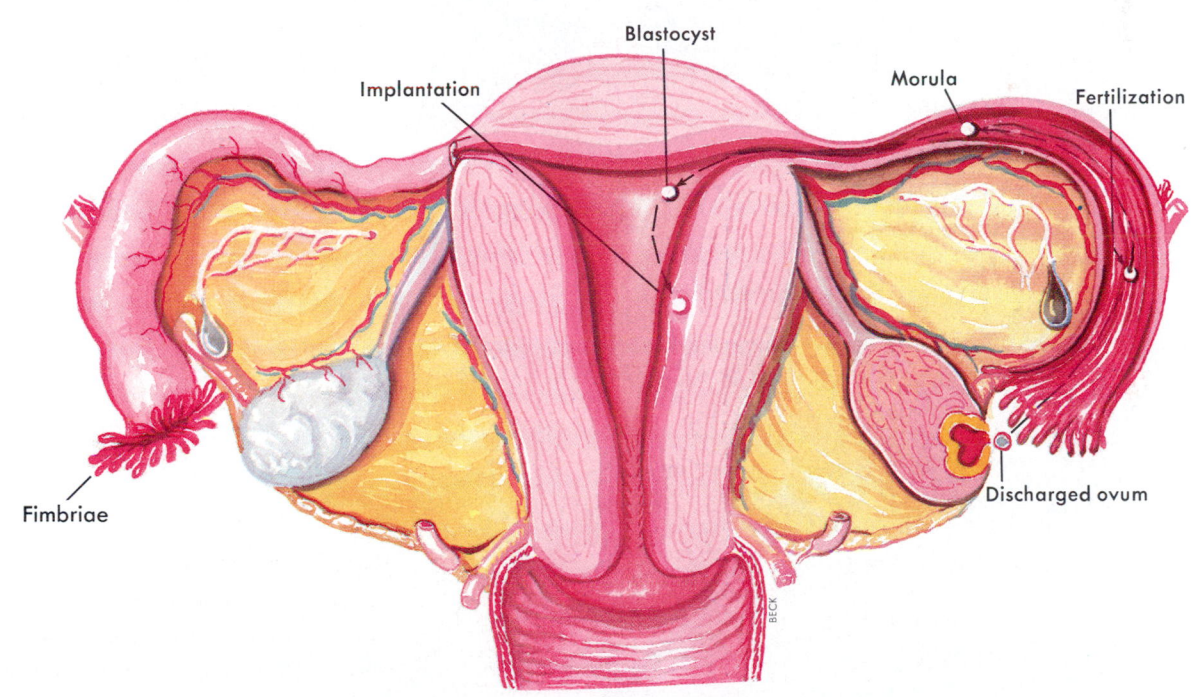

**APPEARANCE OF UTERUS AND UTERINE TUBES FROM FERTILIZATION TO IMPLANTATION**

Fertilization occurs in the outer third of the uterine tube. Development reaches the blastocyst stage after the embryo has entered the uterus.

**A-25**

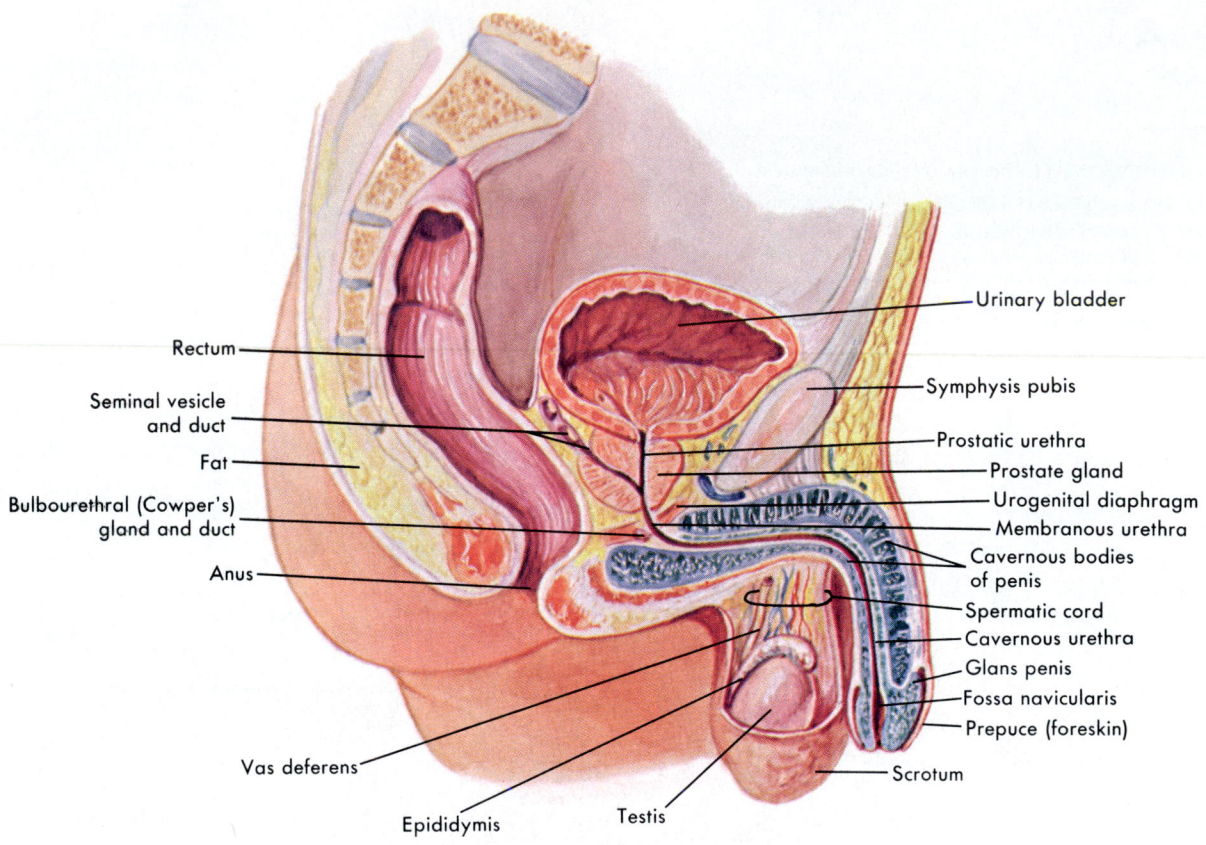

Rectum

Seminal vesicle
and duct

Fat

Bulbourethral (Cowper's)
gland and duct

Anus

Vas deferens

Epididymis

Testis

Urinary bladder

Symphysis pubis

Prostatic urethra

Prostate gland

Urogenital diaphragm

Membranous urethra

Cavernous bodies
of penis

Spermatic cord

Cavernous urethra

Glans penis

Fossa navicularis

Prepuce (foreskin)

Scrotum

**MALE REPRODUCTIVE ORGANS AND
ASSOCIATED STRUCTURES**

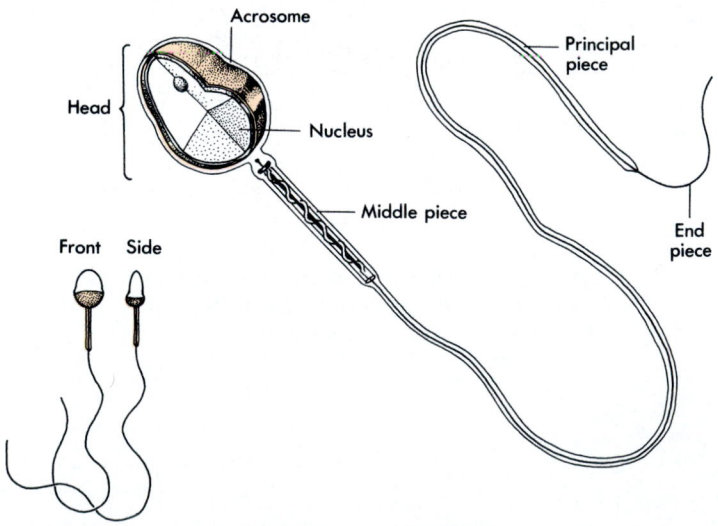

Acrosome

Head

Nucleus

Middle piece

Front   Side

Principal
piece

End
piece

**ANATOMY OF A SPERM**

# URINARY SYSTEM

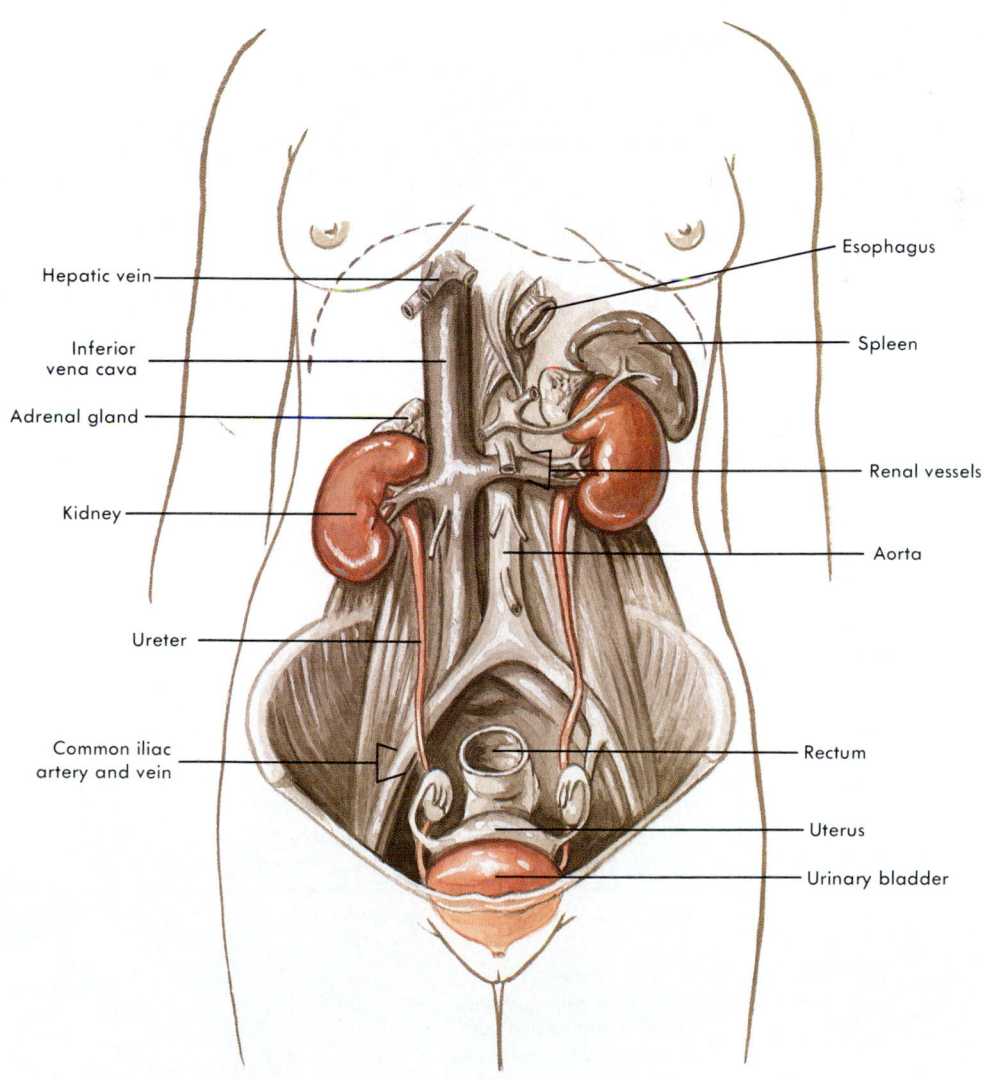

Hepatic vein

Inferior vena cava

Adrenal gland

Kidney

Ureter

Common iliac artery and vein

Esophagus

Spleen

Renal vessels

Aorta

Rectum

Uterus

Urinary bladder

**URINARY SYSTEM AND SOME ASSOCIATED STRUCTURES**

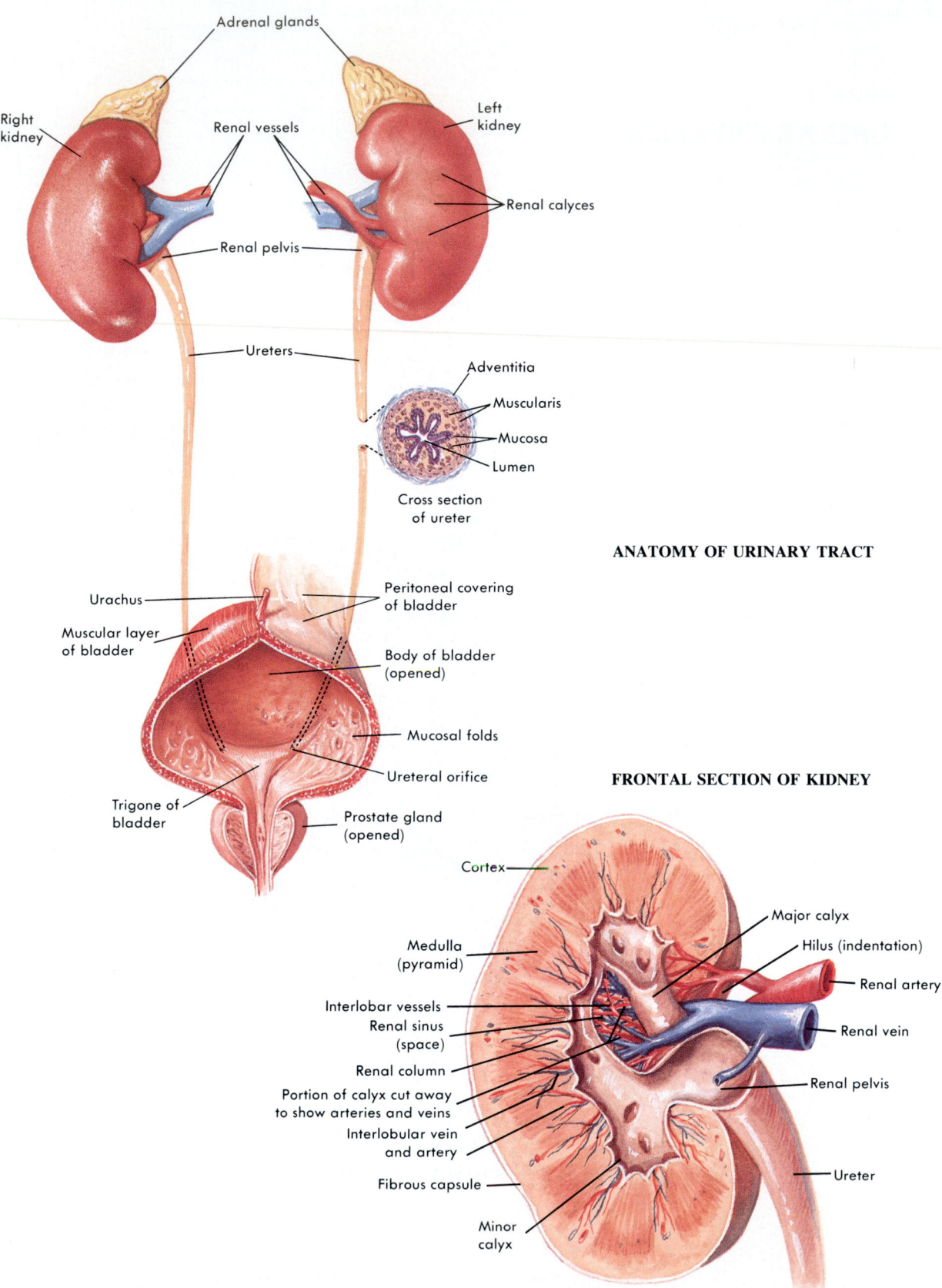

Adrenal glands

Right kidney

Renal vessels

Left kidney

Renal calyces

Renal pelvis

Ureters

Adventitia

Muscularis

Mucosa

Lumen

Cross section of ureter

**ANATOMY OF URINARY TRACT**

Urachus

Peritoneal covering of bladder

Muscular layer of bladder

Body of bladder (opened)

Mucosal folds

Ureteral orifice

**FRONTAL SECTION OF KIDNEY**

Trigone of bladder

Prostate gland (opened)

Cortex

Major calyx

Hilus (indentation)

Renal artery

Medulla (pyramid)

Interlobar vessels

Renal sinus (space)

Renal column

Portion of calyx cut away to show arteries and veins

Interlobular vein and artery

Fibrous capsule

Minor calyx

Renal vein

Renal pelvis

Ureter

# SPECIAL SENSES

## Hearing

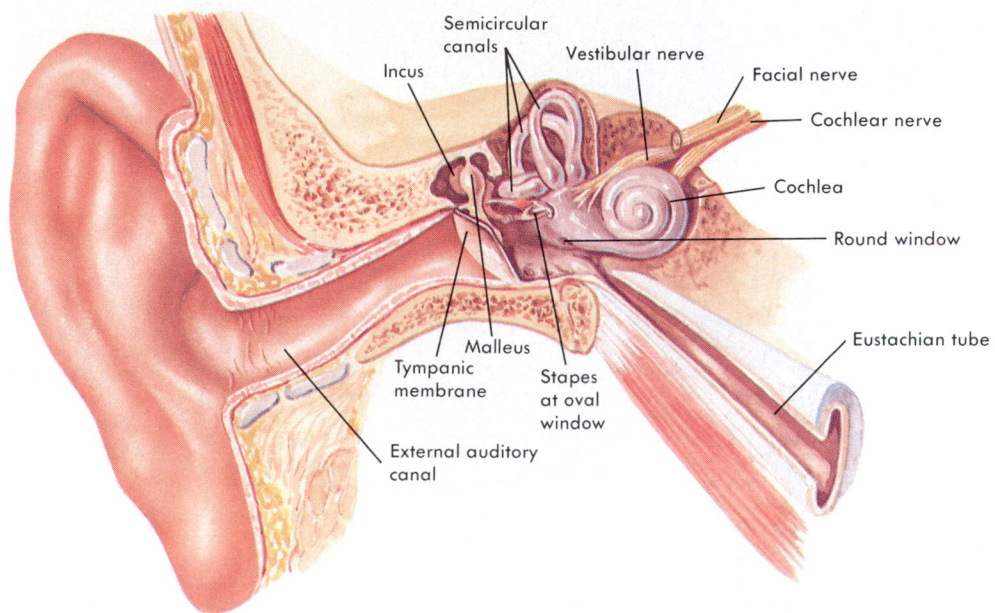

**GROSS ANATOMY OF THE EAR IN FRONTAL SECTION**

Semicircular canals

Incus

Vestibular nerve

Facial nerve

Cochlear nerve

Cochlea

Round window

Eustachian tube

Tympanic membrane

Malleus

Stapes at oval window

External auditory canal

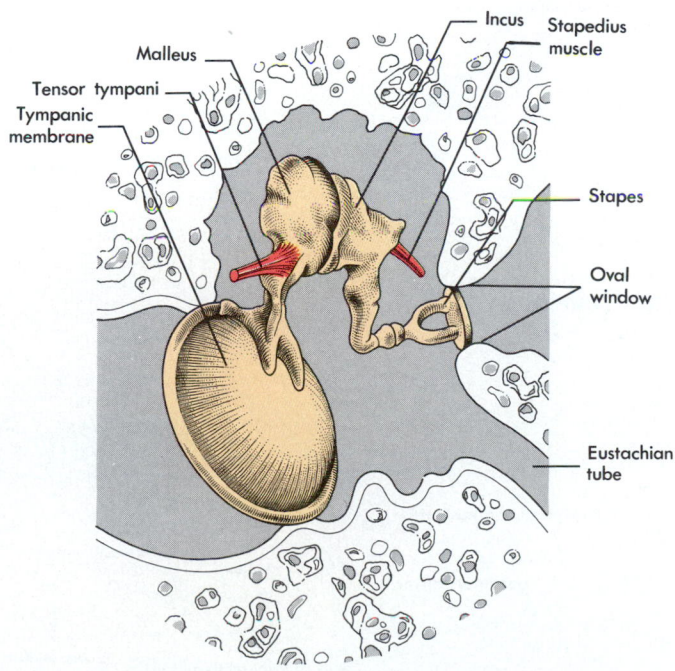

**IMPEDENCE-MATCHING COMPONENTS OF INNER EAR**

Malleus

Incus

Stapedius muscle

Tensor tympani

Tympanic membrane

Stapes

Oval window

Eustachian tube

# Sight

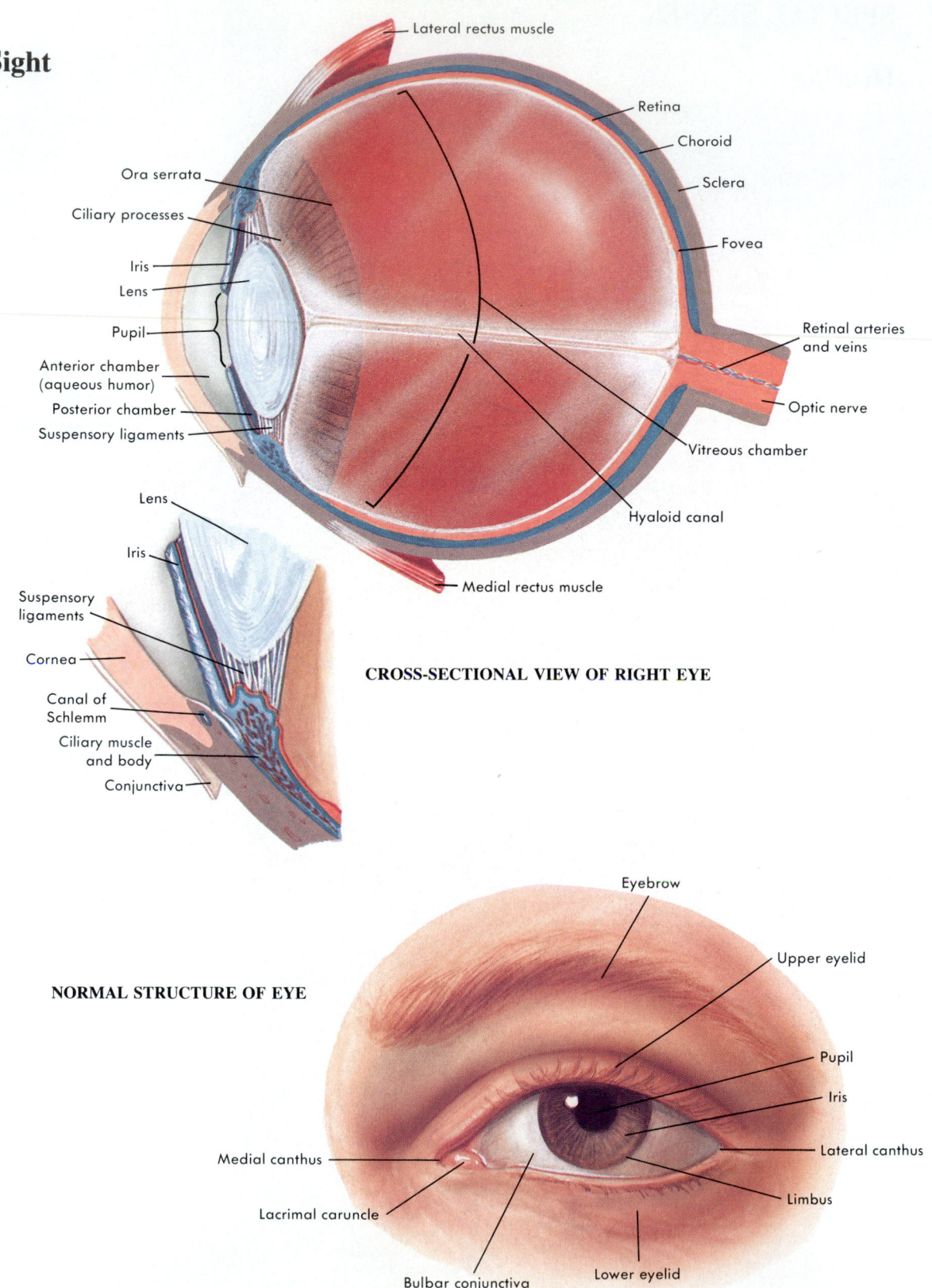

Lateral rectus muscle

Retina

Choroid

Sclera

Fovea

Ora serrata

Ciliary processes

Iris

Lens

Pupil

Anterior chamber (aqueous humor)

Posterior chamber

Suspensory ligaments

Retinal arteries and veins

Optic nerve

Vitreous chamber

Hyaloid canal

Medial rectus muscle

Lens

Iris

Suspensory ligaments

Cornea

Canal of Schlemm

Ciliary muscle and body

Conjunctiva

**CROSS-SECTIONAL VIEW OF RIGHT EYE**

**NORMAL STRUCTURE OF EYE**

Eyebrow

Upper eyelid

Pupil

Iris

Lateral canthus

Limbus

Medial canthus

Lacrimal caruncle

Bulbar conjunctiva

Lower eyelid

**A-30**

# SKIN

## Protection and Touch

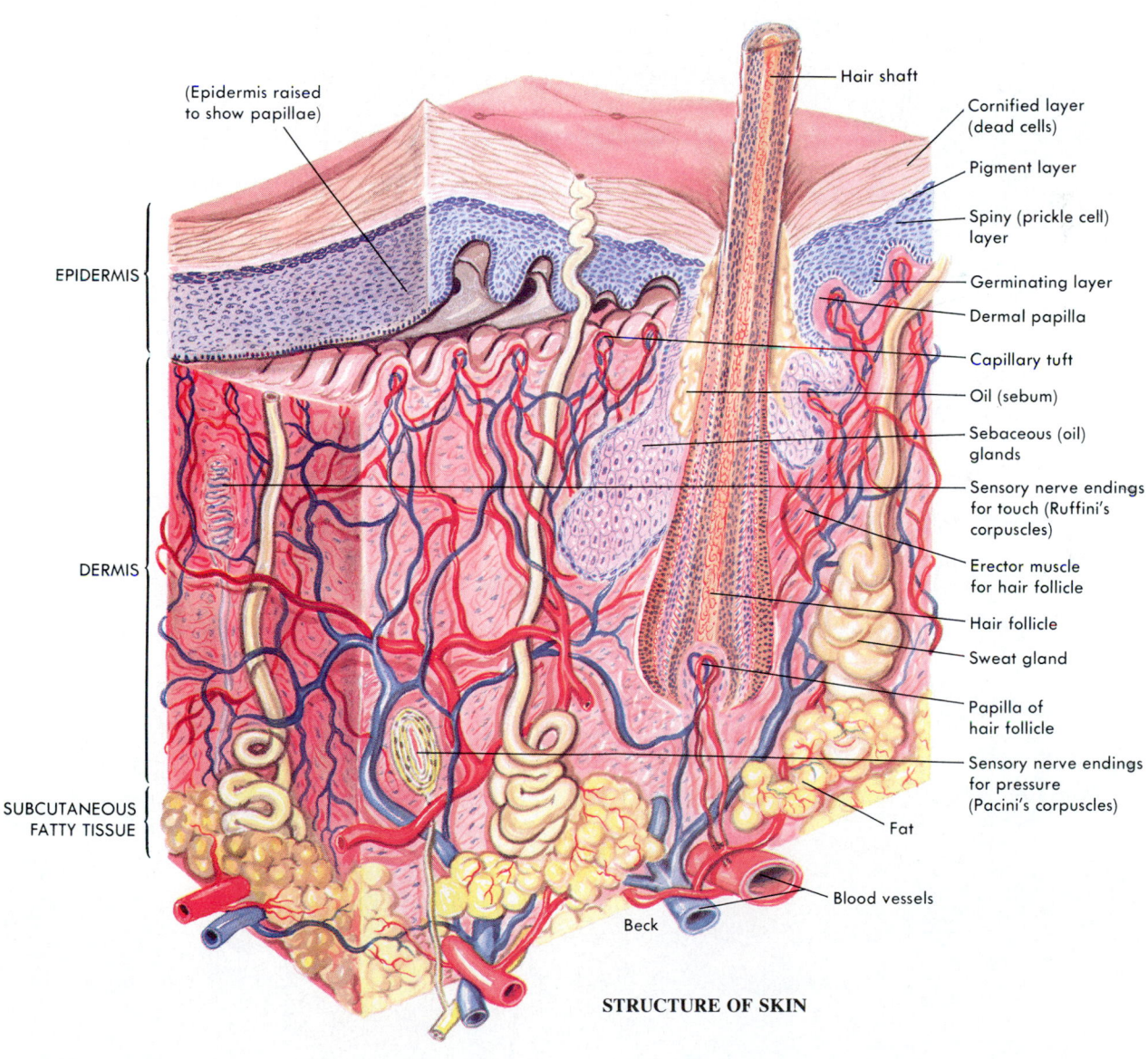

(Epidermis raised to show papillae)

Hair shaft

Cornified layer (dead cells)

Pigment layer

Spiny (prickle cell) layer

Germinating layer

Dermal papilla

Capillary tuft

Oil (sebum)

Sebaceous (oil) glands

Sensory nerve endings for touch (Ruffini's corpuscles)

Erector muscle for hair follicle

Hair follicle

Sweat gland

Papilla of hair follicle

Sensory nerve endings for pressure (Pacini's corpuscles)

Fat

Blood vessels

EPIDERMIS

DERMIS

SUBCUTANEOUS FATTY TISSUE

Beck

**STRUCTURE OF SKIN**

# Common Skin Disorders

**CLINICAL NOTE: Skin disorders**

Skin problems may result from various causes, such as parasitic infestations, fungal, bacterial, or viral infections, reactions to substances encountered externally or taken internally, or new growths. Many of the skin manifestations have no known cause; others are hereditary.

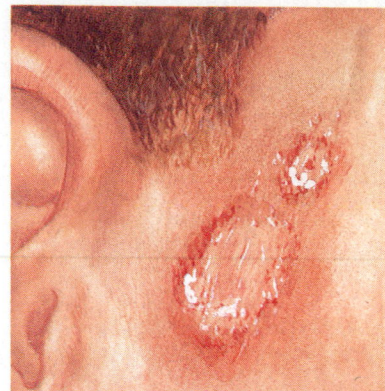

**TINEA CORPORIS (RINGWORM)**

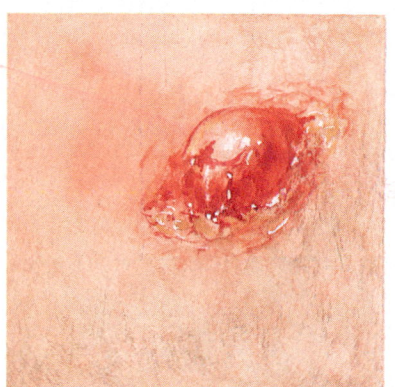

**SQUAMOUS CELL CARCINOMA**

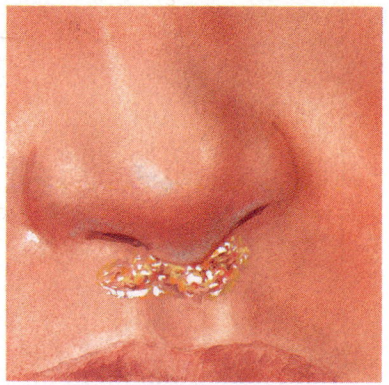

**IMPETIGO CONTAGIOSA**

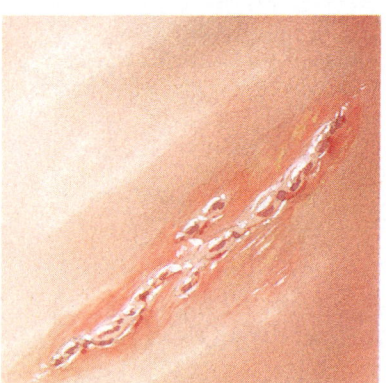

**HERPES ZOSTER (SHINGLES)**

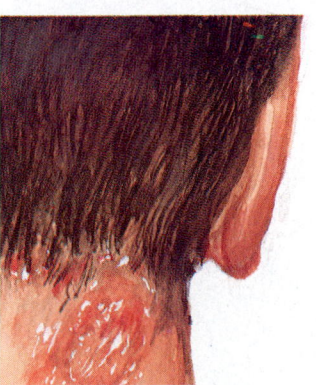

**DERMATITIS**

# 1

# Introduction to Word Parts

## Objectives

**Upon completion of this chapter you will be able to:**

1. **Identify and define the four word parts.**

2. **Identify and define combining forms.**

3. **Analyze and define medical terms**

4. **Build medical terms for given definitions.**

Medicine has a language of its own. Medical language, like the language of a people, possesses a historical development. Current medical vocabulary includes: terms used by Hippocrates and Aristotle 2000 years ago, *eponyms*, words based on the personal names of people, and terms from modern language. With the advancement of medical and scientific knowl-

### Figure 1-1
Origins of medical language.

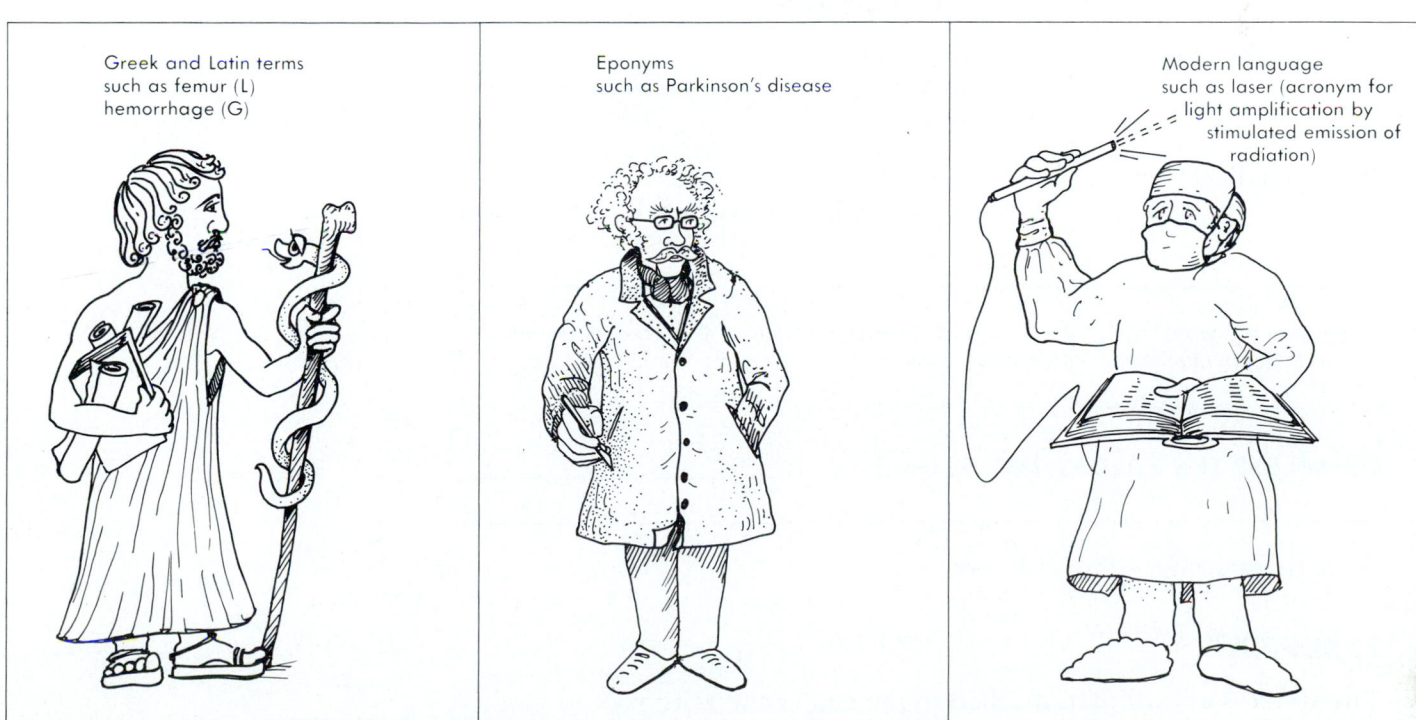

Greek and Latin terms
such as femur (L)
hemorrhage (G)

Eponyms
such as Parkinson's disease

Modern language
such as laser (acronym for
light amplification by
stimulated emission of
radiation)

edge, medical language changes: discarding some words, altering the meaning of the others, and adding new words.

   Still, the majority of medical terms in current use are composed of Greek and Latin word parts. There are two ways to learn the language of medicine: one is memorizing the medical terms, and the other is learning word parts and how they fit together to form medical terms. Because memorization of medical terms can be monotonous this text uses the word part method. Learning word parts and how they fit together provides the key to learning scores of medical words.

# Objective 1   IDENTIFY AND DEFINE THE FOUR WORD PARTS.

## Four Word Parts

Most medical terms consist of some or all of the following word parts:

1. Word roots
2. Suffixes
3. Prefixes
4. Combining vowels

### 1. WORD ROOT

The word root is the word part that is the core of the word. The word root contains the fundamental meaning of the word.

Examples:
In the word . . . . . . . . . . . . . .   play/er,
                                          *play* is the word root.

In the medical term . . . . . . . .   arthr/itis,
                                          *arthr* (which means *joint*) is the word root.

In the medical term . . . . . . . .   hepat/itis,
                                          *hepat* (which means *liver*), is the word root.

> Because the word root contains the fundamental meaning of the word, *each medical term contains one or more word roots.*

**COMPLETE THE FOLLOWING:** A word root is _____

_____

*Answer: the word part that is the core of the word.*

### 2. SUFFIX

The suffix is a word part attached to the end of the word root to modify its meaning.

Examples:

In the word . . . . . . . . . . . . . play/er,
*-er* is the suffix.

In the medical term . . . . . . . hepat/ic,
*-ic* (which means *pertaining to*) is the suffix.

As mentioned above, *hepat* is the word root for *liver;* therefore *hepatic* means *pertaining to the liver*.

In the medical term . . . . . . . hepat/itis,
*-itis* (which means *inflammation*) is the suffix.

The term *hepatitis* means *inflammation of the liver*.

> The suffix is used to modify the meaning of a word; therefore, *not all medical terms have a suffix.*

**COMPLETE THE FOLLOWING:** The suffix is _____

_____

*Answer: a word part attached to the end of the word root to modify its meaning.*

## 3. PREFIX

The prefix is a word part attached to the beginning of a word root to modify its meaning

Examples:

In the word . . . . . . . . . . . . . re/play,
*re-* is the prefix.

In the medical term . . . . . . . sub/hepat/ic,
*sub-* (which means *under*) is the prefix.

*Hepat* is the *word root* for *liver*, and *-ic* is the *suffix* for *pertaining to*. The medical term *subhepatic* means *pertaining to under the liver*.

In the medical term . . . . . . . intra/ven/ous,
*intra-* (which means *within*) is the prefix,
*ven-* (which means *vein*) is the word root, and
*-ous* (which means *pertaining to*) is the suffix.

The word *intravenous* means *pertaining to within the vein*.

> A prefix may be used to modify the meaning of a word; therefore, *not all medical terms have a prefix.*

**COMPLETE THE FOLLOWING:** The prefix is _____

_____

*Answer: a word part attached to the beginning of a word root to modify its meaning.*

## 4. COMBINING VOWEL

The combining vowel is a word part, usually an *o*, and is used between two word roots or between a word root and a suffix to ease pronunciation. The combining vowel is *not* used between a prefix and a word root.

Examples:

In the word . . . . . . . . . . . . . therm/o/meter,
                     *o* is the combining vowel used between two word parts.

In the medical term . . . . . . . arthr/o/pathy,
                     *o* is the combining vowel used between the word root *arthr* and the suffix *-pathy* (which means *disease*).

# Guidelines For Using Combining Vowels

**GUIDELINE ONE:** *When connecting a word root and a suffix, a combining vowel is usually not used if the suffix begins with a vowel.*

Example:

In the medical term . . . . . . . hepat/ic,
                     the suffix *-ic* begins with the vowel *i*; therefore a combining vowel is not used.

**GUIDELINE TWO:** *When connecting two word roots, a combining vowel is usually used even if vowels are present at the junction.*

Example:

In the medical term . . . . . . . oste/o/arthr/itis,
                     *o* is the combining vowel used, even though the word root *oste* (which means *bone*) ends with the vowel *e* and the word root *arthr* begins with the vowel *a*.

> The combining vowel is used to ease pronunciation; therefore, *not all medical terms have combining vowels.* Medical terms introduced throughout the text that have combining vowels other than *o* are highlighted at their introduction.

**COMPLETE THE FOLLOWING:** A combining vowel is _____

_____

*Answer: used between two word roots or between a word root and a suffix to ease pronunciation.*

# Objective 2 IDENTIFY AND DEFINE COMBINING FORMS.

## Combining Form

A combining form is a word root with the combining vowel attached, separated by a diagonal line.

> EXAMPLES: arthr/o
> oste/o
> ven/o

The combining form is not a word part; rather it is a presentation of two word parts. For learning purposes word roots are presented as combining forms throughout the text.

**COMPLETE THE FOLLOWING:** A combining form is _____

_____

*Answer: a word root with the combining vowel attached, separated by a diagonal line.*

Learn the word parts and combining forms by completing the following exercises.

### EXERCISE 1

Match the phrases in the first column with the correct terms in the second column. Check your answers with the correct answers at the end of the chapter.

_b_ 1. attached at the beginning of a word root    a. combining vowel

_a_ 2. usually an o    b. prefix

_d_ 3. all medical terms contain one or more    c. combining form

_e_ 4. attached at the end of word root    d. word root

   e. suffix

_c_ 5. word root with combining vowel attached

### EXERCISE 2

Answer *T* for *true* and *F* for *false*.

_F_ 1. There is always a prefix at the beginning of medical terms.

_F_ 2. A combining vowel is always used when connecting a word root and a suffix.

_T_ 3. A prefix modifies the meaning of the word.

___I___ 4. A combining vowel is used to ease pronunciation.

___F___ 5. *I* is the most commonly used combining vowel.

___I___ 6. The word root is the core of a medical term.

___F___ 7. A combining vowel is used between a prefix and a word root.

___F___ 8. A combining form is a word part.

Place a check mark (√) in the boxes to indicate that you have completed Objectives 1 and 2.

☐ **IDENTIFYAND DEFINE THE FOUR WORD PARTS**

☐ **IDENTIFY AND DEFINE COMBINING FORMS.**

# Objective 3   ANALYZE AND DEFINE MEDICAL TERMS.

# Analyzing and Defining Medical Terms
## ANALYZING

To analyze medical terms divide the medical terms into word parts, label each word part, and label the combining forms. Follow the procedure below:

1. Divide the term into word parts by vertical slashes.

    EXAMPLE:    oste/o/arthr/o/pathy

2. Label each word part by using the following abbreviations.

    WR   word root
    P    prefix
    S    suffix
    CV   combining vowel

                   WR   CV   WR   CV   S

EXAMPLE:    oste / o / arthr / o / pathy

3. Label the combining forms.

                   WR   CV   WR   CV   S

EXAMPLE:    oste / o / arthr / o / pathy

              CF           CF

Analyze the following medical term.

osteopathy

$$
\begin{array}{ccc} WR & CV & S \end{array}
$$
*Answer:* <u>oste</u> / o / pathy
$$\underbrace{\phantom{oste \,/\, o}}_{CF}$$

## DEFINING

To define medical terms apply the meaning of each word part in the term.

> A helpful rule: *Begin by defining the suffix, then move to the beginning of the term to complete the definition.* (Does not apply to all medical terms)

Apply this rule to find the definition of oste/o/arthr/o/pathy.

Write the definition of *osteoarthropathy*. Begin by defining the word *pathy*, then move to the beginning of the term. Use the box to find the meaning of the word parts. _____

_____

*Answer: disease of the bone and joint.*

Practice analyzing and defining medical terms by completing the following exercise.

| COMBINING FORMS | DEFINITION |
|---|---|
| arthr/o | joint |
| hepat/o | liver |
| ven/o | vein |
| oste/o | bone |
| **PREFIXES** | |
| intra- | within |
| sub- | under |
| **SUFFIXES** | |
| -itis | inflammation |
| -ic | pertaining to |
| -ous | pertaining to |
| -pathy | disease |
| **COMBINING VOWEL** | |
| -o- | |

## EXERCISE 3

Using the box to the right to identify the word parts and their meaning, analyze and define the following terms.

$$
\begin{array}{cccccc} & WR & CV & WR & CV & S \end{array}
$$
EXAMPLE:   oste/o/arthr/o/pathy   *disease of bone and joint*
$$\underbrace{\phantom{oste/o}}_{CF}\;\underbrace{\phantom{arthr/o}}_{CF}$$

1. arthritis  *inflamation of the joints*

2. hepatitis  *inflamation of the liver*

3. subhepatic  *pertaining to under the liver*

4. intravenous  *pertaining to within the vein*

5. arthropathy  *disease of the joints*

6. osteitis  *inflamation of the bones*

Place a check mark (√) in the box below to indicate that you have completed Objective 3.

☐ ANALYZE AND DEFINE MEDICAL TERMS.

# Objective 4   BUILD MEDICAL TERMS FOR GIVEN DEFINITIONS.

## Building Medical Terms

Building medical terms means using word parts to build a medical term that matches the definition.

Using the box on p. 7 as a reference, complete the following steps to build the medical term for

*disease of a joint.*

**STEP 1:** Find the word part for *disease*. Write the word part in the space below.

**STEP 2:** Find the word part for *joint*. Write the word part in the space below.

**STEP 3:** The suffix does not begin with a vowel, so a combining vowel is needed. Insert the combining vowel *o* in the correct space below.

$$\underline{\quad \underset{\text{WR}}{arthr} \mid \underset{\text{CV}}{o} \mid \underset{\text{S}}{pathy} \quad}$$

*Answer: arthropathy.*

**COMPLETE THE FOLLOWING:** Building a medical term means _____ _____

*Answer: using word parts to create a medical term that matches the definition.*

Practice building medical terms by completing the following exercises.

### EXERCISE 4

Using the box on p. 7 as a reference, build medical terms for the following definitions.

EXAMPLE:   disease of the joint   $\underset{\text{WR} \mid \text{CV} \mid \text{S}}{arthr \mid o \mid pathy}$

> Keep in mind that the beginning of the definition usually indicates the suffix.

1. inflammation of the joint   $\underset{\text{WR} \mid \text{S}}{arthr \mid itis}$

2. pertaining to the liver   $\underset{\text{WR} \mid \text{S}}{hepat \mid ic}$

3. pertaining to under the liver

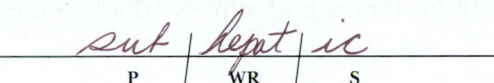

P | WR | S

4. pertaining to within the vein

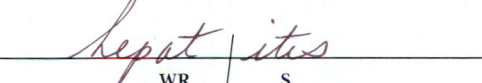

P | WR | S

5. inflammation of the bone

*oste | itis*

WR | S

6. inflammation of the liver

*hepat | itis*

WR | S

7. disease of the bone and joint

*oste | o | arthr | o | pathy*

WR | CV | WR | CV | S

> In a term that has more than one root there is no rule as to which goes first. The order is usually dictated by common practice. You will eventually become accustomed to the accepted order.

Place a check mark (√) in the box to indicate that you have completed Objective 4.

☐ BUILD MEDICAL TERMS FOR GIVEN DEFINITIONS.

## Summary

To complete this chapter successfully, you do not need to know what the word parts, such as *arthr,* mean. You will learn these in subsequent chapters. **It is important that you have met these objectives:**

1. Can you identify and define the four word parts?   yes ☐   no ☐
2. Can you identify and define a combining form?   yes ☐   no ☐
3. Can you use word parts to analyze and define medical terms? yes ☐   no ☐
4. Can you use word parts to build medical terms for a given definition?   yes ☐   no ☐

If you answered *yes* to these questions, move on to Chapter 2 and begin to build your medical vocabulary so that you will be better prepared than

Grimm, in the cartoon (Figure 1-2), to understand and use the language of medicine.

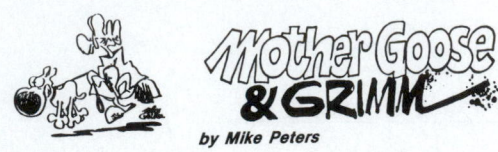

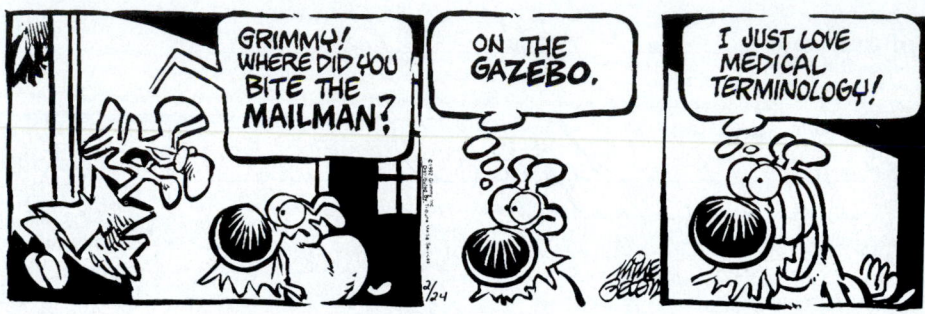

Figure 1-2

Reprinted by permission: Tribune Media Services.

# Answers

### Exercise 1

1. b   2. a   3. d   4. e   5. c

### Exercise 2

1. *F*, a medical term may begin with the root and have no prefix.
2. *F*, if the suffix begins with a vowel, the combining vowel is usually not used.
3. *T*
4. *T*
5. *F*, *O* is the combining vowel most used.
6. *T*
7. *F*, a combining vowel is used between two word roots or between a word root and a suffix beginning with a consonant.
8. *F*, a combining form is not a word part.

### Exercise 3

1. arthr/itis
   WR   S
   inflammation of the joint

2. hepat/itis
   WR   S
   inflammation of the liver

3. sub/hepat/ic
   P   WR   S
   pertaining to under the liver

4. intra/ven/ous
   P   WR   S
   pertaining to within the vein

5. arthr/ o /pathy
   WR  CV   S
   CF
   disease of the joint

6. oste/itis
   WR   S
   inflammation of the bone

### Exercise 4

1. arthr/itis
2. hepat/ic
3. sub/hepat/ic
4. intra/ven/ous
5. oste/itis
6. hepat/itis
7. oste/o/arthr/o/pathy

# Note to Students and Instructors:

To introduce directional terms and anatomical planes and regions, complete Chapter 16 before proceeding to Chapter 2.

# 2

# Structure of the Human Body

## Objectives

Upon completion of this chapter you will be able to:

1. Define the anatomical terms of the human body structure.

2. Write the definitions of the word parts included in this chapter.

3. Build, analyze, define, pronounce, and spell the diagnostic terms related to the human body structure.

4. Build, analyze, define, pronounce, and spell additional terms related to the human body structure.

5. Define, pronounce, and spell the other additional terms related to the human body structure.

## Objective 1    DEFINE THE ANATOMICAL TERMS OF THE HUMAN BODY STRUCTURE.

## Anatomical Terms

### ORGANIZATION OF THE BODY

The structure of the human body falls into four categories: cells, tissues, organs, and systems. Each structure is a highly organized unit of smaller structures (Figure 2-1).

1. cell . . . . . . . . . . . . . . . . . Basic unit of all living things (Figure 2-2). The human body is composed of trillions of cells, which vary in size and shape according to function.

   a. cell membrane. . . . . . Forms the boundary of the cell.

   b. cytoplasm. . . . . . . . . . Makes up the body of the cell.

   c. nucleus . . . . . . . . . . Small, round structure in the center of the cell that contains chromosomes.

   d. chromosomes. . . . . . . Located in the nucleus of the cell. There are 46 chromosomes in all human cells with the exception of the mature sex cell, which has 23.

   e. genes . . . . . . . . . . . . . Regions within the chromosome. Each chromosome has several thousand genes that determine hereditary characteristics.

The cell was named about 300 years ago by Robert Hooke. Upon seeing them through a microscope, he named them **cells** because they reminded him of miniature prison cells.

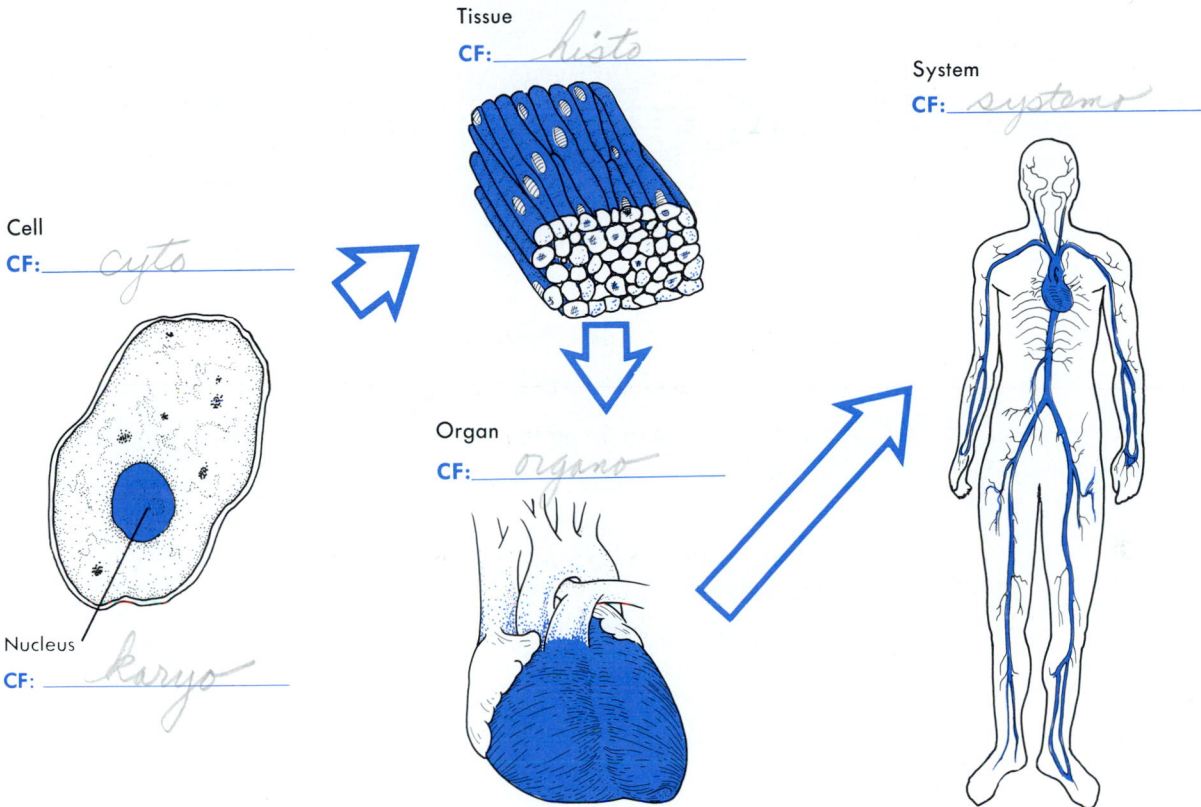

**Cell**
**CF:** _cyto_

**Nucleus**
**CF:** _karyo_

**Tissue**
**CF:** _histo_

**Organ**
**CF:** _organo_

**System**
**CF:** _systemo_

### Figure 2-1

Organization of the body. The abbreviation **CF** preceding the blank lines on this figure means "combining form." In Exercise 3 you will be asked to fill in the blanks on Figures 2-1 and 2-3 with the combining form that corresponds with the body part illustrated.

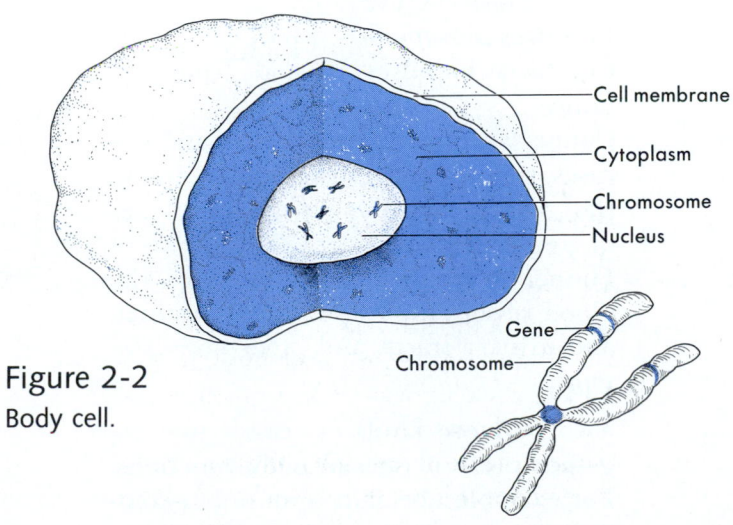

Cell membrane
Cytoplasm
Chromosome
Nucleus
Gene
Chromosome

### Figure 2-2
Body cell.

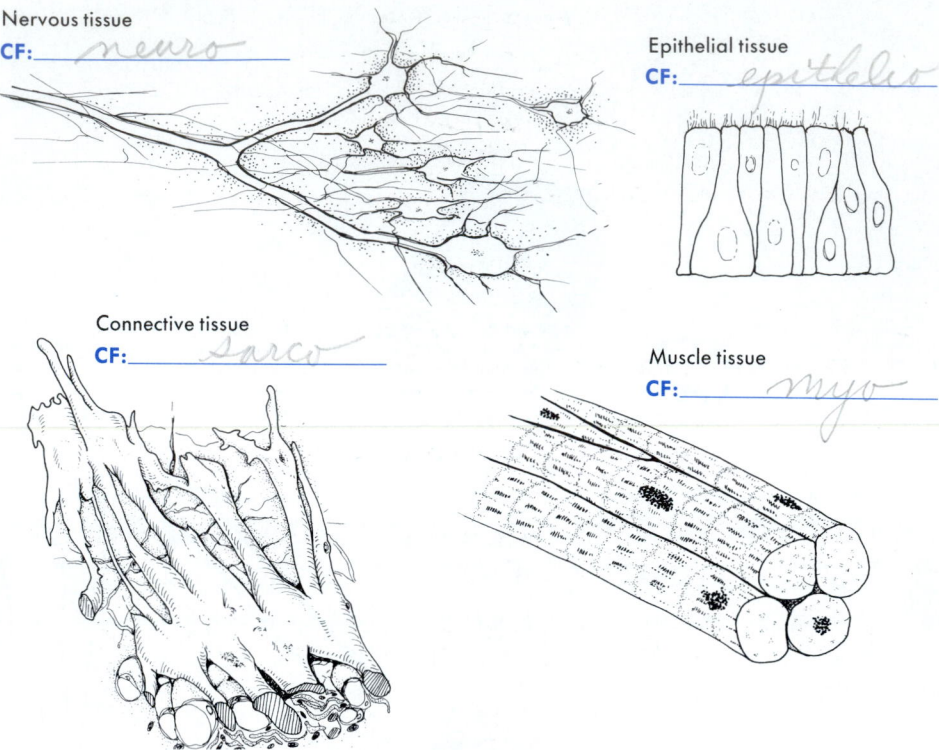

Nervous tissue
CF: _neuro_

Epithelial tissue
CF: _epithelio_

Connective tissue
CF: _sarco_

Muscle tissue
CF: _myo_

Figure 2-3
Types of tissues.

| | | |
|---|---|---|
| f. | DNA (deoxyribonucleic acid)......... | Each gene is composed of DNA, a chemical that regulates the activities of the cell. |
| 2. | tissue ............... | Group of similar cells that performs a specific task (Figure 2-3). |
| a. | muscle tissue ....... | Produces movement. |
| b. | nervous tissue ...... | Conducts impulses to and from the brain. |
| c. | connective tissue .... | Connects, supports, penetrates, and encases various body structures. Adipose (fat) and osseous (bone) tissues are types of connective tissue. |
| d. | epithelial tissue ..... | Found in the skin and lining of the blood vessels, the respiratory, intestinal, and urinary tracts, and other body systems. |
| 3. | organ ............... | Two or more kinds of tissues that together perform special body functions. For example, the skin is an organ composed of epithelial, connective, and nerve tissue. |

4.  system . . . . . . . . . . . . . . .   Group of organs that work together to perform complex body functions. For example, the nervous system is made up of the brain, spinal cord, and nerves; its function is to coordinate and control other body parts.

## BODY CAVITIES

The body is not a solid structure, as it appears on the outside, but has five cavities (Figure 2-4), each containing an orderly arrangement of internal organs.

1.  cranial cavity . . . . . . . . . .   Space inside the skull (cranium), containing the brain.

2.  spinal cavity . . . . . . . . . .   Space inside the spinal column, containing the spinal cord.

3.  thoracic, *or* chest cavity . .   Space containing the heart, lungs, esophagus, trachea, bronchi, and thymus.

4.  abdominal cavity . . . . . . .   Space containing the stomach, intestines, kidneys, liver, gallbladder, pancreas, spleen, and ureters.

5.  pelvic cavity . . . . . . . . . .   Space containing the urinary bladder, certain reproductive organs, part of the large intestine, and the rectum.

Learn the anatomical terms by completing the following exercises.

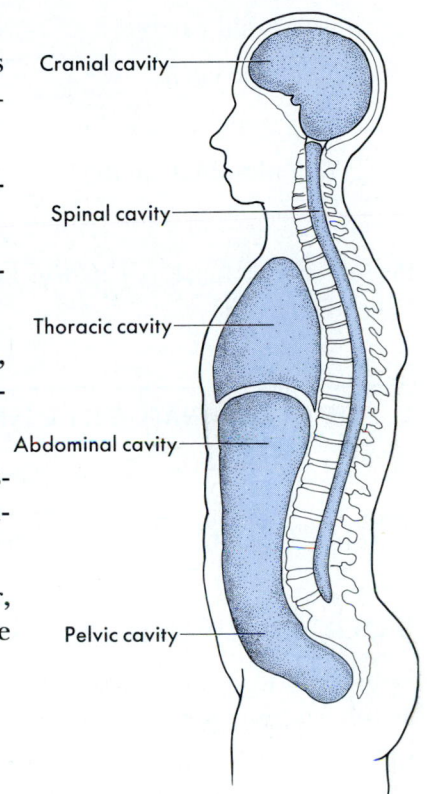

Figure 2-4

## EXERCISE 1

Match the terms in the first column with the correct definitions in the second column.

| | | |
|---|---|---|
| _h_ | 1. chromosomes | a. type of connective tissue |
| _e_ | 2. nucleus | b. regions within the chromosome |
| _d_ | 3. cytoplasm | c. tissue found in the skin |
| _k_ | 4. cell | d. comprises the body of the cell |
| _g_ | 5. muscle | e. contains chromosomes |
| _f_ | 6. nerve | f. conducts impulses |
| _c_ | 7. epithelial | g. produces movement |
| _a_ | 8. bone | h. contains genes |
| _b_ | 9. genes | i. chest cavity |
| _j_ | 10. DNA | j. a chemical that regulates the activities of the cell |
| | | k. basic unit of all living things |

## EXERCISE 2

Match the terms in the first column with the correct definitions in the second column.

_h_ 1. spinal cavity

_b_ 2. thoracic cavity

_c_ 3. organ

_e_ 4. cranial cavity

_g_ 5. pelvic cavity

_a_ 6. system

_f_ 7. abdominal cavity

a. group of organs functioning together

b. chest cavity

c. composed of two or more tissues

d. found in the skin

e. space inside the skull

f. contains the stomach

g. contains the urinary bladder

h. contains the spinal cord

Place a check mark (√) in the box to indicate that you have completed Objective 1.

☐ DEFINE THE ANATOMICAL TERMS OF THE HUMAN BODY STRUCTURE.

## Objective 2    WRITE THE DEFINITIONS OF THE WORD PARTS INCLUDED IN THIS CHAPTER.

## Body Structure Word Parts

Begin building your medical vocabulary by learning the word parts listed as follows. The list may appear long to you; however, the many exercises that follow are designed to ease your learning task.

> Reminder: The word root is the core of the word. The combining form is the word root with the combining vowel attached, separated by a diagonal line.

| COMBINING FORM | DEFINITION |
| --- | --- |
| 1. cyt/o | cell |
| 2. epitheli/o | epithelium |
| 3. hist/o | tissue |
| 4. kary/o | nucleus |
| 5. lip/o | fat |
| 6. my/o | muscle |
| 7. neur/o | nerve |
| 8. organ/o | organ |
| 9. sarc/o | flesh, connective tissue |

**Epithelium** originally meant **surface over the nipple. Epi** means **upon**, and **thela** means **nipple** (or projecting surfaces of many kinds).

10.  system/o . . . . . . . . . . . .  system
11.  viscer/o . . . . . . . . . . . .  internal organs

Learn the anatomical locations and definitions of the combining forms by completing the following exercises.

## EXERCISE 3

Write the combining forms in the spaces marked **CF** on the diagrams in Figures 2-1 and 2-3, pp. 13 and 14.

## EXERCISE 4

Write the definitions of the following combining forms.

1.  sarc/o __flesh, connective tissue__
2.  lip/o __fat__
3.  kary/o __nucleus__
4.  viscer/o __internal organs__
5.  cyt/o __cell__
6.  hist/o __tissue__
7.  my/o __muscle__
8.  neur/o __nerve__
9.  organ/o __organ__
10. system/o __system__
11. epitheli/o __epithelium__

## EXERCISE 5

Write the combining form for each of the following.

1.  internal organs __viscer/o__
2.  epithelium __epitheli/o__
3.  organ __organ/o__
4.  nucleus __kary/o__
5.  cell __cyt/o__
6.  tissue __hist/o__

7. nerve                          _neur/o_

8. muscle                         _my/o_

9. fat                            _lip/o_

10. system                        _system/o_

11. connective tissue,            _sarc/o_
    flesh

# Related Word Parts

| COMBINING FORM | DEFINITION |
|---|---|
| 1. carcin/o<br>cancer/o . . . . . . . . . . . . . | cancer (a disease characterized by the unregulated, abnormal growth of new cells) |
| 2. eti/o . . . . . . . . . . . . . . . | cause (of disease) |
| 3. gno/o . . . . . . . . . . . . . | knowledge |
| 4. iatr/o . . . . . . . . . . . . . . | physician, medicine |
| 5. lei/o . . . . . . . . . . . . . | smooth |
| 6. onc/o . . . . . . . . . . . . . | tumor |
| 7. path/o . . . . . . . . . . . . . . | disease |
| 8. rhabd/o . . . . . . . . . . . . . | rod-shaped, striated |
| 9. somat/o . . . . . . . . . . . . . | body |

> Both **carcin** and **cancer** are derived from Latin and Greek words meaning **crab** and originated before the nature of malignant growth was understood. One explanation is that the swollen veins around the diseased area looked like the claws of a crab.

Learn the related combining forms by completing the following exercises.

## EXERCISE 6

Write the definitions of the following combining forms.

1. onc/o _____tumor_____

2. carcin/o _____cancer_____

3. eti/o _____cause (of disease)_____

4. path/o _____disease_____

5. somat/o _____body_____

6. cancer/o _____cancer_____

7. rhabd/o _____rod-shaped, striated_____

8. lei/o _____smooth_____

9. gno/o _____ *knowledge* _____

10. iatr/o _____ *physician medicine* _____

## EXERCISE 7

Write the combining form for each of the following.

1. disease                          _____ *path/o* _____

2. tumor                            _____ *onc/o* _____

3. cause (of disease)               _____ *eti/o* _____

4. cancer              a.           _____ *carcin/o* _____

                       b.           _____ *cancer/o* _____

5. body                             _____ *somat/o* _____

6. smooth                           _____ *lei/o* _____

7. rod-shaped, striated             _____ *rhabd/o* _____

8. knowledge                        _____ *gno/o* _____

9. physician, medicine              _____ *iatr/o* _____

# Color

| COMBINING FORM | DEFINITION |
| --- | --- |
| 1. chrom/o . . . . . . . . . . . . | color |
| 2. cyan/o. . . . . . . . . . . . . | blue |
| 3. erythr/o . . . . . . . . . . . | red |
| 4. leuk/o. . . . . . . . . . . . . | white |
| 5. melan/o . . . . . . . . . . . | black |
| 6. xanth/o. . . . . . . . . . . . | yellow |

Learn the color combining forms by completing the following exercises.

## EXERCISE 8

Write the definitions of the following combining forms.

1. cyan/o _____ *blue* _____

2. erythr/o _____ *red* _____

3. leuk/o _____ *white* _____

4. xanth/o _____ *yellow* _____

5. chrom/o _____ *color* _____

6. melan/o _____ *black* _____

## EXERCISE 9

Write the combining form for each of the following.

1. blue _____ *cyan/o* _____

2. red _____ *erythr/o* _____

3. white _____ *leuk/o* _____

4. black _____ *melan/o* _____

5. yellow _____ *xanth/o* _____

6. color _____ *chrom/o* _____

# Prefixes

| PREFIX | DEFINITION |
|---|---|
| 1. dia-................. | through, complete |
| 2. dys-................. | difficult, labored, painful, abnormal |
| 3. hyper-............... | above, excessive |
| 4. hypo- ............... | below, incomplete, deficient |
| 5. meta- ............... | after, beyond, change |
| 6. neo- ................. | new |
| 7. pro ................. | before |

> Reminder: Prefixes are placed at the beginning of a word root.

Learn the prefixes by completing the following exercises.

## EXERCISE 10

Write the definitions of the following prefixes.

1. neo- _____ *new* _____

2. hyper- _____ *above, excessive* _____

3. meta- _____ *after, beyond, change* _____

4. hypo- _____ *below, incomplete, deficient* _____

5. dys- _____ *difficult, labored, painful, abnormal* _____

6. dia- _____ *complete, through* _____

7. pro- _____ *before* _____

## EXERCISE 11

Write the prefix for each of the following.

1. new                                          _neo_

2. above, excessive                    _hyper_

3. below, incomplete,               _hypo_
   deficient

4. beyond, after, change          _meta_

5. abnormal, painful,               _dys_
   labored, difficult

6. through, complete                _dia_

7. before                                    _pro_

# Suffixes

| SUFFIX | | DEFINITION |
|---|---|---|
| 1. | -al<br>-ic<br>-ous............... | pertaining to |
| 2. | -cyte ...............<br>(NOTE: *Cyte* ends in an "e" when used as a suffix). | cell |
| 3. | -gen ............... | substance or agent that produces or causes |
| 4. | -genesis............. | origin, cause |
| 5. | -genic.............. | producing, originating, causing |
| 6. | -oid................. | resembling |
| 7. | -ologist ............ | one who studies and practices (specialist, physician) |
| 8. | -ology ............. | study of |
| 9. | -oma............... | tumor, swelling |
| 10. | -osis ............... | abnormal condition (means *increase* when used with blood cell word roots) |
| 11. | -pathy............. | disease |
| 12. | -plasia............. | formation, development, a growth  _(cellular level)_ |
| 13. | -plasm........... | growth, substance, formation  _(tumor)_ |
| 14. | -sarcoma........... | malignant tumor |
| 15. | -sis ............... | state of |
| 16. | -stasis ............. | control, stop |

Reminder: Suffixes are placed at the end of a word.

Some suffixes are made up of a word root plus a suffix; they are presented as suffixes for ease of learning. For example: **-pathy** is made up of the word root **path** and the suffix **y**. When analyzing a word, divide the suffixes as learned. For example, a word such as **somatopathy** should be divided somat/o/pathy and **not** somat/o/path/y

Learn the suffixes by completing the following exercises.

## EXERCISE 12

Match the suffixes in the first column with their correct definitions in the second column.

| | | |
|---|---|---|
| _i_ | 1. -ology | a. producing |
| _l_ | 2. -osis | b. cell |
| _e_ | 3. -pathy | c. specialist |
| _f_ | 4. -plasm | d. new |
| _g_ | 5. -al, -ic, -ous | e. disease |
| _j_ | 6. -stasis | f. substance, growth, formation |
| _h_ | 7. -oid | g. pertaining to |
| _b_ | 8. -cyte | h. resembling |
| _p_ | 9. -genesis | i. study of |
| _c_ | 10. -ologist | j. control, stop |
| _n_ | 11. -oma | k. substance that produces |
| _k_ | 12. -gen | l. abnormal condition |
| _q_ | 13. -sarcoma | m. formation, development, a growth |
| _m_ | 14. -plasia | n. tumor |
| _a_ | 15. -genic | o. state of |
| _o_ | 16. -sis | p. origin, cause |
| | | q. malignant tumor |

> **Sarcoma** has been used since ancient Greece to describe any fleshy tumor. Since the introduction of cellular pathology the term came to be restricted to mean a malignant connective tissue tumor.

## EXERCISE 13

Write the definitions of the following suffixes.

1. -ologist ___one who studies and practices___
2. -pathy ___disease___
3. -ology ___study of___
4. -ic ___pertaining to___
5. -stasis ___control, stop___
6. -cyte ___cell___
7. -osis ___abnormal condition___
8. -ous ___pertaining to___
9. -plasm ___substance, growth, formation___

10. -al ___ *pertaining to* ___

11. -plasia ___ *formation, development, a growth* ___

12. -oid ___ *resembling* ___

13. -gen ___ *substance that produces or causes* ___

14. -genic ___ *producing, originating, causing* ___

15. -oma ___ *tumor, swelling* ___

16. -genesis ___ *origin, cause* ___

17. -sarcoma ___ *malignant tumor* ___

18. -sis ___ *state of* ___

Place a check mark (√) in the box to indicate that you have completed Objective 2.

☐ **WRITE THE DEFINITIONS OF THE WORD PARTS INCLUDED IN THIS CHAPTER.**

# Medical Terms

The terms you need to learn to complete this chapter are listed as follows. Do not be alarmed by the length of this list. You already know the meaning of the word parts, and the following exercises will assist you in learning the definition and spelling of the terms.

## HOW TERMS ARE LISTED

The terms listed under the headings

*Diagnostic Terms*
*Surgical Terms*
*Diagnostic Procedural Terms*
*Additional Terms*

are composed of word parts, and literal translation will give the meaning or the approximate meaning of the terms. Further explanation of terms beyond the literal translation, if needed, is included in brackets following the definition.

The terms listed under the headings

*Other Diagnostic Terms*
*Other Surgical Terms*
*Other Diagnostic Procedural Terms*
*Other Additional Terms*

include terms that cannot be literally translated to find the meaning. Some of these terms are built from word parts, but new knowledge has changed their meanings since they were coined. Some terms are eponyms, and some have no apparent explanation for their names.

The chapters may have lists in some or all of these categories. In this chapter, for example, there is no list of surgical terms.

## Objective 3  BUILD, ANALYZE, DEFINE, PRONOUNCE, AND SPELL THE DIAGNOSTIC TERMS RELATED TO THE HUMAN BODY STRUCTURE.

# Diagnostic Terms

| TERM<br>(built from word parts) | DEFINITION |
|---|---|
| 1. **carcinoma**............<br>(*kar*-si-NŌ-ma) | cancerous tumor (malignant tumor) (Figure 2-5) |
| 2. **epithelioma** .........<br>(*ep*-i-*thē*-lē-Ō-ma) | tumor composed of epithelial cells (malignant tumor) |
| 3. **leiomyoma** .... ....<br>(lī-ō-mī-Ō-ma) | tumor of smooth muscle (benign) |
| 4. **leiomyosarcoma**.......<br>(lī-ō-mī-ō-sar-KŌ-ma) | malignant tumor of smooth muscle |
| 5. **lipoma** .............<br>(li-PŌ-ma) | tumor containing fat (benign tumor) |

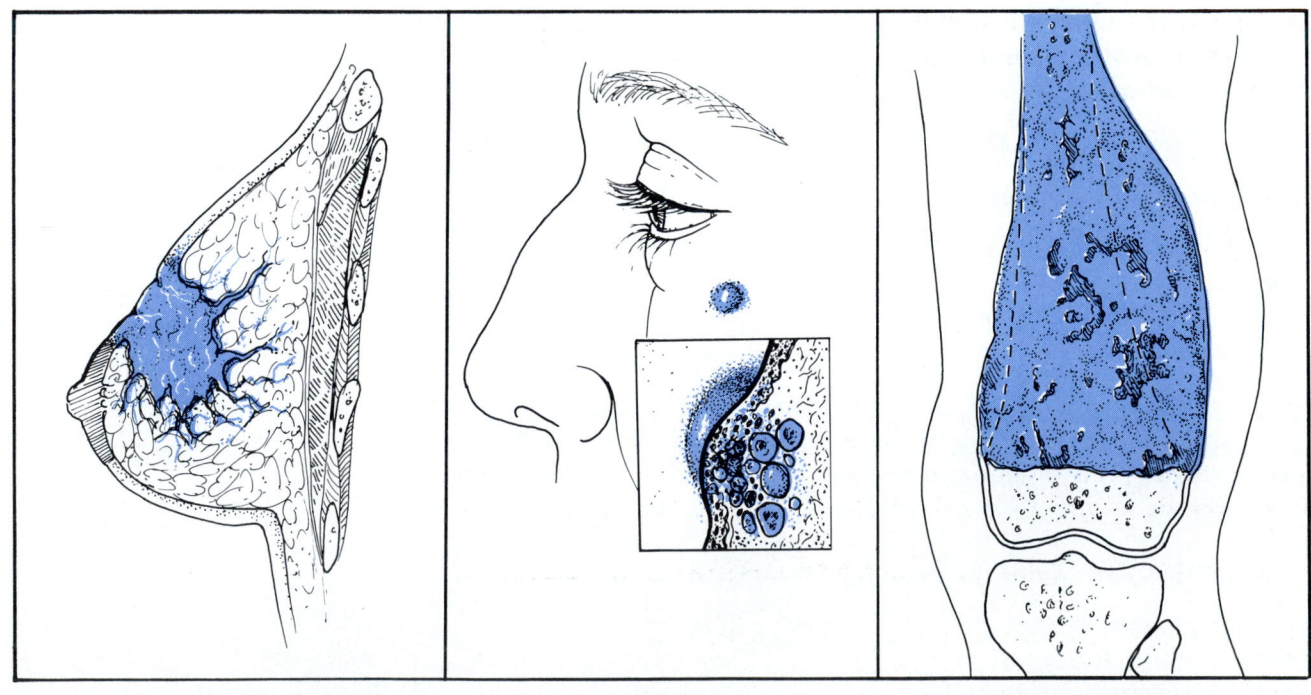

Carcinoma          Melanoma          Sarcoma of the femur

Figure 2-5
Types of cancer.

6.  melanocarcinoma . . . . . .    cancerous (malignant) black tumor
    (*mel*-a-nō-*kar*-si-NŌ-ma)

7.  melanoma . . . . . . . . . . .    black tumor (primarily of the skin) (Fig-
    (*mel*-a-NŌ-ma)                    ure 2-5)

8.  myoma . . . . . . . . . . . . .    tumor formed of muscle tissue
    (mī-Ō-ma)

9.  neoplasm . . . . . . . . . . .    new growth (of abnormal tissue or tu-
    (NĒ-ō-plazm)                       mor)

10. neuroma . . . . . . . . . . . .    tumor made up of nerve cells
    (nū-RŌ-ma)

11. rhabdomyoma . . . . . . . .    tumor of striated muscle (benign)
    (rab-dō-mī-Ō-ma)

12. rhabdomyosarcoma . . . .    malignant tumor of striated muscle
    (rab-dō-mī-ō-sar-KŌ-ma)

13. sarcoma . . . . . . . . . . . .    tumor composed of connective tissue
    (sar-KŌ-ma)                        (such as bone or cartilage) and highly
                                        malignant (Figure 2-5)

Practice saying each of these terms aloud. Refer to "How to Use This
Text," p. xi, for explanation of the pronunciation key. To assist you in
pronunciation, obtain the audiotape designed for use with this text. Learn
the definitions and spellings of the diagnostic terms by completing the following exercises.

## EXERCISE 14

Analyze and define the following diagnostic terms. Refer to Chapter 1,
pp. 6 and 7, to review analyzing and defining techniques. **This is an important exercise; do not skip any portion of it.**

> Note: When you are analyzing terms that have a suffix containing a word root, it
> may appear, as in the word **neoplasm,** that the word is composed of only a prefix
> and a suffix. Keep in mind that the word does have a word root but that it is em-
> bedded in the suffix.

                                         WR  CV  WR    S
            EXAMPLE:    melan/o/carcin/oma    *cancerous black tumor*
                                  CF

1. sarcoma _____ *flesh tumor of connective tissue + highly malignant*

2. melanoma _____ *black tumor*

3. epithelioma _____ *tumor of epithelium*

4. lipoma _____ *fatty tumor*

5. neoplasm _____ *new growth*

6. myoma    WR S    _muscle tumor_

7. neuroma    WR S    _nerve tumor_

8. carcinoma    WR S    _cancerous tumor_

9. leiomyosarcoma    WR CV WR WR S    _malignant tumor of smooth muscle_

10. rhabdomyosarcoma    WR CV WR WR S    _malignant tumor of striated muscle_

11. leiomyoma    WR CV WR S    _tumor of smooth muscle_

12. rhabdomyoma    WR CV WR S    _tumor of striated muscle_

## EXERCISE 15

Build medical terms for the following definitions by using the word parts you have learned. If you need help, refer to p. 8 to review word-building techniques. Once again, this is an integral part of the learning process; do not skip any part of this exercise.

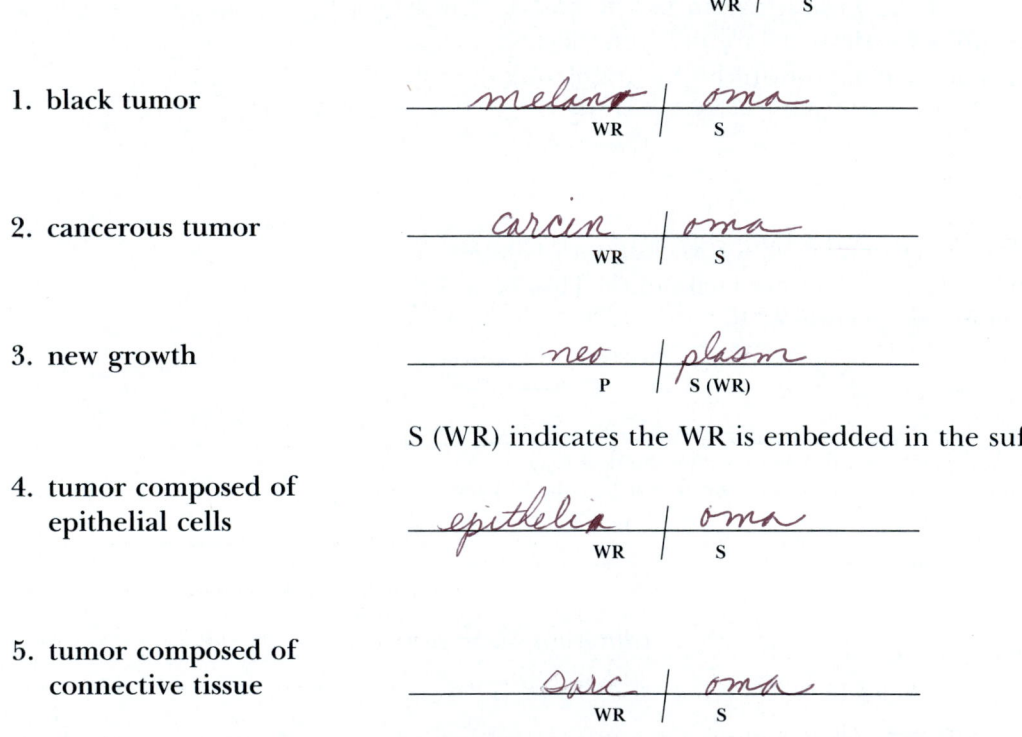

EXAMPLE: a tumor containing fat

$$\frac{lip}{WR} \mid \frac{oma}{S}$$

1. black tumor

$$\frac{melan}{WR} \mid \frac{oma}{S}$$

2. cancerous tumor

$$\frac{carcin}{WR} \mid \frac{oma}{S}$$

3. new growth

$$\frac{neo}{P} \mid \frac{plasm}{S (WR)}$$

S (WR) indicates the WR is embedded in the suffix.

4. tumor composed of epithelial cells

$$\frac{epithelia}{WR} \mid \frac{oma}{S}$$

5. tumor composed of connective tissue

$$\frac{sarc}{WR} \mid \frac{oma}{S}$$

6. cancerous black tumor

$$\frac{melan}{WR} \mid \frac{o}{CV} \mid \frac{carcin}{WR} \mid \frac{oma}{S}$$

7. tumor made up of nerve cells

_neur_ | _oma_
WR | S

8. tumor formed of muscle tissue

_my_ | _oma_
WR | S

9. malignant tumor of striated muscle

_rhabd_ | _o_ | ~~_my_~~ | _o_ | _sarcoma_
WR | CV | WR | CV | S

10. tumor of smooth muscle

_lei_ | _o_ | _my_ | _oma_
WR | CV | WR | S

11. tumor of striated muscle

_rhabd_ | _o_ | _my_ | _oma_
WR | CV | WR | S

12. malignant tumor of smooth muscle

_lei_ | _o_ | _my_ | _o_ | _sarcoma_
WR | CV | WR | CV | S

## EXERCISE 16

Spell each of the diagnostic terms. Have someone dictate the terms on pp. 24 and 25 to you or say the words into a tape recorder; then spell the words from your recording as often as necessary. Think about the word parts before attempting to write the word. Study any you have spelled incorrectly.

1. carcinoma
2. epithelioma
3. leiomyoma
4. leiomyosarcoma
5. lipoma
6. melanocarcinoma
7. melanoma
8. myoma
9. neoplasm
10. neuroma
11. rhabdomyoma
12. rhabdomyosarcoma
13. sarcoma

Place a check mark (√) in the box to indicate that you have completed Objective 3.

☐ **BUILD, ANALYZE, DEFINE, PRONOUNCE, AND SPELL THE DIAGNOSTIC TERMS RELATED TO THE HUMAN BODY STRUCTURE**

# Objective 4  BUILD, ANALYZE, DEFINE, PRONOUNCE, AND SPELL ADDITIONAL TERMS RELATED TO THE HUMAN BODY STRUCTURE.

## Additional Terms

| TERM (built from word parts) | DEFINITION |
|---|---|
| 1. cancerous (KAN-ser-us) | pertaining to cancer |
| 2. carcinogen (kar-SIN-ō-jen) | substance that causes cancer |
| 3. carcinogenic (*kar*-sin-ō-JEN-ik) | producing cancer |
| 4. cyanosis (*sī*-a-NŌ-sis) | abnormal condition of blue (bluish discoloration of the skin caused by inadequate supply of oxygen in the blood) |
| 5. cytogenic (*sī*-tō-JEN-ik) | producing cells |
| 6. cytoid (SĪ-toid) | resembling a cell |
| 7. cytology (sī-TOL-ō-jē) | study of cells |
| 8. cytoplasm (SĪ-tō-plazm) | cell substance |
| 9. diagnosis (*di*-ag-NŌ-sis) | state of complete knowledge (identifying a disease) |
| 10. dysplasia (dis-PLĀ-zhē-a) | abnormal development |
| 11. epithelial (*ep*-i-THĒ-lē-al) | pertaining to epithelium |
| 12. erythrocyte (e-RITH-rō-sīt) | red (blood) cell (RBC) |
| 13. erythrocytosis (e-*rith*-rō-sī-TŌ-sis) | increase in the number of red (blood) cells |
| 14. etiology (*e*-tē-OL-ō-jē) | study of causes (of diseases) |
| 15. histology (his-TOL-ō-jē) | study of tissue |
| 16. hyperplasia (*hī*-per-PLĀ-zhē-a) | excessive development (of cells) (Figure 2-6) |
| 17. hypoplasia (*hī*-pō-PLĀ-zhē-a) | incomplete development (of an organ or tissues) |

Aristotle noted "two colors of blood" and applied the term **erythro** to the dark red blood.

An essential part of a word, such as the word root for **blood,** may be omitted from a medical term, as in **erythrocyte,** by common consent. The practice is called **ellipsis.**

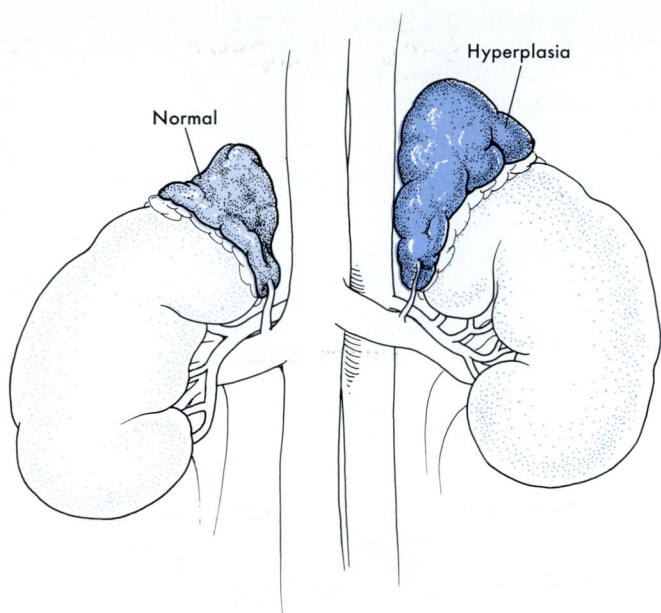

Figure 2-6
Hyperplasia.

18. iatrogenic . . . . . . . . . . .    produced by a physician (adverse condi-
    (ī-at-rō-JEN-ik)                   tion)

19. iatrology . . . . . . . . . . . .    study of medicine
    (ī-a-TROL-ō-jē)

20. karyocyte . . . . . . . . . . .    cell with a nucleus
    (KĀR-ē-ō-sīt)

21. karyoplasm . . . . . . . . . .    substance of a nucleus
    (KAR-ē-ō-*plazm*)

22. leukocyte . . . . . . . . . . .    white (blood) cell (WBC)
    (LŪ-kō-sīt)

23. leukocytosis . . . . . . . . . .    increase in the number of white (blood)
    (*lū*-kō-sī-TŌ-sis)                cells

24. lipoid . . . . . . . . . . . . . .    resembling fat
    (LIP-oid)

25. metastasis . . . . . . . . . . .    beyond control (transfer of disease from
    (me-TAS-ta-sis)                    one organ to another as in the transfer
                                       of malignant tumors)

26. myopathy . . . . . . . . . . .    disease of the muscle
    (mī-OP-a-thē)

27. neopathy . . . . . . . . . . .    new disease
    (nē-OP-a-thē)

28. neuroid. . . . . . . . . . . . .   resembling a nerve
    (NŪ-rōyd)

29. oncogenic. . . . . . . . . . .   causing tumors
    (*ong*-kō-JEN-ik)

30. oncologist. . . . . . . . . . .   physician who specializes in oncology
    (ong-KOL-ō-jist)

31. oncology. . . . . . . . . . . .   study of tumors
    (ong-KOL-ō-jē)

32. pathogenic . . . . . . . . . .   producing disease
    (path-ō-JEN-ik)

33. pathologist . . . . . . . . . .   specialist in pathology
    (pa-THOL-ō-jist)

34. pathology . . . . . . . . . . .   study of body changes caused by disease
    (pa-THOL-ō-jē)

35. prognosis . . . . . . . . . . .   state of before knowledge (forecast of
    (prog-NŌ-sis)                     probable outcome of disease)

36. somatic. . . . . . . . . . . . .   pertaining to the body
    (sō-MAT-ik)

37. somatogenic . . . . . . . . .   originating in the body (as opposed to
    (sō-ma-tō-JEN-ik                  mental)

38. somatopathy . . . . . . . . .   disease of the body
    (sō-ma-TOP-a-thē)

39. somatoplasm . . . . . . . .   body substance
    (sō-MAT-ō-plazm)

40. systemic . . . . . . . . . . . .   pertaining to a body system (or the body
    (sis-TEM-ik)                       as a whole)

41. visceral . . . . . . . . . . . . .   pertaining to the internal organs
    (VIS-er-al)

42. xanthochromic . . . . . . . .   pertaining to yellow color
    (*zan*-tho-KRŌ-mik)

43. xanthosis . . . . . . . . . . .   abnormal condition of yellow (or yellow
    (zan-THŌ-sis)                     discoloration)

Oncology and oncological are used to name the medical specialty and hospital nursing units devoted to the treatment and care of cancer patients.

Practice saying each of these terms aloud. Refer to "How to Use This Text," p. xi, for an explanation of the pronunciation key. To assist you in pronunciation, obtain the audiotape designed for use with this text. Learn the definitions and spellings of the additional terms by completing the following exercises.

## EXERCISE 17

Analyze and define the following additional terms.

                                WR  CV   S
EXAMPLE:   path/o/genic  *producing disease*
                                   CF

      WR   S
1. cytology     *study of cells*

2. histology _____ study of tissues _____

3. pathology _____ study of disease _____

4. pathologist _____ one who studies & practices disease _____

5. visceral _____ pertaining to internal organs _____

6. metastasis _____ beyond control _____

7. oncogenic _____ causing tumors _____

8. oncology _____ study of tumors _____

9. karyocyte _____ cell with a nucleus _____

10. neopathy _____ new disease _____

11. karyoplasm _____ substance of a nucleus _____

12. cytogenic _____ producing cells _____

13. systemic _____ pertaining to a body system _____

14. cancerous _____ pertaining to cancer _____

15. cytoplasm _____ cell substance _____

16. carcinogenic _____ producing cancer _____

17. somatic _____ pertaining to the body _____

18. somatogenic _____ originating in the body _____

19. somatoplasm _____ body substance _____

20. somatopathy _____ disease of the body _____

21. neuroid _____ resembling a nerve _____

22. myopathy _____ disease of the muscle _____

23. erythrocyte _____ red blood cell _____

24. leukocyte _____ white blood cell _____

25. cyanosis _____ abnormal condition of blue _____

26. epithelial _____ pertaining to the epithelium _____

27. lipoid _____ resembling fat _____

28. etiology _____ study of causes of diseases _____

29. xanthosis _____ abnormal condition of yellow _____

30. xanthochromic   *pertaining to yellow color*

31. hyperplasia   *excessive development of cells*

32. erythrocytosis   *increase in the number of RBC*

33. leukocytosis   *increase in the number of white blood cells*

34. carcinogen   *substance that produces cancer*

35. hypoplasia   *incomplete development*

36. cytoid   *resembling a cell*

37. oncologist   *physician who specializes in study of tumors (oncology)*

38. dysplasia   *abnormal development*

39. pathogenic   *producing disease*

40. prognosis   *state of before knowledge*

41. diagnosis   *state of complete knowledge*

42. iatrogenic   *produced by a physician*

43. iatrology   *study of medicine*

## EXERCISE 18

Build medical terms for the following definitions by using the word parts you have learned.

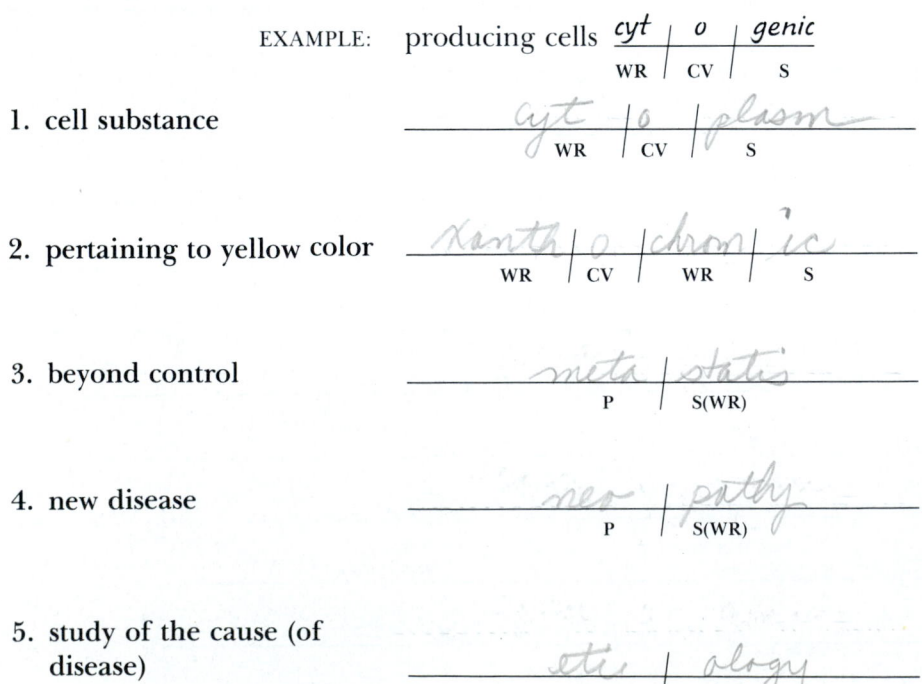

EXAMPLE: producing cells   cyt / o / genic
    WR   CV   S

1. cell substance    cyt / o / plasm
    WR   CV   S

2. pertaining to yellow color    xanth / o / chrom / ic
    WR   CV   WR   S

3. beyond control    meta / stasis
    P   S(WR)

4. new disease    neo / pathy
    P   S(WR)

5. study of the cause (of disease)    eti / ology
    WR   S

6. substance of a nucleus

    _kary_ / _o_ / _plasm_
       WR    CV    S

7. study of tumors

    _onc_ / _ology_
      WR     S

8. study of (body changes caused by) disease

    _path_ / _ology_
      WR     S

9. pertaining to the body

    _somat_ / _ic_
      WR     S

10. specialist in pathology

    _path_ / _ologist_
      WR     S

11. disease of the muscle

    _my_ / _o_ / _pathy_
      WR    CV    S

12. body substance

    _somat_ / _o_ / _plasm_
      WR    CV    S

13. abnormal condition of yellow

    _xanth_ / _osis_
      WR     S

14. pertaining to the internal organs

    _viscer_ / _al_
      WR     S

15. causing tumors

    _onc_ / _o_ / _genic_
      WR    CV    S

16. originating in the body

    _somat_ / _o_ / _genic_
      WR    CV    S

17. disease of the body

    _somat_ / _o_ / _pathy_
      WR    CV    S

18. red (blood) cell

    _eryth_ / _o_ / _cyte_
      WR    CV    S

19. resembling a nerve

        _neur_ | _oid_
         WR     S

20. pertaining to a body
    system

        _system_ic
         WR     S

21. white (blood) cell

        _leuc_ | _o_ | _cyte_
         WR   CV   S

22. cell with a nucleus

        _kary_ | _o_ | _cyte_
         WR   CV   S

23. resembling fat

        _lip_ | _oid_
         WR     S

24. pertaining to cancer

        _cancer_ | _ous_
         WR     S

25. study of cells

        _cyt_ | _ology_
         WR     S

26. excessive development
    (of cells)

        _hyper_ | _plasia_
         P    S(WR)

27. resembling a cell

        _cyt_ | _oid_
         WR     S

28. pertaining to epithelium

        _epitheli_ | _al_
         WR     S

29. abnormal condition of
    blue

        _cyan_ | _osis_
         WR     S

30. producing cancer

        _carcin_ | _o_ | _genic_
         WR   CV   S

31. producing disease

        _path_ | _o_ | _genic_
         WR   CV   S

32. study of tissue

          *hist* | *ology*
           WR     S

33. increase in the number of red (blood) cells

       *erthr* | *o* | *cyt* | *osis*
        WR   CV   WR   S

34. incomplete development (of an organ or tissue)

       *hypo* | *plasia*
         P    S(WR)

35. increase in the number of white (blood) cells

       *leuko* | *o* | *cyt* | *osis*
        WR   CV   WR   S

36. substance that causes cancer

       *carcin* | *o* | *gen*
        WR   CV   S

37. physician who specializes in oncology

       *onc* | *ologist*
        WR    S

38. abnormal development

       *dys* | *plasia*
        P    S(WR)

39. study of medicine

       *iatr* | *ology*
        WR    S

40. state of complete knowledge

       *dia* | *gno* | *sis*
        P   WR   S

41. produced by a physician

       *iatr* | *o* | *genic*
        WR   CV   S

42. state of before knowledge

       *pro* | *gno* | *sis*
        P   WR   S

## EXERCISE 19

Spell each of the additional terms. Have someone dictate the terms on pp. 28-30 to you or say the words into a tape recorder; then spell the words from your recording as often as necessary. Remember to think about the word parts before attempting to write the word. Study any you have spelled incorrectly.

1. cancerous
2. carcinogen
3. carcinogenic
4. cyanosis
5. cytogenic cytogenic
6. cytoid
7. cytology
8. cytoplasm
9. diagnosis
10. dysplasia
11. epithelial
12. erythrocyte
13. erythrocytosis
14. etiology
15. histology
16. hyperplasia
17. hypoplasia
18. iatrogenic
19. iatrology
20. karyocyte
21. karyoplasm
22. leukocyte

23. leukocytosis
24. lipoid
25. metastasis
26. myopathy
27. neopathy
28. neuroid
29. oncogenic
30. oncologist
31. oncology
32. pathogenic
33. pathologist
34. pathology
35. prognosis
36. somatic
37. somatogenic
38. somatopathy
39. somatoplasm
40. systemic
41. visceral
42. xanthochromic
43. xanthosis

Place a check (√) in the box to indicate that you have completed Objective 4.

☐ **BUILD, ANALYZE, DEFINE, PRONOUNCE, AND SPELL THE ADDITIONAL TERMS RELATED TO THE HUMAN BODY STRUCTURE.**

# Objective 5   DEFINE, PRONOUNCE, AND SPELL THE OTHER ADDITIONAL TERMS.

## Other Additional Terms

| TERM | DEFINITION |
|---|---|
| 1. benign .............. <br> (bē-NĪN) | not malignant, nonrecurrent, favorable for recovery |
| 2. cancer chemotherapy.... <br> (kē-mō-THER-a-pē) | treatment of cancer by using drugs |
| 3. cancer radiotherapy..... <br> (rā-dē-ō-THER-a-pē) | treatment of cancer using radioactive substance (x-ray or radiation) |
| 4. idiopathic............ <br> (id-ē-ō-PATH-ik) | disease of unknown origin |
| 5. inflammation ......... <br> (in-fla-MĀ-shun) | response to injury or destruction of tissue. Signs are redness, swelling, and pain |
| 6. malignant............ <br> (ma-LIG-nant) | tending to become progressively worse and to cause death, as in cancer |
| 7. remission ............ <br> (rē-MISH-un) | improvement or absence of signs of disease |

**Benign** is derived from the Latin word root **bene**, meaning well or good, as used in **benefit** or **benefactor**.

**Idiopathic** is derived from the Greek word **idios** meaning "one's own" and "path" or disease. The term probably originated from the idea that disease of unknown origin comes from within oneself and is not acquired from without.

**Inflammatory** and **Inflammation** are spelled with two "m's". Inflame and inflamed have one "m".

**Malignant** is derived from the Latin word root **mal** meaning bad, as used in **malicious**.

Practice saying each of these terms aloud. To assist you in pronunciation, obtain the audiotape designed for use with this text. Learn the definitions and spellings of the other additional terms by completing the following exercises.

## EXERCISE 20

Define the following terms.

1. benign _not malignant, nonrecurrent, favorable for recovery_

2. malignant _tending to become progressively worse and to cause death as in cancer_

3. remission _improvement or absence of signs of disease_

4. idiopathic _disease of unknown origin_

5. inflammation _response to injury or destruction of tissue a. Signs are redness swelling pain_

6. cancer chemotherapy _treatment of cancer by drugs_

7. cancer radiotherapy _treatment of cancer using radioactive substance (X-ray or radiation)_

## EXERCISE 21

Spell each of the other additional terms. Have someone dictate the terms on this page to you or say the words into a tape recorder; then spell the

words from your recording as often as necessary. Study any you have
spelled incorrectly.

1. _benign_    5. _inflamation_
2. _malignant_    6. _cancer chemotherapy_
3. _remission_    7. _cancer radiotherapy_
4. _idiopathic_

Place a check mark (√) in the box to indicate that you have completed Objective 5.

☐ DEFINE, PRONOUNCE, AND SPELL THE OTHER ADDITIONAL TERMS.

## EXERCISE 22

To test your understanding of the terms introduced in this chapter, circle
the words that correctly complete the sentence. The italicized words refer
to the correct answer.

1. Mr. Roberts was diagnosed as having a cancerous _tumor of the bone_, or
   (sarcoma, melanoma, lipoma). The doctor said the tumor was _becoming progressively worse;_ that is, it was (benign, malignant, pathogenic).
2. The blood test showed an _increased amount of red blood cells_, or (erythrocytosis, leukocytosis, cyanosis).
3. (Organic, Visceral, Systemic) means _pertaining to internal organs_.
4. A _tumor containing fat_, or (neuroma, carcinoma, lipoma) is _benign_, or
   (recurrent, nonrecurrent, cancerous).
5. Many substances are thought to be _cancer producing_, or (carcinogenic, carcinogen, cancerous).
6. _Etiology_ is the study of (the causes of disease, tissue disease, the causes of tumors).
7. A _tumor_ may be called a (neopathy, neoplasm, karyoplasm).
8. The pain _originated in the body_, or was (somatogenic, oncogenic, pathogenic).
9. Any _disease of a muscle_ is called (myoma, myopathy, somatopathy).
10. The term for _abnormal development_ is (hypoplasia, dysplasia, hyperplasia).
11. The term that means _produced by a physician_ is (diagnosis, iatrogenic, prognosis).

The following exercise is for those who like an extra challenge.

## EXERCISE 23

Unscramble the following mixed-up terms. The word on the left indicates
the word root in each of the following.

EXAMPLE:  blue  / c / y / a / n / o / s / i / s /
                  s   o   n   a   i   s   y   c

1. tumor    / / / / / / / /
            g o n o c l o y

2. body     / / / / / / /
            m a t o s i c

3. cancer   / / / / / / / /
            a n c c a r i m o

4. black    / / / / / / / /
            n a m o l a e m

5. cell     / / / / / /
            o t c i d y                    *cytoid*

6. medicine / / / / / / / / /
            i y t a r g o l o

## EXERCISE 24

The following are medical terms that did not appear in this chapter but
are composed of word parts studied in the chapter. Find their definitions
by translating the word parts literally. Translate the meaning of the suffix first, and then go back to the beginning of the word.

1.  **epithelioid** (ep-i-THĒ-lē-oyd) _____

2.  **neural** (NŪR-al) _____

3.  **pathogen** (PATH-ō-jen) _____

4.  **myoid** (MĪ-oyd) _____

5.  **leukocytic** (*lūk-ō-CĪT-ik*) _____

6.  **iatric** (ī-AT-rik) _____

## COMBINING FORMS CROSSWORD PUZZLE

### ACROSS CLUES

- 2. tissue
- 4. nerve
- 7. red
- 8. nucleus
- 9. tumor
- 12. epithelium
- 16. disease
- 17. cancer
- 19. body
- 20. muscle
- 21. blue
- 22. black

### DOWN CLUES

- 1. organ
- 3. flesh, connective tissue
- 5. system
- 6. cell
- 7. cause (of disease)
- 10. internal organs
- 11. cancer
- 13. fat
- 14. white
- 15. color
- 18. yellow

# Summary

Can you build, analyze, define, spell, and pronounce the following terms *built from word parts?*   yes ☐   no ☐

| DIAGNOSTIC | ADDITIONAL |
| --- | --- |

**DIAGNOSTIC**

carcinoma
(*kar*-si-NŌ-ma)

epithelioma
(*ep*-i-*thē*-lē-Ō-ma)

leiomyoma
(lī-ō-mī-Ō-ma)

leiomyosarcoma
(li-ō-mī-ō-sar-KŌ-ma)

lipoma
(li-PŌ-ma)

melanocarcinoma
(*mel*-a-nō-*kar*-si-NŌ-ma)

melanoma
(*mel*-a-NŌ-ma)

myoma
(mī-Ō-ma)

neoplasm
(NĒ-ō-plazm)

neuroma
(nū-RŌ-ma)

rhabdomyoma
(rab-dō-mī-Ō-ma)

rhabdomyosarcoma
(rab-dō-mī-ō-sar-KŌ-ma)

sarcoma
(sar-KŌ-ma)

**ADDITIONAL**

cancerous
(KAN-ser-us)

carcinogen
(kar-SIN-ō-jen)

carcinogenic
(*kar*-sin-ō-JEN-ik)

cyanosis
(sī-a-NŌ-sis)

cytogenic
(*si*-tō-JEN-ik)

cytoid
(SĪ-toid)

cytology
(sī-TOL-ō-jē)

cytoplasm
(SĪ-tō-plazm)

diagnosis
(dī-ag-NŌ-sis)

dysplasia
(dis-PLĀ-zhē-a)

epithelial
(*ep*-i-THĒ-lē-al)

erythrocyte
(e-RITH-rō-sīt)

erythrocytosis
(e-*rith*-rō-sī-TŌ-sis)

etiology
(*e*-tē-OL-ō-jē)

histology
(his-TOL-ō-jē)

hyperplasia
(hī-per-PLĀ-zhē-a)

hypoplasia
(hī-pō-PLĀ-zhē-a)

iatrogenic
(ī-*at*-rō-JEN-ik)

iatrology
(ī-a-TROL-ō-jē)

karyocyte
(KĀR-ē-ō-sīt)

karyoplasm
(KAR-ē-ō-*plazm*)

leukocyte
(LŪ-kō-sīt)

leukocytosis
(*lu*-kō-sī-TŌ-sis)

lipoid
(LIP-ōid)

metastasis
(me-TAS-ta-sis)

myopathy
(mī-OP-a-thē)

neopathy
(nē-OP-a-thē)

neuroid
(NŪ-rōyd)

oncogenic
(*ong*-kō-JEN-ik)

oncologist
(ong-KOL-ō-jist)

oncology
(ong-KOL-ō-jē)

pathogenic
(path-ō-JEN-ik)

pathologist
(pa-THOL-ō-jist)

pathology
(pa-THOL-ō-jē)

prognosis
(prog-NŌ-sis)

somatic
(sō-MAT-ik)

somatogenic
(sō-ma-tō-JEN-ik)

somatopathy
(sō-ma-TOP-a-thē)

somatoplasm
(sō-MAT-ō-plazm)

systemic
(sis-TEM-ik)

visceral
(VIS-er-al)

xanthochromic
(*zan*-tho-KRŌ-mik)

xanthosis
(zan-THŌ-sis)

## Summary

Can you define, pronounce, and spell the following terms *not built from word parts?*   yes ☐   no ☐

### ADDITIONAL

benign
(be-NĪN)

cancer radiotherapy
(rā-dē-ō-THER-a-pē)

inflammation
(in-fla-MĀ-shun)

remission
(re-MISH-un)

cancer chemotherapy
(kē-mō-THER-a-pē)

idiopathic
(id-ē-ō-PATH-ik)

malignant
(ma-LIG-nant)

## Answers

### Exercise 1

1. h     3. d     5. g     7. c     9. b
2. e     4. k     6. f     8. a     10. j

### Exercise 2

1. h     3. c     5. g     7. f
2. b     4. e     6. a

### Exercise 3

**Figure 2-1**
Cell: cyt/o              Organ: organ/o
Nucleus: kary/o       System: system/o
Tissue: hist/o
**Figure 2-3**
Nervous tissue: neur/o        Epithelial tissue: epitheli/o
Connective tissue: sarc/o     Muscle tissue: my/o

### Exercise 4

1. flesh, connective tissue      5. cell        9. organ
2. fat                                    6. tissue      10. system
3. nucleus                             7. muscle     11. epithelium
4. internal organs                   8. nerve

### Exercise 5

1. viscer/o      5. cyt/o      9. lip/o
2. epitheli/o    6. hist/o    10. system/o
3. organ/o       7. neur/o    11. sarc/o
4. kary/o        8. my/o

### Exercise 6

1. tumor                      6. cancer
2. cancer                     7. rod-shaped, striated
3. cause (of disease)     8. smooth
4. disease                    9. knowledge
5. body                       10. physician, medicine

### Exercise 7

1. path/o      4. a. cancer/o     6. lei/o
2. onc/o           b. carcin/o     7. rhabd/o
3. eti/o        5. somat/o         8. gno/o
                                    9. iatr/o

### Exercise 8

1. blue     3. white     5. color
2. red      4. yellow     6. black

### Exercise 9

1. cyan/o      3. leuk/o     5. xanth/o
2. erythr/o    4. melan/o    6. chrom/o

### Exercise 10

1. new
2. above, excessive
3. after, beyond, change
4. below, incomplete, deficient
5. difficult, labored, painful, abnormal
6. through, complete
7. before

### Exercise 11

1. neo-     4. meta-     6. dia-
2. hyper-   5. dys-      7. pro-
3. hypo-

### Exercise 12

1. i     4. f     7. h     10. c     13. q     16. o
2. l     5. g     8. b     11. n     14. m
3. e     6. j     9. p     12. k     15. a

## Exercise 13

1. specialist
2. disease
3. study of
4. pertaining to
5. control, stop
6. cell
7. abnormal condition
8. pertaining to
9. growth, substance, formation
10. pertaining to
11. formation, development, a growth
12. resembling
13. substance or agent that produces or causes
14. producing, originating, causing
15. tumor
16. origin, cause
17. malignant tumor
18. state of

## Exercise 14

|   | WR   S |   |
|---|---|---|
| 1. | sarc/oma | tumor composed of connective tissue |
| 2. | melan/oma (WR  S) | black tumor |
| 3. | epitheli/oma (WR   S) | tumor composed of epithelial cells |
| 4. | lip/oma (WR  S) | tumor containing fat |
| 5. | neo/plasm (P  S(WR)) | new growth |
| 6. | my/oma (WR  S) | tumor formed of muscle tissue |
| 7. | neur/oma (WR  S) | tumor made up of nerve cells |
| 8. | carcin/oma (WR   S) | cancerous tumor |
| 9. | lei/ o / my/o / sarcoma (WR CV WR CV   S) (CF  CF) | malignant tumor of smooth muscle |
| 10. | rhabd/ o /my/ o /sarcoma (WR  CV WR CV   S) (CF  CF) | malignant tumor of striated muscle |
| 11. | lei/ o /my/oma (WR CV WR   S) (CF) | tumor of smooth muscle |
| 12. | rhabd/ o /my/oma (WR  CV WR  S) (CF) | tumor of striated muscle |

## Exercise 15

1. melan/oma
2. carcin/oma
3. neo/plasm
4. epitheli/oma
5. sarc/oma
6. melan/o/carcin/oma
7. neur/oma
8. my/oma
9. rhabd/o/my/o/sarcoma
10. lei/o/my/oma
11. rhabd/o/my/oma
12. lei/o/my/o/sarcoma

## Exercise 16

Spelling exercise; *see* text, p. 27

## Exercise 17

|   | WR    S |   |
|---|---|---|
| 1. | cyt/ology | study of cells |
| 2. | hist/ology (WR    S) | study of tissue |
| 3. | path/ology (WR    S) | study of (body changes caused by) disease |
| 4. | path/ologist (WR    S) | specialist in pathology |
| 5. | viscer/al (WR    S) | pertaining to internal organs |
| 6. | meta/stasis (P    S(WR)) | beyond control (transfer of disease) |
| 7. | onc/ o /genic (WR CV   S) (CF) | causing tumors |
| 8. | onc/ology (WR    S) | study of tumors |
| 9. | kary/ o /cyte (WR CV  S) (CF) | cell with a nucleus |
| 10. | neo/pathy (P   S(WR)) | new disease |
| 11. | kary/ o /plasm (WR CV   S) (CF) | substance of a nucleus |
| 12. | cyt/ o /genic (WR CV   S) (CF) | producing cells |
| 13. | system/ic (WR   S) | pertaining to a body system |
| 14. | cancer/ous (WR   S) | pertaining to cancer |
| 15. | cyt/ o /plasm (WR CV   S) (CF) | cell substance |
| 16. | carcin/ o /genic (WR CV   S) (CF) | producing cancer |

WR  S
17. somat/ic — pertaining to the body

WR CV  S
18. somat/ o /genic — originating in the body
　　　CF

WR CV  S
19. somat/ o /plasm — body substance
　　　CF

WR CV  S
20. somat/ o /pathy — disease of the body
　　　CF

WR  S
21. neur/oid — resembling a nerve

WR CV  S
22. my/ o /pathy — disease of the muscle
　　CF

WR CV  S
23. erythr/ o /cyte — red (blood) cell
　　　CF

WR CV  S
24. leuk/ o /cyte — white (blood) cell
　　CF

WR  S
25. cyan/osis — abnormal condition of blue (bluish discoloration of the skin)

WR  S
26. epitheli/al — pertaining to epithelium

WR  S
27. lip/oid — resembling fat

WR  S
28. eti/ology — study of causes (of disease)

WR  S
29. xanth/osis — abnormal condition of yellow

WR CV WR  S
30. xanth/ o /chrom/ic — pertaining to yellow color
　　　CF

P  S(WR)
31. hyper/plasia — excessive development (of cells)

WR CV WR  S
32. erythr/ o /cyt/osis — increase in the number of red (blood) cells
　　　CF

WR CV WR  S
33. leuk/ o /cyt/osis — increase in the number of white (blood) cells
　　　CF

WR CV  S
34. carcin/ o /gen — substance that causes cancer
　　　CF

P  S(WR)
35. hypo/plasia — incomplete development (of an organ or tissue)

WR  S
36. cyt/oid — resembling a cell

WR  S
37. onc/ologist — physician who specializes in oncology

P  S(WR)
38. dys/plasia — abnormal development

WR CV  S
39. path/ o /genic — producing disease
　　CF

P  WR  S
40. pro/gno/sis — state of before knowledge

P  WR  S
41. dia/gno/sis — state of complete knowledge

WR CV  S
42. iatr/ o /genic — produced by a physician (adverse condition)
　　CF

WR  S
43. iatr/ology — study of medicine

## Exercise 18

1. cyt/o/plasm
2. xanth/o/chrom/ic
3. meta/stasis
4. neo/pathy
5. eti/ology
6. kary/o/plasm
7. onc/ology
8. path/ology
9. somat/ic
10. path/ologist
11. my/o/pathy
12. somat/o/plasm
13. xanth/osis
14. viscer/al
15. onc/o/genic
16. somat/o/genic
17. somat/o/pathy
18. erythr/o/cyte
19. neur/oid
20. system/ic
21. leuk/o/cyte
22. kary/o/cyte
23. lip/oid
24. cancer/ous
25. cyt/ology
26. hyper/plasia
27. cyt/oid
28. epitheli/al
29. cyan/osis
30. carcin/o/genic
31. path/o/genic
32. hist/ology
33. erythr/o/cyt/osis
34. hypo/plasia
35. leuk/o/cyt/osis
36. carcin/o/gen
37. onc/ologist
38. dys/plasia
39. iatr/ology
40. dia/gno/sis
41. iatr/o/genic
42. pro/gno/sis

## Exercise 19

Spelling exercise; *see* text, p. 36.

## Exercise 20

1. not malignant, nonrecurrent
2. becoming progressively worse
3. improvement or absence of signs of disease
4. disease of unknown origin
5. response to injury or destruction of tissue. Signs are redness, swelling, and pain.
6. treatment of cancer by using drugs
7. treatment of cancer by using a radioactive substance

## Exercise 21

Spelling exercise; *see* text, pp. 37 and 38.

## Exercise 22

1. sarcoma, malignant
2. erythrocytosis
3. visceral
4. lipoma, nonrecurrent
5. carcinogenic
6. causes of disease
7. neoplasm
8. somatogenic
9. myopathy
10. dysplasia
11. iatrology

## Exercise 23

1. oncology
2. somatic
3. carcinoma
4. melanoma
5. cytoid
6. iatrology

## Exercise 24

1. resembling epithelium
2. pertaining to the nerves
3. agent that produces disease
4. resembling muscle
5. pertaining to white (blood) cells
6. pertaining to a physician or medicine

## Answers

```
      O                   H I S T O
N E U R O             S         A
    G   C       E R Y T H R O
    K A R Y O   T   S         C
    N   T       I   T         O
    O   O N C O     E
    V               M
C   E P I T H E L I O               L
A     S           I       C         E
R     C           P A T H O         U
C A N C E R O     O       R   X     K
I     R             S O M A T O
N   M Y O                 M   N
O           C Y A N O     T
                          H
          M E L A N O
```

# 3

# Integumentary System

## Objective 1    DEFINE THE ANATOMICAL TERMS OF THE INTEGUMENTARY SYSTEM.

## Anatomical Terms

The term *integumentary* is derived from the Latin word *tegere*, meaning *to cover*. Part of the integumentary system is the skin, our body's covering, which serves as a defense against germs, regulates body temperature, excretes wastes through sweat, and acts as a sensor for pain, touch, heat, and cold. Hair, nails, sweat glands, and oil glands are also part of the integumentary system.

### THE SKIN

1. epidermis . . . . . . . . . . . .   Outer layer of skin.
  a.  keratin . . . . . . . . . . .   Horny or cornified layer, composed of protein. It is contained in the hair, skin, and nails.
  b.  melanin . . . . . . . . . .   Color, or pigmentation, of the skin.

**46**

2.  dermis (also called the true skin) . . . . . . . . . . . .    Inner layer of skin.

    a.  sweat glands (also called sudoriferous glands) . . . . . . . . . .    Tiny, coiled, tubular structures that emerge through pores on the skin's surface.

    b.  sebaceous glands . . . .    Secrete sebum (oil) into the hair follicles where the hair shafts pass through the dermis.

## ACCESSORY STRUCTURES OF THE SKIN

1.  hair. . . . . . . . . . . . . . . . .    Compressed, keratinized cells that arise from hair follicles; the sacs that enclose the hair fibers.

2.  nails . . . . . . . . . . . . . . . .    Originate in the epidermis. Nails are found on the upper surface of the ends of the fingers and toes. The white area at the base of the nail is called the lunula, or moon.

Learn the anatomical terms by completing the following exercise.

## EXERCISE 1

Match the anatomical terms in the first column with the correct definitions in the second column.

_c_ 1. dermis

_d_ 2. epidermis

_g_ 3. hair

_b_ 4. melanin

_f_ 5. nail

_h_ 6. sebaceous glands

_a_ 7. sweat glands

a.  coiled, tubular structures

b.  responsible for skin color

c.  true skin

d.  outermost layer of the skin

e.  white area at nail's base

f.  originate in the epidermis

g.  composed of compressed, keratinized cells

h.  secrete sebum

Place a check mark (√) in the box to indicate that you have completed Objective 1.

☐ **DEFINE THE ANATOMICAL TERMS OF THE INTEGUMENTARY SYSTEM.**

# Objective 2   WRITE THE DEFINITIONS OF THE WORD PARTS INCLUDED IN THIS CHAPTER.

## Integumentary System Word Parts

Study the word parts and their definitions listed as follows. Learning will be made easier by completing the exercises that follow.

| COMBINING FORM | DEFINITION |
|---|---|
| 1. cutane/o<br>   derm/o, dermat/o . . . . . . . | skin |
| 2. hidr/o . . . . . . . . . . . . . . . | sweat |
| 3. kerat/o . . . . . . . . . . . . .<br>   (NOTE: *Kerat/o* is also used to refer to the cornea of the eye; see Chapter 11.) | horny tissue, hard |
| 4. onych/o<br>   ungu/o . . . . . . . . . . . . . . | nail |
| 5. seb/o . . . . . . . . . . . . . . . . | sebum (oil) |
| 6. trich/o . . . . . . . . . . . . . . | hair |

Learn the anatomical locations and meanings of these combining forms by completing the following exercises.

## EXERCISE 2

Write the combining forms in the spaces marked **CF** on the diagrams in Figures 3-1 and 3-2.

## EXERCISE 3

Write the definitions of the following combining forms.

1. hidr/o _____ *sweat* _____

2. derm/o _____ *skin* _____

3. onych/o _____ *nail* _____

4. trich/o _____ *hair* _____

5. kerat/o _____ *horny tissue, hard* _____

6. dermat/o _____ *skin* _____

7. seb/o _____ *sebum* _____

8. ungu/o _____ *nail* _____

9. cutane/o _____ *skin* _____

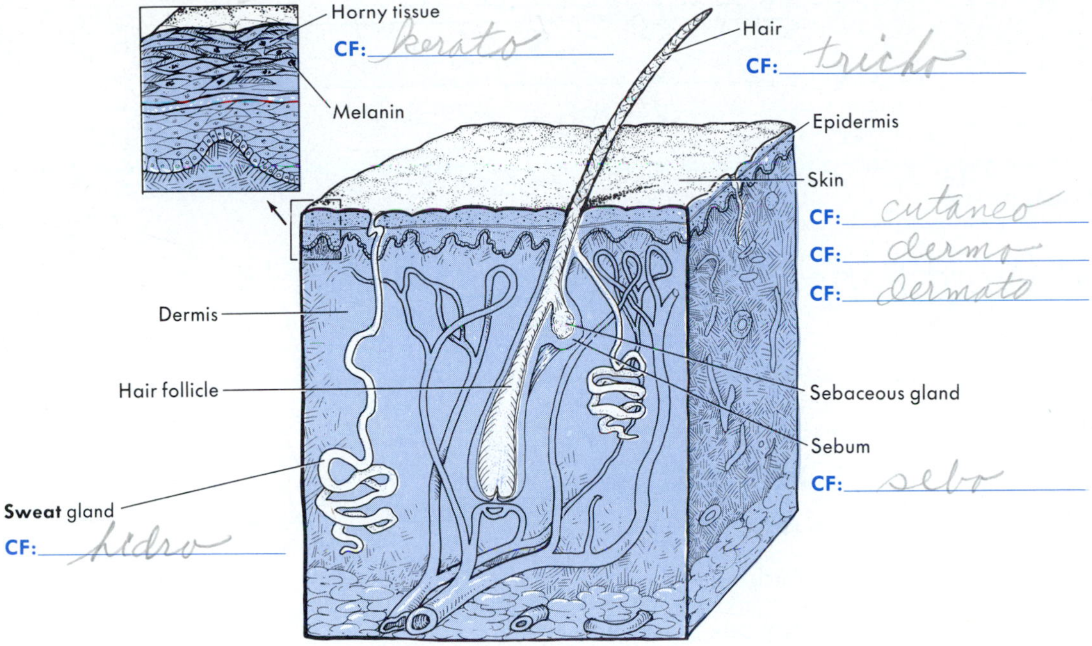
Horny tissue
CF: kerato
Melanin
Hair
CF: tricho
Epidermis
Skin
CF: cutaneo
CF: dermo
CF: dermato
Dermis
Hair follicle
Sebaceous gland
Sebum
CF: sebo
Sweat gland
CF: hidro

Figure 3-1
Cross section of the skin.

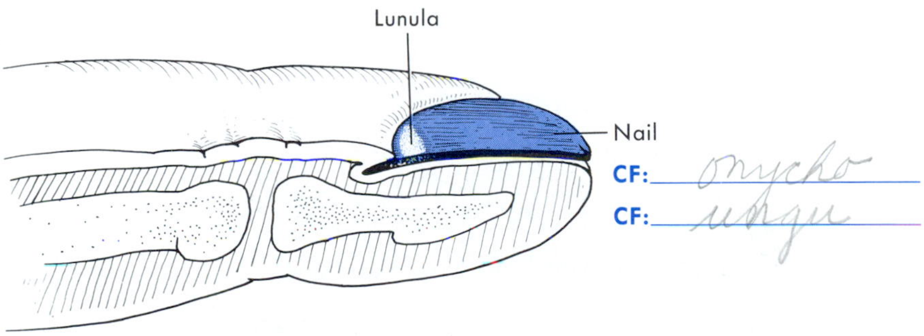
Lunula
Nail
CF: onycho
CF: ungu

Figure 3-2
Cross section of the finger with nail.

## EXERCISE 4

Write the combining form for each of the following.

1. hair _trich/o_
2. sweat _hidr/o_
3. nail a. _onych/o_
   b. _ungu/o_
4. sebum _seb/o_

5. skin

     a. _dermo_

     b. _dermato_

     c. _cutaneo_

6. hard, horny tissue      _kerato_

# Related Word Parts

| COMBINING FORM | DEFINITION |
| --- | --- |
| 1. aden/o . . . . . . . . . . . . . | gland |
| 2. aut/o . . . . . . . . . . . . . . | self |
| 3. bi/o . . . . . . . . . . . . . . | life |
| 4. coni/o . . . . . . . . . . . . . | dust |
| 5. crypt/o . . . . . . . . . . . . | hidden |
| 6. fibr/o . . . . . . . . . . . . . | fibrous tissue, fibers |
| 7. heter/o . . . . . . . . . . . . | other |
| 8. myc/o . . . . . . . . . . . . . | fungus |
| 9. necr/o . . . . . . . . . . . . . | death (cells, body) |
| 10. pachy/o . . . . . . . . . . . . | thick |
| 11. rhytid/o . . . . . . . . . . . | wrinkles |
| 12. staphyl/o . . . . . . . . . . . | grapelike clusters |
| 13. strept/o . . . . . . . . . . . | twisted chains |
| 14. xer/o . . . . . . . . . . . . . | dry |

Learn the combining forms by completing the following exercises.

## EXERCISE 5

Write the definitions of the following combining forms.

1. necr/o _death_

2. fibr/o _fibrous tissues, fibers_

3. staphyl/o _grape-like clusters_

4. crypt/o _hidden_

5. pachy/o _thick_

6. coni/o _dust_

7. myc/o _fungus_

8. bi/o _____ *life* _____

9. heter/o _____ *other* _____

10. aden/o _____ *gland* _____

11. strept/o _____ *twisted chains* _____

12. xer/o _____ *dry* _____

13. aut/o _____ *self* _____

14. rhytid/o _____ *wrinkles* _____

## EXERCISE 6

Write the combining form for each of the following.

1. fungus _____ *myc/o* _____

2. death (cells, body) _____ *necr/o* _____

3. other _____ *heter/o* _____

4. dry _____ *xer/o* _____

5. thick _____ *pachy/o* _____

6. fibrous tissue _____ *fibr/o* _____

7. twisted chains _____ *strept/o* _____

8. wrinkles _____ *rhytid/o* _____

9. grapelike clusters _____ *staphyl/o* _____

10. self _____ *aut/o* _____

11. gland _____ *aden/o* _____

12. hidden _____ *crypt/o* _____

13. dust _____ *coni/o* _____

14. life _____ *bi/o* _____

# Prefixes

| PREFIX | DEFINITION |
| --- | --- |
| 1. epi- | on, upon, over |
| 2. intra- | within |
| 3. para- | beside, beyond, around |

4.  per-................  through

5.  sub-................  under, below

Learn the prefixes by completing the following exercises.

## EXERCISE 7

Write the definitions of the following prefixes.

1.  sub- _____ *under, below* _____

2.  para- _____ *beside, beyond, around* _____

3.  epi- _____ *on, upon, over* _____

4.  intra- _____ *within* _____

5.  per- _____ *through* _____

## EXERCISE 8

Write the prefix for each of the following.

1.  within _____ *per- intra* _____

2.  under, below _____ *sub-* _____

3.  on, upon, over _____ *epi* _____

4.  beside, beyond, around _____ *para* _____

5.  through _____ *per* _____

# Suffixes

| SUFFIX | DEFINITION |
| --- | --- |
| 1. -coccus (*pl.* -cocci) ..... | berry-shaped (form of bacterium) |
| 2. -ectomy............ | excision or surgical removal |
| 3. -ia................ | diseased or abnormal state, condition of |
| 4. -itis............... | inflammation |
| 5. -malacia ........... | softening |
| 6. -opsy.............. | to view |
| 7. -orrhea ............ | flow, excessive discharge |
| 8. -phagia............ | eating or swallowing |
| 9. -plasty............ | plastic or surgical repair |
| 10. -tome ............. | instrument used to cut |

Learn the suffixes by completing the following exercises.

## EXERCISE 9

Match the suffixes in the first column with the correct definitions in the second column.

| | | |
|---|---|---|
| _c_ | 1. -coccus | a. inflammation |
| _e_ | 2. -ectomy | b. plastic or surgical repair |
| _a_ | 3. -itis | c. berry-shaped |
| _j_ | 4. -malacia | d. eating or swallowing |
| _i_ | 5. -opsy | e. excision or surgical removal |
| _h_ | 6. -orrhea | f. instrument used to cut |
| _d_ | 7. -phagia | g. thick |
| _b_ | 8. -plasty | h. flow, excessive discharge |
| _f_ | 9. -tome | i. to view |
| _k_ | 10. -ia | j. softening |
| | | k. diseased or abnormal state, condition of |

## EXERCISE 10

Write the definitions of the following suffixes.

1. -plasty ___plastic or surgical repair___
2. -ectomy ___excision or surgical removal___
3. -malacia ___softening___
4. -itis ___inflamation___
5. -tome ___instrument used to cut___
6. -phagia ___eating or swallowing___
7. -orrhea ___flow, exessive discharge___
8. -coccus ___berry shaped___
9. -opsy ___to view___
10. -ia ___diseased or abnormal state, condition of___

Place a check mark (√) in the box to indicate that you have completed Objective 2.

☐ WRITE THE DEFINITIONS OF THE WORD PARTS INCLUDED IN THIS CHAPTER.

**CLINICAL NOTE: Skin disorders**

Skin problems may result from various causes, such as parasitic infestations, fungal, bacterial, or viral infections, reactions to substances encountered externally or taken internally, or new growths. Many of the skin manifestations have no known cause; others are hereditary.

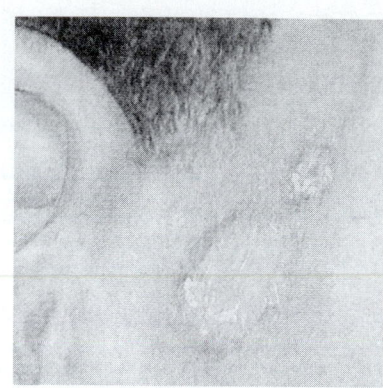

TINEA (RINGWORM)

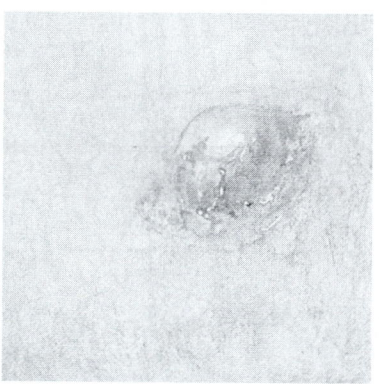

SQUAMOUS CELL CARCINOMA

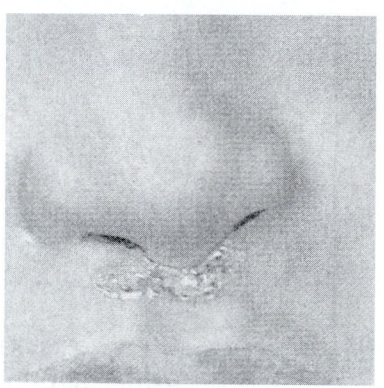

IMPETIGO

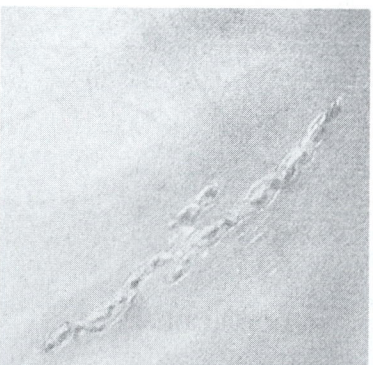

HERPES ZOSTER (SHINGLES)

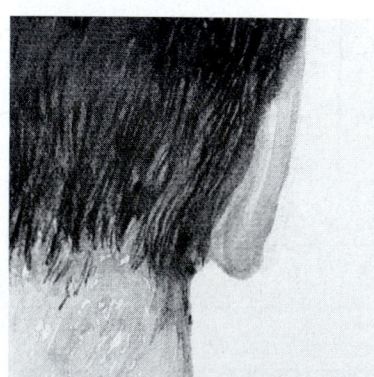

DERMATITIS

Figure 3-3
Common skin disorders.

# Medical Terms

The terms you need to learn to complete this chapter are listed as follows. Now that you know the meaning of the word parts, the exercises at the end of the list will assist you to learn the definition and spelling of each word.

## Objective 3    BUILD, ANALYZE, DEFINE, PRONOUNCE, AND SPELL THE DIAGNOSTIC TERMS RELATED TO THE INTEGUMENTARY SYSTEM.

# Diagnostic Terms

**TERM**
(built from word parts)

**DEFINITION**

1. **dermatitis** . . . . . . . . . . .    inflammation of the skin (Figure 3-3)
   (*der*-ma-TĪ-tis)

2. **dermatoconiosis** . . . . . . .    abnormal condition of the skin caused
   (der-*ma*-tō-kō-nē-Ō-sis)    by dust

3. **dermatofibroma** . . . . . . .    fibrous tumor of the skin
   (*der*-ma-tō-fī-BRŌ-ma)

4. **hidradenitis** . . . . . . . . . .    inflammation of a sweat gland
   (*hī*-drad-e-NĪ-tis)

5. **leiodermia** . . . . . . . . . .    condition of smooth skin
   (lī-ō-DER-mēa)

6. **onychocryptosis** . . . . . . .    abnormal condition of a hidden nail (in-
   (*on*-i-kō-krip-TŌ-sis)    grown nail)

7. **onychomalacia** . . . . . . . .    softening of the nails
   (*on*-i-kō-ma-LĀ-shē-a)

8. **onychomycosis** . . . . . . . . .    abnormal condition of a fungus in the
   (*on*-i-kō-mī-KŌ-sis)    nails

9. **onychophagia** . . . . . . . . .    eating the nails or nail biting
   (*on*-i-kō-FĀ-jē-a)

10. **pachyderma** . . . . . . . . . .    thickening of the skin
    (paki-DER-ma)
    (NOTE: The *a* ending is a noun
    suffix and has no meaning.)

11. **paronychia** . . . . . . . . . .    diseased state around the nail (Figure
    (pār-ō-NIK-ē-a)    3-4)
    (NOTE: The *a* from *para*- has
    been dropped. The final vowel in
    a prefix is dropped when the
    word to which it is added begins
    with a vowel.)

12. **seborrhea** . . . . . . . . . .    excessive discharge of sebum
    (*seb*-ōr-Ē-a)

13. **trichomycosis** . . . . . . . .    abnormal condition of a fungus in the
    (*trik*-ō-mī-KŌ-sis)    hair

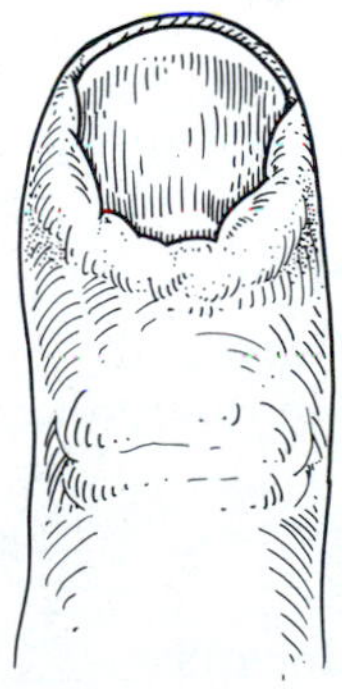

**Figure 3-4**
Paronychia; also called "run around" because the infection runs around the nail.

14. xeroderma . . . . . . . . . . dry skin
(zē-rō-DER-ma)
(NOTE: The *a* ending is a noun
suffix and has no meaning.)

Practice saying each of these terms aloud. To assist you in pronunciation, obtain the audiotape designed for use with this text. Learn the definitions and spellings of the diagnostic terms by completing the following exercises.

## EXERCISE 11

Analyze and define the following diagnostic terms. If you need to, refer to p. 6 for a review.

EXAMPLE:   onych/o/myc/osis   *abnormal condition of a fungus in the nails*

1. dermatoconiosis ___abnormal condition of the skin caused by dust___
2. hidradenitis ___inflamation of the sweat glands___
3. dermatitis ___inflamation of the skin___
4. pachyderma ___thickening of the skin___
5. onychomalacia ___softening of the nails___
6. trichomycosis ___abnormal condition of fungus in the hair___
7. dermatofibroma ___fibrous tumor of the skin___
8. paronychia ___diseased state around the nail___
9. onychocryptosis ___abnormal condition of a hidden nail___
10. seborrhea ___excessive flow of sebum (discharge)___
11. onychophagia ___nail biting___
12. xeroderma ___dry skin___
13. leiodermia ___condition of smooth skin___

## EXERCISE 12

Build diagnostic terms for the following definitions by using the word parts you have learned. If you need help, refer to p. 8 to review word-building techniques.

EXAMPLE:   abnormal condition of a fungus in the hair   trich | o | myc | osis
                                                        WR | CV | WR | S

1. thickening of the skin   ___pachy | derm | a___
                              WR | WR | S

2. abnormal condition of a
   fungus in the nails

   _onych_ / _o_ / _myc_ / _osis_
   WR / CV / WR / S

3. excessive discharge of
   sebum

   _seb_ / _orrhea_
   WR / S

4. inflammation of the skin

   _dermat_ / _itis_
   WR / S

5. fibrous tumor of the skin

   _dermat_ / _o_ / _fibr_ / _oma_
   WR / CV / WR / S

6. softening of the nails

   _onych_ / _o_ / _malacia_
   WR / CV / S

7. inflammation of a sweat
   gland

   _hidr_ / _aden_ / _itis_
   WR / WR / S

8. abnormal condition of a
   hidden nail

   _onych_ / _o_ / _crypt_ / _osis_
   WR / CV / WR / S

9. abnormal condition of
   the skin caused by dust

   _dermat_ / _o_ / _coni_ / _osis_
   WR / CV / WR / S

10. eating the nails

    _onych_ / _o_ / _phagia_
    WR / CV / S

11. diseased state around the
    nail

    _par_ / _onych_ / _ia_
    P / WR / S

12. dry skin

    _xer_ / _o_ / _derm_ / _a_
    WR / CV / WR / S

13. condition of smooth skin

    _lei_ / _o_ / _derm_ / _ia_
    WR / CV / WR / S

## EXERCISE 13

Spell each of the diagnostic terms. Have someone dictate the terms on pp. 55 and 56 to you or say the words into a tape recorder; then spell the words from your recording as often as necessary. Think about the word parts before attempting to write the word. Study any you have spelled incorrectly.

1. *dermatitis*
2. *dermatoconiosis*
3. *dermatofibroma*
4. *hydradenitis*
5. *leiodermia*
6. *onychocryptosis*
7. *onychomalacia*

8. *onychomycosis*
9. *onychophagia*
10. *pachyderma*
11. *paronychia*
12. *seborrhea*
13. *trichomycosis*
14. *xeroderma*

Place a check mark (√) in the box to indicate that you have completed Objective 3.

☐ **BUILD, ANALYZE, DEFINE, PRONOUNCE, AND SPELL THE DIAGNOSTIC TERMS RELATED TO THE INTEGUMENTARY SYSTEM.**

## Objective 4   DEFINE, PRONOUNCE, AND SPELL OTHER DIAGNOSTIC TERMS RELATED TO THE INTEGUMENTARY SYSTEM.

## Other Diagnostic Terms

| TERM | DEFINITION |
|---|---|
| 1. **abrasion** . . . . . . . . . . . .<br>(a-BRĀ-zhun) | scraping away of the skin by mechanical process or injury |
| 2. **abscess** . . . . . . . . . . . . .<br>(AB-ses) | localized collection of pus |
| 3. **acne** . . . . . . . . . . . . . . .<br>(AK-nē) | inflammatory disease of the skin involving the sebaceous glands and hair follicles |
| 4. **actinic keratosis** . . . . . . .<br>(ack-TIN-ik) (ker-a-TŌ-sis) | a precancerous skin condition of horny tissue formation that results from excessive exposure to sunlight |
| 5. **basal cell carcinoma**. . . .<br>(BĀ-sal) (sel) (kar-si-NŌ-ma) | epithelial tumor arising from epidermis. Seldom metastasizes but invades local tissue. Common on face of elderly. |
| 6. **carbuncle** . . . . . . . . . . .<br>(KAR-bung-kl) | skin infection composed of a cluster of boils caused by staphylococcal bacteria |

**Abscess** is derived from the Latin **ab**, meaning **from**, and **cedo**, meaning **to go**. The tissue dies and goes away, with the pus replacing it.

It is believed that **acne** may be derived from **arme**, meaning **point**. Thus it was named for the point on a pimple.

7. cellulitis . . . . . . . . . . . .
(sel-ū-LĪ-tis)

inflammation of the connective tissue caused by infection, leading to redness, swelling, and fever

8. contusion . . . . . . . . . . .
(kon-TŪ-zhun)

injury with no break in the skin, characterized by pain, swelling, and discoloration (also called a *bruise*)

9. eczema . . . . . . . . . . . . .
(EK-ze-ma)

non-infectious, inflammatory skin disease characterized by redness, blisters, scabs, and itching

10. fissure . . . . . . . . . . . . . .
(FISH-ūr)

slit or cracklike sore in the skin

11. furuncle . . . . . . . . . . . .
(FER-ung-kl)

painful skin node caused by staphylococcal bacterial in a hair follicle (also called a *boil*)

12. gangrene . . . . . . . . . . .
(GANG-grēn)

death of tissue caused by loss of blood supply followed by bacteria invasion

13. herpes . . . . . . . . . . . . .
(HER-pēz)

inflammatory skin disease caused by herpes virus, and characterized by small blisters in clusters. There are many types of herpes; herpes simplex, for example, causes fever blisters and herpes zoster, also called shingles, is characterized by painful skin eruptions that follow nerves inflamed by the virus (Figure 3-3).

> **Herpes** is derived from the Greek **herpo,** meaning to **creep along.** It is descriptive of the course and type of skin lesion.

14. impetigo . . . . . . . . . . . .
(im-pe-TĪ-go)

superficial skin infection, characterized by pustules and caused by either staphylococci or streptococci (Figure 3-3).

15. Kaposi's sarcoma . . . . . .
(KAP-o-sēz)(sar-KŌ-ma)

a cancerous condition starting as purple or brown pimples on feet. Spreads through skin to lymph nodes and internal organs. Frequently seen in AIDS (acquired immune deficiency syndrome).

16. laceration . . . . . . . . . . .
(*las*-er-Ā-shun)

torn, ragged-edged wound

17. lesion . . . . . . . . . . . . . .
(LĒ-zhun)

any pathological change in the structure or function of tissue owing to injury or disease

18. pediculosis . . . . . . . . . .
(pe-*dik*-ū-LŌ-sis)

invasion into the skin and hair by lice

19. psoriasis . . . . . . . . . . . .
(so-RĪ-a-sis)

chronic skin condition producing red lesions covered with silvery scales

20. scabies . . . . . . . . . . . .    skin infection caused by the itch mite, a
    (SKĀ-bēz)                          minute animal whose relative is the tick.
                                       The infection causes severe itching with
                                       red papules.

21. scleroderma . . . . . . . . .    a disease characterized by chronic hard-
    (skle-rō-DER-ma)                   ening (induration) of the connective tis-
                                       sue of the skin and other body organs

22. **squamous cell carci-**
    **noma** . . . . . . . . . . . . . .    a malignant growth that develops from
    (SQWĀ-mus)  (sel)  (kar-si-       scale-like epithelial tissue. On the skin it
    NŌ-ma)                             appears like a firm, red, painless bump.
                                       It is also found in other body sites. (Fig-
                                       ure 3-3)

23. **systemic lupus erythema-**
    **tosus (SLE)** . . . . . . . . . .    inflammatory disease of the joints and
    (sis-TEM-ik) (LŪ-pus) (er-i-       the protein in the white fibers (collagen)
    thē-ma-TŌ-sus)                     of the connective tissue of the skin. It
                                       may also affect other organs.

24. tinea . . . . . . . . . . . . . .    fungus infection of the skin commonly
    (TIN-ē-a)                          called "ringworm" (Figure 3-3)

25. urticaria . . . . . . . . . . .    an itching skin eruption composed of
    (ūr-ti-KA-rē-a)                    wheals of varying size and shape

Practice saying each of these terms aloud. To assist you in pronunciation,
obtain the audiotape designed for use with this text. Learn the definitions
and spellings of the other diagnostic terms by completing the following
exercises.

## EXERCISE 14

Fill in the blanks with the correct terms.

1. An inflammatory disease affecting joints and the collagen of connective tissue is _systemic_ _lupus_
   _erythematosus_ .

2. A(n) _abscess_ is a localized collection of pus.

3. A cracklike sore in the skin is called a(n) _fissure_ .

4. The scraping away of the skin by mechanical process or injury is called
   a(n) _abrasion_ .

5. _psoriasis_ is a chronic skin condition characterized by
   red lesions covered with silvery scales.

6. An inflammatory skin disease characterized by small blisters in clusters is called _herpes_ .

7. _pediculosis_ is the name given to the invasion of the skin
   and hair by lice.

8. A fungus infection of the skin, also known as ringworm, is called ___tinea___ .

9. An injury with no break in the skin and characterized by pain, swelling, and discoloration is called a(n) ___contusion___ .

10. ___gangrene___ is the name given to tissue death caused by a loss of blood supply followed by bacterial invasion.

11. Any pathological change in the structure or function of tissue owing to injury or disease is called a ___lesion___ .

12. ___Kaposi's___ ___sarcoma___ is a cancerous condition starting as purple or brown pimples on the feet.

13. A horny tissue formation that results from excessive exposure to sunlight and is precancerous is called ___actinic___ ___keratosis___ .

14. A cluster of boils caused by staphylococcal bacteria is a ___carbuncle___ .

15. An inflammatory skin disease that involves the oil glands and hair follicles is called ___acne___ .

16. ___Laceration___ is the name given to a torn, ragged-edge wound.

17. A painful skin node caused by staphylococcal bacteria in a hair follicle is called a(n) ___furuncle___ .

18. A malignant growth that develops from scale-like epithelial tissue is known as ___squamous___ ___cell___ _____ carcinoma.

19. Inflammation of the connective tissue caused by infection and creating redness, swelling, and fever is called ___cellulitis___ .

20. ___Impetigo___ is the name given to a superficial skin infection characterized by pustules and caused by either staphylococci or streptococci.

21. ___eczema___ is a noninfectious inflammatory skin disease characterized by redness, blisters, scabs, and itching.

22. A skin infection caused by the itch mite is called ___scabies___ .

23. ___Urticaria___ is an itching skin eruption composed of wheals.

24. An epithelial tumor commonly found on the face of elderly is ___basal___ ___cell___ _____ carcinoma.

25. ___Scleroderma___ is a disease characterized by induration of the connective tissue.

## EXERCISE 15A

Match the words in the first column with their correct definitions in the second column.

f  1. abrasion
j  2. abscess
g  3. acne
l  4. actinic keratosis
m  5. basal cell carcinoma
c  6. carbuncle
i  7. cellulitis
k  8. contusion
e  9. eczema
b  10. fissure
h  11. furuncle
a  12. gangrene
d  13. scleroderma

a. death of tissue caused by loss of blood supply and entry of bacteria

b. cracklike sore in the skin

c. cluster of boils

d. induration of connective tissue

e. noninfectious inflammatory skin disease having redness, blisters, scabs, and itching.

f. scraped-away skin

g. involves sebaceous glands and hair follicles

h. painful skin node caused by staphylococci in a hair follicle

i. inflammation of connective tissue with redness, swelling, and fever

j. localized collection of pus

k. injury characterized by pain, swelling, and discoloration

l. precancerous skin condition owing to excessive exposure to sunlight

m. epithelial tumor commonly found on face of elderly

n. red lesions with silvery scales

## EXERCISE 15B

Match the words in the first column with their correct definitions in the second column.

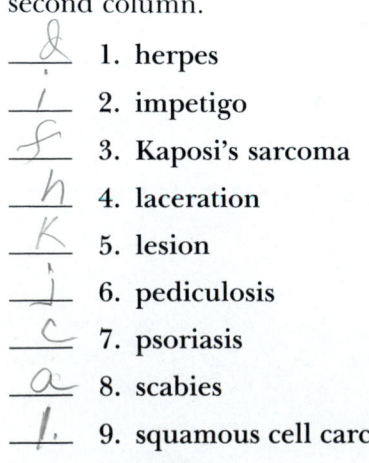

d  1. herpes
l  2. impetigo
f  3. Kaposi's sarcoma
h  4. laceration
k  5. lesion
j  6. pediculosis
c  7. psoriasis
a  8. scabies
l  9. squamous cell carcinoma

a. skin infection caused by the itch mite

b. fungus infection of the skin

c. red lesions covered by silvery scales

d. inflammatory skin disease having clusters of blisters

e. inflammatory disease of joints and collagen of the connective tissue of the skin

f. a cancerous condition that starts as brown or purple pimples on feet

g. composed of wheals

_e_ 10. systemic lupus ery-
       thematosus

_b_ 11. tinea

_g_ 12. urticaria

h.  torn, ragged-edged wound

i.  superficial skin condition having pustules and caused by staphylococci or streptococci

j.  invasion of the hair and skin by lice

k.  pathological change in tissue structure or function owing to injury or disease

l.  a malignant growth that develops from scale-like epithelial tissue

m.  cracklike sore in the skin

## EXERCISE 16

Spell each of the other diagnostic terms. Have someone dictate the terms on pp. 55 and 56 to you or say the words into a tape recorder; then spell the words from your recording as often as necessary. Study any you have spelled incorrectly.

1. _____
2. _____
3. _____
4. _____
5. _____
6. _____
7. _____
8. _____
9. _____
10. _____
11. _____
12. _____
13. _____

14. _____
15. _____
16. _____
17. _____
18. _____
19. _____
20. _____
21. _____
22. _____
23. _____
24. _____
25. _____

Place a check mark (√) in the box to indicate that you have completed Objective 4.

**DEFINE, PRONOUNCE, AND SPELL OTHER DIAGNOSTIC TERMS RELATED TO THE INTEGUMENTARY SYSTEM.**

# Objective 5

**BUILD, ANALYZE, DEFINE, PRONOUNCE, AND SPELL THE SURGICAL TERMS RELATED TO THE INTEGUMENTARY SYSTEM**

## Surgical Terms

| TERM (built from word parts) | DEFINITION |
|---|---|
| 1. **biopsy**............ (BĪ-op-sē) | view of life (the removal of living tissue from the body to be viewed under the microscope) |
| 2. **dermatoautoplasty**...... (*der*-ma-tō-AW-tō-*plas*-tē) | plastic repair using patient's own skin for the skin graft |
| 3. **dermatoheteroplasty**.... (*der*-ma-tō-HET-er-ō-*plas*-tē) | plastic repair using skin from others for the skin graft |
| 4. **dermatoplasty**......... (DER-ma-tō-*plas*-tē) | plastic repair on the skin |
| 5. **onychectomy**......... (on-i-KEK-tō-mē) | excision of a nail |
| 6. **rhytidectomy**......... (*rit*-i-DEK-tō-mē) | excision of wrinkles |
| 7. **rhytidoplasty**......... (RĪT-i-dō-*plas*-tē) | plastic repair of wrinkles |

Practice saying each of these terms aloud. To assist you in the pronunciation, obtain the audiotape designed for use with this text. Learn the definitions and spellings of the surgical terms by completing the following two exercises.

## EXERCISE 17

Analyze and define the following surgical terms.

EXAMPLE:   dermat/o/plasty/   *plastic repair of the skin*

1. rhytidectomy ___ excision of wrinkles
2. biopsy ___ view of life
3. dermatoautoplasty ___ plastic repair using patient's own skin as skin graft
4. onychectomy ___ excision of a nail
5. rhytidoplasty ___ plastic repair of wrinkles
6. dermatoheteroplasty ___ plastic repair using skin from others for skin graft

## EXERCISE 18

Build surgical terms for the following definitions by using the word parts you have learned.

EXAMPLE: plastic repair using one's own skin $\underset{\text{WR}}{dermat}\,|\,\underset{\text{CV}}{o}\,|\,\underset{\text{WR}}{aut}\,|\,\underset{\text{CV}}{o}\,|\,\underset{\text{S}}{plasty}$

1. excision of wrinkles

rhytid | ectomy
WR | S

2. view of life (removal of living tissue from the body)

bi | opsy
WR | S

3. plastic repair using skin from others

dermat o | hetero o | plasty
WR | CV | WR | CV | S

4. excision of a nail

onych | ectomy
WR | S

5. plastic repair of wrinkles

rhytid | o | plasty
WR | CV | S

6. plastic repair on the skin

dermat o | plasty
WR | CV | S

## EXERCISE 19

Spell each of the surgical terms. Have someone dictate the terms on p. 64 to you or say the words into a tape recorder; then spell the words from your recording as often as necessary. Think about the word parts before attempting to write the word. Study any you have spelled incorrectly.

1. _____  5. _____
2. _____  6. _____
3. _____  7. _____
4. _____

Place a check mark (√) in the box to indicate that you have completed Objective 5.

☐ BUILD, ANALYZE, DEFINE, PRONOUNCE, AND SPELL THE SURGICAL TERMS RELATED TO THE INTEGUMENTARY SYSTEM.

# Objective 6 — BUILD, ANALYZE, DEFINE, PRONOUNCE, AND SPELL ADDITIONAL TERMS RELATED TO THE INTEGUMENTARY SYSTEM.

## Additional Terms

**TERM**
(built from word parts)

**DEFINITION**

1. dermatologist . . . . . . . . . physician who specializes in skin diseases
   (*der*-ma-TOL-ō-jist)

2. dermatology . . . . . . . . . study of the skin
   (*der*-ma-TOL-ō-jē)

3. dermatome . . . . . . . . . . instrument used to cut skin
   (DER-ma-tōm)
   (NOTE: When two consonants of the same letter come together, one is sometimes dropped.)

4. epidermal . . . . . . . . . . . pertaining to upon the skin
   (*ep*-i-DER-mal)

5. erythroderma . . . . . . . . red skin (abnormal redness of the skin)
   (ē-rith-rō-DER-ma)
   (NOTE: The a ending is a noun suffix and has no meaning.)

6. hypodermic . . . . . . . . . pertaining to under the skin
   (*hī*-po-DER-mik)

7. intradermal . . . . . . . . . pertaining to within the skin
   (*in*-tra-DER-mal)

8. keratogenic . . . . . . . . . . originating in horny tissue
   (*ker*-a-TO-jen-ik)

9. leukoderma . . . . . . . . . white skin (less color than normal)
   (lū-kō-DER-ma)
   (NOTE: The a ending is a noun suffix and has no meaning.)

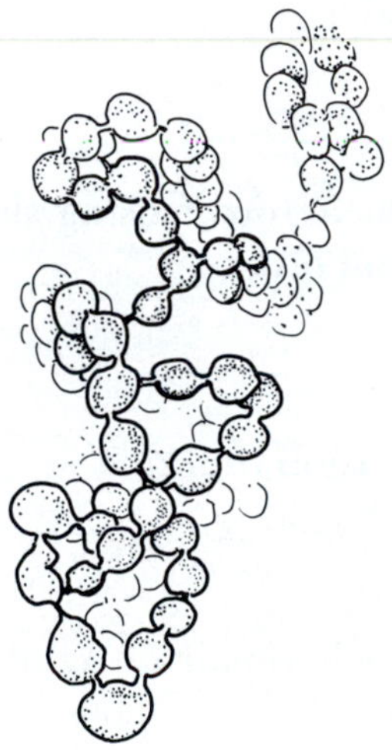

Figure 3-5
Staphylococci.

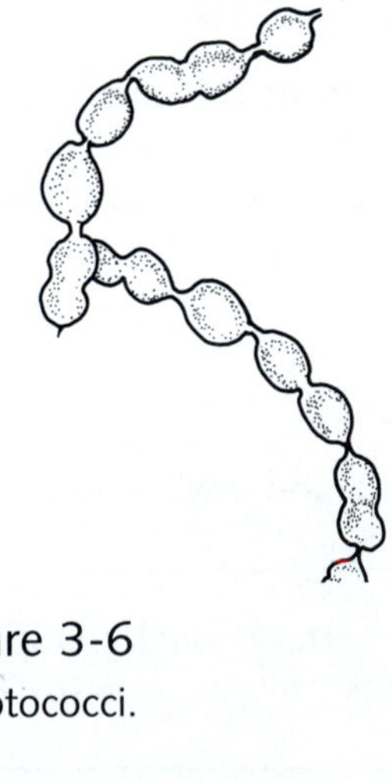

10. necrosis . . . . . . . . . . . abnormal condition of death (cells and tissue die because of disease)
    (ne-KRŌ-sis)

11. percutaneous . . . . . . . . pertaining to through the skin
    (per-kū-TĀ-nē-us)

12. staphylococcus
    (pl. **staphylococci**) . . . . . berry-shaped bacteria in grapelike clusters (these bacteria cause many skin diseases) (Figure 3-5)
    (*staf*-il-ō-KOK-us, *staf*-il-ō-KOK-sē)

13. streptococcus
    (pl. **streptococci**) . . . . . . berry-shaped bacteria in twisted chains (Figure 3-6)
    (*strep*-tō-KOK-us, *strep*-tō-KOK-sē)

Figure 3-6
Streptococci.

14. **subcutaneous** . . . . . . . .     pertaining to under the skin
    (*sub*-kū-TĀ-nē-us)

15. **ungual** . . . . . . . . . . . . .     pertaining to the nail
    (UNG-gwal)

16. **xanthoderma** . . . . . . . .     yellow skin (also called jaundice)
    (zan-thō-DER-ma)
    (Note: The a ending is a noun
    suffix and has no meaning.)

Practice saying each of these terms aloud. To assist you in pronunciation, obtain the audiotape designed for use with this text. Learn the definitions and spellings of the additional terms by completing the following exercises.

## EXERCISE 20

Analyze and define the following additional terms.

EXAMPLE:   intra/derm/al *pertaining to within the skin*

1. ungual _____ *pertaining to the nail*

2. dermatome _____ *instrument used to cut skin*

3. streptococcus _____ *berry-shaped bacteria in twisted chains*

4. hypodermic _____ *pertaining to under the skin*

5. dermatology _____ *study of the skin*

6. subcutaneous _____ *pertaining to under the skin*

7. staphylococcus _____ *berry-shaped bacteria in grape-like clusters*

8. keratogenic _____ *originating in horny tissue*

9. dermatologist _____ *Physician who specializes in skin diseases*

10. necrosis _____ *abnormal condition of death*

11. epidermal _____ *pertaining to upon the skin*

12. xanthoderma _____ *yellow skin (jaundice)*

13. erythroderma _____ *red skin (abnormal redness of the skin)*

14. leukoderma _____ *white skin*

15. percutaneous _____ *pertaining to through the skin*

## EXERCISE 21

Build additional terms related to the integumentary system by using the word parts you have learned.

EXAMPLE:   pertaining to under the skin   $\dfrac{hypo}{P}$ | $\dfrac{derm}{WR}$ | $\dfrac{ic}{S}$

1. study of the skin

   _____ / _____
   WR          S

2. abnormal condition of death (of cells and tissue)

   _____ / _____
   WR          S

3. instrument used to cut skin

   _____ / _____
   WR          S

4. pertaining to the nail

   _____ / _____
   WR          S

5. berry-shaped bacteria in grapelike clusters

   _____ / ____ / _____
   WR        CV        S

6. specialist in skin diseases

   _____ / _____
   WR          S

7. pertaining to within the skin

   _____ / ____ / _____
   P         WR         S

8. pertaining to upon the skin

   _____ / ____ / _____
   P         WR         S

9. pertaining to under the skin

   _____ / ____ / _____
   P         WR         S

10. berry-shaped bacteria in twisted chains

    _____ / ____ / _____
    WR        CV        S

11. originating in the horny
    tissue

    _____/_____/_____
         WR      CV      S

12. white skin

    _____/_____/_____/_____
      WR    CV    WR      S

13. red skin

    _____/_____/_____/_____
      WR    CV    WR      S

14. yellow skin

    _____/_____/_____/_____
      WR    CV    WR      S

15. pertaining to through the
    skin

    _____/_____/_____
       P     WR     S

## EXERCISE 22

Spell each of the additional terms. Have someone dictate the terms on p.
68 to you or say the words into a tape recorder; then spell the words from
your recording as often as necessary. Think about the word parts before
attempting to write the word. Study any you have spelled incorrectly.

1. _____     9. _____
2. _____    10. _____
3. _____    11. _____
4. _____    12. _____
5. _____    13. _____
6. _____    14. _____
7. _____    15. _____
8. _____    16. _____

Place a check mark (√) in the box to indicate that you have completed Objective 6.

☐ **BUILD, ANALYZE, DEFINE, PRONOUNCE, AND SPELL ADDITIONAL TERMS RELATED
TO THE INTEGUMENTARY SYSTEM.**

# Objective 7 DEFINE, PRONOUNCE, AND SPELL THE OTHER ADDITIONAL TERMS RELATED TO THE INTEGUMENTARY SYSTEM.

## Other Additional Terms

| TERM | DEFINITION |
|---|---|
| 1. adipose (AD-i-pōs) | fat |
| 2. albino (al-BĪ-nō) | white |
| 3. allergy (AL-er-jē) | hypersensitivity to a substance |
| 4. alopecia (al-ō-PĒ-shē-a) | baldness |
| 5. cicatrix (SIK-a-triks) | scar |
| 6. cytomegalovirus (CMV) (sī-tō-*meg*-a-lō-VĪ-rus) | a herpes type virus that usually causes disease when the immune system is compromised |
| 7. debridement (da-BRĒD-mon) | removal of contaminated or dead tissue and foreign matter from an open wound |
| 8. decubitus ulcer (de-KŪ-bi-tus) (UL-ser) | bedsore; an open area of skin caused by pressure or irritation |
| 9. dermabrasion (*derm*-a-BRĀ-zhun) | procedure to remove skin scars with abrasive material, such as sandpaper |
| 10. diaphoresis (*dī*-a-fō-RĒ-sis) | profuse sweating |
| 11. disseminate (dis-SEM-i-nāt) | to scatter over a considerable area |
| 12. ecchymosis (*ek*-i-MŌ-sis) | escape of blood into the tissues, causing superficial discoloration; a "black and blue" mark |
| 13. edema (e-DĒ-ma) | puffy swelling of tissue from the accumulation of fluid |
| 14. emollient (e-MOL-yent) | agent that softens or soothes the skin |
| 15. erythema (*er*-i-THĒ-ma) | redness |
| 16. induration (in-dū-RĀ-shun) | abnormal hard spot(s) |
| 17. jaundice (JAWN-dis) | condition characterized by a yellow tinge to the skin (xanthoderma) |
| 18. keloid (KĒ-loyd) | overgrowth of scar tissue (Figure 3-7) |

**Alopecia** is derived from the Greek **alopex,** meaning **fox.** One was thought to bald like a mangy fox.

**Decubitus** is derived from **de,** meaning **down,** and **cubere, meaning to lie. Decubitus** is a term also used in x-ray terminology to denote the recumbent (lying-down) position.

**Diaphoresis** is derived from the Greek **dia,** meaning **through,** and **phoreo,** meaning **I carry.** Translated, it means the carrying through of perspiration.

**Ecchymosis** is derived from the Greek **ek,** meaning **out of,** and **chumos,** meaning **juice.** Extended, it means to pour out juice of the body, or blood.

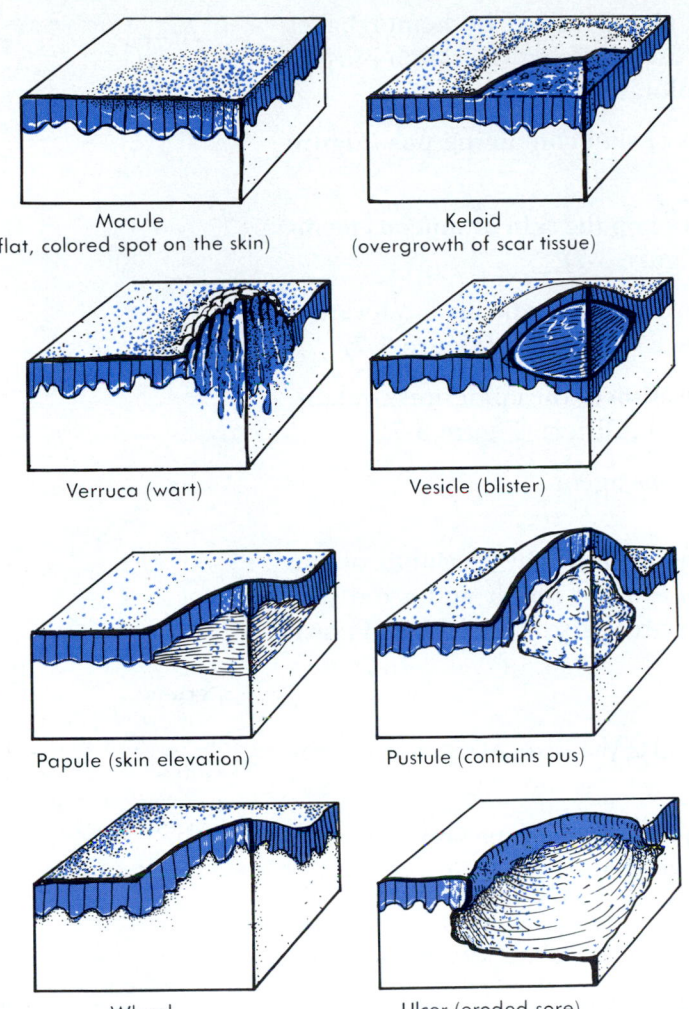

**Figure 3-7**
Cutaway sections of some common skin conditions.

Macule
(flat, colored spot on the skin)

Keloid
(overgrowth of scar tissue)

Verruca (wart)

Vesicle (blister)

Papule (skin elevation)

Pustule (contains pus)

Wheal

Ulcer (eroded sore)

19. leukoplakia . . . . . . . . . .   condition characterized by white spots
    (lū-kō-PLĀ-kē-a)              or patches on mucous membrane which
                                   may be precancerous

20. macule . . . . . . . . . . . .   flat, colored spot on the skin (Figure 3-7)
    (MAK-ūl)

21. nevus, (*pl.* nevi) . . . . . . .   circumscribed pigmented area present at
    (NĒ-vus, nē-vī)              birth; mole, birthmark

22. pallor . . . . . . . . . . . . .   paleness
    (PAL-ōr)

23. papule . . . . . . . . . . . . .   small, solid skin elevation (pimple)
    (PAP-ūl)                      (Figure 3-7)

24. petechia (*pl.* petechiae) .   pinpoint skin hemorrhages
    (pe-TĒ-kē-a, pe-TĒ-kē-e)

25. pruritus . . . . . . . . . . . .   severe itching
    (prū-RĪ-tus)

**Macule** is probably derived from the ancient language of Sanskrit: **mala,** meaning **dirt.**

**Petechia** is originally from the Italian **petechio,** meaning **flea bite.** The small hemorrhagic spot resembles the mark made by a flea.

26. **purpura** . . . . . . . . . . . .     disorder characterized by hemorrhages
    (PER-pū-ra)                              into the tissue, giving the skin a purple-
                                             red discoloration

27. **pustule** . . . . . . . . . . . .     elevation of skin containing pus (Figure
    (PUS-tūl)                                3-7)

28. **ulcer** . . . . . . . . . . . . .     eroded sore on the skin or mucous mem-
    (UL-ser)                                 brane (Figure 3-7)

29. **verruca** . . . . . . . . . . . .     circumscribed     cutaneous     elevation
    (ver-RŪ-ka)                              caused by a virus; wart (Figure 3-7)

30. **vesicle** . . . . . . . . . . . .     small elevation of the epidermis contain-
    (VES-i-kl)                               ing a liquid (blister) (Figure 3-7)

31. **virus** . . . . . . . . . . . . .     an infectious agent
    (VĪ-ras)

32. **wheal** . . . . . . . . . . . . .     transitory, round itchy elevation of the
    (hwēl)                                   skin with a white center and a red sur-
                                             rounding area, also called hive (Figure
                                             3-7)

# Dermatology
## *or*
## Give Me a Man
## Who Calls a Spade a Geotome

I wish the *dermatologist*
Were less a firm apologist
For all the terminology
That's used in *dermatology*.

Something you or I would deem a
Redness he calls *erythema;*
If it's blistered, raw and warm he
Has to call it *multiforme*.

Things to him are never simple;
*Papule* is his word for pimple
What's a *macule*, clearly stated?
Just a spot that's over-rated!

Over the skin that looks unwell
He chants Latin like a spell;
What he's labeled and obscured
Looks to him as good as cured.

Julia Bess Frank, M.D.

Reprinted with permission from The New England Journal of
Medicine, ©1977; 297(12):660.

Practice saying each of these terms aloud. To assist you in pronunciation,
obtain the audiotape designed for use with this text. Learn the definitions
and spellings of the other additional terms by completing the following
exercises.

## EXERCISE 23

Fill in the blanks with the correct terms.

1. Another name for a scar is _____*cicatrix*_____ .

2. Profuse sweating is called _____*diaphoresis*_____ .

3. The term for an agent that softens or soothes the skin is
   _____*emollient*_____ .

4. The medical term for wart is ___verruca___ .

5. ___Macule___ is the name for a flat, colored skin spot.

6. A yellow skin condition is known as ___jaundice___ .

7. The condition of white spots or patches on mucous membrane is called ___leukoplakia___ .

8. ___petechia___ are pinpoint hemorrhages of the skin.

9. An eroded sore is called a(n) ___ulcer___ .

10. A(n) ___keloid___ is an overgrowth of scar tissue.

11. Another name for paleness is ___pallor___ .

12. Superficial skin discoloration caused by escaping blood is referred to as ___ecchymosis___ .

13. Another name for white is ___albino___ .

14. A bedsore caused by prolonged lying down is called a(n) ___Decubitus ulcer___ .

15. Another name for fat is ___adipose___ .

16. ___disseminated___ means scattered over a considerable area.

17. Severe itching is called ___pruritus___ .

18. Another name for redness is ___erythema___ .

19. The condition of tissue hemorrhages giving the skin a purple-red discoloration is known as ___purpura___ .

20. ___nevus___ is another name for mole or birthmark.

21. The removal of dead or contaminated tissue from an open wound is called ___Debridement___ .

22. The term for baldness is ___alopecia___ .

23. Hypersensitivity to a substance is called a(n) ___allergy___ .

24. A small, solid skin elevation is called a(n) ___papule___ .

25. A transitory, round skin elevation with a white center and a red surrounding area is a(n) ___wheal___ .

26. A(n) ___pustule___ is a skin elevation containing pus.

27. A blister is also called a(n) ___vesicle___ .

28. ___dermabrasion___ is the name of the procedure using abrasive material to remove scars.

29. ___virus___ is an infectious agent.

30. An abnormal hard spot(s) is called ___induration___ .

31. ___edema___ is the swelling of tissue.

32. ___cytomegalovirus___ is a herpes type virus.

## EXERCISE 24A

Match the items in the first column with the correct definitions in the second column.

_m_ 1. adipose

_o_ 2. albino

_h_ 3. allergy

_a_ 4. alopecia

_j_ 5. cicatrix

_e_ 6. debridement

_n_ 7. decubitus ulcer

_l_ 8. dermabrasion

_g_ 9. diaphoresis

_d_ 10. disseminated

_b_ 11. ecchymosis

_f_ 12. emollient

_k_ 13. erythema

_c_ 14. jaundice

_q_ 15. edema

_i_ 16. induration

a.  baldness

b.  superficial discoloration caused by blood escaping into the tissues

c.  yellow color to the skin

d.  spread over a considerable area

e.  removal of dead tissue from an open wound

f.  agent that softens or soothes the skin

g.  profuse sweating

h.  hypersensitivity to a substance

i.  hard spot(s)

j.  scar

k.  redness

l.  procedure to remove skin scars by using abrasive material

m.  fat

n.  bedsore

o.  white

p.  patches on the mucous membrane

q.  swelling of tissue

## EXERCISE 24B

Match the terms in the first column with the correct definitions in the second column.

_g_ 1. keloid

_d_ 2. leukoplakia

_j_ 3. macule

_a_ 4. nevus

_l_ 5. pallor

_k_ 6. papule

_h_ 7. petechiae

_b_ 8. pruritus

_e_ 9. purpura

_f_ 10. pustule

a.  mole

b.  severe itching

c.  wart

d.  condition of white spots or patches on mucous membranes

e.  hemorrhages in tissue giving skin a red-purple color

f.  skin elevation containing pus

g.  overgrowth of scar tissue

h.  small elevation of epidermis containing liquid

___o___ 11. ulcer

___c___ 12. verruca

___h___ 13. vesicle

___i___ 14. wheal

___m___ 15. virus

___q___ 16. cytomegalovirus

i.   transitory elevation of skin with a white center and a red surrounding area

j.   flat, colored spot on skin

k.   small, solid skin elevation

l.   paleness

m.  an infectious agent

n.   pinpoint hemorrhages

o.   eroded sore on the skin or mucous membrane

p.   profuse sweating

q.   herpes type virus

## EXERCISE 25

Spell each of the other additional terms. Have someone dictate the terms on pp. 70-72 to you or say the words into a tape recorder; then spell the words from your recording as often as necessary. Study any you have spelled incorrectly.

1. _____    17. _____

2. _____    18. _____

3. _____    19. _____

4. _____    20. _____

5. _____    21. _____

6. _____    22. _____

7. _____    23. _____

8. _____    24. _____

9. _____    25. _____

10. _____   26. _____

11. _____   27. _____

12. _____   28. _____

13. _____   29. _____

14. _____   30. _____

15. _____   31. _____

16. _____   32. _____

Place a check mark (√) in the box to indicate that you have completed Objective 7.

☐ **DEFINE, PRONOUNCE, AND SPELL THE OTHER ADDITIONAL TERMS RELATED TO THE INTEGUMENTARY SYSTEM.**

**Case History:** 50-year-old white female presents in the dermatologist's office with a complaint of changes in nevus located in medial aspect of left eyebrow. Changes include hair loss, "crusty" surface, and some enlargement of lesion. Nevus has been present for approximately 3 years. Hair loss present for 2 years. Patient has past history of actinic keratosis and current case of nonrelated eczema bilaterally on both forearms. Biopsy revealed basal cell carcinoma, nodular, transected at base.

**Operative Report:** Patient's operative site was prepped with betadine. Xylocaine 1% with epinephrine was used as local anesthesia. Skin was incised at superior pole of lesion. Lesion was then excised as diagnosed, including a margin of clinical normal dermis. Specimen submitted to pathology. The superior pole was sutured. Hemostasis achieved with electrocautery. Two "A" to "T" flaps were then constructed on superior aspect of upper eyelid. Flaps and upper eyelid undermined 2 to 3 mm. Flaps sutured with 6/0 vicryl, followed by 6/0 nylon for closure. Pressure dressing applied.

## EXERCISE 26

To test your understanding of the terms introduced in this chapter, circle the words that correctly complete the sentences. The italicized words refer to the correct answer.

1. The physician called the *injury with pain, swelling, and discoloration with no break in the skin* a (fissure, contusion, laceration).
2. *Berry-shaped bacteria in grapelike clusters* are (streptococci, staphylococci, pediculosis).
3. The physician ordered lotions applied to the patient's *skin* to alleviate *dryness* or (pachyderma, dermatoconiosis, xeroderma).
4. The injection given *within the skin* is called a(n) (intradermal, epidermal, hypodermic) injection.
5. The diagnosis of *onychomalacia* was given by the physician for (ingrown nails, nail biting, softening of the nails).
6. The *pinpoint hemorrhages,* or (nevi, verrucae, petechiae), were distributed over the patient's entire body.
7. The primary symptom of the disease was *profuse sweating,* or (diaphoresis, ecchymosis, pruritus).
8. The patient had an *abnormal condition of fungus in the hair;* therefore the doctor recorded the diagnosis as (onychocryptosis, trichomycosis, onychomycosis).
9. The student nurse learned that the medical name for a *blister* was (verruca, keloid, vesicle).
10. The patient was to receive a *skin graft from her mother,* so the operation was listed as a (dermoplasty, dermatoautoplasty, dermatoheteroplasty).
11. An *abnormal hard spot* is called (edema, induration, virus).

12. Another word for *jaundice* is (erythroderma, leukoderma, xantho-derma).

13. *Leiodermia* is a condition of (striated, smooth, sweaty) skin.

The following exercise is for the student who likes an extra challenge.

## EXERCISE 27

Unscramble the following mixed-up terms. The word(s) on the left hint at the meaning of the word in each of the opposite scrambled words.

EXAMPLE:  skin  / d / e / r / m / a / t / i / t / i / s /
t   t   m   i   s   r   e   d   a   i

1. bad habit  / / / / / h / / h / / / /
p  o  n  a  a  g  y  o  i  h  h  c

2. examination  / / / / / /
s  i  b  y  o  p

3. skin needs fluids  / / / r / / / / r / / /
m  e  d  o  x  r  r  e  a

4. face-lift  / / / / t / / / / / / o / / /
m  e  c  t  o  r  t  y  h  i  d  y

5. hidden nail  / / / / c / / / c / / / / / o / / / /
p  o  t  h  o  s  s  y  c  o  n  c  r  i  y

6. herpes type virus  / / / / o / / / / / / / v / / / /
m  e  a  g  o  l  r  v  i  c  s  o  y  u  t

## EXERCISE 28

The following words did not appear in this chapter but are composed of word parts studied in this or the previous chapters. Find their definitions by translating the word parts literally.

1.  **dermatopathic** (*der*-ma-tō-PATH-ik) _____

2.  **fibroma** (fi-BRŌ-ma) _____

3.  **keratosis** (*kār*-a-TŌ-sis) _____

4.  **lipocyte** (LIP-ō-sīt) _____

5.  **onychoid** (ON-i-koyd) _____

6.  **trichoid** (TRIK-oyd) _____

# COMBINING FORMS CROSSWORD PUZZLE

## Across Clues

4. dust
5. skin
7. hair
11. grapelike clusters
13. death (cell, body)
17. wrinkles
19. self
20. other

## Down Clues

1. horny tissue, hard
2. fibrous tissue
3. dry
6. sebum (oil)
8. skin
9. fungus
10. thick
12. twisted chains
14. hidden
15. nail
16. life
18. sweat

# Summary

Can you build, analyze, define, pronounce, and spell the following terms *built from word parts?*    yes ☐    no ☐

### DIAGNOSTIC

dermatitis
(*der*-ma-TĪ-tis)

dermatoconiosis
(der-*ma*-tō-kō-nē-Ō-sis)

dermatofibroma
(*der*-ma-tō-fī-BRŌ-ma)

hidradenitis
(*hī*-drad-e-NĪ-tis)

leiodermia
(lī-ō-DER-mē-a)

onychocryptosis
(*on*-i-kō-krip-TŌ-sis)

onychomalacia
(on-i-kō-ma-LĀ-shē-a)

onychomycosis
(*on*-i-kō-mi-KŌ-sis)

onychophagia
(*on*-i-kō-FĀ-jē-a)

pachyderma
(paki-DER-ma)

paronychia
(pār-ō-NIK-ē-a)

seborrhea
(*seb*-ōr-Ē-a)

trichomycosis
(*trik*-ō-mī-KŌ-sis)

xeroderma
(zē-rō-DER-ma)

### SURGICAL

biopsy
(BĪ-op-sē)

dermatoautoplasty
(*der*-ma-tō-AW-tō-*plas*-tē)

dermatoheteroplasty
(*der*-ma-tō-HET-er-ō-*plas*-tē)

dermatoplasty
(DER-ma-tō-*plas*-tē)

onychectomy
(on-i-KEK-tō-mē)

rhytidectomy
(*rit*-i-DEK-tō-mē)

rhytidoplasty
(RĪT-i-dō-*plas*-tē)

### ADDITIONAL

dermatologist
(*der*-ma-TOL-ō-jist)

dermatology
(*der*-ma-TOL-ō-jē)

dermatome
(DER-ma-tōm)

epidermal
(*ep*-i-DER-mal)

erythroderma
(e-rith-rō-DER-ma)

hypodermic
(*hī*-po-DER-mik)

intradermal
(*in*-tra-DER-mal)

keratogenic
(*ker*-a-TŌ-jen-ik)

leukoderma
(lū-kō-DER-ma)

necrosis
(ne-KRŌ-sis)

percutaneous
(per-kū-TĀ-nē-us)

staphylococcus
(***pl. staphylococci***)
(*staf*-il-ō-KOK-us, *staf*-il-ō-KOK-sē)

streptococcus
(***pl. streptococci***)
(*strep*-tō-KOK-us, *strep*-tō-KOK-sē)

subcutaneous
(*sub*-kū-TĀ-nē-us)

ungual
(UNG-gwal)

xanthoderma
(zan-thō-DER-ma)

# Summary

Can you define, pronounce, and spell the following terms *not built from word parts?*   yes ☐   no ☐

## DIAGNOSTIC

abrasion
(a-BRĀ-zhun)

abscess
(AB-ses)

acne
(AK-nē)

actinic keratosis
(ack-TIN-ik)
(ker-a-TŌ-sis)

basal cell carcinoma
(BĀ-sal) (sel)
(kar-si-NŌ-ma)

carbuncle
(KAR-bung-kl)

cellulitis
(*sel*-ū-LĪ-tis)

contusion
(kon-TŪ-zhun)

eczema
(EK-ze-ma)

fissure
(FISH-ūr)

furuncle
(FER-ung-kl)

gangrene
(GANG-grēn)

herpes
(HER-pēz)

impetigo
(im-pe-TĪ-go)

Kaposi's sarcoma
(KAP-o-sēz)(sar-KŌ-ma)

laceration
(*las*-er-Ā-shun)

lesion
(LĒ-zhun)

pediculosis
(pe-*dik*-ū-LŌ-sis)

psoriasis
(so-RĪ-a-sis)

scabies
(SKĀ-bēz)

scleroderma
(skle-rō-DER-ma)

squamous cell
carcinoma
(SQWĀ-mus) (sel)
(kar-si-NŌ-ma)

systemic lupus
erythematosus
(sis-TEM-ik) (LŪ-pus)
(er-i-thē-ma-TŌ-sus)

tinea
(TIN-ē-a)

urticaria
(ūr-ti-KĀ-rē-a)

## ADDITIONAL

adipose
(AD-i-pōs)

albino
(al-BĪ-nō)

allergy
(AL-er-jē)

alopecia
(al-ō-PĒ-shē-a)

cicatrix
(SIK-a-triks)

cytomegalovirus
(si-to-*meg*-a-lō-VĪ-rus)

debridement
(da-BRĒD-mon)

decubitus ulcer
(de-KŪ-bi-tus) (UL-ser)

dermabrasion
(*derm*-a-BRĀ-zhun)

diaphoresis
(*di*-a-fō-RĒ-sis)

disseminate
(dis-SEM-i-nāt)

ecchymosis
(*ek*-i-MŌ-sis)

edema
(e-DĒ-ma)

emollient
(e-MOL-yent)

erythema
(*er*-i-THĒ-ma)

induration
(in-dū-RĀ-shun)

jaundice
(JAWN-dis)

keloid
(KĒ-loyd)

leukoplakia
(*lū*-kō-PLĀ-kē-a)

macule
(MAK-ūl)

nevus, (*pl.* nevi)
(NĒ-vus, nē-vī)

pallor
(PAL-ōr)

papule
(PAP-ūl)

petechia (*pl.* petechiae)
(pe-TĒ-kē-a) (pe-TĒ-kē-e)

pruritus
(prū-RĪ-tus)

purpura
(PER-pū-ra)

pustule
(PUS-tūl)

ulcer
(UL-ser)

verruca
(ver-RŪ-ka)

vesicle
(VES-i-kl)

virus
(VĪ-rus)

wheal
(hwēl)

# Answers

### Exercise 1

1. c     5. f
2. d     6. h
3. g     7. a
4. b

### Exercise 2

**Figure 3-1**
Horny tissue: kerat/o
Sweat gland; hidr/o
Hair: trich/o
Skin: cutane/o, dermat/o, derm/o
Sebum: seb/o

**Figure 3-2**
Nail: onych/o, ungu/o

### Exercise 3

1. sweat     4. hair               7. sebum (oil)
2. skin      5. horny tissue, hard 8. nail
3. nail      6. skin               9. skin

### Exercise 4

1. trich/o        5. a. derm/o
2. hidr/o            b. dermat/o
3. a. onych/o       c. cutane/o
   b. ungu/o     6. kerat/o
4. seb/o

### Exercise 5

1. death                  8. life
2. fibrous tissue, fibers 9. other
3. grapelike clusters    10. gland
4. hidden                11. twisted chains
5. thick                 12. dry
6. dust                  13. self
7. fungus                14. wrinkles

### Exercise 6

1. myc/o     6. fibr/o      11. aden/o
2. necr/o    7. strept/o    12. crypt/o
3. heter/o   8. rhytid/o    13. coni/o
4. xer/o     9. staphyl/o   14. bi/o
5. pachy/o  10. aut/o

### Exercise 7

1. under, below           4. within
2. beside, beyond, around 5. through
3. on, upon, over

### Exercise 8

1. intra-    4. para-
2. sub-      5. per-
3. epi-

### Exercise 9

1. c    3. a    5. i    7. d    9. f
2. e    4. j    6. h    8. b   10. k

### Exercise 10

1. plastic or surgical    6. eating, swallowing
   repair                 7. excessive discharge,
2. excision or surgical      flow
   removal                8. berry-shaped
3. softening              9. to view
4. inflammation          10. diseased or abnormal
5. instrument used to        state, condition of
   cut

### Exercise 11

```
      WR  CV WR  S
1. dermat/ o /coni/osis     abnormal condition of the
          ‾‾                   skin caused by dust
          CF

      WR   WR  S
2. hidr/aden/itis           inflammation of the sweat
                               glands

      WR    S
3. dermat/itis              inflammation of the skin

      WR    WR S
4. pachy/derm/a             thickening of the skin

      WR  CV    S
5. onych/ o /malacia        softening of the nails
         ‾‾
         CF

      WR CV WR  S
6. trich/ o /myc/osis       abnormal condition of a
         ‾‾                    fungus in the hair
         CF

      WR   CV WR  S
7. dermat/ o /fibr/oma      fibrous tumor of the skin
          ‾‾
          CF

      P   WR    S
8. par/onych/ia             diseased state around the
                               nail

      WR   CV WR  S
9. onych/ o /crypt/osis     abnormal condition of a
         ‾‾                    hidden nail
         CF

      WR    S
10. seb/orrhea              excessive discharge of se-
                               bum

       WR CV   S
11. onych/ o /phagia        eating the nails, or nail
          ‾‾                   biting
          CF
```

WR CV   WR  S
12. xer/ o /derm/a          dry skin
      ‾‾CF‾‾

WR CV  WR  S
13. lei/ o /derm/ia          condition of smooth skin
      ‾‾CF‾‾

## Exercise 12

1. pachy/derm/a
2. onych/o/myc/osis
3. seb/orrhea
4. dermat/itis
5. dermat/o/fibr/oma
6. onych/o/malacia
7. hidr/aden/itis
8. onych/o/crypt/osis
9. dermat/o/coni/osis
10. onych/o/phagia
11. par/onych/ia
12. xer/o/derm/a
13. lei/o/derm/ia

## Exercise 13

Spelling exercise; *see* text, p. 58.

## Exercise 14

1. systemic lupus erythe-matosus
2. abscess
3. fissure
4. abrasion
5. psoriasis
6. herpes
7. pediculosis
8. tinea
9. contusion
10. gangrene
11. lesion
12. Kaposi's sarcoma
13. actinic keratosis
14. carbuncle
15. acne
16. laceration
17. furuncle
18. squamous cell
19. cellulitis
20. impetigo
21. eczema
22. scabies
23. urticaria
24. basal cell
25. scleroderma

## Exercise 15A

1. f    3. g    5. m    7. i    9. e    11. h
2. j    4. l    6. c    8. k    10. b   12. a
                                        13. d

## Exercise 15B

1. d    3. f    5. k    7. c    9. l    11. b
2. i    4. h    6. j    8. a    10. e   12. g

## Exercise 16

Spelling exercise; *see* text, pp. 55 and 56.

## Exercise 17

WR        S
1. rhytid/ectomy          excision of wrinkles

WR  S
2. bi /opsy          view of life (removal of living tissue)

WR   CV  WR CV   S
3. dermat/ o /aut/ o /plasty          plastic repair using
      ‾‾CF‾‾    ‾‾CF‾‾                patient's own skin
                                      for the skin graft

WR        S
4. onych/ectomy          excision of a nail

WR  CV  S
5. rhytid/ o/ plasty          plastic repair of wrin-kles
        ‾‾CF‾‾

WR   CV  WR CV   S
6. dermat/ o /heter/ o /plasty          plastic repair using
      ‾‾CF‾‾    ‾‾CF‾‾                  skin from others for
                                        the skin graft

## Exercise 18

1. rhytid/ectomy
2. bi/opsy
3. dermat/o/heter/o/plasty
4. onych/ectomy
5. rhytid/o/plasty
6. dermat/o/plasty

## Exercise 19

Spelling exercise; *see* text p. 65.

## Exercise 20

WR   S
1. ungu/al          pertaining to the nail

WR       S
2. derma/tome          instrument used to cut skin

WR  CV   S
3. strept/ o /coccus          berry-shaped bacteria in
        ‾‾CF‾‾                chains

P      WR  S
4. hypo/derm/ic          pertaining to under the skin

WR        S
5. dermat/ology          study of the skin

P       WR   S
6. sub/cutane/ous          pertaining to under the skin

WR   CV   S
7. staphyl/ o /coccus          berry-shaped bacteria in
         ‾‾CF‾‾                clusters

WR  CV  S
8. kerat/ o /genic          originating in horny tis-sue
        ‾‾CF‾‾

WR        S
9. dermat/ologist          physician who specializes in skin diseases

WR  S
10. necr/osis          abnormal condition of death

P    WR  S
11. epi/derm/al          pertaining to upon the skin

12. 
```
   WR   CV  WR  S
xanth/ o /derm/a
      ⌣
      CF
```
yellow skin

13. 
```
   WR    CV  WR  S
erythro/ o /derm/a
        ⌣
        CF
```
red skin

14. 
```
 WR CV WR  S
leuk/ o /derm/a
     ⌣
     CF
```
white skin

15. 
```
   P    WR    S
per/cutane/ous/
```
pertaining to
   through the skin

## Exercise 21

| | |
|---|---|
| 1. dermat/ology | 8. epi/derm/al |
| 2. necr/osis | 9. sub/cutane/ous |
| 3. derma/tome | 10. strept/o/coccus |
| 4. ungu/al | 11. kerat/o/genic |
| 5. staphyl/o/coccus | 12. leuk/o/derm/a |
| 6. dermat/ologist | 13. erythr/o/derm/a |
| 7. intra/derm/al | 14. xanth/o/derm/a |
| | 15. per/cutane/ous |

## Exercise 22

Spelling exercise; *see* text, pp. 66-67.

## Exercise 23

| | | |
|---|---|---|
| 1. cicatrix | 12. ecchymosis | 23. allergy |
| 2. diaphoresis | 13. albino | 24. papule |
| 3. emollient | 14. decubitus ulcer | 25. wheal |
| 4. verruca | 15. adipose | 26. pustule |
| 5. macule | 16. disseminated | 27. vesicle |
| 6. jaundice | 17. pruritus | 28. dermabrasion |
| 7. leukoplakia | 18. erythema | 29. virus |
| 8. petechiae | 19. purpura | 30. induration |
| 9. ulcer | 20. nevus | 31. edema |
| 10. keloid | 21. debridement | 32. cytomegalovirus |
| 11. pallor | 22. alopecia | |

## Exercise 24A

| | | | | |
|---|---|---|---|---|
| 1. m | 5. j | 8. l | 11. b | 14. c |
| 2. o | 6. e | 9. g | 12. f | 15. q |
| 3. h | 7. n | 10. d | 13. k | 16. i |
| 4. a | | | | |

## Exercise 24B

| | | | | | |
|---|---|---|---|---|---|
| 1. g | 4. a | 7. n | 10. f | 13. h | 16. q |
| 2. d | 5. l | 8. b | 11. o | 14. i | |
| 3. j | 6. k | 9. e | 12. c | 15. m | |

## Exercise 25

Spelling exercise; *see* text, pp. 70 to 72.

## Exercise 26

| | |
|---|---|
| 1. contusion | 8. trichomycosis |
| 2. staphylococci | 9. vesicle |
| 3. xeroderma | 10. dermatoheteroplasty |
| 4. intradermal | 11. induration |
| 5. softening of the nails | 12. xanthoderma |
| 6. petechiae | 13. smooth |
| 7. diaphoresis | |

## Exercise 27

| | | |
|---|---|---|
| 1. onychophagia | 3. xeroderma | 5. onychocryptosis |
| 2. biopsy | 4. rhytidectomy | 6. cytomegalovirus |

## Exercise 28

1. pertaining to disease of the skin
2. fibrous tumor
3. abnormal condition of horny tissue
4. fat cell
5. resembling a nail
6. resembling hair

# Answers

# 4

# Respiratory System

## Objectives

Upon completion of this chapter you will be able to:

1. Define the anatomical terms of the respiratory system.

2. Write the definitions of the word parts included in this chapter.

3. Build, analyze, define, pronounce, and spell the diagnostic terms related to the respiratory system.

4. Define, pronounce, and spell other diagnostic terms related to the respiratory system.

5. Build, analyze, define, pronounce, and spell the surgical terms related to the respiratory system.

6. Build, analyze, define, pronounce, and spell the diagnostic procedural terms related to the respiratory system.

7. Build, analyze, define, pronounce, and spell additional terms related to the respiratory system.

8. Define, pronounce, and spell the other additional terms related to the respiratory system.

## Objective 1  DEFINE THE ANATOMICAL TERMS OF THE RESPIRATORY SYSTEM.

## Anatomical Terms

Most humans do not consciously think about breathing. We take in oxygen from the air while we talk, eat, walk, and sleep. We also exhale carbon dioxide, a waste product of cell function, while doing other things. The organs of the respiratory system function to bring about this exchange of gases in the body.

### ORGANS OF THE RESPIRATORY SYSTEM (Figure 4-1)

1. nose . . . . . . . . . . . . . . . . Lined with mucous membrane and fine hairs. It acts as a filter and also moistens the entering air.
   a. nasal septum . . . . . . . Partition separating the right and left nasal cavities.
   b. paranasal sinuses . . . . Air cavities within the cranial bones that open into the nasal cavities.

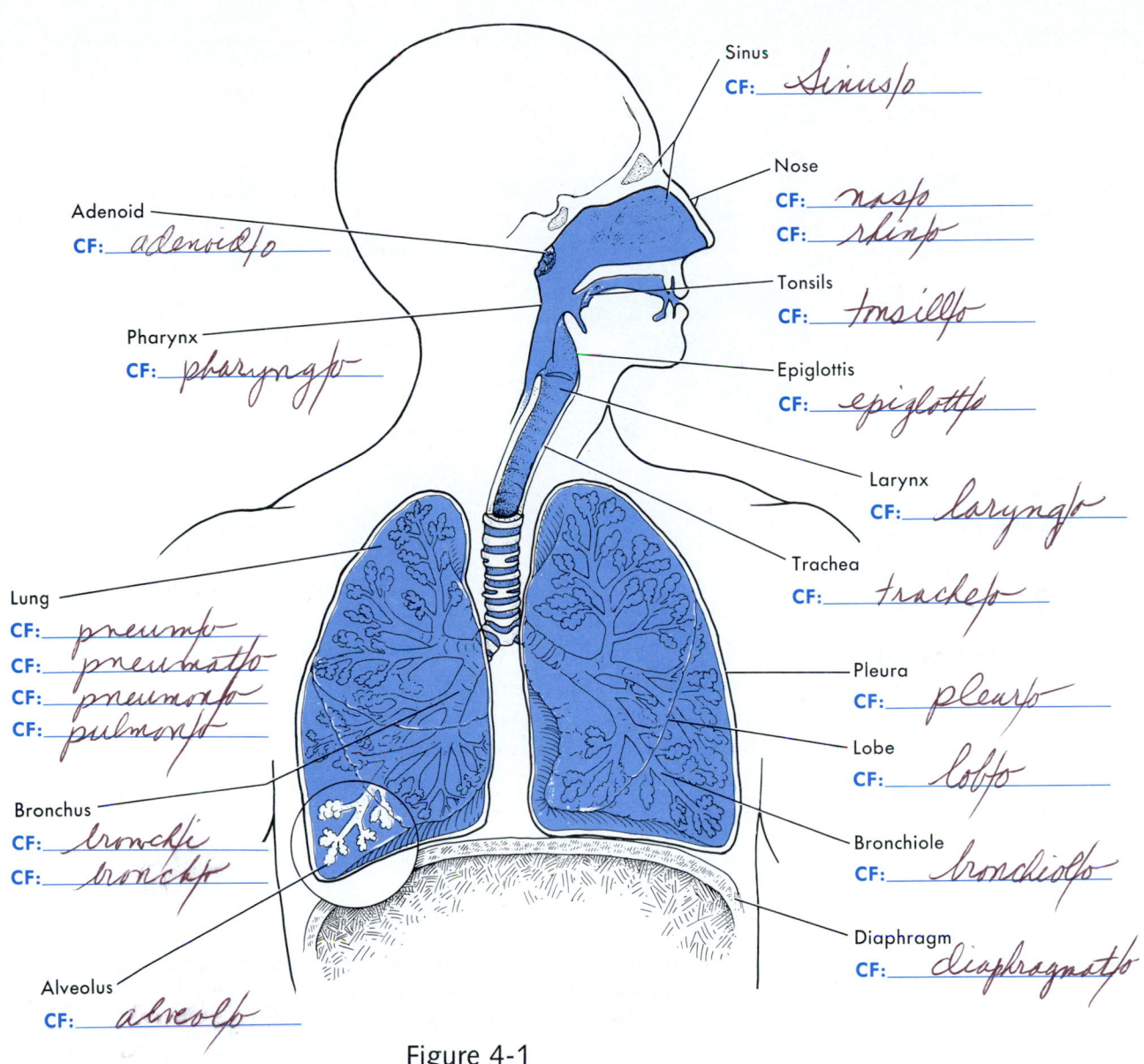

**Figure 4-1**
Diagram of the respiratory system.

Labels and combining forms (CF) shown in the figure:

- Sinus — CF: _Sinus/o_
- Nose — CF: _nas/o_ — CF: _rhin/o_
- Tonsils — CF: _tonsill/o_
- Epiglottis — CF: _epiglott/o_
- Larynx — CF: _laryng/o_
- Trachea — CF: _trache/o_
- Pleura — CF: _pleur/o_
- Lobe — CF: _lob/o_
- Bronchiole — CF: _bronchiol/o_
- Diaphragm — CF: _diaphragmat/o_
- Adenoid — CF: _adenoid/o_
- Pharynx — CF: _pharyng/o_
- Lung — CF: _pneum/o_ — CF: _pneumat/o_ — CF: _pneumon/o_ — CF: _pulmon/o_
- Bronchus — CF: _bronchi_ — CF: _bronch/o_
- Alveolus — CF: _alveol/o_

2. **pharynx (also called the throat)** . . . . . . . . . . . . . . Serves as a food and air passageway. Air enters from the nasal cavities and passes through the pharynx to the larynx. Food enters the pharynx from the mouth and passes into the esophagus.

   a. **adenoids** . . . . . . . . . Lymphoid tissue located behind the nasal cavity.

   b. **tonsils** . . . . . . . . . . . Lymphoid tissue located behind the mouth.

> The largest ring of cartilage in the larynx is known as the thyroid cartilage, also called the **Adam's apple.** The name came from the belief that Adam, realizing he had sinned when he ate the forbidden fruit, was unable to swallow the apple lodged in his throat.

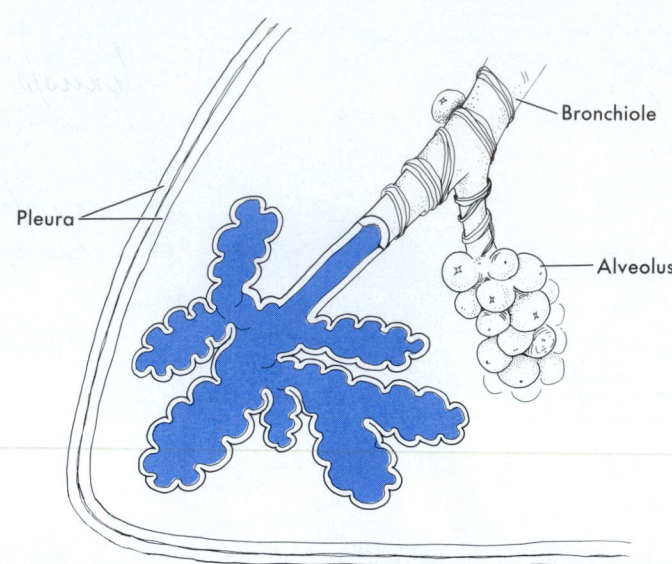

Pleura

Bronchiole

Alveolus

**Figure 4-2**
Bronchioles and alveoli.

3.  larynx (also called the
    voice box) . . . . . . . . . . . .    Location of the vocal cords. Air enters
                                           from the pharynx.

    a.  epiglottis . . . . . . . . .       Flap of cartilage that automatically cov-
                                           ers the opening of the larynx during
                                           swallowing and keeps food from enter-
                                           ing.

4.  trachea (also called the
    windpipe) . . . . . . . . . . . .      Passageway for air to the bronchi.

5.  bronchus (*pl.* bronchi) . . .         Has two branches, which carry the air
                                           from the trachea into the lungs, where
                                           the branches divide and subdivide. The
                                           branchings resemble a tree and there-
                                           fore are referred to as the *bronchial tree.*

    a.  bronchioles . . . . . . . .        Smallest subdivisions of the bronchial
                                           tree.

    b.  alveolus (*pl.* alveoli) . .       Air sacs at the end of the bronchioles.
                                           Oxygen and carbon dioxide are ex-
                                           changed through the alveolar walls and
                                           the capillaries (Figure 4-2).

6.  lungs . . . . . . . . . . . . . . .    Two sponge-like organs in the thoracic
                                           cavity. The right lung consists of three
                                           lobes, and the left lung has two lobes.

    a.  pleura . . . . . . . . . . .       Serous membrane covering each lung
                                           and lining the thoracic cavity.

7.  diaphragm . . . . . . . . . . .        Muscular partition that separates the
                                           thoracic cavity from the abdominal cav-
                                           ity. It aids in the breathing process.

**Bronchi** originated from the Greek **brecho,** meaning **to pour** or **wet.** An ancient belief was that the esophagus carried solid food to the stomach while the bronchi carried liquids.

8.  mediastinum . . . . . . . . .    Space between the lungs. It contains the heart, esophagus, trachea, and other structures.

> **Mediastinum** literally means **to stand in the middle**, since it is derived from the Latin **medius**, meaning **middle**, and **stare**, meaning **to stand.**

Learn the anatomical terms by completing the following exercises.

## EXERCISE 1

Match the anatomical terms in the first column with the correct definitions in the second column.

*h* 1. alveoli

*a* 2. bronchi

*g* 3. larynx

*c* 4. lungs

*f* 5. pharynx

*d* 6. pleura

*e* 7. adenoids

*b* 8. trachea

a. tubes carrying air between the trachea and lungs

b. also called the *windpipe*

c. located in the thoracic cavity

d. membrane covering the lung

e. lymphoid tissue located behind the nasal cavity

f. acts as food and air passageway

g. also called the *voice box*

h. air sacs at the end of the bronchioles

i. keeps food out of windpipe

## EXERCISE 2

Fill in the blanks with the correct terms.

1.  The partition that separates the right and left nasal cavities is called the _nasal septum_ .

2.  The _epiglottis_ is a flap of cartilage that prevents food from entering the larynx.

3.  The smallest subdivisions of the bronchial tree are the _bronchioles_ .

4.  The _nose_ serves as a filter and moistener of air entering the body.

5.  The thoracic cavity is separated from the abdominal cavity by the _diaphragm_ .

6.  The space between the lungs is called the _mediastinum_ .

7.  The lymphoid tissues located in the pharynx behind the mouth are called the _tonsils_ .

Place a check mark (√) in the box to indicate that you have completed Objective 1.

☐ **DEFINE THE ANATOMICAL TERMS OF THE RESPIRATORY SYSTEM.**

# Objective 2   WRITE THE DEFINITIONS OF THE WORD PARTS INCLUDED IN THIS CHAPTER.

## Respiratory System Word Parts

Study the word parts and their definitions listed as follows. Learning will be made easier by completing the exercises that follow.

| COMBINING FORM | DEFINITION |
| --- | --- |
| 1.  adenoid/o . . . . . . . . . . . | adenoids |
| 2.  alveol/o . . . . . . . . . . . . | alveolus |
| 3.  bronch/i, bronch/o<br>(NOTE: Both *i* and *o* combining vowels are used with the word root *bronch.*) | bronchus |
| 4.  bronchiol/o . . . . . . . . . . | bronchiole |
| 5.  diaphragmat/o . . . . . . . . | diaphragm |
| 6.  epiglott/o . . . . . . . . . . . | epiglottis |
| 7.  laryng/o . . . . . . . . . . . . | larynx |
| 8.  lob/o . . . . . . . . . . . . . . | lobe |
| 9.  nas/o<br>rhin/o . . . . . . . . . . . . . . | nose |
| 10.  pharyng/o . . . . . . . . . . . | pharynx |
| 11.  pleur/o . . . . . . . . . . . . . | pleura |
| 12.  pneum/o<br>pneumat/o<br>pneumon/o . . . . . . . . . . . | lung, air |
| 13.  pulmon/o . . . . . . . . . . . | lung |
| 14.  sinus/o . . . . . . . . . . . . . | sinus |
| 15.  sept/o . . . . . . . . . . . . . | septum (wall off, fence) |
| 16.  thorac/o . . . . . . . . . . . . | thorax (chest) |
| 17.  tonsill/o . . . . . . . . . . . .<br>(NOTE: *Tonsil* has one *l*, and the combining form has two *l*'s.) | tonsil |
| 18.  trache/o . . . . . . . . . . . . | trachea |

**Adenoid** is derived from the Greek **aden**, meaning **gland** and **eidos**, meaning **like**. The word was once used for the prostate gland. The first adenoid surgery was performed in 1868.

**Lobe** literally means **the part that hangs down**, although it comes from the Greek **lobos**, meaning **capsule** or **pod**. Also applied to the lobe of an ear, liver, or brain.

Learn the anatomical locations and meanings of the combining forms by completing the following exercises.

## EXERCISE 3

Write the combining forms in the spaces marked **CF** on the diagram in Figure 4-1, p. 85.

## EXERCISE 4

Write the definitions of the following combining forms.

1. laryng/o _____ larynx
2. bronch/o, bronch/i _____ bronchus
3. pleur/o _____ pleura
4. pneum/o _____ lung, air
5. tonsill/o _____ tonsil
6. bronchiol/o _____ bronchiole
7. pulmon/o _____ lung
8. diaphragmat/o _____ diaphragm
9. trache/o _____ trachea
10. alveol/o _____ alveolus
11. pneumon/o _____ lung, air
12. thorac/o _____ thorax
13. adenoid/o _____ adenoids
14. pharyng/o _____ pharynx
15. rhin/o _____ nose
16. sinus/o _____ sinus
17. lob/o _____ lobe
18. epiglott/o _____ epiglottis
19. pneumat/o _____ lung, air
20. nas/o _____ nose
21. sept/o _____ septum

## EXERCISE 5

Write the combining form for each of the following terms.

1. nose  a. _____ nas/o
   b. _____ rhin/o
2. larynx  _____ laryng/o

3. lung, air     a. _pneum/o_

              b. _pneumat/o_

              c. _pneumon/o_

4. lung           _pulmon/o_

5. tonsils         _tonsill/o_

6. trachea        _trache/o_

7. adenoids       _adenoid/o_

8. bronchiole      _bronchiol/o_

9. pleura         _pleur/o_

10. diaphragm     _diaphragmat/o_

11. sinus          _sinus/o_

12. thorax         _thorac/o_

13. alveolus       _alveol/o_

14. pharynx       _pharyng/o_

15. bronchi-    a. _bronchi_
      _us_

              b. _bronch/o_

16. lobe           _lob/o_

17. epiglottis      _epiglott/o_

18. septum        _sept/o_

# Related Word Parts

| COMBINING FORM | DEFINITION |
|---|---|
| 1. atel/o . . . . . . . . . . . . . . . | imperfect, incomplete |
| 2. hem/o, hemat/o . . . . . . . . | blood |
| 3. muc/o . . . . . . . . . . . . . . . | mucus |
| 4. orth/o . . . . . . . . . . . . . . . | straight |
| 5. ox/o, ox/i . . . . . . . . . . . . | oxygen |
| (NOTE: The combining vowels *o* and *i* are used with the word root *ox*.) | |
| 6. py/o . . . . . . . . . . . . . . . . | pus |
| 7. spir/o . . . . . . . . . . . . . . | breathe, breathing |

Learn the other combining forms by completing the following exercises.

**Oxygen** was discovered in 1774 by Joseph Priestly. In 1775 Antoine-Laurent Lavoisier, a French chemist, noted that all the acids he knew contained oxygen. Since he thought it was an acid producer, he named it, using the Greek **oxys**, meaning **sour**, and the suffix **gen**, meaning **to produce.**

## EXERCISE 6

Write the definitions of the following combining forms.

1. ox/o, ox/i _____ *oxygen* _____

2. spir/o _____ *breathe, breathing* _____

3. muc/o _____ *mucus* _____

4. atel/o _____ *imperfect, incomplete* _____

5. orth/o _____ *straight* _____

6. py/o _____ *pus* _____

7. hem/o, hemat/o _____ *blood* _____

## EXERCISE 7

Write the combining form for each of the following.

1. breathe, breathing _____ *spir/o* _____

2. oxygen a. _____ *ox/o* _____

   b. _____ *ox/i* _____

3. imperfect, incomplete _____ *atel/o* _____

4. straight _____ *orth/o* _____

5. pus _____ *py/o* _____

6. mucus _____ *muc/o* _____

7. blood a. _____ *hem/o* _____

   b. _____ *hemat/o* _____

# Prefixes

| PREFIX | DEFINITION |
|---|---|
| 1. a-, an-............... (NOTE: *An* is used when the word root begins with a vowel.) | without or absence of |
| 2. endo- ............... (NOTE: The prefix *intra*, introduced in Chapter 3, also means *within*.) | within |
| 3. eu- ................ | normal, good |
| 4. pan- ................ | all, total |

Learn the prefixes by completing the following exercises.

## EXERCISE 8

Write the definitions of the following prefixes.

1. endo- _____ *within*

2. a-, an- _____ *without absence of*

3. pan- _____ *all, total*

4. eu- _____ *normal, good*

## EXERCISE 9

Write the prefix for each of the following.

1. within _____ *endo*

2. normal, good _____ *eu*

3. without or absence of   a. _____ *a*

                        b. _____ *an*

4. all, total _____ *pan*

# Suffixes

| SUFFIX | DEFINITION |
| --- | --- |
| 1. -algia | pain |
| 2. -ar, -ary | pertaining to |
| 3. -capnia | carbon dioxide |
| 4. -cele | hernia or protrusion |
| 5. -centesis | surgical puncture to aspirate fluid (with a sterile needle) |
| 6. -eal | pertaining to |
| 7. -ectasis | stretching-out, dilatation, expansion |
| 8. -emia | blood condition |
| 9. -gram | record, x-ray film |
| 10. -graphy | process of recording, x-ray filming |
| 11. -meter | instrument used to measure |
| 12. -metry | measurement |
| 13. -orrhagia | rapid flow of blood |
| 14. -ostomy | creation of an artificial opening |

**Capnia** is derived from the Greek **kapnos,** meaning **smoke.** It now refers to carbon dioxide.

15. -otomy . . . . . . . . . . . . . cut into or incision
16. -oxia . . . . . . . . . . . . . . . oxygen
17. -pexy . . . . . . . . . . . . . . surgical fixation, suspension
18. -phonia . . . . . . . . . . . . sound or voice
19. -pnea . . . . . . . . . . . . . breathing
20. -scope . . . . . . . . . . . . . instrument used for visual examination
21. -scopy, -scopic . . . . . . . . visual examination
22. -spasm . . . . . . . . . . . . . sudden, involuntary muscle contraction (spasmodic contraction)
23. -stenosis . . . . . . . . . . . . constriction or narrowing
24. -thorax . . . . . . . . . . . . . chest

Learn the suffixes by completing the following exercises.

## EXERCISE 10A

Match the suffixes in the first column with their correct definitions in the second column.

_K_ 1. -algia
_f_ 2. -ar, -ary, -eal
_e_ 3. -capnia
_g_ 4. -cele
_c_ 5. -centesis
_b_ 6. -ectasis
_j_ 7. -emia
_a_ 8. -gram
_l_ 9. -graphy
_h_ 10. -meter
_d_ 11. -metry

a. record, x-ray film
b. stretching-out, dilatation, expansion
c. surgical puncture to aspirate fluid
d. measurement
e. carbon dioxide
f. pertaining to
g. hernia or protrusion
h. instrument used to measure
i. rapid flow of blood
j. blood condition
k. pain
l. process of recording

## EXERCISE 10B

Match the suffixes in the first column with their correct definitions in the second column.

_c_ 1. -orrhagia
_f_ 2. -ostomy
_a_ 3. -otomy
_i_ 4. -oxia

a. cut into or incision
b. instrument used for visual examination
c. rapid flow of blood

_K_ 5. -pexy
_e_ 6. -phonia
_j_ 7. -pnea
_b_ 8. -scope
_m_ 9. -scopy,-scopic
_g_ 10. -spasm
_d_ 11. -stenosis
_h_ 12. -thorax

d. constriction, narrowing
e. sound or voice
f. creation of an artificial opening
g. sudden, involuntary muscle contraction
h. chest
i. oxygen
j. breathing
k. surgical fixation, suspension
l. carbon dioxide
m. visual examination

## EXERCISE 11

Write the definitions of the following suffixes.

1. -thorax _chest_

2. -ar, -ary, -eal _pertaining to_

3. -stenosis _constriction or narrowing_

4. -cele _hernia, or protrusion_

5. -ostomy _creation of an artifical opening_

6. -pexy _surgical fixation, suspension_

7. -meter _instrument used to measure_

8. -spasm _sudden involuntary muscle contraction_

9. -algia _pain_

10. -scopy, -scopic _visual examination_

11. -centesis _surgical puncture to aspirate fluid_

12. -otomy _cut into or incision_

13. -scope _instrument used for visual exam_

14. -orrhagia _rapid flow of blood_

15. -ectasis _stretching out, dialation, expansion_

16. -gram _record, or x-ray film_

17. -pnea _breathing_

18. -graphy *process of recording, x-ray filming*

19. -metry *measurement*

20. -emia *blood condition*

21. -oxia *oxygen*

22. -capnia *carbon dioxide*

23. -phonia *sound or voice*

Place a check mark (√) in the box to indicate that you have completed Objective 2.

☐ **WRITE THE DEFINITIONS OF THE WORD PARTS INCLUDED IN THIS CHAPTER.**

## Medical Terms

The terms you need to learn to complete this chapter are listed as follows. Now that you know the meaning of the word parts, the exercises found at the end of the list will assist you to learn the definition and the spelling of each word.

## Objective 3   BUILD, ANALYZE, DEFINE, PRONOUNCE, AND SPELL THE DIAGNOSTIC TERMS RELATED TO THE RESPIRATORY SYSTEM.

## Diagnostic Terms

**TERM**
(built from word parts)

**DEFINITION**

1. adenoiditis . . . . . . . . . . . . inflammation of the adenoids
   (ad-e-noyd-Ī-tis)

2. atelectasis . . . . . . . . . . . . incomplete expansion (of the lung of a
   (at-e-LEK-ta-sis)    newborn or collapsed lung) (Figure 4-3)

3. bronchiectasis . . . . . . . . dilatation of the bronchi (Figure 4-4)
   (bron-ki-EK-ta-sis)
   (NOTE: i is the combining vowel)

4. bronchitis . . . . . . . . . . . inflammation of the bronchi
   (bron-KĪ-tis)

5. bronchogenic
   carcinoma . . . . . . . . . . . cancerous tumor originating in the
   (bron-kō-JEN-ik) (kar-si-NŌ-ma)    bronchus

6. bronchopneumonia . . . . diseased state of the bronchi and lungs
   (bron-kō-nū-MŌ-nē-a)

> **Atelectasis** is derived from the Greek **ateles**, meaning **not perfect**, and **ektasis**, meaning **expansion**. It denotes an incomplete expansion of lungs, especially at birth.

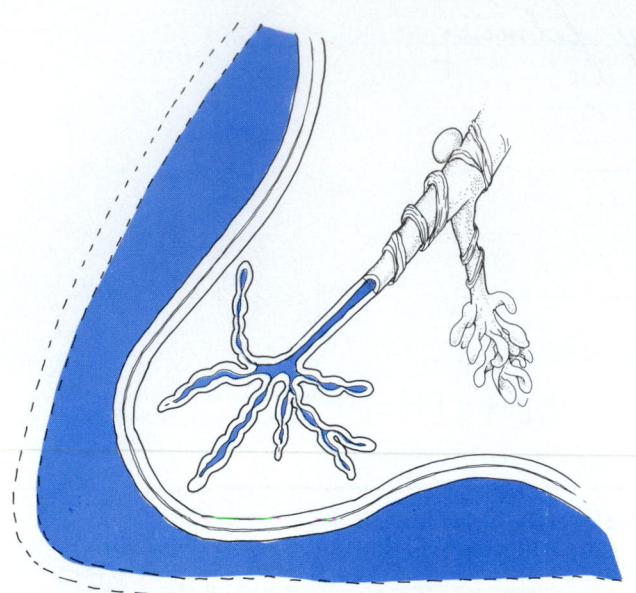

**Figure 4-3**
Atelectasis showing the alveoli.

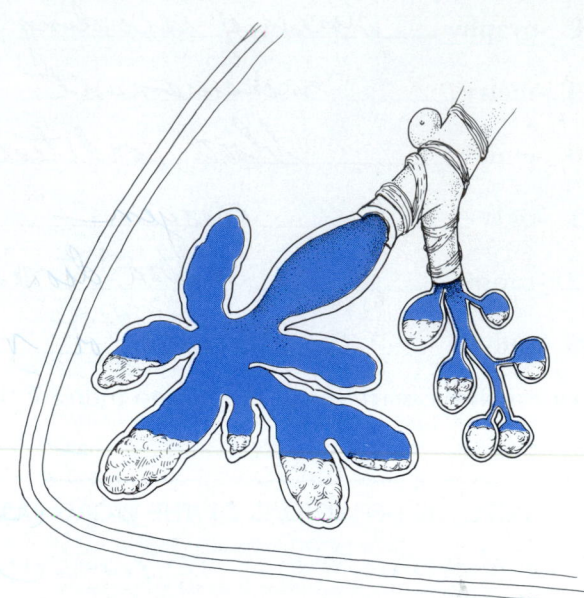

**Figure 4-4**
Bronchiectasis showing the alveoli.

7.  **diaphragmatocele**. . . . . .        hernia of the diaphragm
    (*dī*-a-frag-MAT-ō-sēl)

8.  **epiglottitis** . . . . . . . . . .        inflammation of the epiglottis
    (*ep*-i-glot-Ī-tis)

9.  **hemothorax** . . . . . . . . . .        blood in the chest (pleural space)
    (hē-mo-THŌ-raks)

10. **laryngitis** . . . . . . . . . . .        inflammation of the larynx
    (*lār*-in-JĪ-tis)

11. **laryngotracheobronchi-**
    **tis** . . . . . . . . . . . . . . . .        inflammation of the larynx, trachea, and
    (lār-*ing*-go-*trā*-kē-ō-bron-        bronchi; the acute form is called *croup*
    KĪ-tis)

12. **lobar pneumonia** . . . . . .        diseased state of a lobe(s) of the lung
    (LŌ-bar) (nū-MŌ-nē-a)

13. **nasopharyngitis** . . . . . . .        inflammation of the nose and pharynx
    (*nā*-zō-fār-in-JĪ-tis)

14. **pansinusitis** . . . . . . . . .        inflammation of all sinuses
    (*pan*-sī-nū-SĪ-tis)

15. **pharyngitis** . . . . . . . . . .        inflammation of the pharynx
    (fār-in-JĪ-tis)

16. **pleuritis** . . . . . . . . . . . .        inflammation of the pleura (also called
    (plū-RĪ-tis)        *pleurisy*)

17. **pneumatocele** . . . . . . . .        hernia of lung (lung tissue protrudes
    (nū-MAT-ō-sēl)        through opening in chest)

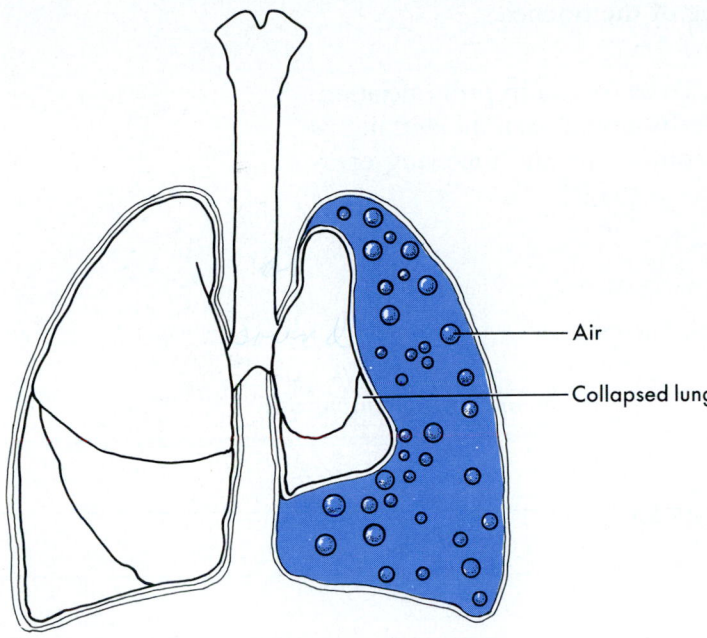

Figure 4-5
Pneumothorax.

18. **pneumonitis** . . . . . . . . . . inflammation of the lung
    (*nū*-mō-NĪ-tis)

19. **pneumoconiosis** . . . . . . . abnormal condition of dust in the lungs
    (*nū*-mō-*kō*-nē-Ō-sis)

20. **pneumothorax** . . . . . . . . air in the chest (pleural space) which
    (*nū*-mō-THŌ-raks)         causes collapse of the lung (Figure 4-5)

21. **pulmonary neoplasm** . . . new growth (tumor) in the lung
    (PUL-mō-nār-ē)
    (NĒ-ō-plazm)

22. **pyothorax** . . . . . . . . . . . pus in the chest (pleural space) (also
    (pī-ō-THŌ-raks)           called *empyema*)

23. **rhinitis** . . . . . . . . . . . . . inflammation of the (mucous mem-
    (rī-NĪ-tis)               branes) nose

24. **rhinomycosis** . . . . . . . . abnormal condition of fungus in the
    (*rī*-nō-mī-KŌ-sis)       nose

25. **rhinorrhagia** . . . . . . . . . rapid flow of blood from the nose (also
    (rī-nō-RĀ-jē-a)           called *epistaxis*)

26. **thoracalgia** . . . . . . . . . . pain in the chest
    (thō-rak-AL-jē-a)

27. **tonsillitis** . . . . . . . . . . . inflammation of the tonsils
    (*ton*-sil-Ī-tis)

28. **tracheitis** . . . . . . . . . . . inflammation of the trachea
    (trā-kē-Ī-tis)

**Pneumoconiosis** is the general name given for chronic inflammatory disease of the lung caused by excessive inhalation of mineral dust. When the disease is caused by a specific dust, it is named for the dust; for example, the disease caused by silica dust is called **silicosis**.

29. tracheostenosis........    narrowing of the trachea
    (tră-kĕ-ō-sten-Ō-sis)

Practice saying each of these terms aloud. To assist you in pronunciation, obtain the audiotape designed for use with this text. Learn the definitions and spellings of the diagnostic terms by completing the following exercises.

## EXERCISE 12

Analyze and define the following diagnostic terms.

EXAMPLE:  diaphragmat/o/cele  *hernia of the diaphragm*

(WR CV S above; CF below)

1. pleuritis _____

2. nasopharyngitis _____

3. pneumothorax _____

4. pansinusitis _____

5. atelectasis _____

6. rhinomycosis _____

7. tracheostenosis _____

8. epiglottitis _____

9. thoracalgia _____

10. pulmonary neoplasm _____

11. bronchiectasis _____

12. tonsillitis _____

13. pneumoconiosis _____

14. bronchopneumonia _____

15. pneumonitis _____

16. laryngitis _____

17. pneumatocele _____

18. pyothorax _____

19. rhinorrhagia _____

20. bronchitis _____

21. pharyngitis _____

22. tracheitis _____

23. laryngotracheobronchitis _____

24. adenoiditis _____

25. hemothorax _____

26. lobar pneumonia _____

27. rhinitis _____

28. bronchogenic carcinoma _____

## EXERCISE 13

Build diagnostic terms for the following definitions by using the word parts you have learned.

EXAMPLE: inflammation of the tonsils $\dfrac{tonsill}{WR} \Big| \dfrac{itis}{S}$

1. pain in the chest

$\dfrac{thorac}{WR} \Big| \dfrac{algia}{S}$

2. abnormal condition of fungus (infection) in the nose

$\dfrac{rhin}{WR} \Big| \dfrac{o}{CV} \Big| \dfrac{myc}{WR} \Big| \dfrac{osis}{S}$

3. hernia of the lung

$\dfrac{pneumat}{WR} \Big| \dfrac{o}{CV} \Big| \dfrac{cele}{S}$

4. new growth (tumor) in the lung

$\dfrac{pulmon}{WR} \Big| \dfrac{ary}{S}$   $\dfrac{neo}{P} \Big| \dfrac{plasm}{S(WR)}$

5. inflammation of the larynx

$\dfrac{laryng}{WR} \Big| \dfrac{itis}{S}$

6. incomplete expansion (of the lung)

$\dfrac{atel}{WR} \Big| \dfrac{ectasis}{S}$

7. inflammation of the adenoids

   <u>adenoid / itis</u>
         WR    S

8. inflammation of the larynx, trachea, and bronchi

   laryng / o / trache / o / bronch / itis
    WR  CV  WR  CV  WR  S

9. dilatation of the bronchi

   bronch / i / ectasis
     WR  CV  S

10. inflammation of the pleu-
    ra

    pleur / itis
       WR  S

11. abnormal condition of
    dust in the lung

    pneum / o / coni / osis
      WR  CV  WR  S

12. inflammation of the lung

    pneumon / itis
       WR  S

13. inflammation of all si-
    nuses

    pan / sinus / itis
      P  WR  S

14. narrowing of the trachea

    trache / o / stenosis
      WR  CV  S

15. inflammation of the nose
    and pharynx

    nas / o / pharyng / itis
      WR  CV  WR  S

16. pus in the chest (pleural
    space)

    py / o / thorax
      WR  CV  S

17. inflammation of the epi-
    glottis

    epiglott / itis
       WR  S

18. hernia of the diaphragm

diaphragmat / o / cele
WR    CV    S

19. air in the chest (pleural space)

pneum / o / thorax
WR    CV    S

20. diseased state of the bronchi and the lungs

bronch / o / pneumon / ia
WR    CV    WR    S

21. rapid flow of blood from the nose

rhin / orrhagia
WR    S

22. inflammation of the pharynx

pharyng / itis
WR    S

23. blood in the chest (pleural space)

hem / o / thorax
WR    CV    S

24. inflammation of the trachea

trache / itis
WR    S

25. inflammation of the bronchi

bronch / itis
WR    S

26. pertaining to disease state of lobe(s) of the lung(s)

lob / ar      pneumon / ia
WR    S      WR    S

27. inflammation of the (mucous membranes) nose

rhin / itis
WR    S

28. cancerous tumor originating in a bronchus

bronch / o / genic carcin / oma
WR    CV    S    WR    S

## EXERCISE 14

Spell each of the diagnostic terms. Have someone dictate the terms on pp. 95-98 to you or say the words into a tape recorder; then spell the words from your recording as often as necessary. Think about the word parts before attempting to write the word. Study any you have spelled incorrectly.

1. _____
2. _____
3. _____
4. _____
5. _____
6. _____
7. _____
8. _____
9. _____
10. _____
11. _____
12. _____
13. _____
14. _____
15. _____

16. _____
17. _____
18. _____
19. _____
20. _____
21. _____
22. _____
23. _____
24. _____
25. _____
26. _____
27. _____
28. _____
29. _____

Place a check mark (√) in the box to indicate that you have completed Objective 3.

☐ **BUILD, ANALYZE, DEFINE, PRONOUNCE, AND SPELL THE DIAGNOSTIC TERMS RELATED TO THE RESPIRATORY SYSTEM.**

# Objective 4  DEFINE, PRONOUNCE, AND SPELL OTHER DIAGNOSTIC TERMS RELATED TO THE RESPIRATORY SYSTEM.

**Adult respiratory distress syndrome** (ARDS) is respiratory failure in an adult as a result of disease(s) or injury(ies). Symptoms include dyspnea, rapid breathing, and cyanosis. In newborns the condition is referred to as **infant respiratory distress syndrome** (RDS) or **hyaline membrane disease.**

# Other Diagnostic Terms

| TERM | DEFINITION |
|------|------------|
| 1. **asthma** . . . . . . . . . . . . . (AZ-ma) | respiratory disease characterized by paroxysms of coughing, wheezing, and shortness of breath |
| 2. **chronic obstructive pulmonary disease (COPD)**. (KRON-ik) (ob-STRUK-tiv) (PUL-mō-nār-ē) (di-ZĒZ) | any persistent lung disease that obstructs the bronchial airflow, such as asthma, chronic bronchitis, and emphysema |
| 3. **coccidioidomycosis** . . . . . (kok-*sid*-ē-oyd-ō-mī-KŌ-sis) | fungal disease affecting the lungs and sometimes other organs of the body (also called *valley fever or cocci*) |
| 4. **cor pulmonale** . . . . . . . (kōr) (*pul*-mō-NAL) | serious cardiac disease associated with chronic lung disorders, such as emphysema |
| 5. **croup** . . . . . . . . . . . . . . (krūp) | condition resulting from acute obstruction of the larynx, which occurs in children |
| 6. **cystic fibrosis** . . . . . . . . (SIS-tik) (fī-BRŌ-sis) | generalized hereditary disorder of infants and children characterized by excess mucus production in the respiratory tract |
| 7. **deviated septum** . . . . . . (SEP-tum) | one part of the nasal cavity is smaller because of malformation or injury |
| 8. **emphysema** . . . . . . . . . (em-fi-SĒ-ma) | stretching of lung tissue caused by the alveoli becoming distended and losing elasticity (Figure 4-6) |

**Asthma** is derived from the Greek **astma,** meaning to **pant.**

Figure 4-6
Emphysema showing the alveoli.

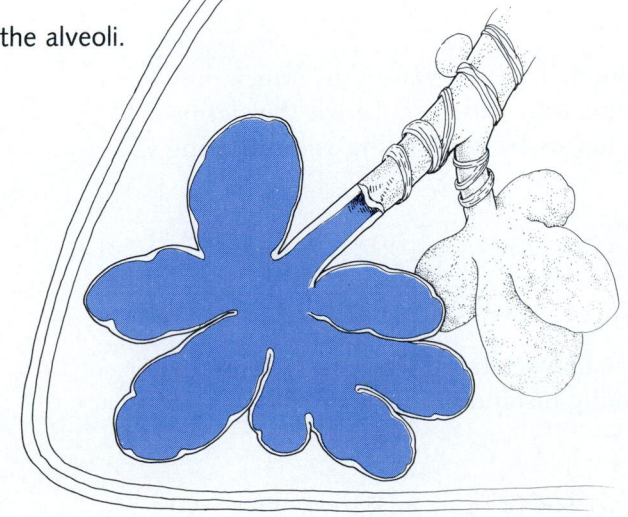

9. epistaxis . . . . . . . . . . . .    nosebleed
   (ep-i-STAK-sis)

10. influenza . . . . . . . . . . .    highly infectious respiratory disease
    (*in*-flū-EN-za)                   caused by a virus (also called *flu*)

11. Legionnaires' disease . . .   a lobar pneumonia caused by the bacte-
    (Lē-JE-narz)                   rium *Legionella pneumophila*

12. obstructive sleep apnea
    (OSA) . . . . . . . . . . . . . .   repetitive pharyngeal collapse during
    (AP-nē-a)                          sleep which leads to absence of breath-
                                       ing (Figure 4-7)

13. pertussis . . . . . . . . . . . .   respiratory disease characterized by an
    (per-TUS-sis)                      acute crowing inspiration, or whoop
                                       (also called *whooping cough*)

14. pleural effusion . . . . . . .    escape of a fluid into the pleural space
    (PLŪ-ral) (e-FŪ-zhun)             as a result of inflammation

15. Pneumocystis    carinii         a pneumonia caused by *P. carinii*, a mi-
    (*P. carinii*) pneumonia         croorganism of uncertain status. Com-
    (PCP) . . . . . . . . . . . . . .  mon disease of AIDS patients
    (nū-mō-SIS-tis) (car-Ē-nī)

16. pulmonary edema . . . . .      fluid accumulation in the alveoli and
    (PUL-mō-nār-ē) (e-DĒ-ma)       bronchioles

17. pulmonary embolism . . .      foreign matter, such as a blood clot, air,
    (PUL-mō-nār-ē)                 or fat clot carried in the circulation to
    (EM-bō-lizm)                   the pulmonary artery, where it acts as a
                                   block.

18. tuberculosis (TB) . . . . . .   an infectious disease, caused by an acid-
    (tū-ber-kū-LŌ-sis)             fast bacillus, most commonly spread by
                                   inhalation of infected droplets, and usu-
                                   ally affecting the lungs.

19. upper respiratory infec-       infection of the nose, larynx, and bron-
    tion (URI) . . . . . . . . . . .  chi
    (RE-spi-ra-tō-rē)

> Before the 1980s, **Pneumocystis carinii pneumonia** was rare. During the 1980s it became the most common opportunistic infection of AIDS patients. Now 60% to 80% of AIDS patients develop Pneumocystis carinii pneumonia.

Practice saying each of these terms aloud. To assist you in pronunciation, obtain the audio tape designed for use with this text. Learn the definitions and spellings of the diagnostic terms by completing the following exercises.

## EXERCISE 15

Fill in the blanks with the correct terms.

1. A disease characterized by lung tissue stretching that results from the alveoli losing elasticity and becoming distended is called

   _____emphysema_____.

2. _____pleural_____ _____effusion_____ is the name given to the escape of fluid into the pleural space as a result of inflammation.

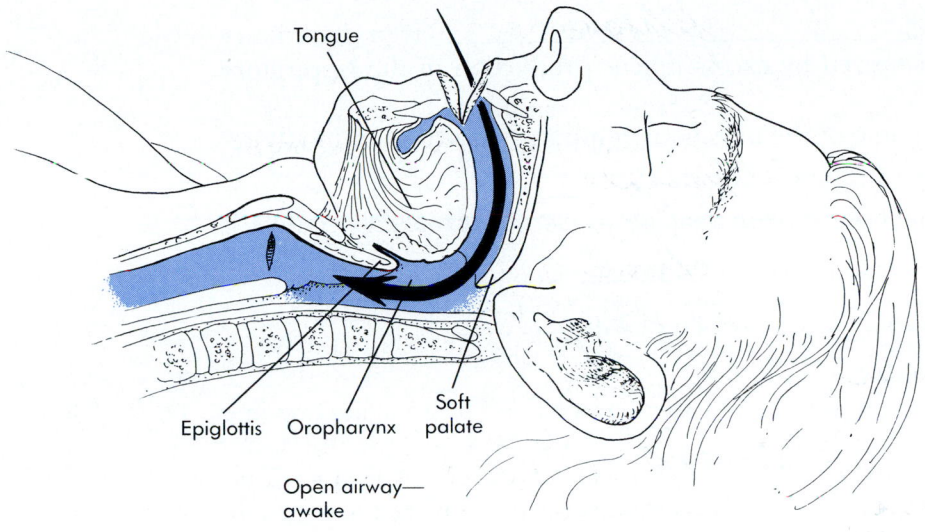

Tongue

Epiglottis    Oropharynx    Soft palate

Open airway—
awake

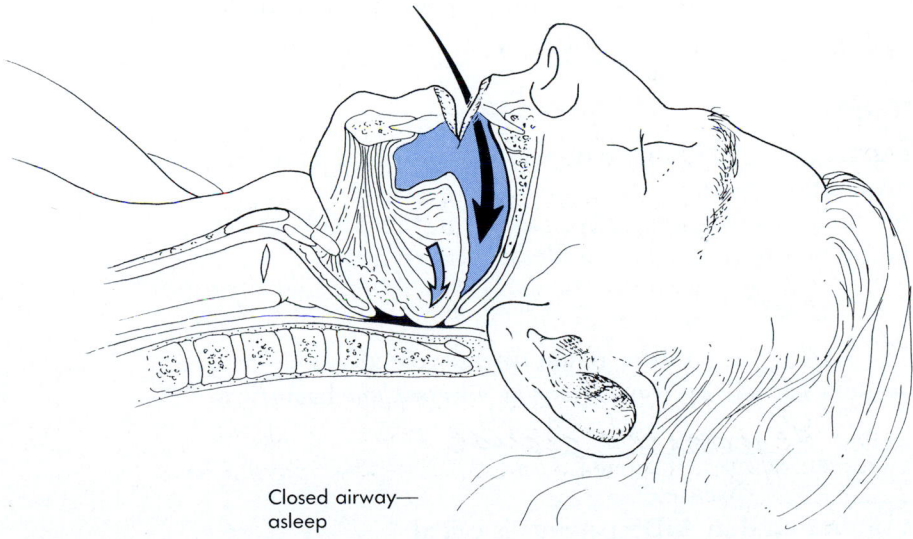

Closed airway—
asleep

## Figure 4-7

Obstructive sleep apnea. During sleep the absence of activity of the pharyngeal muscle structure allows the airway to close.

Courtesy artist May S. Cheney.

3. A cardiac condition that is associated with chronic lung disorders is called ___*cor pulmonale*___

4. A fungal disease affecting the lungs is called ___*coccidioidomycosis*___

5. ___*cystic*___ ___*fibrosis*___ is a hereditary disease characterized by excess mucus production in the respiratory tract.

6. The medical name of the infectious respiratory disease commonly referred to as *flu* is ___*influenza*___.

7. Any persistent lung disease that obstructs the bronchial air flow is known by the general term ___*chronic*___ ___*obstructive*___ ___*pulmonary*___ ___*disease*___.

8. The medical name for the disease characterized by an acute crowing inspiration is ___*pertussis*___.

9. ___*Croup*___ is a condition resulting from an acute obstruction of the larynx.

10. A chronic respiratory disease characterized by shortness of breath, wheezing, and paroxysmal coughing is called ___*asthma*___.

11. A condition in which fluid accumulates in the alveoli and bronchioles is called ___*pulmonary edema*___.

12. A(n) ___*upper*___ ___*respiratory*___ ___*infection*___ generally refers to an infection involving the nose, larynx, and trachea.

13. Foreign matter, such as a clot, air, or fat, carried in the circulation to the pulmonary artery where it acts as a block is called a(n) ___*pulmonary embolism*___.

14. ___*epistaxis*___ is another name for nosebleed.

15. A lobar pneumonia caused by the *Legionella pneumophila* bacterium commonly is called ___*Legionnaire's disease*___ disease.

16. A pneumonia often found in AIDS patients is called ___*Pneumocystis carinii pneumonia*___.

17. ___*Deviated Septum*___ is one part of the nasal cavity smaller than the other because of malformation or injury.

18. The diagnosis for repetitive pharyngeal collapse is ___*obstructive sleep apnea*___.

19. An infectious disease usually affecting the lungs is ___*tuberculosis*___.

## EXERCISE 16

Match the terms in the first column with the correct definitions in the second column.

_h_ 1. asthma

_t_ 2. chronic obstructive pulmonary disease

_o_ 3. coccidioidomycosis

_k_ 4. cor pulmonale

_n_ 5. croup

_e_ 6. cystic fibrosis

_a_ 7. emphysema

_j_ 8. epistaxis

_b_ 9. influenza

_p_ 10. Legionnaires' disease

_g_ 11. pertussis

_d_ 12. pleural effusion

_f_ 13. pulmonary edema

_i_ 14. pulmonary embolism

_l_ 15. upper respiratory infection

_q_ 16. deviated septum

_s_ 17. obstructive sleep apnea

_m_ 18. *P. carinii* pneumonia

_c_ 19. tuberculosis

a. alveoli become distended and lose elasticity

b. caused by virus (commonly called *flu*)

c. an infectious disease usually affecting the lungs

d. escape of fluid into pleural cavity

e. hereditary disorder characterized by excess mucus in the respiratory tract

f. fluid accumulation in alveoli and bronchioles

g. whooping cough

h. characterized by wheezing, paroxysmal coughing, and shortness of breath

i. foreign material, moved by circulation, that blocks pulmonary artery

j. nosebleed

k. cardiac disease associated with chronic lung disorders

l. infection of trachea, larynx, and nose

m. common in AIDS patients

n. condition resulting from obstruction of the larynx

o. also called *valley fever*

p. a lobar pneumonia caused by bacterium *Legionella pneumophila*

q. unequal size of nasal cavities

r. narrowing of the trachea

s. repetitive pharyngeal collapse

t. name given to any persistent lung disease that obstructs the bronchial air flow

## EXERCISE 17

Spell each of the other diagnostic terms. Have someone dictate the terms on pp. 103-104 to you or say the words into a tape recorder; then spell the words from your recording as often as necessary. Study any you have spelled incorrectly.

1. _____     11. _____
2. _____     12. _____
3. _____     13. _____
4. _____     14. _____
5. _____     15. _____
6. _____     16. _____
7. _____     17. _____
8. _____     18. _____
9. _____     19. _____
10. _____

Place a check mark (√) in the box to indicate that you have completed Objective 4.

☐ DEFINE, PRONOUNCE, AND SPELL OTHER DIAGNOSTIC TERMS RELATED TO THE RESPIRATORY SYSTEM.

# Objective 5    BUILD, ANALYZE, DEFINE, PRONOUNCE, AND SPELL THE SURGICAL TERMS RELATED TO THE RESPIRATORY SYSTEM.

## Surgical Terms

**TERM**
(built from word parts)                     **DEFINITION**

1. adenoidectomy . . . . . . . .    excision of the adenoids (Figure 4-8)
   (ad-e-noyd-EK-tō-mē)

2. bronchoplasty . . . . . . . .    surgical repair of a bronchus
   (BRON-kō-plas-tē)

3. laryngectomy . . . . . . . .    excision of the larynx
   (lār-in-JEK-tō-mē)

4. laryngocentesis . . . . . . . .    surgical puncture of the larynx to aspirate fluid
   (lār-in-gō-sen-TĒ-sis)

5. laryngoplasty . . . . . . . .    surgical repair of the larynx
   (lār-IN-gō-plas-tē)

6. laryngostomy . . . . . . . .    creation of an artificial opening into the larynx
   (lār-in-GOS-tō-mē)

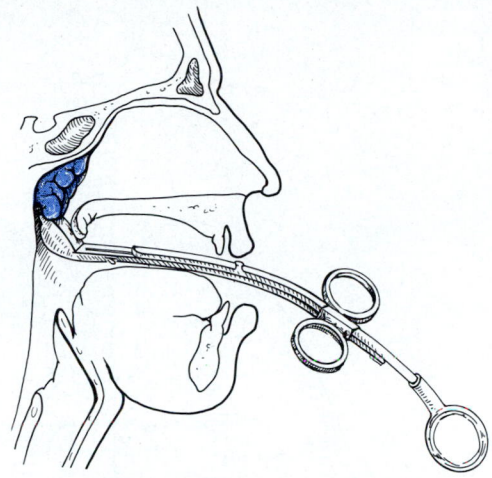

Figure 4-8

Adenoidectomy, performed with adenotome.

7. laryngotracheotomy . . . .      incision of the larynx and trachea
   (lār-in-gō-*trā*-kē-OT-ō-mē)

8. lobectomy . . . . . . . . . . .      excision of a lobe of the lung (Figure
   (lō-BEK-tō-mē)                     4-9)

9. pleurocentesis . . . . . . .      surgical puncture to aspirate fluid from
   (*plūr*-ō-sen-TĒ-sis)             pleural space

10. pleuropexy . . . . . . . . . .     surgical fixation of the pleura
    (plū-rō-PEK-sē)

11. pneumobronchotomy . . .     incision of lung and bronchus
    (*nū*-mō-bron-KOT-ō-mē)

12. pneumonectomy . . . . . . .     excision of a lung (Figure 4-9)
    (*nū*-mon-EK-tō-mē)

13. rhinoplasty . . . . . . . . . .     surgical repair of the nose (Figure 4-10)
    (RĪ-nō-plast-ē)

14. septoplasty . . . . . . . . . .     surgical repair of the (nasal) septum
    (*sep*-tō-PLAS-tē)

15. septotomy . . . . . . . . . . .     incision into the (nasal) septum
    (*sep*-TOT-ō-mē)

16. sinusotomy . . . . . . . . . .     incision of a sinus
    (sī-nū-SOT-ō-mē)

17. thoracocentesis . . . . . . .     surgical puncture of chest cavity to aspi-
    (thō-rak-ō-sen-TĒ-sis)          rate fluid (also called *thoracentesis*)

18. thoracotomy . . . . . . . . .     incision into the chest cavity
    (thō-rak-OT-ō-mē)

**Endoscopic thoracotomy,** and *thoracoscopy*, are current terms used to describe the use of an endoscope (thoracoscope) to perform a *thorocotomy*.

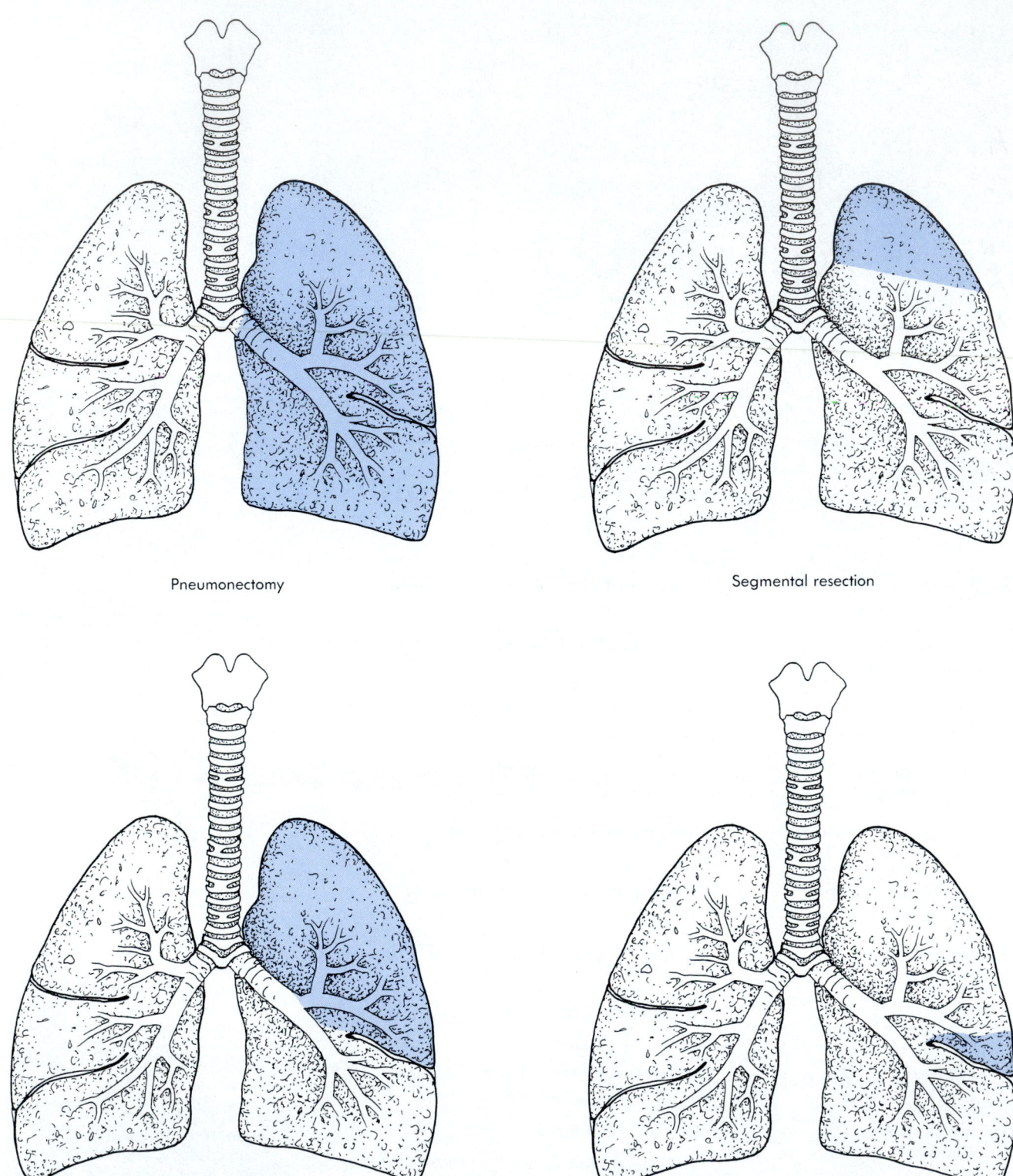

Pneumonectomy

Segmental resection

Lobectomy

Wedge resection

## Figure 4-9

Lung resection types. The diagrams illustrate the amount of lung tissue re-moved with each type of surgery.

Courtesy artist May S. Cheney.

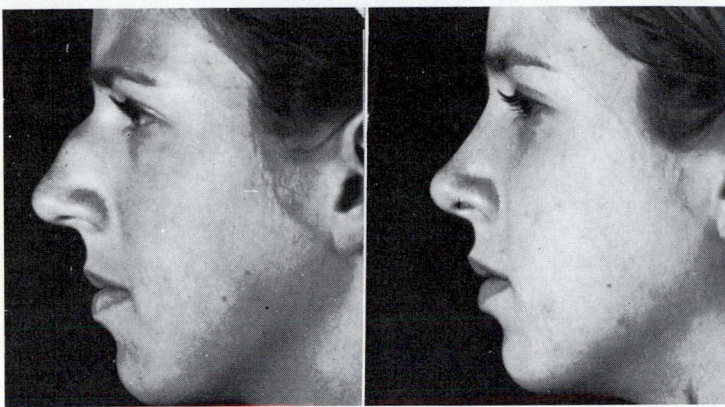

## Figure 4-10

**A,** Side view of a young woman with nasal convexity and chin retrusion. **B,** Appearance after rhinoplasty and chin augmentation.

From Saunders WH and others: *Nursing care in eye, ear, nose and throat disorders,* ed 4, St. Louis, 1979, Mosby.

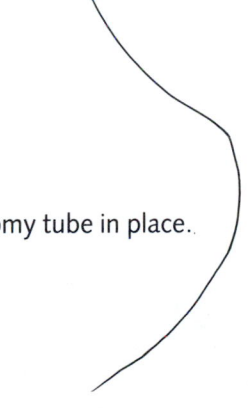
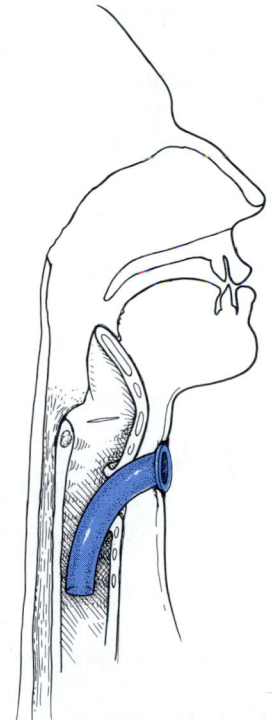

## Figure 4-11

Tracheostomy, with tracheostomy tube in place.

19.  tonsillectomy . . . . . . . .    excision of the tonsils
     (*ton*-sil-EK-tō-mē)

20.  tracheoplasty . . . . . . . .    surgical repair of the trachea
     (TRĀ-kē-ō-*plas*-tē)

21.  tracheostomy . . . . . . . .    creation of an artificial opening into the
     (*trā*-kē-OS-tō-mē)              trachea (Figure 4-11)

22.  tracheotomy . . . . . . . . .    incision of the trachea
     (*trā*-kē-OT-ō-mē)

Practice saying each of these terms aloud. To assist you in pronunciation, obtain the audiotape designed for use with this text. Learn the definitions and spellings of the surgical terms by completing the following exercises.

## EXERCISE 18

Analyze and define the following surgical terms.

EXAMPLE:   pneumon/ectomy *removal of lung*
(WR = pneumon, S = ectomy)

1. tracheotomy _____

2. laryngostomy _____

3. adenoidectomy _____

4. rhinoplasty _____

5. pleurocentesis _____

6. tracheostomy _____

7. sinusotomy _____

8. laryngoplasty _____

9. pneumobronchotomy _____

10. bronchoplasty _____

11. lobectomy _____

12. laryngotracheotomy _____

13. tracheoplasty _____

14. thoracotomy _____

15. laryngectomy _____

16. thoracocentesis _____

17. tonsillectomy _____

18. laryngocentesis _____

19. pleuropexy _____

20. septoplasty _____

21. septotomy _____

## EXERCISE 19

Build surgical terms for the following definitions by using the word parts you have learned.

EXAMPLE:   
$$\underset{\text{WR}}{pleur} \mid \underset{\text{CV}}{o} \mid \underset{\text{S}}{pexy}$$

1. surgical repair of the trachea

$$\underset{\text{WR}}{trachea} \mid \underset{\text{CV}}{o} \mid \underset{\text{S}}{plasty}$$

2. incision of larynx and trachea

$$\underset{\text{WR}}{laryng} \mid \underset{\text{CV}}{o} \mid \underset{\text{WR}}{trache} \mid \underset{\text{S}}{otomy}$$

3. surgical puncture of the pleural cavity to remove fluid

$$\underset{\text{WR}}{pleur} \mid \underset{\text{CV}}{o} \mid \underset{\text{S}}{centesis}$$

4. incision into the chest cavity

$$\underset{\text{WR}}{thorac} \mid \underset{\text{S}}{otomy}$$

5. creation of an artificial opening into the trachea

$$\underset{\text{WR}}{trache} \mid \underset{\text{S}}{ostomy}$$

6. excision of the tonsils

$$\underset{\text{WR}}{tonsill} \mid \underset{\text{S}}{ectomy}$$

7. incision of the trachea

$$\underset{\text{WR}}{trache} \mid \underset{\text{S}}{otomy}$$

8. surgical repair of a bronchus

$$\underset{\text{WR}}{bronch} \mid \underset{\text{CV}}{o} \mid \underset{\text{S}}{plasty}$$

9. excision of the larynx

$$\underset{\text{WR}}{laryng} \mid \underset{\text{S}}{ectomy}$$

10. surgical puncture of the larynx to aspirate fluid

$$\underset{\text{WR}}{laryng} \mid \underset{\text{CV}}{o} \mid \underset{\text{S}}{centesis}$$

11. surgical repair of the nose

rhin / o / plasty
WR / CV / S

12. incision of a sinus

sinus / otomy
WR / S

13. surgical puncture of a chest cavity to aspirate fluid

thorac / o / centesis    or
WR / CV / S

thora / centesis
WR / S

14. excision of the adenoids

adenoid / ectomy
WR / S

15. surgical repair of the larynx

laryng / o / plasty
WR / CV / S

16. excision of a lobe of the lung

lob / ectomy
WR / S

17. incision of lung and bronchus

pneum / o / bronch / otomy
WR / CV / WR / S

18. creation of an artificial opening into the larynx

laryng / ostomy
WR / S

19. excision of a lung

pneumon / ectomy
WR / S

20. incision into the septum

sept / otomy
WR / S

21. surgical repair of the septum

sept / o / plasty
WR / CV / S

## EXERCISE 20

Spell each of the surgical terms. Have someone dictate the terms on pp. 108-111 to you or say the words into a tape recorder; then spell the words from your recording as often as necessary. Think about the word parts before attempting to write the word. Study any you have spelled incorrectly.

1. _____    12. _____
2. _____    13. _____
3. _____    14. _____
4. _____    15. _____
5. _____    16. _____
6. _____    17. _____
7. _____    18. _____
8. _____    19. _____
9. _____    20. _____
10. _____   21. _____
11. _____   22. _____

Place a check mark (√) in the box to indicate that you have completed Objective 5.

☐ BUILD, ANALYZE, DEFINE, PRONOUNCE, AND SPELL THE SURGICAL TERMS RELATED TO THE RESPIRATORY SYSTEM.

## Objective 6  BUILD, ANALYZE, DEFINE, PRONOUNCE, AND SPELL THE DIAGNOSTIC PROCEDURAL TERMS RELATED TO THE RESPIRATORY SYSTEM.

# Diagnostic Procedural Terms

**TERM**
(built from word parts)

**DEFINITION**

1. bronchogram . . . . . . . . . x-ray film of the bronchi
   (BRON-kō-gram)

2. bronchography . . . . . . . . process of x-ray filming the bronchi
   (bron-KOG-ra-fē)

3. bronchoscope . . . . . . . . instrument used for visual examination
   (BRON-kō-skōp)       of the bronchi (Figure 4-12)

4. bronchoscopy . . . . . . . . visual examination of the bronchi (Fig-
   bron-KOS-kō-pē)      ure 4-13)

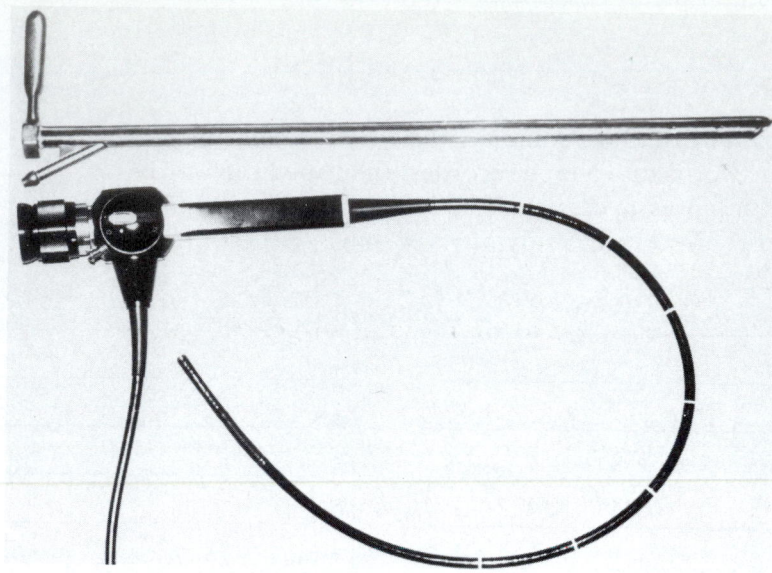

## Figure 4-12

Bronchoscopes. **Top,** rigid bronchoscope. **Bottom,** flexible fiberoptic bronchoscope.

From Saunders WH and others: *Nursing care in eye, ear, nose, and throat disorders,* ed 4, St. Louis, 1979, Mosby.

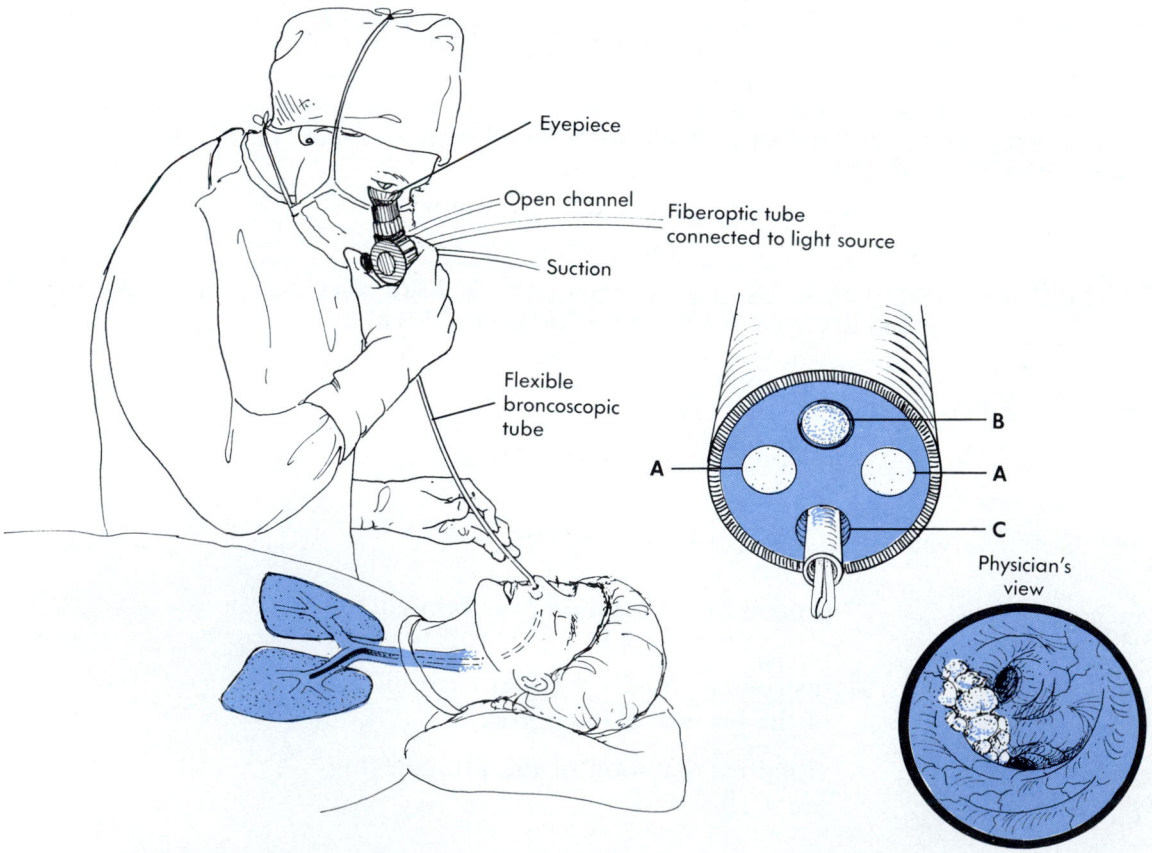

Eyepiece

Open channel

Fiberoptic tube
connected to light source

Suction

Flexible
broncoscopic
tube

A

B

A

C

Physician's
view

## Figure 4-13

Bronchoscopy. The bronchoscope is inserted through the nostril into the bronchi. The tube has four channels: **A,** light source (2); **B,** viewing channel; **C,** channel to hold biopsy forceps and other instruments.

Courtesy artist May S. Cheney.

5.  endoscope . . . . . . . . . . .    instrument used for visual examination
    (EN-dō-skōp)                       within a hollow organ or body cavity
                                       (Current trend is to use endoscopes for
                                       surgical procedures as well as for view-
                                       ing.)

6.  endoscopic . . . . . . . . . .     visual examination of a hollow organ or
    (en-dō-SKOP-ic)                    body cavity (Used to describe the current
                                       practice of performing surgeries using
                                       endoscopes.)

7.  laryngoscope . . . . . . . . .     instrument used for visual examination
    (lār-IN-gō-skōp)                   of the larynx

8.  laryngoscopy . . . . . . . . .     visual examination of the larynx
    (lār-in-GOS-kō-pē)

9.  oximeter . . . . . . . . . . . .   instrument used to measure oxygen
    (ok-SIM-e-ter)                     (saturation in the blood)
    (NOTE: The combining vowel
    is *i*.)

10. spirometer . . . . . . . . . .     instrument used to measure breathing
    (spī-ROM-e-ter)                    (or lung volumes)

11. spirometry . . . . . . . . . .     a measurement of breathing (or lung
    (spī-ROM-e-trē)                    volumes)

12. thoracoscope . . . . . . . . .     instrument used for visual examination
    (tho-RA-kō-skōp)                   of the thorax

13. thoracoscopy . . . . . . . . .     visual examination of the thorax
    (tho-ra-KOS-kō-pē)

Practice saying each of these words aloud. To assist you in pronunciation, obtain the audiotape designed for use with this text. Learn the definitions and spellings of the diagnostic procedural terms by completing the following exercises.

## EXERCISE 21

Analyze and define the following diagnostic procedural terms.

EXAMPLE:  WR  CV  S
          bronch/o/scopy   *visual examination of the bronchi*
              ‿
              CF

1. spirometer _____

2. laryngoscope _____

3. bronchogram _____

4. spirometry _____

5. oximeter _____

6. bronchography _____

7. laryngoscopy _____

8. bronchoscope _____

9. thoracoscope _____

10. endoscope _____

11. thoracoscopy _____

12. endoscopic _____

## EXERCISE 22

Build diagnostic procedural terms for the following definitions by using the word parts you have learned.

EXAMPLE:  instrument used to measure oxygen  $\underset{\text{WR} \quad \text{CV} \quad \text{S}}{\underline{ox \mid i \mid meter}}$

1. visual examination of the larynx

$\underset{\text{WR} \quad \text{CV} \quad \text{S}}{\underline{laryng \mid o \mid scopy}}$

2. instrument used to measure breathing

$\underset{\text{WR} \quad \text{CV} \quad \text{S}}{\underline{ox \mid i \mid meter}}$

3. x-ray film of the bronchi

$\underset{\text{WR} \quad \text{CV} \quad \text{S}}{\underline{bronch \mid o \mid gram}}$

4. instrument used for visual examination of the larynx

$\underset{\text{WR} \quad \text{CV} \quad \text{S}}{\underline{laryng \mid o \mid scope}}$

5. visual examination of the bronchi

$\underset{\text{WR} \quad \text{CV} \quad \text{S}}{\underline{bronch \mid o \mid scopy}}$

6. measurement of breathing

$\underset{\text{WR} \quad \text{CV} \quad \text{S}}{\underline{spir \mid o \mid metry}}$

7. instrument used for visual examination of the bronchi

$\underset{\text{WR} \quad \text{CV} \quad \text{S}}{\underline{bronch \mid o \mid scope}}$

8. process of x-ray filming the bronchi

<u>broncho / o / graphy</u>
      WR    CV    S

9. visual examination of a hollow organ or body cavity

<u>endo / scopy</u>
      P    S(WR)

10. instrument for visual examination of the thorax

<u>thorac / o / scope</u>
      WR    CV    S

11. instrument used for visual examination of a hollow organ or body cavity

<u>endo / scope</u>
      P    S(WR)

12. visual examination of the thorax

<u>thorac / o / scopy</u>
      WR    CV    S

## EXERCISE 23

Spell each of the diagnostic procedural terms. Have someone dictate the terms on pp. 115-117 to you or say the words into a tape recorder; then spell the words from your recording as often as necessary. Study any you have spelled incorrectly.

1. _____  8. _____
2. _____  9. _____
3. _____  10. _____
4. _____  11. _____
5. _____  12. _____
6. _____  13. _____
7. _____

Place a check mark (✓) in the box to indicate that you have completed Objective 6.

☐ BUILD, ANALYZE, DEFINE, PRONOUNCE, AND SPELL THE DIAGNOSTIC PROCEDURAL TERMS RELATED TO THE RESPIRATORY SYSTEM.

# Objective 7    BUILD, ANALYZE, DEFINE, PRONOUNCE, AND SPELL ADDITIONAL TERMS RELATED TO THE RESPIRATORY SYSTEM.

## Additional Terms

| TERM (built from word parts) | DEFINITION |
|---|---|
| 1. acapnia. . . . . . . . . . . . .<br>(a-CAP-nē-a) | absence (less than normal level) of carbon dioxide (in the blood) |
| 2. adenotome. . . . . . . . . .<br>(AD-e-nō-tōm)<br>(NOTE: The word root *aden* is used instead of *adenoid* because *adenoid* means *resembling a gland*) | surgical instrument used to cut the adenoids |
| 3. anoxia. . . . . . . . . . . . .<br>(a-NOK-sē-a) | absence (deficiency) of oxygen |
| 4. aphonia . . . . . . . . . . . .<br>(a-FŌ-nē-a) | absence of voice |
| 5. apnea . . . . . . . . . . . . . .<br>(ĂP-nē-a) | absence of breathing |
| 6. bronchoalveolar . . . . . . .<br>(*bron*-kō-al-VĒ-ō-lar) | pertaining to the bronchi and alveoli |
| 7. bronchospasm . . . . . . . .<br>(BRON-kō-spazm) | spasmodic contraction in the bronchi |
| 8. diaphragmatic . . . . . . . .<br>(*dī*-a-frag-MAT-ik) | pertaining to the diaphragm |
| 9. dysphonia. . . . . . . . . . .<br>(dis-FŌ-nē-a) | difficulty in speaking (voice) |
| 10. dyspnea . . . . . . . . . . . .<br>(DĬSP-nē-a) | difficult breathing |
| 11. endotracheal . . . . . . . .<br>(*en*-dō-TRĀ-kē-al) | pertaining to within the trachea |
| 12. eupnea . . . . . . . . . . . . .<br>(YŪP-nē-a) | normal breathing |
| 13. hypercapnia. . . . . . . . .<br>(*hī*-per-KĂP-nē-a) | excessive carbon dioxide (in the blood) |
| 14. hyperpnea . . . . . . . . . .<br>(hī-perp-NĒ-a) | excessive breathing |
| 15. hypocapnia. . . . . . . . . .<br>(hī-pō-KĂP-nē-a) | deficient in carbon dioxide (in the blood) |
| 16. hypopnea . . . . . . . . . . .<br>(hī-pop-NĒ-a) | deficient breathing |

The literal meaning of **anoxia** is **without oxygen** or **absence of oxygen.** The term actually denotes an oxygen deficiency in the body tissues.

17. **hypoxemia** . . . . . . . . . .    deficient oxygen in the blood
    (hī-pok-SĒ-mē-a)
    (NOTE: The *o* from *hypo* has
    been dropped. The final vowel in
    a prefix may be dropped when
    the word to which it is added be-
    gins with a vowel.)

18. **hypoxia** . . . . . . . . . . . .    deficient oxygen (to the tissues)
    (hī-POK-sē-a)
    (*See* NOTE for hypoxemia)

19. **laryngeal** . . . . . . . . . . .    pertaining to the larynx
    lār-IN-jē-al)

20. **laryngospasm** . . . . . . . .    spasmodic contraction of the larynx
    (lar-ING-gō-spazm)

21. **mucoid** . . . . . . . . . . . .    resembling mucus
    (MŪ-koyd)

22. **mucous** . . . . . . . . . . . .    pertaining to mucus
    (MŪ-kus)

23. **orthopnea** . . . . . . . . . . .    able to breathe only in a straight (up-
    (or-thop-NĒ-a)                        right) position

24. **nasopharyngeal** . . . . . . .    pertaining to the nose and pharynx
    (*nā*-zō-fa-RIN-jē-al)

25. **rhinorrhea** . . . . . . . . . .    discharge from the nose (as in a cold)
    (rī-nō-RĒ-a)

Practice saying each of these terms aloud. To assist you in pronunciation, obtain the audiotape designed for use with this text. The following exercises will assist you to learn the definitions and spellings of the additional terms related to the respiratory system.

## EXERCISE 24

Analyze and define the following additional terms.

>                            P    S(WR)
> EXAMPLE:    hyper/capnia    *excessive carbon dioxide (in the blood)*

1. laryngeal _____

2. eupnea _____

3. mucoid _____

4. apnea _____

5. hypoxia _____

6. laryngospasm _____

7. endotracheal _____

8. anoxia _____

9. dysphonia _____

10. bronchoalveolar _____

11. dyspnea _____

12. hypocapnia _____

13. bronchospasm _____

14. orthopnea _____

15. hyperpnea _____

16. acapnia _____

17. hypopnea _____

18. hypoxemia _____

19. aphonia _____

20. rhinorrhea _____

21. adenotome _____

22. mucous _____

23. nasopharyngeal _____

24. diaphragmatic _____

## EXERCISE 25

Build the additional terms for the following definitions by using the word parts you have learned.

EXAMPLE: pertaining to bronchi and alveoli  _bronch_ / _o_ / _alveol_ / _ar_
                                                                  WR / CV / WR / S

1. deficient oxgyen      _hyp_ / _oxemia_
                                              P / S(WR)

2. resembling mucus      _muc_ / _oid_
                                              WR / S

3. able to breathe only in straight (upright) position      _orth_ / _o_ / _pnea_
                                              WR / CV / S

4. pertaining to within the trachea

*endo | troche· al*
P    WR    S

5. absence of oxygen

*an oxia*
~~*a pnea*~~
P    S(WR)

6. difficult breathing

*dys | pnea*
P    S(WR)

7. pertaining to the larynx

*laryng | eal*
WR    S

8. excessive carbon dioxide

*hyper | capnia*
P    S(WR)

9. normal breathing

*eu | pnea*
P    S(WR)

10. absence of voice

*a | phonia*
P    S(WR)

11. spasmodic contraction of the larynx

*laryng | o | spasm*
WR    CV    S

12. deficient in carbon dioxide

*hypo | capnia*
P    WR

13. pertaining to the nose and pharynx

*naso | o | pharyng | eal*
WR    CV    WR    S

14. pertaining to the diaphragm

*diaphragm | atic*
WR    S

15. absence of breathing

*a | pnea*
P    S(WR)

16. deficient oxygen in the blood

*hyp | o | oxemia*
P    WR    S

17. excessive breathing _____ *hyper* | *pnea* _____
                                         P    S(WR)

18. spasmodic contraction in
    the bronchi          _____ *bronch* | *o* | *spasm* _____
                                      WR       CV     S

19. deficient breathing _____ *hypo* | *pnea* _____
                                      P      S(WR)

20. absence of carbon diox-
    ide                 _____ *a* | *capnia* _____
                                    P    S(WR)

21. difficulty in speaking
    (voice)             _____ *dys* | *phonia* _____
                                    P       S(WR)

22. discharge from the nose _____ *rhin* | *orrhea* _____
                                         WR       S

23. pertaining to mucus _____ *muc* | *ous* _____
                                     WR      S

24. instrument used to cut
    the adenoids        _____ *adeno* | *o* | *tome* _____
                                     WR       CV     S

## EXERCISE 26

Spell each of the additional terms. Have someone dictate the terms on pp. 120 and 121 to you or say the words into a tape recorder; then spell the words from your recording as often as necessary. Think about the word parts before attempting to write the word. Study any you have spelled incorrectly.

1. _____        9. _____
2. _____       10. _____
3. _____       11. _____
4. _____       12. _____
5. _____       13. _____
6. _____       14. _____
7. _____       15. _____
8. _____       16. _____

17. _____      22. _____
18. _____      23. _____
19. _____      24. _____
20. _____      25. _____
21. _____

Place a check mark (√) in the box to indicate that you have completed Objective 7.

☐ BUILD, ANALYZE, DEFINE, PRONOUNCE, AND SPELL ADDITIONAL TERMS RELATED TO THE RESPIRATORY SYSTEM.

## Objective 8 — DEFINE, PRONOUNCE, AND SPELL THE OTHER ADDITIONAL TERMS RELATED TO THE RESPIRATORY SYSTEM.

## Other Additional Terms

**TERM** / **DEFINITION**

1. airway (ĀR-wā) — *a*, mechanical device used to keep the air passageway unobstructed; *b*, passageway by which air enters and leaves the lungs

2. asphyxia (as-FIK-sē-a) — deprivation of oxygen for tissue usage; suffocation

3. aspirate (AS-per-āt) — *a*, to withdraw fluid or to suction; *b*, to draw foreign material into respiratory tract

4. bronchoconstrictor (*bron*-kō-kon-STRIK-tor) — agent causing narrowing of the bronchi

5. bronchodilator (*bron*-kō-dī-LĀ-tor) — agent causing the bronchi to widen

6. cough (kawf) — sudden, noisy expulsion of air from the lungs

7. hiccup (HIK-up) — sudden catching of breath with a spasmodic contraction of the diaphragm (also called *hiccough*)

8. hyperventilation (*hī*-per-ven-ti-LĀ-shun) — ventilation of lungs beyond normal body needs

9. hypoventilation (*hī*-pō-ven-ti-LĀ-shun) — ventilation of lungs, which does not fulfill the body's gas exchange needs

10. mucopurulent (*mū*-kō-PŪR-u-lent) — containing both mucus and pus

11. mucus (MŪ-kus) — slimy fluid secreted by the mucous membranes

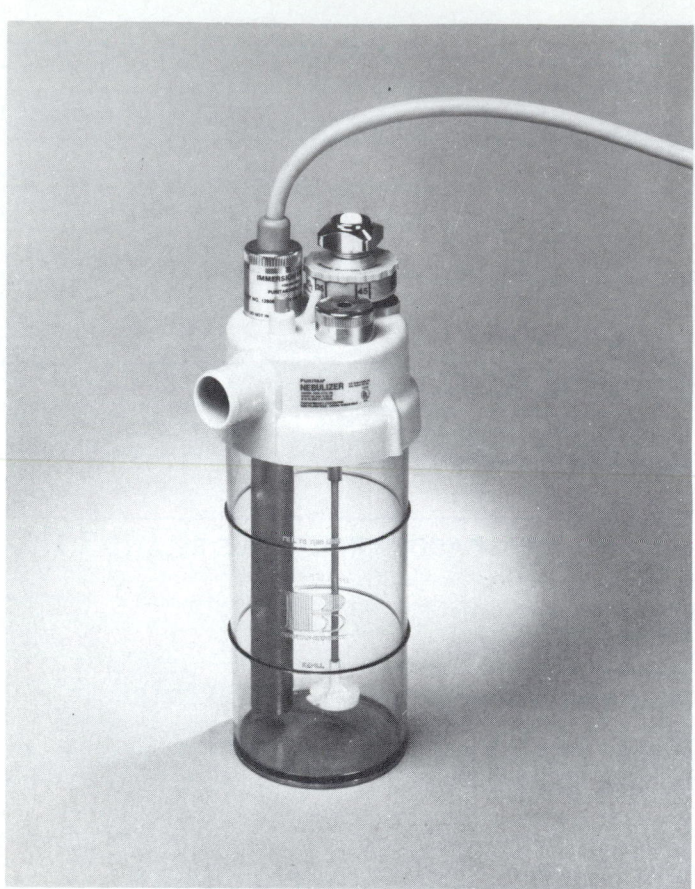

## Figure 4-14
Nebulizer.

Courtesy Puritan-Bennett Corp., Kansas
City, Mo.

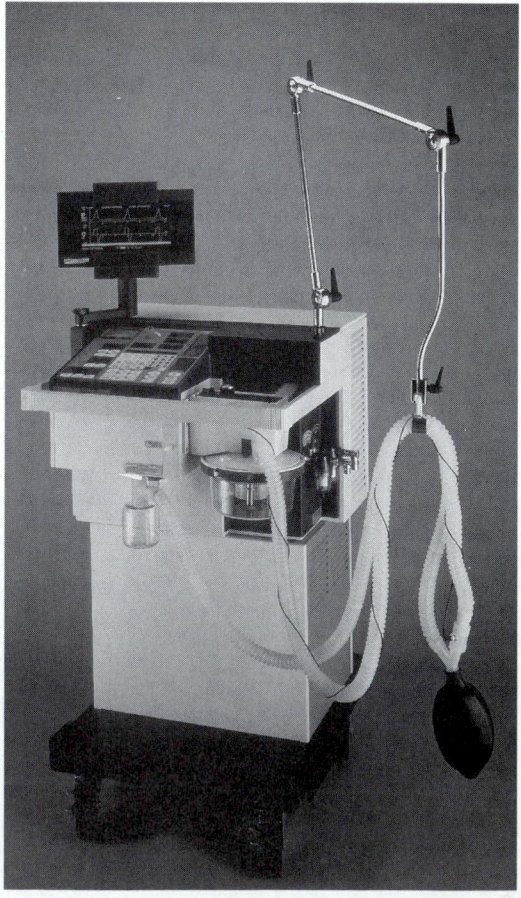

## Figure 4-15
BP7200² ventilator.

Courtesy Puritan-Bennett Corp., Kansas
City, Mo.

12. nebulizer . . . . . . . . . . .  device that creates a fine spray (used for
    (neb-ū-LĪZ-er)                   giving respiratory treatment) (Figure
                                      4-14)

13. paroxysm . . . . . . . . . . .  periodic, sudden attack
    (PĂR-ok-sizm)

14. patent . . . . . . . . . . . . .  open (an airway must be patent)
    (PĀ-tent)

15. sputum . . . . . . . . . . . . .  mucous secretion from the lungs, bron-
    (SPŪ-tum)                         chi, and trachea expelled through the
                                      mouth

16. ventilator . . . . . . . . . . .  mechanical device used to assist with or
    (VEN-ti-lā-tor)                   substitute for breathing when patient
                                      cannot breathe unassisted (Figure 4-15)

> **Sputum** is derived from the Latin **spuere**, meaning **to spit**. In a 1693 dictionary it is defined as a "secretion thicker than ordinary spittle."

Practice saying each of these terms aloud. To assist you in pronunciation, obtain the audiotape designed for use with this text. Learn the definitions and spellings of the other additional terms by completing the following exercises.

## EXERCISE 27

Fill in the blanks with the correct terms.

1. Another term for ventilation of the lungs beyond normal body needs
   is ___hyperventilation___
2. A device that creates a fine spray for respiratory treatment is a(n)
   ___nebulizer___.
3. A(n) ___bronchodilator___ is an agent that causes the air passages
   to widen.
4. A patient who has difficulty breathing may be attached to a mechanical breathing device called a(n) ___ventilator___.
5. Another term for suffocation is ___asphyxiation___.
6. Material made up of mucous secretions from the lungs, bronchi, and
   trachea is called ___sputum___.
7. To withdraw fluid or suction is to ___aspirate___.
8. A(n) ___airway___ is a mechanical device that keeps the
   air passageways unobstructed.
9. A sudden catching of breath with spasmodic contraction of the diaphragm is called a(n) ___hiccup___.
10. A sudden, noisy expulsion of air from the lung is a(n)
    ___cough___.
11. Material containing both mucus and pus is referred to as being
    ___mucopurulent___.
12. ___hypoventilation___ is the name given to ventilation of the lungs
    that does not fulfill the body's gas exchange needs.

13. The term that applies to a periodic sudden attack of coughing is
    ___*paroxysm*___ coughing.
14. An airway must be kept ___*patent*___ (open) for the patient to breathe.
15. An agent that causes bronchi to narrow is called a ___*bronchoconstrictor*___
16. ___*mucus*___ is the name given to the slimy fluid secreted by the mucous membranes.

## EXERCISE 28A

Match the terms in the first column with the correct definitions in the second column.

*b* 1. airway
*f* 2. asphyxia
*h* 3. aspirate
*c* 4. bronchoconstrictor
*i* 5. bronchodilator
*a* 6. cough
*d* 7. hiccup
*g* 8. hyperventilation

a. sudden, noisy expulsion of air from lungs

b. mechanical device used to keep the air passageway unobstructed

c. agent that narrows the bronchi

d. catching of breath with spasmodic contraction of diaphragm

e. mucus from throat and lungs

f. suffocation

g. ventilation of lungs beyond normal body needs

h. to draw foreign material into the respiratory tract

i. agent that widens bronchi

## EXERCISE 28B

Match the terms in the first column with the correct definitions in the second column.

*e* 1. hypoventilation
*h* 2. mucopurulent
*i* 3. mucus
*c* 4. nebulizer
*f* 5. paroxysm
*a* 6. patent
*b* 7. sputum
*d* 8. ventilator

a. open

b. mucous secretion from lungs, bronchi, and trachea expelled through the mouth

c. respiratory treatment device that sends a fine spray

d. mechanical breathing device

e. ventilation of lungs, which does not fulfill the body's gas exchange needs

f. periodic, sudden attack

g. agent that widens air passages

h. containing both mucus and pus

i. slimy fluid secreted by mucous membranes

## EXERCISE 29

Spell each of the other additional terms. Have someone dictate the terms on pp. 125-127 to you or say the words into a tape recorder; then spell the words from your recording as often as necessary. Study any you have spelled incorrectly.

1. _____      9. _____
2. _____      10. _____
3. _____      11. _____
4. _____      12. _____
5. _____      13. _____
6. _____      14. _____
7. _____      15. _____
8. _____      16. _____

Place a check mark (√) in the box to indicate that you have completed Objective 8.

☐ **DEFINE, PRONOUNCE, AND SPELL THE OTHER ADDITIONAL TERMS RELATED TO THE RESPIRATORY SYSTEM.**

---

**Case History:** This 55-year-old Asian male was admitted to the hospital with complaints of recent cough, dyspnea, and shortness of breath. He denies hemoptysis, chest pain, or night sweats. Complains of weight loss and chronic cough of 6 months duration. Moderate clubbing of fingers. History of smoking 2 packs/day for 40 years. Referred for pulmonary consult.

---

**Pulmonary Consultation:** Chest x-ray reveals a suspicious lesion in the left upper lobe proximal to the left bronchus, and diffuse interstitial fibrotic lesions. Indirect laryngoscopy shows edematous vocal cords with no obvious nodules; however at entry of the left bronchus a lesion is observed which partially obstructs the opening. Blood gases show alveolar hypoventilation of moderate degree and significant hypoxemia for age. Evaluating the overall situation for this man, it is my feeling this patient may have bronchogenic carcinoma. My approach to the workup would be to obtain full pulmonary function tests, including lung volumes and diffusing capacity, and to obtain a biopsy of the lesion in the bronchus. The question also arises as to his having pulmonary hypertension, but he doesn't seem to demonstrate any overt evidence of cor pulmonale at this time. I will also obtain a gallium scan to see if there is active inflammation in other locations in the lung not shown in the above workup.

## EXERCISE 30

To test your understanding of the terms introduced in this chapter, circle the words that correctly complete the sentences. The italicized words refer to the correct answer.

1. The patient in the emergency room was admitted with a *severe nosebleed,* or (rhinomycosis, rhinorrhagia, nasopharyngitis).
2. The accident caused damage to the *larynx,* necessitating *a surgical repair,* or a (laryngectomy, laryngostomy, laryngoplasty).
3. Mr. Prince was *able to breathe only in an upright position,* so the nurse recorded that he had (orthopnea, eupnea, dyspnea).
4. The pulmonary function study indicated the patient was *deficient in oxygen,* or had (dysphonia, hypoxia, hypocapnia).
5. The physician informed the patient that a heart attack was not the cause of the *chest pain,* or (thoracalgia, pneumothorax, thoracentesis).
6. The patient complained of dizziness brought on by *ventilation of the lungs beyond normal body needs,* or (hyperventilation, hypoventilation, dysphonia).
7. The physician wished the patient to have the medication given by a *device that delivers a fine spray,* so he ordered that the treatment be given by (airway, nebulizer, ventilator).
8. The patient with *blood in the chest* was diagnosed as having a (pneumothorax, pleuritis, hemothorax).
9. Following surgery the patient developed *a block in the circulation to the pulmonary artery* or (pleural effusion, pulmonary edema, pulmonary embolism).
10. The patient was diagnosed as having *a fungal disease affecting the lung,* or (obstructive sleep apnea, *P. carinii* pneumonia, coccidioidomycosis).

## EXERCISE 31

Unscramble the following mixed-up terms. The words on the left hint at the meaning in each of the following.

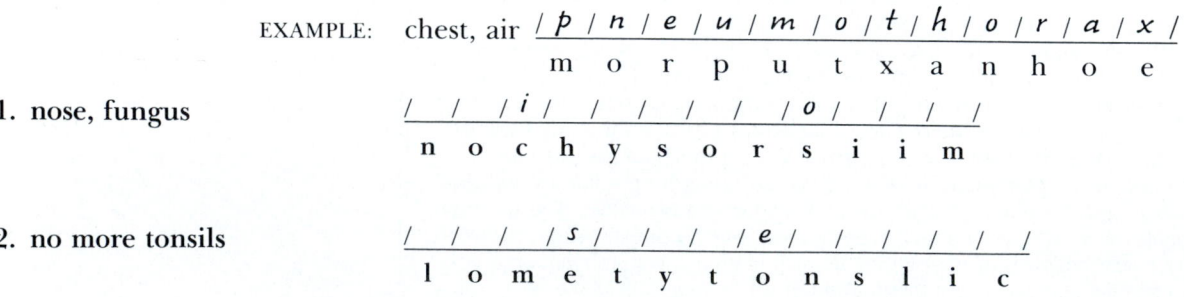

EXAMPLE:  chest, air  / p / n / e / u / m / o / t / h / o / r / a / x /
                          m  o  r  p  u  t  x  a  n  h  o  e

1. nose, fungus  / / / i / / / / / o / / / /
                  n  o  c  h  y  s  o  r  s  i  i  m

2. no more tonsils  / / / / s / / / / e / / / / /
                      l  o  m  e  t  y  t  o  n  s  l  i  c

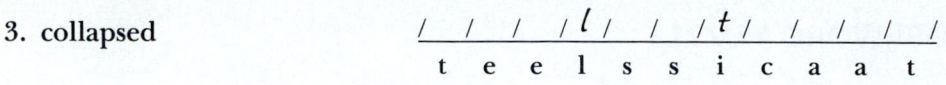

3. collapsed　　　　/ / / / l / / / t / / / / /
　　　　　　　　　　t　e　e　l　s　s　i　c　a　a　t

4. all sinuses affected　　/ / / / / n / / / i / / / /
　　　　　　　　　　　　s　t　u　s　i　i　n　a　p　s　i　n

5. to lose one of the five found
　in thorax　　　　　/ / / / / t / / / /
　　　　　　　　　　　t　o　o　m　y　b　e　c　l

6. x-ray film of part of tree　/ / / n / / / / / r / / /
　　　　　　　　　　　　　m　o　o　n　h　r　r　b　a　g　c

7. inside the windpipe　/ / / / / r / / / e / / /
　　　　　　　　　　　h　e　e　l　d　a　t　c　a　n　r　o

# EXERCISE 32

The following terms did not appear in this chapter but are composed of prefixes, word roots, and suffixes that have appeared in this or the previous chapters. Find their definitions by translating the word parts literally.

1. dermatogenic(*der*-ma-tō-JEN-ik) _____

2. erythrocytometer(e-*rith*-rō-sī-TOM-e-ter) _____

3. melanonychia (*mel*-a-nō-NIK-ē-a) _____

4. mycology (mī-KOL-ō-jē) _____

5. myomalacia (*mī*-ō-ma-LĀ-shē-a) _____

6. myonecrosis (mī-ō-nē-KRŌ-sis) _____

7. tonsillomycosis (ton-*sil*-ō-mī-KŌ-sis) _____

8. viscerosomatic (*vis*-er-ō-sō-MAT-ik) _____

# COMBINING FORMS CROSSWORD PUZZLE

## Across Clues

1. pleura
3. tonsil
5. mucus
6. sinus
7. pus
8. nose
11. pharynx
13. trachea
15. alveolus
17. straight
18. nose

## Down Clues

1. lung
2. lung, air
4. larynx
10. lobe
12. adenoids
14. breathe
16. oxygen

# Summary

Can you build, analyze, define, pronounce, and spell the following terms *built from word parts?*   yes ☐   no ☐

| DIAGNOSTIC | SURGICAL | PROCEDURAL | ADDITIONAL |
|---|---|---|---|
| adenoiditis<br>(*ad*-e-noyd-Ī-tis) | adenoidectomy<br>(*ad*-e-noyd-EK-tō-mē) | bronchogram<br>(BRON-kō-gram) | acapnia<br>(a-CAP-nē-a) |
| atelectasis<br>(at-e-LEK-ta-sis) | bronchoplasty<br>(BRON-kō-plas-tē) | bronchography<br>(bron-KOG-ra-fē) | adenotome<br>(AD-e-nō-tōm) |
| bronchiectasis<br>(*bron*-ki-EK-ta-sis) | laryngectomy<br>(lār-in-JEK-tō-mē) | bronchoscope<br>(BRON-kō-skōp) | anoxia<br>(a-NOK-sē-a) |
| bronchitis<br>(bron-KĪ-tis) | laryngocentesis<br>(lār-*in*-gō-sen-TĒ-sis) | bronchoscopy<br>(bron-KOS-kō-pē) | aphonia<br>(a-FŌ-nē-a) |
| bronchogenic<br>carcinoma<br>(bron-kō-JEN-ik)<br>(kar-si-NŌ-ma) | laryngoplasty<br>(lār-IN-gō-*plas*-tē) | endoscope<br>(EN-dō-scōpe) | apnea<br>(ĂP-nē-a) |
|  | laryngostomy<br>(lār-in-GOS-tō-mē) | endoscopic<br>(en-dō-SKOP-ic) | bronchoalveolar<br>(*bron*-kō-al-VĒ-ō-lar) |
| bronchopneumonia<br>(*bron*-kō-nū-MŌ-nē-a) | laryngotracheotomy<br>(lār-in-gō-*trā*-kē-OT-ō-mē) | laryngoscope<br>(*lār*-IN-gō-skōp) | bronchospasm<br>(BRON-kō-spazm) |
| diaphragmatocele<br>(*dī*-a-frag-MAT-ō-sēl) | lobectomy<br>(lō-BEK-tō-mē) | laryngoscopy<br>(lār-in-GOS-kō-pē) | diaphragmatic<br>(*dī*-a-frag-MAT-ik) |
| epiglottitis<br>(*ep*-i-glot-Ī-tis) | pleurocentesis<br>(*plūr*-ō-sen-TĒ-sis) | oximeter<br>(ok-SIM-e-ter) | dysphonia<br>(dis-FŌ-nē-a) |
| hemothorax<br>(hē-mo-THŌ-raks) | pleuropexy<br>(plū-rō-PEK-sē) | spirometer<br>(spī-ROM-e-ter) | dyspnea<br>(DISP-nē-a) |
| laryngitis<br>(*lar*-in-JĪ-tis) | pneumobronchotomy<br>(*nū*-mō-bron-KOT-ō-mē) | spirometry<br>(spi-ROM-e-trē) | endotracheal<br>(*en*-dō-TRĀ-kē-al) |
| laryngotracheobronchitis<br>(lār-*ing*-go-trā-kē-ō-bron-<br>KĪ-tis) | pneumonectomy<br>(*nū*-mon-EK-tō-mē) | thoracoscope<br>(tho-RA-ko-skōp) | eupnea<br>(YŪP-nē-a) |
| lobar pneumonia<br>(LŌ-bar) (nū-MŌ-nē-a) | rhinoplasty<br>(RĪ-nō-plast-ē) | thoracoscopy<br>(tho-ra-KOS-kō-pē) | hypercapnia<br>(*hī*-per-KAP-nē-a) |
| nasopharyngitis<br>(*nā*-zō-făr-in-JĪ-tis) | septoplasty<br>(*sep*-tō-PLAS-tē) |  | hyperpnea<br>(hī-perp-NĒ-a) |
| pansinusitis<br>(*pan*-sī-nū-SĪ-tis) | septotomy<br>(sep-TOT-ō-mē) |  | hypocapnia<br>(hī-pō-KAP-nē-a) |
| pharyngitis<br>(făr-in-JĪ-tis) | sinusotomy<br>(*sī*-nū-SOT-ō-mē) |  | hypopnea<br>(hī-pop-NĒ-a) |
| pleuritis<br>(plū-RĪ-tis) | thoracocentesis<br>(*thō*-rak-ō-sen-TĒ-sis) |  | hypoxemia<br>(hī-pok-SĒ-mē-a) |
| pneumatocele<br>(nū-MAT-ō-sēl) | thoracotomy<br>(*thō*-rak-OT-ō-mē) |  | hypoxia<br>(hī-POK-sē-a) |
| pneumonitis<br>(*nū*-mō-NĪ-tis) | tonsillectomy<br>(*ton*-sil-EK-tō-mē) |  | laryngeal<br>(lār-IN-jē-al) |

## DIAGNOSTIC

pneumoconiosis
(*nū*-mō-*kō*-nē-Ō-sis)

pneumothorax
(*nū*-mō-THŌ-raks)

pulmonary neoplasm
(PUL-mō-năr-ē)
(NĒ-ō-plazm)

pyothorax
(pī-ō-THŌ-raks)

rhinitis
(rī-NĪ-tis)

rhinomycosis
(*rī*-nō-mī-KŌ-sis)

rhinorrhagia
(ri-nō-RĀ-jē-a)

thoracalgia
(thō-rak-AL-jē-a)

tonsillitis
(*ton*-sil-Ī-tis)

tracheitis
(trā-kē-Ī-tis)

tracheostenosis
(*trā*-kē-ō-sten-Ō-sis)

## SURGICAL

tracheoplasty
(*TRĀ*-kē-ō-*plas*-tē)

tracheostomy
(*trā*-kē-OS-tō-mē)

tracheotomy
(*trā*-kē-OT-ō-mē)

## PROCEDURAL

## ADDITIONAL

laryngospasm
(lar-ING-gō-spazm)

mucoid
(MŪ-koyd)

mucous
(MŪ-kus)

orthopnea
(or-thop-NĒ-a)

nasopharyngeal
(*nā*-zō-fa-RIN-jē-al)

rhinorrhea
(rī-nō-RĒ-a)

# Summary

Can you define, pronounce, and spell the following terms *not built from word parts?* yes □ no □

## DIAGNOSTIC

asthma
(AZ-ma)

chronic obstructive
pulmonary disease
(KRON-ik) (ob-STRUK-tiv)
(PUL-mō-nār-ē) (di-ZĒZ)

coccidioidomycosis
(kok-*sid*-ē-oyd-ō-mī-KŌ-sis)

cor pulmonale
(kōr) (*pul*-mō-NAL)

croup
(krūp)

cystic fibrosis
(SIS-tik) (fī-BRŌ-sis)

deviated septum
(SEP-tum)

emphysema
(em-fi-SĒ-ma)

epistaxis
(ep-i-STAK-sis)

influenza
(*in*-flū-EN-za)

Legionnaires' disease
(Lē-JE-narz)

obstructive sleep apnea
(AP-nē-a)

pertussis
(per-TUS-sis)

pleural effusion
(PLŪ-ral) (e-FŪ-zhun)

Pneumocystis carinii
pneumonia
(*nū*-mō-SIS-tis) (car-Ē-ni)

pulmonary edema
(PUL-mō-nār-ē) (e-DĒ-ma)

pulmonary embolism
(PUL-mō-nār-ē)
(EM-bō-lizm)

tuberculosis
(tu-ber-ku-LŌ-sis)

upper respiratory
infection
(RE-spi-ra-tō-rē)

## ADDITIONAL

airway
(ĀR-wā)

asphyxia
(as-FIK-sē-a)

aspirate
(AS-per-āt)

bronchoconstrictor
(*bron*-kō-kon-STRIK-tor)

bronchodilator
(*bron*-kō-dī-LĀ-tor)

cough
(kawf)

hiccup
(HIK-up)

hyperventilation
(*hī*-per-ven-ti-LĀ-shun)

hypoventilation
(*hī*-pō-ven-ti-LĀ-shun)

mucopurulent
(*mū*-kō-PUR-u-lent)

mucus
(MŪ-kus)

nebulizer
(*neb*-ū-LĪZ-er)

paroxysm
(PĀR-ok-sizm)

patent
(PĀ-tent)

sputum
(SPŪ-tum)

ventilator
(VEN-ti-lā-tor)

# Answers

## Exercise 1

| | | | |
|---|---|---|---|
| 1. h | 3. g | 5. f | 7. e |
| 2. a | 4. c | 6. d | 8. b |

## Exercise 2

| | | |
|---|---|---|
| 1. septum | 4. nose | 7. tonsils |
| 2. epiglottis | 5. diaphragm | |
| 3. bronchioles | 6. mediastinum | |

## Exercise 3

**Figure 4-1**

Adenoid: adenoid/o
Pharynx: pharyng/o
Lung: pneum/o, pneumat/o,
    pneumon/o, pulmon/o
Bronchus: bronch/i,
        bronch/o
Alveolus: alveol/o
Sinus: sinus/o
Nose: nas/o, rhin/o

Tonsils: tonsill/o
Epiglottis: epiglott/o
Larynx: laryng/o
Trachea: trache/o
Pleura: pleur/o
Lobe: lob/o
Bronchiole: bronchiol/o
Diaphragm: diaphragmat/o

## Exercise 4

| | | |
|---|---|---|
| 1. larynx | 8. diaphragm | 15. nose |
| 2. bronchus | 9. trachea | 16. sinus |
| 3. pleura | 10. alveolus | 17. lobe |
| 4. air, lung | 11. air, lung | 18. epiglottis |
| 5. tonsil | 12. thorax (chest) | 19. air, lung |
| 6. bronchiole | 13. adenoid | 20. nose |
| 7. lung | 14. pharynx | 21. septum |

## Exercise 5

| | | |
|---|---|---|
| 1. a. nas/o | 5. tonsill/o | 12. thorac/o |
|    b. rhin/o | 6. trache/o | 13. alveol/o |
| 2. laryng/o | 7. adenoid/o | 14. pharyng/o |
| 3. a. pneum/o | 8. bronchiol/o | 15. a. bronch/o |
|    b. pneumat/o | 9. pleur/o |     b. bronch/i |
|    c. pneumon/o | 10. diaphragmat/o | 16. lob/o |
| 4. pulmon/o | 11. sinus/o | 17. epiglott/o |
| | | 18. sept/o |

## Exercise 6

| | |
|---|---|
| 1. oxygen | 5. straight |
| 2. breathe, breathing | 6. pus |
| 3. mucus | 7. blood |
| 4. imperfect, incomplete | |

## Exercise 7

| | | |
|---|---|---|
| 1. spir/o | 3. atel/o | 6. muc/o |
| 2. a. ox/o | 4. orth/o | 7. a. hem/o |
|    b. ox/i | 5. py/o |     b. hemat/o |

## Exercise 8

| | |
|---|---|
| 1. within | 3. all, total |
| 2. without or absence of | 4. normal, good |

## Exercise 9

| | |
|---|---|
| 1. endo- | 3. a. a- |
| 2. eu- |     b. an- |
| | 4. pan- |

## Exercise 10A

| | | | |
|---|---|---|---|
| 1. k | 4. g | 7. j | 10. h |
| 2. f | 5. c | 8. a | 11. d |
| 3. e | 6. b | 9. l | |

## Exercise 10B

| | | | |
|---|---|---|---|
| 1. c | 4. i | 7. j | 10. g |
| 2. f | 5. k | 8. b | 11. d |
| 3. a | 6. e | 9. m | 12. h |

## Exercise 11

| | |
|---|---|
| 1. chest | 12. cut into or incision |
| 2. pertaining to | 13. instrument used for visual examination |
| 3. constriction, narrowing | 14. rapid flow of blood |
| 4. hernia or protrusion | 15. stretching-out, dilatation, or expansion |
| 5. creation of artificial opening | 16. record, x-ray film |
| 6. surgical fixation or suspension | 17. breathing |
| 7. instrument used to measure | 18. process of recording |
| 8. sudden, involuntary muscle contraction | 19. measurement |
| 9. pain | 20. blood condition |
| 10. visual examination | 21. oxygen |
| 11. surgical puncture to aspirate fluid | 22. carbon dioxide |
| | 23. sound or voice |

## Exercise 12

```
        WR   S
1. pleur/itis                      inflammation of the
                                       pleura

      WR CV  WR   S
2. nas/ o /pharyng/itis            inflammation of the
   CF                                  nose and pharynx

       WR  CV   S
3. pneum/ o /thorax                air in the chest
         CF

     P   WR   S
4. pan/sinus/itis                  inflammation of all
                                       sinuses
```

WR   S
5. atel/ectasis       incomplete expansion or collapsed lung

WR CV WR  S
6. rhin/ o /myc/osis      abnormal condition
     CF                  of fungus in the nose

WR  CV  S
7. trache/ o /stenosis      narrowing of the
     CF                  trachea

WR    S
8. epiglott/itis       inflammation of the epiglottis

WR    S
9. thorac/algia       pain in the chest

WR    S  P  S(WR)
10. pulmon/ary neo/plasm       new growth (tumor) in the lung

WR  CV  S
11. bronch/ i /ectasis       dilatation of the
     CF                  bronchi

WR    S
12. tonsill/itis       inflammation of the tonsils

WR  CV WR  S
13. pneum/ o /coni/osis       abnormal condition of
     CF                  dust in the lungs

WR  CV  WR   S
14. bronch/ o /pneumon/ia       diseased state (inflammation) of bronchi and
     CF                  lungs

WR    S
15. pneumon/itis       inflammation of the lung

WR    S
16. laryng/itis       inflammation of the larynx

WR   CV S
17. pneumat/ o /cele       hernia of the lung
       CF

WR CV  S
18. py/ o /thorax       pus in the chest (pleural
     CF                  space)

WR    S
19. rhin/orrhagia       rapid flow of blood from nose (nosebleed)

WR    S
20. bronch/itis       inflammation of the bronchi

WR    S
21. pharyng/itis       inflammation of the pharynx

WR    S
22. trache/itis       inflammation of the trachea

WR  CV WR CV  WR  S
23. laryng/ o /trache/ o /bronch/itis       inflammation of the larynx, trachea, and bronchi
     CF       CF

WR    S
24. adenoid/itis       inflammation of the adenoids

WR CV  S
25. hem/ o /thorax       blood in the chest (pleural space)
     CF

WR S   WR    S
26. lob/ar pneumon/ia       diseased state of the lobe(s) of a lung

WR  S
27. rhin/itis       inflammation of the nose

WR  CV S   WR   S
28. bronch/ o /genic carcin/oma       cancerous tumor originating in a bronchus
     CF

## Exercise 13

1. thorac/algia
2. rhin/o/myc/osis
3. pneumat/o/cele
4. pulmon/ary neo/plasm
5. laryng/itis
6. atel/ectasis
7. adenoid/itis
8. laryng/o/trache/o/bronch/itis
9. bronch/i/ectasis
10. pleur/itis (or pleurisy)
11. pneum/o/coni/osis
12. pneumon/itis
13. pan/sinus/itis
14. trache/o/stenosis
15. nas/o/pharyng/itis
16. py/o/thorax
17. epiglott/itis
18. diaphragmat/o/cele
19. pneum/o/thorax
20. bronch/o/pneumon/ia
21. rhin/orrhagia
22. pharyng/itis
23. hem/o/thorax
24. trache/itis
25. bronch/itis
26. lob/ar pneumon/ia
27. rhin/itis
28. bronch/o/genic carcin/oma

## Exercise 14

Spelling exercise; *see* text, p. 102.

## Exercise 15

1. emphysema
2. pleural effusion
3. cor pulmonale
4. coccidioidomycosis
5. cystic fibrosis
6. influenza
7. chronic obstructive pulmonary disease
8. pertussis
9. croup
10. asthma
11. pulmonary edema
12. upper respiratory infection
13. pulmonary embolism
14. epistaxis
15. Legionnaires' disease
16. Pneumocystis carinii pneumonia
17. deviated septum
18. obstructive sleep apnea
19. tuberculosis

## Exercise 16

1. h    4. k    7. a    10. p    13. f    16. q
2. t    5. n    8. j    11. g    14. i    17. s
3. o    6. e    9. b    12. d    15. l    18. m
                                                    19. c

## Exercise 17

Spelling exercise; *see* text, p. 108.

## Exercise 18

      WR     S
1. trache/otomy              incision of the trachea

      WR     S
2. laryng/ostomy         creation of an artificial opening into the larynx

      WR     S
3. adenoid/ectomy       excision of the adenoids

    WR CV  S
4. rhin/ o /plasty          surgical repair of the nose
      CF

    WR CV  S
5. pleur/ o /centesis       surgical puncture of the pleural space to aspirate fluid
      CF

      WR     S
6. trache/ostomy        creation of an artificial opening into the trachea

      WR     S
7. sinus/otomy              incision of a sinus

    WR CV  S
8. laryng/ o /plasty       surgical repair of the larynx
      CF

    WR CV WR  S
9. pneum/ o /bronch/otomy   incision of lung and bronchus
      CF

     WR CV  S
10. bronch/ o /plasty       surgical repair of a bronchus
       CF

     WR     S
11. lob/ectomy            excision of a lobe of the lung

     WR CV WR  S
12. laryng/ o /trache/otomy   incision of larynx and trachea
       CF

     WR CV  S
13. trache/ o /plasty       surgical repair of the trachea
       CF

     WR     S
14. thorac/otomy        incision into the chest cavity

     WR     S
15. laryng/ectomy       excision of the larynx

     WR CV  S
16. thorac/ o /centesis     puncture of chest cavity to aspirate fluid
       CF

     WR     S
17. tonsill/ectomy       excision of the tonsils

     WR CV  S
18. laryng/ o /centesis     puncture of larynx to aspirate fluid
       CF

     WR CV  S
19. pleur/ o /pexy         surgical fixation of the pleura
       CF

     WR CV  S
20. sept/ o /plasty        surgical repair of the septum
       CF

     WR     S
21. sept/otomy           incision into the septum

## Exercise 19

1. trache/o/plasty
2. laryng/o/trache/otomy
3. pleur/o/centesis
4. thorac/otomy
5. trache/ostomy
6. tonsill/ectomy
7. trache/otomy
8. bronch/o/plasty
9. laryng/ectomy
10. laryng/o/centesis
11. rhin/o/plasty
12. sinus/otomy
13. thorac/o/centesis or thora/centesis
14. adenoid/ectomy
15. laryng/o/plasty
16. lob/ectomy
17. pneum/o/bronch/otomy
18. laryng/ostomy
19. pneumon/ectomy
20. sept/otomy
21. sept/o/plasty

## Exercise 20

Spelling exercise; *see* text, p. 115.

## Exercise 21

    WR CV  S
1. spir/ o /meter        instrument used to measure breathing
      CF

    WR CV  S
2. laryng/ o /scope      instrument used for visual examination of the larynx
      CF

    WR CV  S
3. bronch/ o /gram      x-ray film of the bronchi
      CF

    WR CV  S
4. spir/ o /metry        measurement of breathing
      CF

    WR CV  S
5. ox/ i /meter          instrument used to measure oxygen
      CF

    WR CV  S
6. bronch/ o /graphy     process of x-ray filming the bronchi
      CF

    WR CV  S
7. laryng/ o /scopy      visual examination of the larynx
      CF

    WR CV  S
8. bronch/ o /scope      instrument used for visual examination of the bronchi
      CF

    WR CV  S
9. thorac/ o /scope      instrument used for visual examination of the thorax
      CF

P    S(WR)
10. endo/scope      instrument used for visual examination of a hollow organ or body cavity

WR  CV  S
11. thorac/ o /scopy      visual examination of the thorax
    CF

P    S(WR)
12. endo/scopic      Visual examination of a hollow organ or body cavity

## Exercise 22

1. laryng/o/scopy
2. spir/o/meter
3. bronch/o/gram
4. laryng/o/scope
5. bronch/o/scopy
6. spir/o/metry
7. bronch/o/scope
8. bronch/o/graphy
9. endo/scopic
10. thorac/o/scope
11. endo/scope
12. thorac/o/scopy

## Exercise 23

Spelling exercise; *see* text, p. 119.

## Exercise 24

WR   S
1. laryng/eal      pertaining to the larynx

P  S(WR)
2. eu/pnea      normal breathing

WR  S
3. muc/oid      resembling mucus

P S(WR)
4. a/pnea      absence of breathing

P  S(WR)
5. hyp/ oxia      deficient oxygen to tissues

WR  CV   S
6. laryng/ o /spasm      spasmodic contraction of the larynx
    CF

P    WR   S
7. endo/trach/eal      pertaining to within the trachea

P  S(WR)
8. an/ oxia      absence of oxygen

P  S(WR)
9. dys/phonia      difficulty in speaking (voice)

WR   CV  WR  S
10. bronch/ o /alveol/ar      pertaining to the bronchi and alveoli
    CF

P  S(WR)
11. dys/pnea      difficult breathing

P    S(WR)
12. hypo/capnia      deficient in carbon dioxide

WR   CV   S
13. bronch/ o /spasm      spasmodic contraction in the bronchus(i)
    CF

WR  CV   S
14. orth/ o /pnea      able to breathe only in straight position
    CF

P    S(WR)
15. hyper/pnea      excessive breathing
P  S(WR)
16. a/capnia      absence of carbon dioxide

P    S(WR)
17. hypo/pnea      deficient breathing

P   WR   S
18. hyp/ ox/emia      deficient oxygen in the blood

P  S(WR)
19. a/phonia      absence of voice

WR    S
20. rhin/orrhea      discharge from the nose

WR  CV   S
21. aden/ o /tome      surgical instrument used to cut and remove the adenoids
    CF

WR   S
22. muc/ous      pertaining to mucus

WR  CV   WR   S
23. nas/ o /pharyng/eal      pertaining to the nose and pharynx
    CF

WR     S
24. diaphragmat/ic      pertaining to the diaphragm

## Exercise 25

1. hyp/oxia
2. muc/oid
3. orth/o/pnea
4. endo/trache/al
5. an/oxia
6. dys/pnea
7. laryng/eal
8. hyper/capnia
9. eu/pnea
10. a/phonia
11. laryng/o/spasm
12. hypo/capnia
13. nas/o/pharyng/eal
14. diaphragmat/ic
15. a/pnea
16. hyp/ox/emia
17. hyper/pnea
18. bronch/o/spasm
19. hypo/pnea
20. a/capnia
21. dys/phonia
22. rhin/orrhea
23. muc/ous
24. aden/o/tome

## Exercise 26

Spelling exercise; *see* text, pp. 124 and 125.

## Exercise 27

1. hyperventilation
2. nebulizer
3. bronchodilator
4. ventilator
5. asphyxia
6. sputum
7. aspirate
8. airway
9. hiccup (hiccough)
10. cough
11. mucopurulent
12. hypoventilation
13. paroxysmal
14. patent
15. bronchoconstrictor
16. mucus

## Exercise 28A

1. b   3. h   5. i   7. d
2. f   4. c   6. a   8. g

## Exercise 28B

1. e   3. i   5. f   7. b
2. h   4. c   6. a   8. d

## Exercise 29

Spelling exercise; *see* text, p. 129.

## Exercise 30

1. rhinorrhagia
2. laryngoplasty
3. orthopnea
4. hypoxia
5. thoracalgia
6. hyperventilation
7. nebulizer
8. hemothorax
9. pulmonary embolism
10. coccidioidomycosis

## Exercise 31

1. rhinomycosis
2. tonsillectomy
3. atelectasis
4. pansinusitis
5. lobectomy
6. bronchogram
7. endotracheal

## Exercise 32

1. originating in the skin
2. instrument used for measuring or counting red blood cells
3. abnormal state of black nail
4. study of fungi
5. softening of a muscle
6. death of muscle tissue
7. abnormal condition of fungus in the tonsils
8. pertaining to the body and internal organs

# Answers

# 5

# Urinary System

## Objectives

Upon completion of this chapter you will be able to:

1. Define the anatomical terms of the urinary system.

2. Write the definitions of the word parts included in this chapter.

3. Build, analyze, define, pronounce, and spell the diagnostic terms related to the urinary system.

4. Define, pronounce, and spell other diagnostic terms related to the urinary system.

5. Build, analyze, define, pronounce, and spell the surgical terms related to the urinary system.

6. Build, analyze, define, pronounce, and spell the diagnostic procedural terms related to the urinary system.

7. Build, analyze, define, pronounce, and spell additional terms related to the urinary system.

8. Define, pronounce, and spell the other additional terms related to the urinary system.

## Objective 1    DEFINE THE ANATOMICAL TERMS OF THE URINARY SYSTEM.

## Anatomical Terms

The body must have a means to eliminate waste products to sustain life. The kidneys are the main organs of excretion; the kidney, ureters, urinary bladder, and urethra comprise the urinary, or excretory, system.

### ORGANS OF THE URINARY SYSTEM (Figure 5-1)

1. kidneys . . . . . . . . . . . . . .    Two brownish bean-shaped organs located on either side of the spinal column on the posterior wall of the abdominal cavity. Their function is to remove waste products from the blood, to aid in maintaining water and acid-base balances.

   a.  nephron . . . . . . . . . .    Urine-producing unit within the kidney.

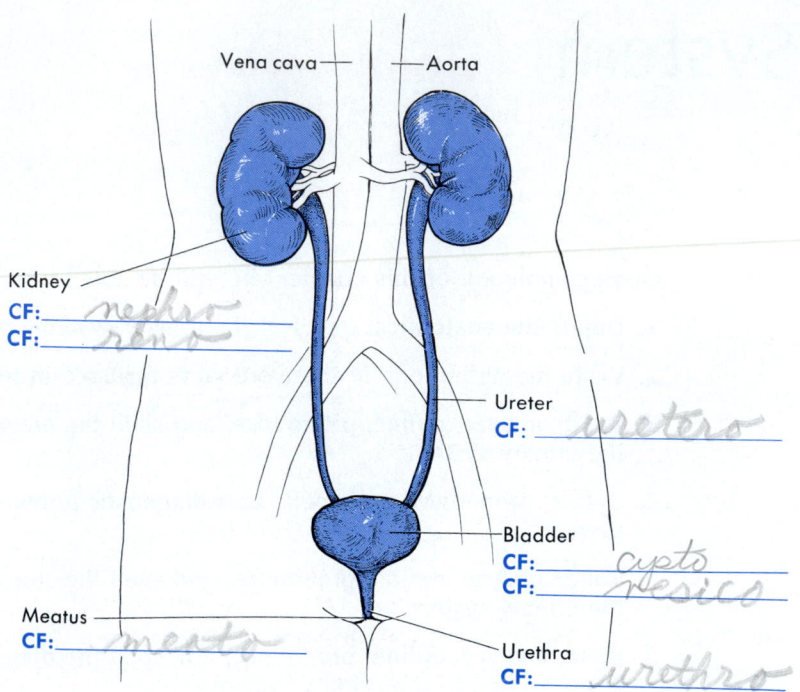

Vena cava — — Aorta

Kidney
**CF:** *nephro*
**CF:** *reno*

Ureter
**CF:** *uretero*

Bladder
**CF:** *cysto*
**CF:** *vesico*

Meatus
**CF:** *meato*

Urethra
**CF:** *urethro*

Figure 5-1
Urinary system.

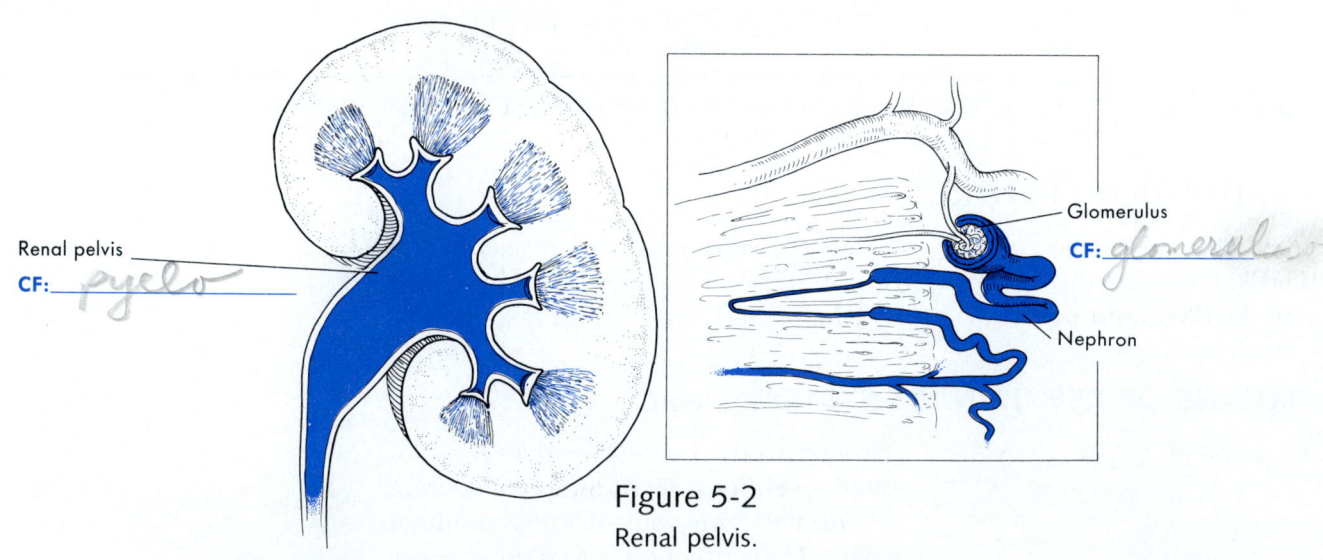

Renal pelvis
**CF:** *pyelo*

Glomerulus
**CF:** *glomerulo*

Nephron

Figure 5-2
Renal pelvis.

b.  glomerulus (*pl.* glo-
    meruli). . . . . . . . . . .       Cluster of capillaries at the entrance of
                                       the nephron. The process of filtering the
                                       blood, thereby forming urine, begins
                                       here.

c.  renal pelvis . . . . . . .         Funnel-shaped reservoir that collects the
                                       urine and passes it to the ureter (Figure
                                       5-2).

2.  ureters . . . . . . . . . . . . .  Two slender tubes, approximately 10 to
                                       13 inches (30 cm) long, that receive the
                                       urine from the kidneys and carry it to
                                       the posterior portion of the bladder.

3.  urinary bladder . . . . . . .      Muscular, hollow organ that temporarily
                                       holds the urine. As it fills, the thick,
                                       muscular wall becomes thinner, and the
                                       organ increases in size.

4.  urethra. . . . . . . . . . . . .   Lowest part of the urinary tract, through
                                       which the urine passes from the urinary
                                       bladder to the outside of the body. This
                                       narrow tube varies in length in each sex.
                                       It is 1.5 inches (3.5 cm) long in the fe-
                                       male and 8 inches (20 cm) in the male,
                                       in whom it is also part of the reproduc-
                                       tive system. It serves to carry the sperm
                                       during intercourse.

a.  urinary meatus . . . . .           Opening through which the urine passes
                                       to the outside.

5.  urine . . . . . . . . . . . . . .  Pale yellow liquid waste product made
                                       up of 95% water and 5% nitrogenous
                                       wastes and mineral salts.

> **Bladder** is a derivative of the Anglo-Saxon **blaeddre**, meaning a **blister** or **windbag**.

Learn the anatomical terms by completing the following exercise.

## EXERCISE 1

Match the terms in the first column with the anatomical terms in the second column.

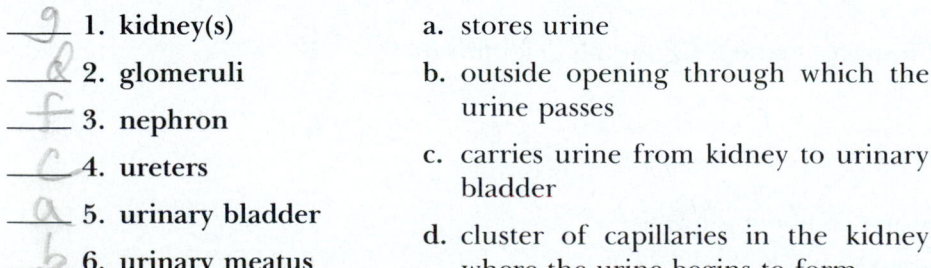

_ _9_ _ 1. **kidney(s)**          a. stores urine

_ _d_ _ 2. **glomeruli**          b. outside opening through which the
                                     urine passes
_ _f_ _ 3. **nephron**

_ _c_ _ 4. **ureters**            c. carries urine from kidney to urinary
                                     bladder
_ _a_ _ 5. **urinary bladder**

_ _b_ _ 6. **urinary meatus**     d. cluster of capillaries in the kidney
                                     where the urine begins to form

_e_ 7. urethra

    e. carries urine from the bladder to the urinary meatus

    f. kidney's urine-producing unit

    g. organs that remove waste products from the blood

Place a check mark (√) in the box to indicate that you have completed Objective 1.

☐ **DEFINE THE ANATOMICAL TERMS OF THE URINARY SYSTEM.**

# Objective 2   WRITE THE DEFINITIONS OF THE WORD PARTS INCLUDED IN THIS CHAPTER.

## Urinary System Word Parts

Study the word parts and their definitions listed as follows. Learning will be made easier by completing the exercises that follow.

| COMBINING FORM | DEFINITION |
|---|---|
| 1. cyst/o<br>   vesic/o . . . . . . . . . . . . . . .<br>   (NOTE: These refer to the urinary bladder unless otherwise identified.) | bladder, sac |
| 2. glomerul/o . . . . . . . . . . . | glomerulus |
| 3. meat/o . . . . . . . . . . . . . | meatus (opening) |
| 4. nephr/o<br>   ren/o . . . . . . . . . . . . . . . | kidney |
| 5. pyel/o . . . . . . . . . . . . . | renal pelvis |
| 6. ureter/o . . . . . . . . . . . . | ureter |
| 7. urethr/o . . . . . . . . . . . . | urethra |

> **Glomerulus** is derived from the Latin **glomus**, which means **ball of thread**. It was thought that the rounded cluster of capillary loops at the nephron's entrance resembled thread in a ball.

> **Meatus** is derived from the Latin **meare**, meaning **to pass** or **to go**. Other anatomical passages share the same name, for instance, the auditory meatus.

> **Pyelos** is the Greek word for **tub-shaped vessel**, which describes the kidney's shape.

Learn the anatomical locations and definitions of the combining forms by completing the following exercises.

### EXERCISE 2

Write the combining forms in the spaces marked **CF** on the diagrams in Figures 5-1 and 5-2, p. 142.

### EXERCISE 3

Write the definitions of the following combining forms.

1. glomerul/o _____ _glomerulus_ _____

2. vesic/o _____ _bladder, sac_ _____

3. nephr/o ___*kidney*___

4. pyel/o ___*renal pelvis*___

5. ureter/o ___*ureter*___

6. cyst/o ___*bladder sac*___

7. urethr/o ___*urethra*___

8. ren/o ___*kidney*___

9. meat/o ___*meatus (opening)*___

## EXERCISE 4

Write the combining form for each of the following.

1. kidney

   a. ___*nephr/o*___

   b. ___*ren/o*___

2. bladder, sac

   a. ___*cyst/o*___

   b. ___*vesic/o*___

3. ureter ___*ureter/o*___

4. renal pelvis ___*pyel/o*___

5. glomerulus ___*glomerul/o*___

6. urethra ___*urethr/o*___

7. meatus ___*meat/o*___

# Related Word Parts

| COMBINING FORM | DEFINITION |
|---|---|
| 1. albumin/o . . . . . . . . . . . . | albumin |
| 2. azot/o . . . . . . . . . . . . . | urea, nitrogen |
| 3. blast/o . . . . . . . . . . . . . | developing cell, germ cell |
| 4. glyc/o, glycos/o . . . . . . . . | sugar |
| 5. hydr/o . . . . . . . . . . . . . | water |
| 6. lith/o . . . . . . . . . . . . . | stone, calculus |
| 7. noct/i . . . . . . . . . . . . . (NOTE: The combining vowel is *i*.) | night |
| 8. olig/o . . . . . . . . . . . . . | scanty, few |

9. son/o . . . . . . . . . . . . . .    sound

10. tom/o . . . . . . . . . . . . .    cut, section

11. trachel/o . . . . . . . . . . . .    neck, necklike

12. urin/o, ur/o . . . . . . . . . .    urine, urinary tract

13. ven/o . . . . . . . . . . . . . .    vein

Learn the related combining forms by completing the following exercises.

## EXERCISE 5

Write the definitions of the following combining forms.

1. hydr/o _____ water _____

2. ven/o _____ vein _____

3. azot/o _____ urea, nitrogen _____

4. trachel/o _____ neck, necklike _____

5. noct/i _____ night _____

6. lith/o _____ stone, calculus _____

7. tom/o _____ cut, section _____

8. albumin/o _____ albumin _____

9. urin/o _____ urine, urinary tract _____

10. son/o _____ sound _____

11. glyc/o _____ sugar _____

12. blast/o _____ developing cell, germ cell _____

13. olig/o _____ scanty, few _____

14. ur/o _____ urine, urinary tract _____

15. glycos/o _____ sugar _____

## EXERCISE 6

Write the combining form for each of the following.

1. sugar    a. _____ glyc/o _____
            b. _____ glycos/o _____

2. neck, necklike    _____ trachel/o _____

3. sound _____ *sono*

4. urine, urinary tract    a. _____ *ur/o*

                         b. _____ *urin/o*

5. water _____ *hydr/o*

6. developing cell, germ cell _____ *blast/o*

7. cut, section _____ *tom/o*

8. albumin _____ *albumin/o*

9. night _____ *noct/i*

10. urea, nitrogen _____ *azot/o*

11. stone, calculus _____ *lith/o*

12. vein _____ *ven/o*

13. scanty _____ *olig/o*

# Prefix

| PREFIX | DEFINITION |
| --- | --- |
| 1. poly- . . . . . . . . . . . . . . . . | many, much |

Learn the prefix by completing the following exercises.

## EXERCISE 7

Write the definitions of the following prefix.

1. poly- _____ *many, much* _____

## EXERCISE 8

Write the prefix for the following.

1. many, much _____ *poly* _____

# Suffixes

| SUFFIX | DEFINITION |
| --- | --- |
| 1. -iasis, -esis . . . . . . . . . . . . . . | condition |
| 2. -lysis . . . . . . . . . . . . . . | loosening, dissolution, separating |
| 3. -megaly . . . . . . . . . . . . . . | enlargement |
| 4. -orrhaphy . . . . . . . . . . . | suturing, repairing |

5.  -ptosis . . . . . . . . . . . . . .     drooping, sagging, prolapse
6.  -tripsy . . . . . . . . . . . . .     surgical crushing
7.  -trophy . . . . . . . . . . . . .     nourishment, development
8.  -uria . . . . . . . . . . . . . .     urine, urination

Learn the suffixes by completing the following exercises.

## EXERCISE 9

Match the terms in the first column with the correct definitions in the second column.

_c_ 1. -iasis, -esis         a. nourishment, development

_i_ 2. -lysis               b. urine, urination

_d_ 3. -megaly              c. condition

_f_ 4. -orrhaphy            d. enlargement

_g_ 5. -ptosis              e. surgical crushing

_e_ 6. -tripsy              f. suturing, repairing

_a_ 7. -trophy              g. drooping, sagging, prolapse

_b_ 8. -uria                h. stretching out

                            i. loosening, dissolution, separating

## EXERCISE 10

Write the definitions of the following suffixes.

1. -orrhaphy _____ suturing, repairing

2. -lysis _____ loosening, dissolution, separating

3. -iasis, -esis _____ condition

4. -trophy _____ nourishment, development

5. -uria _____ urine, urination

6. -megaly _____ enlargement

7. -ptosis _____ drooping, sagging prolapse

8. -tripsy _____ surgical crushing

Place a check mark (√) in the box to indicate that you have completed Objective 2.

☐ **WRITE THE DEFINITIONS OF THE WORD PARTS INCLUDED IN THIS CHAPTER.**

## Medical Terms

The terms you need to learn to complete this chapter are listed as follows. Now that you know the meaning of the word parts, the exercises found at the end of this list will assist you to learn the definition and the spelling of each word.

## Objective 3    BUILD, ANALYZE, DEFINE, PRONOUNCE, AND SPELL THE DIAGNOSTIC TERMS RELATED TO THE URINARY SYSTEM.

## Diagnostic Terms

| TERM (built from word parts) | DEFINITION |
|---|---|
| 1. cystitis.............<br>(sis-TĪ-tis) | inflammation of the bladder |
| 2. cystocele...........<br>(SIS-tō-sēl) | protrusion of the bladder |
| 3. cystolith...........<br>(SIS-tō-lith) | stone in the bladder (Figure 5-3) |
| 4. glomerulonephritis ....<br>(glo-*mer*-ū-lō-ne-FRĪ-tis) | inflammation of the glomeruli of the kidney |
| 5. hydronephrosis .......<br>(hī-drō-ne-FRŌ-sis) | abnormal condition of water in the kidney (distention of the kidney pelvis with urine because of an obstruction) |
| 6. nephritis............<br>(ne-FRĪ-tis) | inflammation of a kidney |

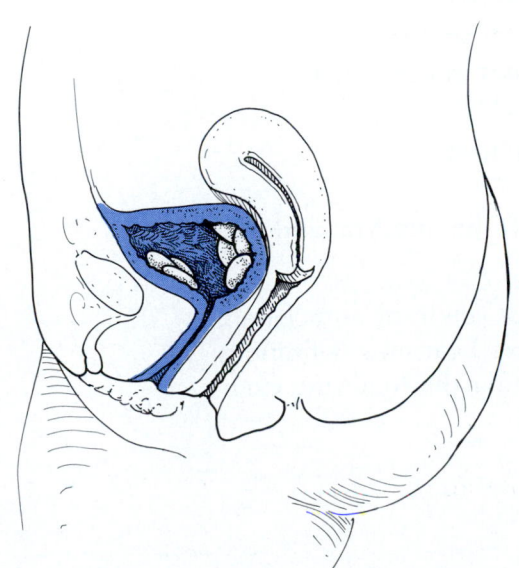

Figure 5-3
Cystolith.

7. **nephroblastoma** . . . . . . .
(nef-rō-blas-TŌ-ma)
kidney tumor containing developing cell (embryonic) tissue. Also known as *Wilms' tumor*.

8. **nephrohypertrophy** . . . .
(*nef*-rō-hī-PER-trō-fē)
(NOTE: The prefix *hyper-* appears in the middle of this term.)
excessive development of the kidney

9. **nephrolithiasis** . . . . . . .
(nef-rō-lith-Ī-a-sis)
condition of stone(s) in the kidney

10. **nephroma**. . . . . . . . . . .
(nef-RŌ-ma)
tumor of the kidney

11. **nephromegaly** . . . . . . . .
(*nef*-rō-MEG-a-lē)
enlargement of a kidney

12. **nephroptosis**. . . . . . . . .
(*nef*-rop-TŌ-sis)
drooping kidney

13. **pyelitis** . . . . . . . . . . . .
(*pī*-e-LĪ-tis)
inflammation of the renal pelvis

14. **pyelonephritis** . . . . . . .
(*pī*-e-lō-ne-FRĪ-tis)
inflammation of the renal pelvis and the kidney

15. **trachelocystitis** . . . . . . .
(*trā*-kel-ō-sis-TĪ-tis)
inflammation of the neck of the bladder

16. **uremia** . . . . . . . . . . . .
(ū-RĒ-mē-a)
condition of urine in the blood (toxic condition resulting from the retention of by-products of the kidney in the blood)

17. **ureteritis**. . . . . . . . . . . .
(ū-rē-ter-Ī-tis)
inflammation of a ureter

18. **ureterocele** . . . . . . . . . .
(ū-RĒ-ter-ō-sēl)
protrusion of a ureter

19. **ureterolithiasis** . . . . . . .
(ū-rē-ter-ō-lith-Ī-a-sis)
condition of stones in the ureters

20. **ureterostenosis** . . . . . . .
(ū-rē-ter-ō-sten-Ō-sis)
narrowing of the ureter

21. **urethrocystitis** . . . . . . .
(ū-*rē*-thrō-sis-TĪ-tis)
inflammation of the urethra and the bladder

Practice saying each of these terms aloud. To assist you in pronunciation, obtain the audiotape designed for use with this text. Learn the definitions and spellings of the diagnostic terms by completing the following exercises.

## EXERCISE 11

Analyze and define the following diagnostic terms.

EXAMPLE:    glomerul/o/nephr/itis  *inflammation of the glomeruli of the kidney*

1. nephroma _____

2. cystolith _____

3. nephrolithiasis _____

4. uremia _____

5. nephroptosis _____

6. cystocele _____

7. nephrohypertrophy _____

8. trachelocystitis _____

9. cystitis _____

10. pyelitis _____

11. ureterocele _____

12. hydronephrosis _____

13. nephromegaly _____

14. ureterolithiasis _____

15. pyelonephritis _____

16. ureteritis _____

17. nephritis _____

18. urethrocystitis _____

19. ureterostenosis _____

20. nephroblastoma _____

## EXERCISE 12

Build diagnostic terms for the following definitions by using the word parts you have learned.

EXAMPLE:    inflammation of the ureter    $\dfrac{ureter}{WR} \Big| \dfrac{itis}{S}$

1. enlargement of the kidney

   $\dfrac{nephr}{WR} \Big| \dfrac{o}{CV} \Big| \dfrac{megaly}{S}$

2. inflammation of the bladder

   $\dfrac{cyst}{WR} \Big| \dfrac{itis}{S}$

3. overdevelopment of the
   kidney

   $\dfrac{nephr}{WR} \Big| \dfrac{o}{CV} \Big| \dfrac{hyper}{P} \Big| \dfrac{trophy}{S}$

4. inflammation of the urethra and bladder

   $\dfrac{urethr}{WR} \Big| \dfrac{o}{CV} \Big| \dfrac{cyst}{WR} \Big| \dfrac{itis}{S}$

5. protrusion of the bladder

   $\dfrac{cyst}{WR} \Big| \dfrac{o}{CV} \Big| \dfrac{cele}{S}$

6. inflammation of the neck
   of the bladder

   $\dfrac{trachel}{WR} \Big| \dfrac{o}{CV} \Big| \dfrac{cyst}{WR} \Big| \dfrac{itis}{S}$

7. abnormal condition of
   water in the kidney

   $\dfrac{hydr}{WR} \Big| \dfrac{o}{CV} \Big| \dfrac{nephr}{WR} \Big| \dfrac{osis}{S}$

8. stone in the bladder

   $\dfrac{cyst}{WR} \Big| \dfrac{o}{CV} \Big| \dfrac{lith}{WR}$

9. inflammation of the glomeruli of the kidney

   $\dfrac{glomerul}{WR} \Big| \dfrac{o}{CV} \Big| \dfrac{nephr}{WR} \Big| \dfrac{itis}{S}$

10. tumor of the kidney

    $\dfrac{nephr}{WR} \Big| \dfrac{oma}{S}$

11. abnormal condition of a
drooping kidney

*nephr / o / ptosis*
WR      CV      S

12. inflammation of a kidney

*nephr / itis*
WR      S

13. condition of stones in the
kidney

*nephr / o / lith / iasis*
WR      CV      WR      S

14. protrusion of a ureter

*ureter / o / cele*
WR      CV      S

15. inflammation of the renal pelvis

*pyel / itis*
WR      S

16. condition of urine in the
blood

*ur / emia*
WR      S

17. narowing of the ureter

*ureter / o / stenosis*
WR      CV      S

18. inflammation of the renal pelvis and the kidney

*pyel / o / nephr / itis*
WR      CV      WR      S

19. condition of stones in the
ureters

*ureter / o / lith / iasis*
WR      CV      WR      S

20. kidney tumor containing
developing cell tissue

*nephr / o / blast / oma*
WR      CV      WR      S

## EXERCISE 13

Spell each of the diagnostic terms. Have someone dictate the terms on
pp. 149 and 150 to you or say the words into a tape recorder; then spell
the words from your recording as often as necessary. Think about the

word parts before attempting to write the word. Study any you have
spelled incorrectly.

1. _____     12. _____
2. _____     13. _____
3. _____     14. _____
4. _____     15. _____
5. _____     16. _____
6. _____     17. _____
7. _____     18. _____
8. _____     19. _____
9. _____     20. _____
10. _____     21. _____
11. _____

Place a check mark (√) in the box to indicate that you have completed Objective 3.

☐ BUILD, ANALYZE, DEFINE, PRONOUNCE, AND SPELL THE DIAGNOSTIC TERMS RELATED TO THE URINARY SYSTEM.

# Objective 4    DEFINE, PRONOUNCE, AND SPELL OTHER DIAGNOSTIC TERMS RELATED TO THE URINARY SYSTEM.

## Other Diagnostic Terms

| TERM | DEFINITION |
|---|---|
| 1. epispadias<br>(*ep*-i-SPĀ-dē-as) | congenital defect in which the urinary meatus is located on the upper surface of the penis; a similar defect can occur in the female. |
| 2. hypospadias<br>(*hī*-pō-SPĀ-dē-as) | congenital defect in which the urinary meatus is located on the underside of the penis; a similar defect can occur in the female (Figure 5-4) |
| 3. polycystic kidney<br>(*pol*-i-SIS-tik) (KID-nē) | condition in which the kidney contains many cysts and is enlarged (Figure 5-5) |
| 4. renal calculi<br>(RĒ-nal) (KAL-kū-lī) | stones in the kidney |
| 5. renal hypertension<br>(RĒ-nal) (hī-per-TEN-shun) | elevated blood pressure resulting from kidney disease |
| 6. urinary retention<br>(Ū-rin-*ā*-rē) (rē-TEN-shun) | abnormal accumulation of urine in the bladder because of an inability to urinate |

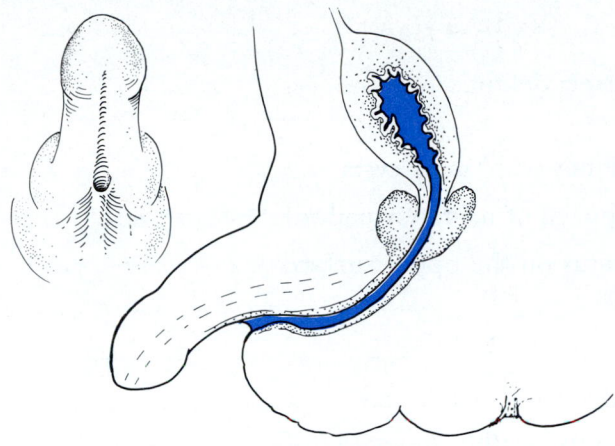

**Figure 5-4**
Hypospadias.

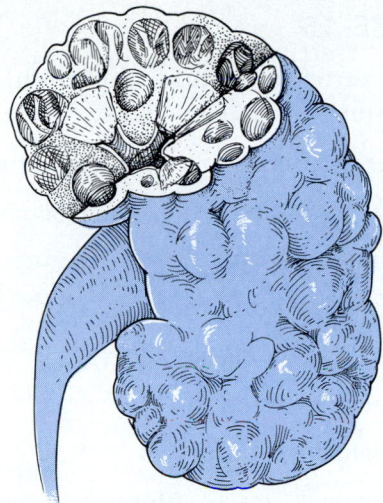

**Figure 5-5**
Polycystic kidney.

7. **urinary suppression** . . . . .     sudden stoppage of urine formation
   (Ū-rin-*ā*-rē) (sū-PRESH-un)

8. **urinary tract infection** . . .     infection of one or more organs of the
   (UTI)                                  urinary tract

Practice saying each of these terms aloud. To assist you in pronunciation, obtain the audiotape designed for use with this text. Learn the definitions and spellings of the other diagnostic terms by completing the following exercises.

## EXERCISE 14

Fill in the blanks with the correct terms.

1. Stones in the kidney are also called ____renal____ ____calculi____.

2. The inability to urinate, which results in an abnormal amount of urine in the bladder, is known as ____urinary____ ____retention____.

3. The name given to a kidney that is enlarged and contains may cysts is ____polycyptic kidney____

4. The condition in which the urinary meatus is located on the underside of the penis is called ____hypospadias____.

5. Elevated blood pressure resulting from kidney disease is ____renal____ ____hypertension____.

6. Sudden stoppage of urine formation is referred to as ____urinary____ ____suppression____.

7. ____epispadias____ is a condition in which the urinary meatus is located on the upper surface of the penis.

8. Infection of one or more urinary system organs is called ____urinary____ ____tract infection____.

## EXERCISE 15

Match the terms in the first column with the correct definitions in the second column.

_c_ 1. epispadias
_f_ 2. hypospadias
_d_ 3. renal calculi
_h_ 4. renal hypertension
_a_ 5. polycystic kidney
_e_ 6. urinary retention
_b_ 7. urinary suppression
_g_ 8. urinary tract infection

a. enlarged kidney with many cysts
b. sudden stoppage of urine formation
c. urinary meatus on the upper surface of the penis
d. kidney stones
e. inability to urinate
f. urinary meatus on the underside of the penis
g. infection of one or more organs of the urinary system
h. characterized by elevated blood pressure
i. excessive amount of urine

## EXERCISE 16

Spell each of the other diagnostic terms. Have someone dictate the terms on pp. 154 and 155 to you or say the words into a tape recorder; then spell the words from your recording as often as necessary. Think about the word parts before attempting to write the word. Study any you have spelled incorrectly.

1. _____    5. _____
2. _____    6. _____
3. _____    7. _____
4. _____    8. _____

Place a check mark (√) in the box to indicate that you have completed Objective 4.

☐ DEFINE, PRONOUNCE, AND SPELL OTHER DIAGNOSTIC TERMS RELATED TO THE URINARY SYSTEM.

# Objective 5

**BUILD, ANALYZE, DEFINE, PRONOUNCE, AND SPELL THE SURGICAL TERMS RELATED TO THE URINARY SYSTEM.**

## Surgical Terms

| **TERM** (built from word parts) | **DEFINITION** |
|---|---|
| 1. **cystectomy** . . . . . . . . . . (sis-TEK-tō-mē) | excision of the bladder |
| 2. **cystolithotomy** . . . . . . . (*sis*-tō-li-THOT-ō-mē) | incision of the bladder to remove a stone |
| 3. **cystoplasty** . . . . . . . . . . (SIS-tō-plas-tē) | plastic repair of the bladder |
| 4. **cystorrhaphy** . . . . . . . . (sist-ŌR-a-fē) | suturing the bladder |
| 5. **cystostomy** . . . . . . . . . . (sis-TOS-tō-mē) | creation of an artificial opening into the bladder (Figure 5-6) |
| 6. **cystotomy** (sis-TOT-ō-mē) or **vesicotomy** . . . . . . . . (*ves*-i-KOT-ō-mē) | incision of bladder |
| 7. **cystotrachelotomy** . . . . . (*sis*-tō-*trā*-ke-LOT-ō-mē) | incision of the neck of the bladder |
| 8. **lithotripsy** . . . . . . . . . . . (LITH-ō-trip-sē) | surgical crushing of a stone (Figure 5-7) |
| 9. **meatotomy** . . . . . . . . . . (*mē*-a-TOT-ō-mē) | incision of the meatus |

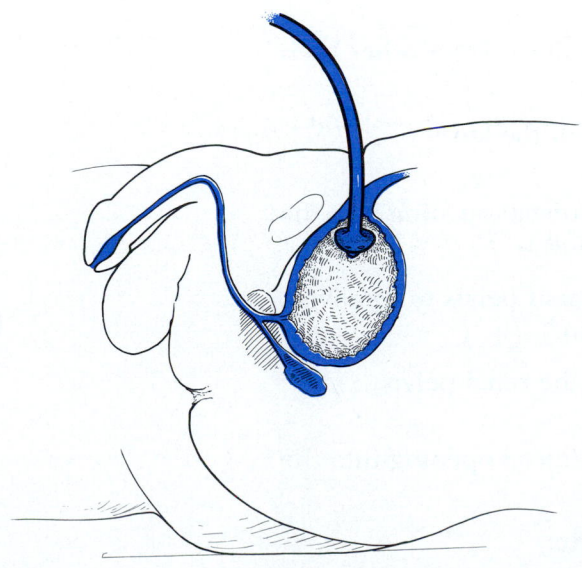

**Figure 5-6**
Cystostomy.

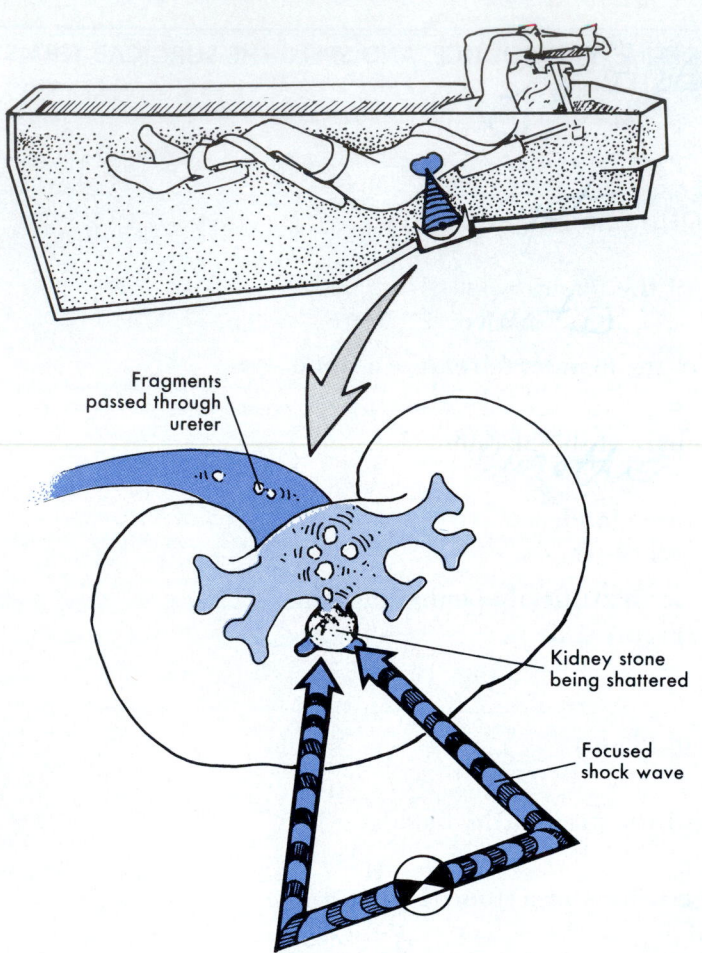

Figure 5-7

Extracorporeal shock-wave lithotripsy (ESWL). ESWL may be carried out by entering the body or by noninvasive procedures. ESWL breaks down the kidney stones into tiny pieces from outside the body. The broken pieces of the kidney stone are then eliminated from the kidney through the urine. Another lithotripsy procedure is percutaneous ultrasonic lithotripsy (PUL—not shown). An ultrasonic probe, which generates high frequency sound waves, is used to shatter the calculi. PUL is useful for treatment of radiolucent calculi lodged in the kidney that cannot be treated by ESWL.

Fragments passed through ureter

Kidney stone being shattered

Focused shock wave

10. nephrectomy . . . . . . . .     excision of a kidney
    (ne-FREK-tō-mē)

11. nephrolysis . . . . . . . . . .     separating the kidney (from other body
    (ne-FROL-i-sis)     structures)

12. nephropexy . . . . . . . . .     surgical fixation of the kidney
    (NEF-rō-*peks*-ē)

13. nephrostomy . . . . . . . .     creation of an artificial opening into the
    (nef-ROS-tō-mē)     kidney (Figure 5-8)

14. pyelolithotomy . . . . . . . .     incision of the renal pelvis to remove a
    (pī-el-ō-lith-OT-ō-mē)     stone (Figure 5-9)

15. pyeloplasty . . . . . . . . . .     plastic repair of the renal pelvis
    (PĪ-el-ō-*plas*-tē)

16. pyelostomy . . . . . . . . . .     creation of an artificial opening into the
    (*pī*-el-OS-tō-mē)     renal pelvis

17. ureterectomy . . . . . . . .     excision of a ureter
    (ū-*rē*-ter-EK-tō-mē)

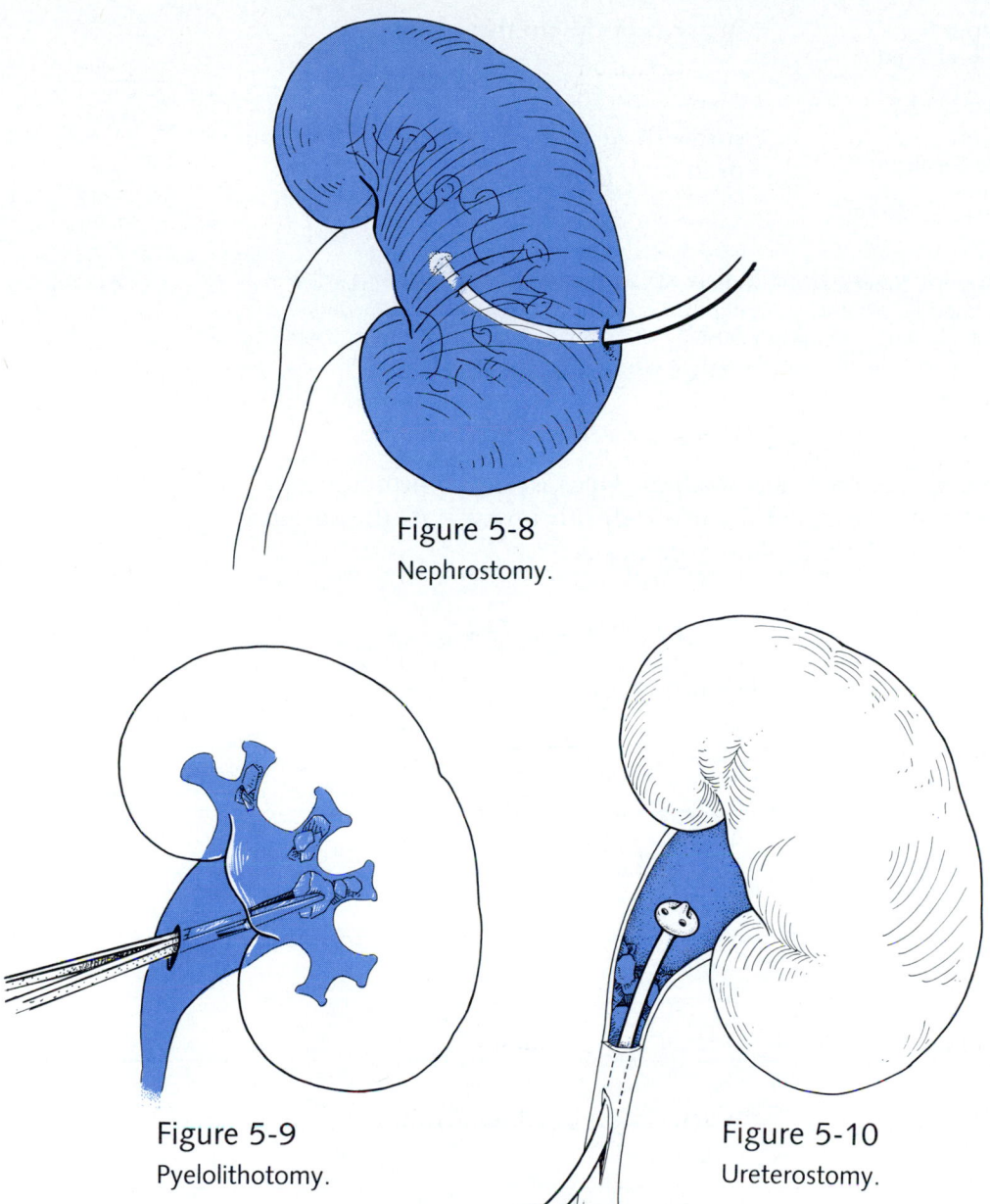

Figure 5-8
Nephrostomy.

Figure 5-9
Pyelolithotomy.

Figure 5-10
Ureterostomy.

18. **ureterostomy** . . . . . . . .    creation of an artificial opening into the
    (ū-rē-ter-OS-tō-mē)              ureter (Figure 5-10)

19. **ureterotomy** . . . . . . . . .    incision of a ureter
    (ū-rē-ter-ŌT-ō-mē)

20. **urethropexy** . . . . . . . . .    surgical fixation of the urethra
    (ū-RĒ-thrō-pek-sē)

21. **urethroplasty** . . . . . . . .    plastic repair of the urethra
    (ū-RĒ-thrō-*plas*-tē)

22. **urethrostomy** . . . . . . . .    creation of an artificial opening into the
    (ū-rē-THROS-tō-mē)              urethra

23. urethrotomy . . . . . . . . .      incision in the urethra
    (ū-rē-THROT-ō-mē)

24. vesicourethral
    suspension . . . . . . . . . .      surgical suspension pertaining to the
    (ves-i-kō-ū-RĒ-thral)              urethra and bladder

> **Marshall-Marchette Krantz,** or vesicourethral suspension, is a bladder suspension surgery performed on patients suffering from stress incontinence. Stress incontinence is the involuntary intermittent leakage of urine as a result of pressure, from a cough or a sneeze, on the weakened area around the urethra and bladder.

Practice saying each of these terms aloud. To assist you in pronunciation, obtain the audiotape designed for use with this text. Learn the surgical terms by completing the following exercises.

## EXERCISE 17

Analyze and define the following surgical terms.

1. vesicotomy _____

2. nephrostomy _____

3. nephrolysis _____

4. cystectomy _____

5. ureterotomy _____

6. pyelolithotomy _____

7. cystotrachelotomy _____

8. nephropexy _____

9. ureterostomy _____

10. cystolithotomy _____

11. nephrectomy _____

12. pyelostomy _____

13. urethropexy _____

14. ureterectomy _____

15. cystostomy _____

16. pyeloplasty _____

17. cystorrhaphy _____

18. urethrostomy _____

19. cystoplasty _____

20. meatotomy _____

21. lithotripsy _____

22. cystotomy _____

23. urethroplasty _____

24. vesicourethral suspension _____

## EXERCISE 18

Build surgical terms for the following definitions by using the word parts you have learned.

1. incision of the urethra

   _urethr_ / _otomy_
   WR       S

2. excision of a kidney

   _nephr_ / _ectomy_
   WR       S

3. incision of the renal pelvis to remove a stone

   _pyel_ / _o_ / _lith_ / _otomy_
   WR  CV  WR  S

4. surgical fixation of the urethra

   _urethr_ / _o_ / _pexy_
   WR  CV  S

5. suturing of the bladder

   _cyst_ / _orrhaphy_
   WR       S

6. separating the kidney (from other structures)

   _nephr_ / _o_ / _lysis_
   WR  CV  S

7. creation of an artificial opening into the kidney

   _nephr_ / _ostomy_
   WR       S

8. incision of a ureter

   _ureter_ / _otomy_
   WR       S

9. plastic repair of the urethra

_urethr_ / _o_ / _plasty_
WR    CV    S

10. excision of the bladder

_cyst_ / _ectomy_
WR    S

11. incision of the meatus

_meat_ / _otomy_
WR    S

12. creation of an artificial opening into the urethra

_urethr_ / _ostomy_
WR    S

13. incision of the bladder

a. _cyst_ / _otomy_
WR    S

b. _vesic_ / _otomy_
WR    S

14. plastic repair of the renal pelvis

_pyel_ / _o_ / _plasty_
WR    CV    S

15. incision of the neck of the bladder

_cyst_ / _o_ / _trachel_ / _otomy_
WR    CV    WR    S

16. excision of the ureter

_ureter_ / _ectomy_
WR    S

17. surgical fixation of the kidney

_nephr_ / _o_ / _pexy_
WR    CV    S

18. creation of an artificial opening into the renal pelvis

_pyel_ / _ostomy_
WR    S

19. incision into the bladder to remove a stone

     _cyst_ / _o_ / _lith_ / _otomy_
      WR    CV    WR    S

20. creation of an artificial opening into the ureter

     _ureter_ / _ostomy_
      WR     S

21. plastic repair of the bladder

     _cyst_ / _o_ / _plasty_
      WR    CV    S

22. surgical crushing of a stone

     _lith_ / _o_ / _tripsy_
      WR    CV    S

23. surgical suspension of the bladder and urethra

     _vesic_ / _o_ / _urethr_ / _al_
      WR    CV    WR    S
     suspension

24. creation of an artificial opening into the bladder

     _cyst_ / _ostomy_
      WR     S

## EXERCISE 19

Spell each of the surgical terms. Have someone dictate the terms on pp. 57 to 60 to you or say the words into a tape recorder; then spell the words from your recording as often as necessary. Think about the word parts before attempting to write the word. Study any you have spelled incorrectly.

1. _____  10. _____
2. _____  11. _____
3. _____  12. _____
4. _____  13. _____
5. _____  14. _____
6. _____  15. _____
7. _____  16. _____
8. _____  17. _____
9. _____  18. _____

| 19. _____ | 22. _____ |
| 20. _____ | 23. _____ |
| 21. _____ | 24. _____ |

Place a check mark (√) in the box to indicate that you have completed Objective 5.

☐ **BUILD, ANALYZE, DEFINE, PRONOUNCE, AND SPELL SURGICAL TERMS RELATED TO THE URINARY SYSTEM.**

# Objective 6 — BUILD, ANALYZE, DEFINE, PRONOUNCE, AND SPELL DIAGNOSTIC PROCEDURAL TERMS RELATED TO THE URINARY SYSTEM.

## Diagnostic Procedural Terms

| TERM (built from word parts) | DEFINITION |
|---|---|
| 1. cystogram (SIS-tō-gram) | x-ray film of the bladder |
| 2. cystography (sis-TOG-ra-fē) | process of x-ray filming the bladder |
| 3. cystopyelogram (sis-to-pī-EL-ō-gram) | x-ray film of the bladder and the renal pelvis |
| 4. cystopyelography (sis-to-pī-e-LOG-ra-fē) | process of x-ray filming the bladder and the renal pelvis |
| 5. cystoscope (SIS-tō-skōp) | instrument used for visual examination of the bladder |
| 6. cystoscopy (sis-TOS-kō-pē) | visual examination of the bladder |
| 7. cystoureterogram (sis-tō-ū-RĒ-ter-ō-gram) | x-ray film of the bladder and the ureters |
| 8. cystourethrogram (sis-to-ū-RĒ-thrō-gram) | x-ray film of the bladder and the urethra |
| 9. intravenous pyelogram (in-tra-VĒ-nus) (PĪ-e-lō-gram) (IVP) | x-ray film of the renal pelvis with contrast medium injected intravenously |
| 10. meatoscope (mē-ĀT-ō-skōp) | instrument used for the visual examination of a meatus |
| 11. meatoscopy (me-ā-TOS-kō-pē) | visual examination of a meatus |
| 12. nephrogram (NEF-rō-gram) | x-ray film of the kidney |
| 13. nephrography (ne-FROG-ra-fē) | process of x-ray filming the kidney |

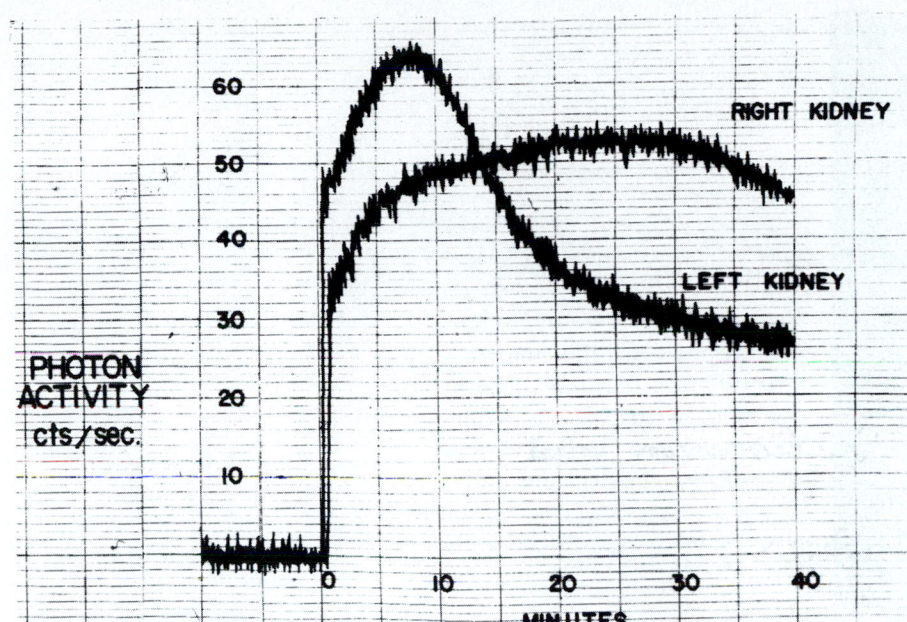

**Figure 5-11**

Renogram, made after injection of a radiopharmaceutical into the body, shows normal left kidney. Tracing of right kidney is characteristic of renal dysfunction caused by stenosis of renal artery.

From Winter C and Morel A: *Nursing care of patients with urologic disease*, ed 4, St. Louis, 1977, Mosby.

14. nephroscopy . . . . . . . . . .     visual examination of the kidney
    (ne-FROS-kō-pē)

15. nephrosonography . . . . .     process of recording the kidney with (ultra) sound
    (*nef*-rō-so-NOG-ra-fē)

16. nephrotomogram . . . . . .     sectional x-ray film of the kidney
    (*nef*-rō-TŌ-mō-gram)

17. pyelogram . . . . . . . . . . .     x-ray film of the renal pelvis
    (PĪ-el-ō-gram)

18. renal biopsy . . . . . . . . .     to view a portion of living kidney tissue
    (RĒ-nal) (BĪ-op-sē)

19. renogram . . . . . . . . . . .     (graphic) record of the kidney (produced by radioactivity after injecting a radiopharmaceutical, or radioactive, material into the blood) (Figure 5-11)
    (RĒ-nō-gram)

20. retrograde pyelogram . .     x-ray film of the renal pelvis (*retrograde* means to move in a direction opposite from normal) with contrast medium injected through the urethra (Figure 5-12)
    (RET-rō-grād) (PĪ-e-lō-gram)

21. ureterogram . . . . . . . . . .     x-ray film of the ureters
    (ū-RĒ-ter-ō-gram)

22. urethrometer . . . . . . . .     instrument used to measure the urethra
    (ū-rē-THROM-e-ter)

23. urethroscope . . . . . . . .     instrument used for visual examination of the urethra
    (ū-RĒ-thrō-skōp)

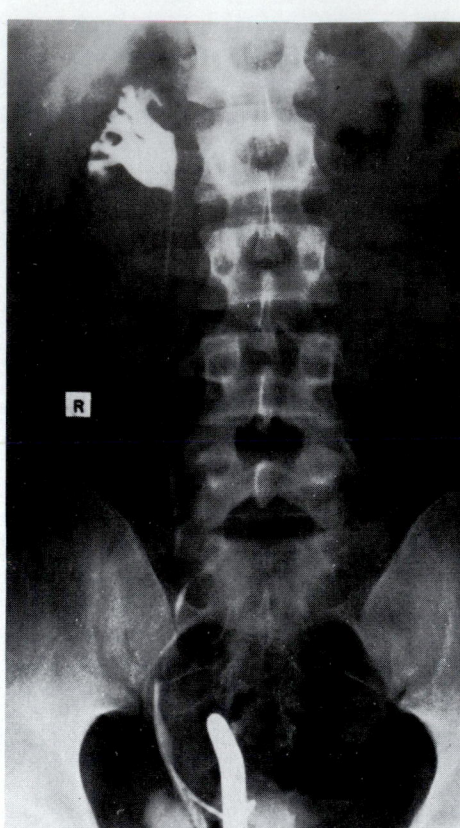

## Figure 5-12

Retrograde pyelogram. Ureteral catheter (white, tube-shaped structure at bottom) is passed by means of cystoscope, and contrast material is injected to show right *(R)* renal pelvis and ureter.

From Winter C and Morel A: *Nursing care of patients with urologic disease,* ed 4, St. Louis, 1977, Mosby.

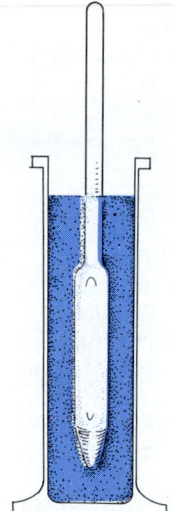

## Figure 5-13

Urinometer.

24.  urinometer . . . . . . . . . .    instrument used to measure (for deter-
     (ū-ri-NOM-e-ter)                  mining the specific gravity of) urine
                                       (Figure 5-13)

Practice saying each of these terms aloud. To assist you in pronunciation, obtain the audiotape designed for use with this text. Learn the definitions and spellings of the diagnostic procedural terms by completing the following exercises.

## EXERCISE 20

Analyze and define the following diagnostic procedural terms.

1. urethrometer _____

2. cystourethrogram _____

3. meatoscope _____

4. cystopyelogram _____

5. cystography _____

6. urethroscope _____

7. nephrosonography _____

8. cystoscope _____

9. pyelogram _____

10. nephrotomogram _____

11. cystogram _____

12. cystoureterogram _____

13. meatoscopy _____

14. nephrogram _____

15. ureterogram _____

16. cystoscopy _____

17. nephrography _____

18. urinometer _____

19. intravenous pyelogram _____

20. (retrograde) pyelogram _____

21. cystopyelography _____

22. renogram _____

23. nephroscopy _____

24. renal biopsy _____

## EXERCISE 21

Build diagnostic terms for the following definitions by using the word
parts you have learned.

1. visual examination of the
   bladder

   _____ cyst _/_ o _/_ scopy _____
        WR    CV    S

2. x-ray film of the bladder
   and ureters

   _____ cyst _/_ o _/_ ureter _/_ o _/_ gram _____
      WR   CV   WR   CV   S

3. instrument used to measure the urethra

   _____ urethr _/_ o _/_ meter _____
        WR    CV    S

4. sectional x-ray film of the kidney

_nephr_ / _o_ / _tom_ / _o_ / _gram_
WR / CV / WR / CV / S

5. x-ray film of the bladder and the renal pelvis

_cysto_ / _o_ / _pyel_ / _o_ / _gram_
WR / CV / WR / CV / S

6. x-ray film of the renal pelvis with contrast medium injected intravenously

_intra_ / _ven_ / _ous_
P / WR / S

_pyel_ / _o_ / _gram_
WR / CV / S

7. instrument used for visual examination of a meatus

_meat_ / _o_ / _scope_
WR / CV / S

8. instrument used for visual examination of the urethra

_urethr_ / _o_ / _scope_
WR / CV / S

9. process of x-ray recording the kidney using (ultra) sound

_nephr_ / _o_ / _son_ / _o_ / _graphy_
WR / CV / WR / CV / S

10. x-ray film of the bladder

_cyst_ / _o_ / _gram_
WR / CV / S

11. visual examination of a meatus

_meat_ / _o_ / _scopy_
WR / CV / S

12. x-ray film of the ureters

_____ / _____ / _____
WR / CV / S

13. x-ray film of the renal pelvis

_____ / _____ / _____
WR / CV / S

14. instrument used for visual examination of the bladder

cyst | o | scope
WR | CV | S

15. x-ray film of the bladder and the urethra

cyst | o | uretr | o | gram
WR | CV | WR | CV | S

16. process of x-ray filming the bladder

cyst | o | graphy
WR | CV | S

17. x-ray film of the kidney

nephr | o | gram
WR | CV | S

18. instrument used to measure (for determing the specific gravity of) urine

urin | o | meter
WR | CV | S

19. (graphic) record of the kidney (produced by radioactivity after injecting a radiopharmaceutical material into the blood)

ren | o | gram
WR | CV | S

20. process of x-ray filming the bladder and the renal pelvis

cyst | o | pyel | o | graphy
WR | CV | WR | CV | S

21. process of x-ray filming the kidney

nephr | o | graphy
WR | CV | S

22. x-ray film of the renal pelvis (with contrast medium injected through the urethra in a direction opposite from normal)

retrograde

pyel | o | gram
WR | CV | S

23. (a procedure) to view a
portion of living kidney
tissue

_ren_ _al_
WR | S

_bi_ _opsy_
WR | S

24. visual examination of the
kidney

_nephr_ _o_ _scopy_
WR | CV | S

## EXERCISE 22

Spell each of the diagnostic procedural terms. Have someone dictate the
terms on pp. 64 to 66 to you or say the words into a tape recorder; then
spell the words from your recording as often as necessary. Think about
the word parts before attempting to write the word. Study any you have
spelled incorrectly.

1. _____   13. _____
2. _____   14. _____
3. _____   15. _____
4. _____   16. _____
5. _____   17. _____
6. _____   18. _____
7. _____   19. _____
8. _____   20. _____
9. _____   21. _____
10. _____  22. _____
11. _____  23. _____
12. _____  24. _____

Place a check mark (√) in the box to indicate that you have completed Objective 6.

☐ BUILD, ANALYZE, DEFINE, PRONOUNCE, AND SPELL DIAGNOSTIC PROCEDURAL TERMS
RELATED TO THE URINARY SYSTEM.

# Objective 7

**BUILD, ANALYZE, DEFINE, PRONOUNCE, AND SPELL ADDITIONAL TERMS RELATED TO THE URINARY SYSTEM.**

## Additional Terms

| TERM (built from word parts) | DEFINITION |
|---|---|
| 1. **albuminuria** (*al*-bū-min-Ū-rē-a) | albumin in the urine (albumin is an important protein in the blood, but when found in the urine it indicates a kidney problem) |
| 2. **anuria** (an-Ū-rē-a) | absence of urine (failure of the kidney to excrete urine) |
| 3. **azoturia** (az-ō-TŪ-rē-a) | (excessive) urea and nitrogenous substances in the urine |
| 4. **diuresis** (dī-ū-RĒ-sis) (NOTE: The *a* is dropped before a word root beginning with a vowel.) | condition of urine passing through (increased excretion of urine) |
| 5. **dysuria** (dis-Ū-rē-a) | difficult or painful urination |
| 6. **glycosuria** (glī-kō-SŪ-rē-a) | sugar (glucose) in the urine |
| 7. **hematuria** (*hēm*-a-TŪ-rē-a) | blood in the urine |
| 8. **meatal** (mē-Ā-tal) | pertaining to the meatus |
| 9. **nocturia** (nok-TŪ-rē-a) | night urination |
| 10. **oliguria** (ol-ig-Ū-rē-a) | scanty urine |
| 11. **polyuria** (pol-ē-Ū-rē-a) | much (excessive) urine |
| 12. **pyuria** (pī-Ū-rē-a) | pus in the urine |
| 13. **urinary** (Ū-rin-*a*-rē) | pertaining to urine |
| 14. **urologist** (ū-ROL-ō-jist) | physician who specializes in the diagnosis and treatment of diseases of the male and female urinary systems and the reproductive system of the male |
| 15. **urology** (ū-ROL-ō-jē) | study of the male and female urinary system and the reproductive system in the male |

Practice saying each of these terms aloud. To assist you in pronunciation, obtain the audiotape designed for use with this text. Learn the definitions and spellings of the additional terms by completing the following exercises.

## EXERCISE 23

Analyze and define the following additional terms

1. nocturia _____

2. urologist _____

3. oliguria _____

4. azoturia _____

5. hematuria _____

6. urology _____

7. polyuria _____

8. albuminuria _____

9. anuria _____

10. diuresis _____

11. pyuria _____

12. urinary _____

13. glycosuria _____

14. meatal _____

15. dysuria _____

## EXERCISE 24

Build additional terms for the following definitions by using the word parts you have learned.

1. night urination
   _____ / _____
          WR            S

2. scanty urination
   _____ / _____
          WR            S

3. pus in the urine
   _____ / _____
          WR            S

4. physician who specializes in the diagnosis and treatment of diseases of the male and female urinary systems and of the reproductive system of the male

_____ / _____
WR              S

5. much (excessive) urine

_____ / _____
P              S(WR)

6. (excessive) urea and nitrogenous substances in the urine

_____ / _____
WR              S

7. pertaining to urine

_____ / _____
WR              S

8. blood in the urine

_____ / _____
WR              S

9. study of the male and female urinary systems and the reproductive system of the male

_____ / _____
WR              S

10. condition of urine passing through (increased excretion of urine)

_____ / _____ / _____
P              WR              S

11. absence of urine

_____ / _____
P              S(WR)

12. sugar in the urine

_____ / _____
WR              S

13. difficult or painful urination

_____ / _____
P              S(WR)

14. albumin in the urine        _____ / _____
                                      WR        S

15. pertaining to the meatus    _____ / _____
                                      WR        S

## EXERCISE 25

Spell each of the additional terms. Have someone dictate the terms on p. 171 to you or say the words into a tape recorder; then spell the words from your recording as often as necessary. Think about the word parts before attempting to write the word. Study any you have spelled incorrectly.

1. _____        9. _____

2. _____        10. _____

3. _____        11. _____

4. _____        12. _____

5. _____        13. _____

6. _____        14. _____

7. _____        15. _____

8. _____

Place a check mark (√) in the box to indicate that you have completed Objective 7.

☐ BUILD, ANALYZE, DEFINE, PRONOUNCE, AND SPELL ADDITIONAL TERMS RELATED TO THE URINARY SYSTEM.

# Objective 8    DEFINE, PRONOUNCE, AND SPELL THE OTHER ADDITIONAL TERMS RELATED TO THE URINARY SYSTEM.

## Other Additional Terms

| TERM | DEFINITION | |
|------|------------|---|
| 1. catheter <br> (KATH-e-ter) | flexible, tubelike device, such as a urinary catheter, for withdrawing or instilling fluids | **Catheter** is derived from the Greek **katheter**, meaning a **thing let down**. A catheter lets down the urine from the bladder. |
| 2. urinary catheterization <br> (kath-e-ter-i-ZĀ-shun) | passage of a catheter into the urinary bladder to withdraw urine (Figure 5-14) | |
| 3. distended <br> (dis-TEN-ded) | stretched out (a bladder is distended when filled with urine) | |
| 4. diuretic <br> (dī-ū-RET-ik) | agent that increases the amount of urine | |

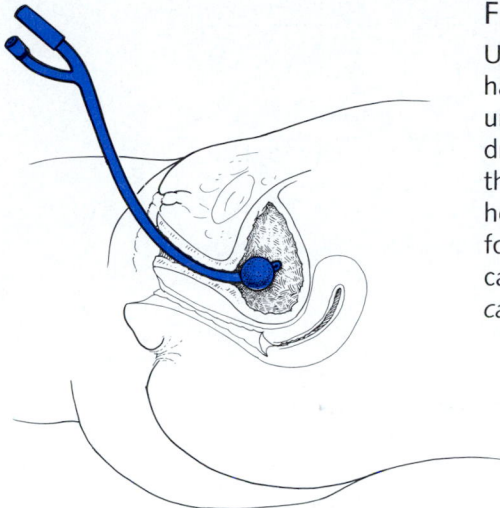

Figure 5-14

Urinary catheterization. Catheter has been inserted through the urethra, and urine has been drained. Balloon on the end of the catheter has been inflated to hold the catheter in the bladder for a period of time. This type of catheter is called a *retention catheter.*

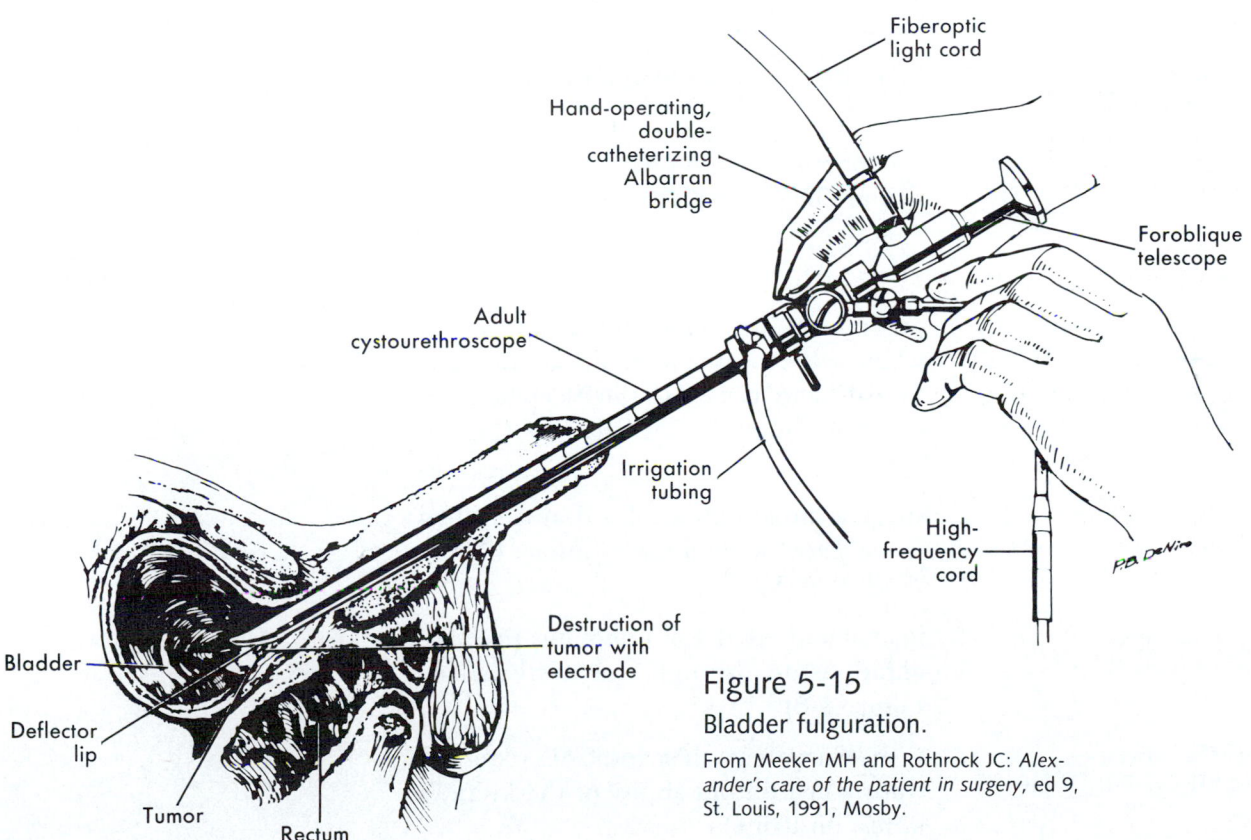

Fiberoptic light cord

Hand-operating, double-catheterizing Albarran bridge

Foroblique telescope

Adult cystourethroscope

Irrigation tubing

High-frequency cord

Destruction of tumor with electrode

Bladder

Deflector lip

Tumor

Rectum

Figure 5-15

Bladder fulguration.

From Meeker MH and Rothrock JC: *Alexander's care of the patient in surgery,* ed 9, St. Louis, 1991, Mosby.

5. enuresis . . . . . . . . . . . .     involuntary urination (bed wetting)
   (en-ū-RĒ-sis)

6. fulguration . . . . . . . . . .     destruction of living tissue with an elec-
   (ful-gū-RĀ-shun)                    tric spark (a method commonly used to
                                       remove bladder growths) (Figure 5-15)

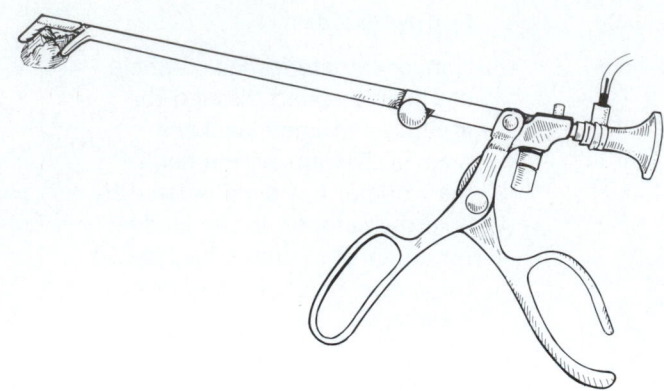

Figure 5-16
Lithotrite.

7.  hemodialysis . . . . . . . . .          procedure for removing impurities from
    (*hē*-mō-dī-AL-i-sis)                the blood because of an inability of the
                                         kidneys to do so

8.  incontinence . . . . . . . . .         inability to control bladder and/or bow-
    (in-KON-ti-nens)                     els

9.  lithotrite . . . . . . . . . . . .     instrument used to crush a stone in the
    (LITH-ō-trīt)                        urinary bladder (Figure 5-16)

10. micturate . . . . . . . . . . .        to urinate or void
    (MIK-tū-rāt)

11. peritoneal dialysis . . . . .          procedure for removing toxic wastes
    (pār-i-tō-NĒ-al) (dī-AL-i-sis)       when kidney is unable to do so; the peri-
                                         toneal cavity is used as the receptacle for
                                         the fluid used in the dialysis (Figure
                                         5-17)

12. renal transplant . . . . . . .         surgical inplantation of a donor kidney
    (RĒ-nal) (trans-PLANT)               to replace a non-functioning kidney
                                         (Figure 5-18)

13. resectoscope . . . . . . . . .         instrument used for removing prostate
    (rē-SEK-tō-skōp)                     gland tissue through the urethra (see
                                         Figure 6-8)

14. specific gravity . . . . . . .         a measurement that indicates concen-
    (spe-SIF-ik) (GRAV-i-tē)             trating or diluting ability of the kidneys
                                         (a test on urine)

15. stricture . . . . . . . . . . . .      abnormal narrowing, such as a urethral
    (STRIK-chūr)                         stricture

16. urinal . . . . . . . . . . . . . .     receptacle for urine
    (Ū-rin-al)

17. urinalysis . . . . . . . . . . .       laboratory examination of urine
    (ū-rin-AL-is-is)

**Micturate** is derived from the Latin **mictus**, meaning **a making of water**.

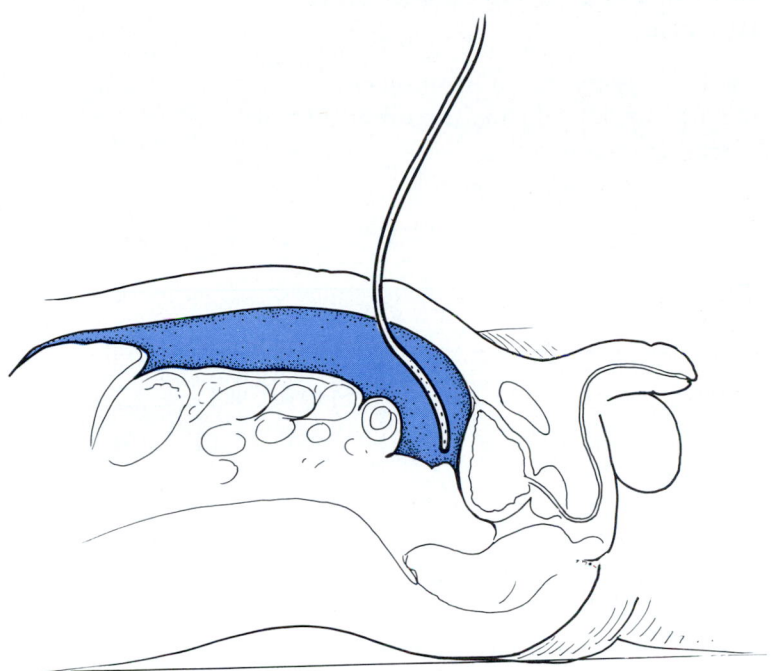

**Figure 5-17**
Peritoneal dialysis. A sterile dialyzing fluid is installed into the peritoneal cavity over a period of time. In 10 to 30 minutes the fluid, containing the nitrogenous wastes and excess water that a healthy kidney normally removes, is drained from the cavity.

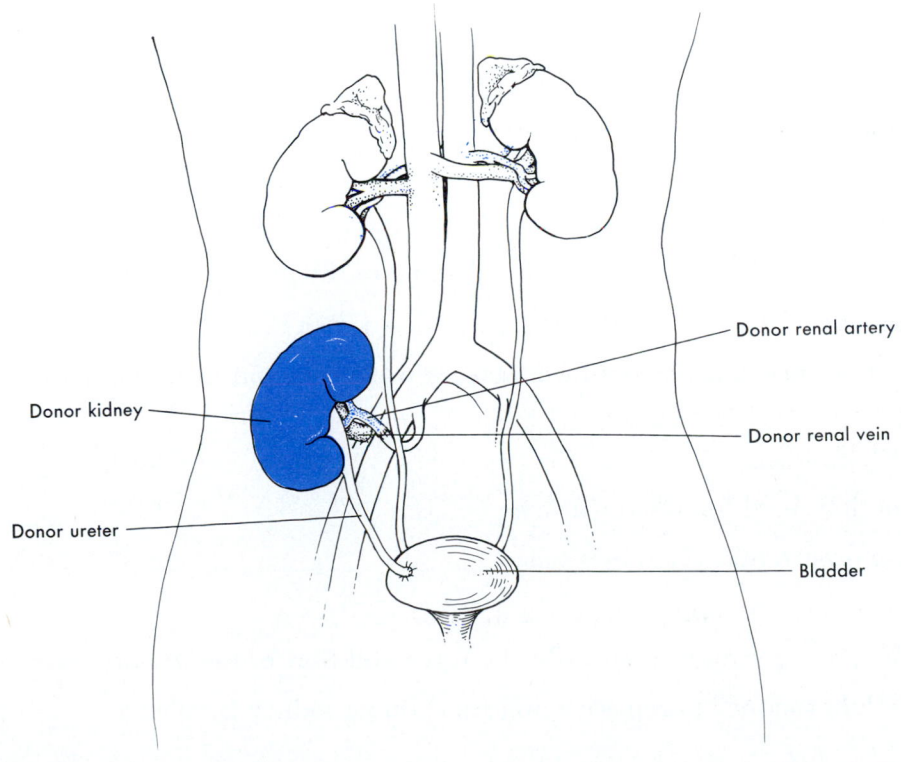

Donor renal artery

Donor kidney

Donor renal vein

Donor ureter

Bladder

**Figure 5-18**
Renal transplant showing donor kidney and blood vessels in place. Recipient's kidney is not always removed unless it is infected or is a cause of hypertension.

18. urodynamics. . . . . . . . .     pertaining to the force and flow of urine
    (ū-rō-dī-NAM-iks)               within the urinary tract

19. void . . . . . . . . . . . . . .     to empty or evacuate waste material, es-
    (voyd)                         pecially urine

Practice saying each of these terms aloud. To assist you in pronunciation, obtain the audiotape designed for use with this text. Learn the other additional terms by completing the following exercises.

## EXERCISE 26

Fill in the blanks with the correct terms.

1. A receptacle for urine is a(n) _____ .

2. The destruction of living tissue with an electric spark is _____ .

3. The procedure for removing impurities from the blood because of the inability of the kidneys to do so is called _____ .

4. When the bladder is stretched out it is called _____ .

5. A(n) _____ is a laboratory examination of urine.

6. A flexible tubelike device for withdrawing or instilling fluids is a(n) _____ .

7. The inability to control bladder and/or bowels is called _____ .

8. The passage of a catheter into the urinary bladder to withdraw urine is a(n)

   _____ _____ .

9. To remove toxic wastes caused by kidney insufficiency by placing dialyzing fluid in the peritoneal cavity is called _____ _____ .

10. To void is to _____ _____ _____ .

11. An abnormal narrowing is a(n) _____ .

12. A(n) _____ is an instrument used to crush a stone in the urinary bladder.

13. An agent that increases the amount of urine is called a(n) _____ .

14. A(n) _____ is an instrument used for removing prostate gland tissue through the urethra.

15. Involuntary urination is called _____ .

16. _____ is another word for void or urinate.

17. A measurement that indicates concentration of urine is called _____

   _____ .

18. _____ is the name given to the study of the force and flow of the urinary tract.

19. The surgical implantation of a donor kidney to replace a non-functioning kidney is called a

   _____ _____ .

## EXERCISE 27A

Match the terms in the first column with the correct definitions in the second column.

_____ 1. catheter

_____ 2. urinary catheterization

_____ 3. distended

_____ 4. diuretic

_____ 5. fulguration

_____ 6. hemodialysis

_____ 7. incontinent

_____ 8. void

_____ 9. renal transplant

a. increases the amount of urine

b. overdevelopment of the kidney

c. inability to control bladder and/or bowels

d. process for removing impurities from the blood when the kidneys are unable to do so.

e. flexible, tubelike device for removing urine from the bladder

f. stretched out

g. surgical implantation of a donor kidney

h. passage of a tubelike device into the urinary bladder

i. evacuation or empty waste material, especially urine

j. destruction of living tissue with an electric spark

## EXERCISE 27B

Match the terms in the first column with the correct definitions in the second column.

_____ 1. lithotrite

_____ 2. micturate, or urinate

_____ 3. peritoneal dialysis

_____ 4. resectoscope

_____ 5. stricture

_____ 6. urinal

_____ 7. urinalysis

_____ 8. enuresis

_____ 9. specific gravity

_____ 10. urodynamics

a. to void liquid waste

b. receptacle for urine

c. instrument used for crushing a stone in the urinary bladder

d. laboratory examination of urine

e. force and flow of urine within urinary tract

f. instrument used for removing prostate gland tissue through the urethra

g. indicates concentration of urine

h. absence of urine

i. use of peritoneal cavity to hold dialyzing fluid in the removal of toxic wastes

j. involuntary urination

k. narrowing

## EXERCISE 28

Spell each of the other additional terms. Have someone dictate the terms on pp. 174 to 178 to you or say the words into a tape recorder; then spell the words from your recording as often as necessary. Study any you have spelled incorrectly.

1. _____     11. _____

2. _____     12. _____

3. _____     13. _____

4. _____     14. _____

5. _____     15. _____

6. _____     16. _____

7. _____     17. _____

8. _____     18. _____

9. _____     19. _____

10. _____

Place a check mark (√) in the box to indicate that you have completed Objective 8.

☐ **DEFINE, PRONOUNCE, AND SPELL THE OTHER ADDITIONAL TERMS RELATED TO THE URINARY SYSTEM.**

**Case History:** This 32-year-old married white male, appearing his stated age, was admitted to the hospital after presenting himself to the emergency room in acute distress. He complained of intermittent pain in the right posterior lumbar area radiating to the right flank. He has a family history of pyelolithiasis and has been treated for this condition several times in the past 10 years.

**Discharge Summary:** This patient was admitted to the urology unit from emergency room, complaining of severe intermittent pain in the back and right flank. His KUB showed a calculus in the region of the right renal pelvis. Laboratory data were all normal except for slight microscopic hematuria. Intravenous pyelography showed three stones in the right kidney with minimal hydronephrosis. Cystoscopy with a right retrograde pyelogram confirmed presence of three stones in the right kidney. Minimal ureteral obstruction was present. Pyelolithotomy was completed with no complication. A ureteral catheter was inserted as was an indwelling Foley catheter. Drainage from the right kidney was pale yellow in forty-eight hours. The Foley and ureteral catheters were removed three days postoperatively. At discharge, the patient is voiding without difficulty, is afebrile, and ambulatory. The stones were sent to the laboratory for analysis. The report indicated that they were calcium oxalate. He is discharged to his home on restricted activity for the next two weeks. He is advised to drink copious amounts of fluids. He will be followed in the office in 3 weeks.

## EXERCISE 29

To test your understanding of the terms introduced in this chapter, circle the words that correctly complete the sentences. The italicized phrase is the definition of the term.

1. The patient was admitted with a *drooping kidney,* or (nephromegaly, nephrohypertrophy, nephroptosis).
2. The patient's x-ray film showed a *stone in the ureter,* or a condition known as (ureterocele, ureterolithiasis, ureterostenosis).
3. The physician ordered an *x-ray film of the renal pelvis,* or a (pyelogram, nephrogram, cystogram).
4. The physician first suspected diabetes when told of the *excessive amounts of urine* voided, or (oliguria, polyuria, dysuria).
5. The physician told the patient with the drooping kidney that it was necessary to put the *kidney back in place* by performing a (nephropexy, nephrolysis, nephrotripsy).
6. The patient experienced a *sudden stoppage of urine formation,* or (urinary suppression, urinary retention, azoturia).
7. The patient was scheduled for an *x-ray film of the urinary bladder,* or a (cystoscopy, cystogram, cystography).
8. The patient informed the doctor of her son's involuntary urination, or (diuresis, dysuria, enuresis).
9. The patient was admitted to the hospital for *kidney and ureter infection,* or (polycystic kidney, urinary retention, urinary tract infection).

## EXERCISE 30

Unscramble the following mixed-up terms. The word(s) on the left indicate the word root in each of the opposite scrambled words.

1. bladder

/  /  /  /  / o /  /  /  /  /
p  o  s  c  c  t  o  y  s  y

2. urine

/  /  /  /  /  /  /
r  a  a  i  u  n

3. renal pelvis

/  /  /  /  / i /  /  /  /
y  i  t  p  e  l  s  i

4. kidney

/  /  /  /  /  / o /  /  /
h  o  p  m  e  n  a  r

5. urine

/  /  /  /  /  /  /
m  e  r  a  u  i

6. ureter

/  /  /  /  /  /  /  / c /  /  /  /
c  u  l  t  e  r  e  o  r  e  e

## EXERCISE 31

The following words did not appear in this chapter but are composed of word parts found in this or the previous chapters. Find their definitions by translating the word parts literally.

1.  **hyperlipemia** (hī-per-li-PĒ-mē-a) _____

2.  **hypoglycemia** (hī-po-glī-SĒ-mē-a) _____

3.  **leukonychia** (lū-kō-NIK-ē-a) _____

4.  **neurocutaneous** (nū-rō-kū-TĀ-nē-us) _____

5.  **oncotomy** (ong-KOT-ō-mē) _____

6.  **phonogram** (FŌ-nō-gram) _____

7.  **somatalgia** (sō-ma-TAL-jē-a) _____

8.  **trichology** (tri-KOL-ō-jē) _____

## COMBINING FORMS CROSSWORD PUZZLE

### Across Clues

1. urine, urinary tract
5. glomerulus
6. sound
9. albumin
11. scanty
14. bladder
15. bladder
18. ureter
22. kidney
23. opening
24. sugar

### Down Clues

2. cut, section
3. blood
4. night
5. sugar
7. neck, necklike
8. urine, urinary tract
10. urethra
12. stone
13. water
16. urea, nitrogen
17. kidney
19. vein
20. renal pelvis
21. blood

# Summary

Can you build, analyze, define, and spell the following terms *built from word parts?* yes ☐ no ☐

| DIAGNOSTIC | SURGICAL | PROCEDURAL | ADDITIONAL |
|---|---|---|---|
| cystitis<br>(sis-TĪ-tis) | cystectomy<br>(sis-TEK-tō-mē) | cystogram<br>(SIS-tō-gram) | albuminuria<br>(*al*-bū-min-Ū-rē-a) |
| cystocele<br>(SIS-tō-sēl) | cystolithotomy<br>(*sis*-tō-li-THOT-ō-mē) | cystography<br>(sis-TOG-ra-fē) | anuria<br>(an-Ū-rē-a) |
| cystolith<br>(SIS-tō-lith) | cystoplasty<br>(SIS-tō-plas-tē) | cystopyelogram<br>(*sis*-to-pī-EL-ō-gram) | azoturia<br>(az-ō-TŪ-rē-a) |
| glomerulonephritis<br>(glo-*mer*-ū-lō-ne-FRĪ-tis) | cystorrhaphy<br>(sist-OR-a-fē) | cystopyelography<br>(sis-to-*pī*-e-LOG-ra-fē) | diuresis<br>(*dī*-ū-RĒ-sis) |
| hydronephrosis<br>(*hī*-drō-ne-FRŌ-sis) | cystostomy<br>(sis-TOS-tō-mē) | cystoscope<br>(SIS-tō-skōp) | dysuria<br>(dis-Ū-rē-a) |
| nephritis<br>(ne-FRĪ-tis) | vesicotomy<br>(*ves*-i-KOT-ō-mē) | cystoscopy<br>(sis-TOS-kō-pē) | glycosuria<br>(glī-kō-SŪ-rē-a) |
| nephroblastoma<br>(nef-rō-blas-TŌ-ma) | cystotrachelotomy<br>(*sis*-tō-*trā*-ke-LOT-ō-mē) | cystoureterogram<br>(*sis*-tō-ū-RĒ-ter-ō-gram) | hematuria<br>(*hēm*-a-TŪ-rē-a) |
| nephrohypertrophy<br>(*nef*-rō-hī-PER-trō-fē) | lithotripsy<br>(LITH-ō-trip-sē) | cystourethrogram<br>(*sis*-to-ū-RĒ-thrō-gram) | meatal<br>(mē-Ā-tal) |
| nephrolithiasis<br>(*nef*-rō-lith-Ī-a-sis) | meatotomy<br>(*mē*-a-TOT-ō-mē) | intravenous pyelogram<br>(in-tra-VĒ-nus)<br>(PĪ-e-lō-gram) | nocturia<br>(nok-TŪ-rē-a) |
| nephroma<br>(nef-RŌ-ma) | nephrectomy<br>(ne-FREK-tō-mē) | meatoscope<br>(mē-ĀT-ō-skōp) | oliguria<br>(ol-ig-Ū-rē-a) |
| nephromegaly<br>(*nef*-rō-MEG-a-lē) | nephrolysis<br>(ne-FROL-i-sis) | meatoscopy<br>(me-ā-TOS-kō-pē) | polyuria<br>(pol-ē-Ū-rē-a) |
| nephroptosis<br>(*nef*-rop-TŌ-sis) | nephropexy<br>(NEF-rō-*peks*-ē) | nephrogram<br>(NEF-rō-gram) | pyuria<br>(pī-Ū-rē-a) |
| pyelitis<br>(*pī*-e-LĪ-tis) | nephrostomy<br>(nef-ROS-tō-mē) | nephrography<br>(ne-FROG-ra-fē) | urinary<br>(Ū-rin-*ā*-rē) |
| pyelonephritis<br>(*pī*-e-lō-ne-FRĪ-tis) | pyelolithotomy<br>(pī-el-ō-lith-OT-ō-mē) | nephroscopy<br>(ne-FROS-kō-pē) | urologist<br>(ū-ROL-ō-jist) |
| trachelocystitis<br>(*trā*-kel-ō-sis-TĪ-tis) | pyeloplasty<br>(PĪ-el-ō-*plas*-tē) | nephrosonography<br>(*nef*-rō-so-NOG-ra-fē) | urology<br>(ū-ROL-ō-jē) |
| uremia<br>(ū-RĒ-mē-a) | pyelostomy<br>(*pī*-el-OS-tō-mē) | nephrotomogram<br>(*nef*-rō-TŌ-mō-gram) | |
| ureteritis<br>(ū-rē-ter-Ī-tis) | ureterectomy<br>(ū-*rē*-ter-EK-tō-mē) | pyelogram<br>(PĪ-el-ō-gram) | |
| ureterocele<br>(ū-RĒ-ter-ō-sēl) | ureterostomy<br>(ū-rē-ter-OS-tō-mē) | renal biopsy<br>(RĒ-nal) (BĪ-op-sē) | |
| ureterolithiasis<br>(ū-rē-ter-ō-lith-Ī-a-sis) | ureterotomy<br>(ū-rē-ter-OT-ō-mē) | renogram<br>(RĒ-nō-gram) | |

| DIAGNOSTIC | SURGICAL | PROCEDURAL |
|---|---|---|
| ureterostenosis<br>(ū-rē-ter-ō-sten-Ō-sis) | urethropexy<br>(ū-RĒ-thrō-pek-sē) | retrograde pyelogram<br>(RET-rō-grād)<br>(PĪ-e-lō-gram) |
| urethrocystitis<br>(ū-rē-thrō-sis-TĪ-tis) | urethroplasty<br>(ū-RĒ-thrō-*plas*-tē) | ureterogram<br>(ū-RĒ-ter-ō-gram) |
| | urethrostomy<br>(ū-rē-THROS-tō-mē) | urethrometer<br>(ū-rē-THROM-e-ter) |
| | urethrotomy<br>(ū-rē-THROT-ō-mē) | urethroscope<br>(ū-RĒ-thrō-skōp) |
| | vesiculorethral<br>suspension<br>(*ves-i-kō-ū-RĒ-thr-al*) | urinometer<br>(ū-ri-NOM-e-ter) |

# Summary

Can you define, pronounce, and spell the following terms *not built from word parts?*   yes □   no □

| DIAGNOSTIC | ADDITIONAL | | |
|---|---|---|---|
| epispadias<br>(*ep*-i-SPĀ-dē-as) | catheter<br>(KATH-eter) | incontinence<br>(in-KON-ti-nens) | specific gravity<br>(spe-SIF-ik) (GRAV-i-tē) |
| hypospadias<br>(*hī*-pō-SPĀ-dē-as) | urinary catheterization<br>(*kath*-e-ter-ī-ZĀ-shun) | lithotrite<br>(LITH-ō-trīt) | stricture<br>(STRIK-chūr) |
| polycystic kidney<br>(*pol*-i-SIS-tik) (KID-nē) | distended<br>(dis-TEN-ded) | micturate<br>(MIK-tū-rāt) | urinal<br>(Ū-rin-al) |
| renal calculi<br>(RĒ-nal) (KAL-kū-lī) | diuretic<br>(dī-ū-RET-ik) | peritoneal dialysis<br>(pār-i-tō-NĒ-al) (dī-AL-i-sis) | urinalysis<br>(ū-rin-AL-is-is) |
| renal hypertension<br>(RĒ-nal) (hī-per-TEN-shun) | enuresis<br>(en-ū-RĒ-sis) | renal transplant<br>(RĒ-nal) (trans-PLANT) | urodynamics<br>(ū-rō-dī-NAM-iks) |
| urinary retention<br>(Ū-rin-*a*-rē) (rē-TEN-shun) | fulguration<br>(ful-gū-RĀ-shun) | resectoscope<br>(rē-SEK-tō-skōp) | void<br>(voyd) |
| urinary suppression<br>(Ū-rin-*a*-rē) (sū-PRESH-un) | hemodialysis<br>(*hē*-mō-dī-AL-i-sis) | | |
| urinary tract infection | | | |

# Answers

## Exercise 1

1. g  3. f  5. a  7. e
2. d  4. c  6. b

## Exercise 2

**Figure 5-1**
Kidney: nephr/o, ren/o  Bladder: cyst/o, vesic/o
Meatus: meat/o  Urethra: urethr/o
Ureter: ureter/o

**Figure 5-2**
Renal pelvis: pyel/o
Glomerulus: glomerul/o

## Exercise 3

1. glomerulus  4. renal pelvis  7. urethra
2. sac, bladder  5. ureter  8. kidney
3. kidney  6. sac, bladder  9. meatus

## Exercise 4

1. a. nephr/o  4. pyel/o
   b. ren/o  5. glomerul/o
2. a. cyst/o  6. urethr/o
   b. vesic/o  7. meat/o
3. ureter/o

## Exercise 5

1. water  9. urine, urinary tract
2. vein  10. sound
3. urea, nitrogen  11. sugar
4. neck, necklike  12. developing cell, germ
5. night      cell
6. stone  13. scanty, few
7. cut, section  14. urine, urinary tract
8. albumin  15. sugar

## Exercise 6

1. a. glyc/o  5. hydr/o  10. azot/o
   b. glycos/o  6. blast/o  11. lith/o
2. trachel/o  7. tom/o  12. ven/o
3. son/o  8. albumin/o  13. olig/o
4. a. urin/o  9. noct/i
   b. ur/o

## Exercise 7

1. many, much

## Exercise 8

1. poly-

## Exercise 9

1. c  3. d  5. g  7. a
2. i  4. f  6. e  8. b

## Exercise 10

1. suturing, repairing  6. enlargement
2. loosening, dissolution,  7. drooping, sagging,
   separating      prolapse
3. condition  8. surgical crushing
4. nourishment, develop-
   ment
5. urine, urination

## Exercise 11

|  |  |
|---|---|
| WR    S<br>1. nephr/oma | tumor of the kidney |
| WR CV WR<br>2. cyst/ o /lith<br>    CF | stone in the urinary bladder |
| WR CV WR S<br>3. nephr/ o /lith/iasis<br>    CF | condition of stone(s) in the kidney |
| WR   S<br>4. ur/emia | condition of urine in the blood |
| WR CV  S<br>5. nephr/ o /ptosis<br>    CF | a drooping kidney |
| WR CV S<br>6. cyst/ o /cele<br>    CF | protrusion of the bladder |
| WR CV P    S<br>7. nephr/ o /hyper/trophy<br>    CF | overdevelopment of the kidney |
| WR CV WR S<br>8. trachel/ o /cyst/itis<br>    CF | inflammation of the neck of the bladder |
| WR  S<br>9. cyst/itis | inflammation of the bladder |
| WR  S<br>10. pyel/itis | inflammation of the renal pelvis |
| WR CV S<br>11. ureter/ o /cele<br>    CF | protrusion of a ureter |
| WR CV WR  S<br>12. hydr/ o /nephr/osis<br>    CF | abnormal condition of water in the kidneys |
| WR CV  S<br>13. nephr/ o /megaly<br>    CF | enlargement of a kidney |

14. WR CV WR S
    ureter/ o /lith/iasis
    CF
    condition of stone(s) in the ureters

15. WR CV WR S
    pyel/ o /nephr/itis
    CF
    inflammation of the renal pelvis and the kidney

16. WR S
    ureter/itis
    inflammation of a ureter

17. WR S
    nephr/itis
    inflammation of a kidney

18. WR CV WR S
    urethr/ o /cyst/itis
    CF
    inflammation of the bladder and urethra

19. WR CV S
    ureter/ o /stenosis
    CF
    narrowing of the ureter

20. WR CV WR S
    nephr/ o /blast/oma
    CF
    kidney tumor containing developing cell tissue

## Exercise 12

1. nephr/o/megaly
2. cyst/itis
3. nephr/o/hyper/trophy
4. urethr/o/cyst/itis
5. cyst/o/cele
6. trachel/o/cyst/itis
7. hydr/o/nephr/osis
8. cyst/o/lith
9. glomerul/o/nephr/itis
10. nephr/oma
11. nephr/o/ptosis
12. nephr/itis
13. nephr/o/lith/iasis
14. ureter/o/cele
15. pyel/itis
16. ur/emia
17. ureter/o/stenosis
18. pyel/o/nephr/itis
19. ureter/o/lith/iasis
20. nephr/o/blast/oma

## Exercise 13

Spelling exercise; *see* text, pp. 153 and 154

## Exericse 14

1. renal calculi
2. urinary retention
3. polycystic kidney
4. hypospadias
5. renal hypertension
6. urinary suppression
7. epispadias
8. urinary tract infection

## Exercise 15

1. c  3. d  5. a  7. b
2. f  4. h  6. e  8. g

## Exercise 16

Spelling exercise; *see* text, p. 156.

## Exercise 17

1. WR S
   vesic/otomy
   incision of the bladder

2. WR S
   nephr/ostomy
   creation of an artificial opening into the kidney

3. WR CV S
   nephr/ o /lysis
   CF
   separating the kidney

4. WR S
   cyst/ectomy
   excision of the bladder

5. WR S
   ureter/otomy
   incision of a ureter

6. WR CV WR S
   pyel/ o /lith/otomy
   CF
   incision of the renal pelvis to remove a stone

7. WR CV WR S
   cyst/ o /trachel/otomy
   CF
   incision of the neck of the bladder

8. WR CV S
   nephr/ o /pexy
   CF
   surgical fixation of the kidney

9. WR S
   ureter/ostomy
   creation of an artificial opening in the ureter

10. WR CV WR S
    cyst/ o /lith/otomy
    CF
    incision of the bladder to remove a stone

11. WR S
    nephr/ectomy
    excision of a kidney

12. WR S
    pyel/ostomy
    creation of an artificial opening in the renal pelvis

13. WR CV S
    urethr/ o /pexy
    CF
    surgical fixation of the urethra

14. WR S
    ureter/ectomy
    excision of the ureter

15. WR S
    cyst/ostomy
    creation of an artificial opening into the bladder

16. WR CV S
    pyel/ o /plasty
    CF
    plastic repair of the renal pelvis

17. WR S
    cyst/orrhaphy
    suturing or repairing of the bladder

18. WR S
    urethr/ostomy
    creation of an artificial opening into the urethra

19. WR CV S
    cyst/ o /plasty
    CF
    plastic repair of the bladder

20. WR S
    meat/otomy
    incision of the urinary meatus

WR CV   S
21. lith/ o /tripsy        surgical crushing of a
     CF                       stone

WR   S
22. cyst/otomy         incision of the bladder

WR  CV   S
23. urethr/ o /plasty      plastic repair of the ure-
      CF                      thra

WR  CV  WR  S
24. vesic/ o /urethr/al/    surgical suspension per-
      CF                      taining to the urethra
                                and bladder

## Exercise 18

| | |
|---|---|
| 1. urethr/otomy | 13. a. cyst/otomy |
| 2. nephr/ectomy |       b. vesic/otomy |
| 3. pyel/o/lith/otomy | 14. pyel/o/plasty |
| 4. urethr/o/pexy | 15. cyst/o/trachel/otomy |
| 5. cyst/orrhaphy | 16. ureter/ectomy |
| 6. nephr/o/lysis | 17. nephr/o/pexy |
| 7. nephr/ostomy | 18. pyel/ostomy |
| 8. ureter/otomy | 19. cyst/o/lith/otomy |
| 9. urethr/o/plasty | 20. ureter/ostomy |
| 10. cyst/ectomy | 21. cyst/o/plasty |
| 11. meat/otomy | 22. lith/o/tripsy |
| 12. urethr/ostomy | 23. vesic/o/urethr/al |
| | 24. cyst/ostomy |

## Exercise 19

Spelling exercise; *see* text, p. 163.

## Exercise 20

WR  CV   S
1. urethr/ o /meter      instrument used to mea-
     CF                     sure the urethra

WR CV  WR  CV  S
2. cyst/ o /urethr/ o /gram    x-ray film of the bladder
     CF       CF               and the urethra

WR CV   S
3. meat/ o /scope       instrument used for vi-
     CF                     sual examination of a
                               meatus

WR CV  WR  CV  S
4. cyst/ o /pyel/ o /gram    x-ray film of the bladder
     CF       CF               and the renal pelvis

WR CV   S
5. cyst/ o /graphy       process of x-ray filming
     CF                     the bladder

WR  CV   S
6. urethr/ o /scope       instrument used for vi-
      CF                      sual examination of
                                the urethra

WR  CV  WR CV   S
7. nephr/ o /son/ o /graphy    process of recording the
      CF      CF               kidney using (ultra)
                               sound

WR CV   S
8. cyst/ o /scope       instrument used for vi-
     CF                     sual examination of
                               the bladder

WR  CV   S
9. pyel/ o /gram       x-ray film of the renal
     CF                     pelvis

WR  CV  WR CV   S
10. nephr/ o /tom/ o /gram    sectional x-ray film of
      CF      CF               the kidney

WR CV   S
11. cyst/ o /gram       x-ray film of the bladder
     CF

WR CV  WR  CV  S
12. cyst/ o /ureter/ o /gram    x-ray film of the bladder
     CF       CF               and ureters

WR  CV   S
13. meat/ o /scopy       visual examination of a
     CF                     meatus

WR  CV   S
14. nephr/ o /gram       x-ray film of the kidney
      CF

WR  CV   S
15. ureter/ o /gram       x-ray film of the ureters
      CF

WR CV   S
16. cyst/ o /scopy       visual examination of
     CF                     the bladder

WR CV   S
17. nephr/ o /graphy       process of x-ray filming
      CF                     the kidney

WR CV   S
18. urin/ o /meter       instrument used to mea-
     CF                     sure urine

P   WR  S  WR CV   S
19. intra/ven/ous pyel/ o /gram    x-ray film of the renal
                    CF         pelvis with contrast
                                medium injected
                                within the vein

WR CV   S
20. retrograde pyel/ o /gram    x-ray film of the renal
                CF            pelvis (contrast me-
                                dium injected in a
                                direction opposite
                                from normal through
                                the urethra)

WR CV  WR  CV   S
21. cyst/ o /pyel/ o /graphy    process of x-ray filming
     CF       CF              the bladder and the
                                renal pelvis

WR CV   S
22. ren/ o /gram       (graphic) record of the
     CF                     kidney

WR CV   S
23. nephr/ o /scopy       visual examination of
     CF                     the kidney

WR  S  WR   S
24. ren/al bi /opsy       to view a portion of liv-
                                ing kidney tissue

## Exercise 21

1. cyst/o/scopy
2. cyst/o/ureter/o/gram
3. urethr/o/meter
4. nephr/o/tom/o/gram
5. cyst/o/pyel/o/gram
6. intra/ven/ous pyel/o/gram
7. meat/o/scope
8. urethr/o/scope
9. nephr/o/son/o/graphy
10. cyst/o/gram
11. meat/o/scopy
12. ureter/o/gram
13. pyel/o/gram
14. cyst/o/scope
15. cyst/o/urethr/o/gram
16. cyst/o/graphy
17. nephr/o/gram
18. urin/o/meter
19. ren/o/gram
20. cyst/o/pyel/o/graphy
21. nephr/o/graphy
22. retrograde pyel/o/gram
23. ren/al bi/opsy
24. nephr/o/scopy

## Exercise 22

Spelling exercise; *see* text, p. 170.

## Exercise 23

|  |  |  |
|---|---|---|
| WR  S | | |
| 1. noct/uria | night urination | |
| WR  S | | |
| 2. ur/ologist | physician who specializes in the diagnosis and treatment of diseases of the male and female urinary systems and in the reproductive system of the male | |
| WR  S | | |
| 3. olig/uria | scanty urination | |
| WR  S | | |
| 4. azot/uria | (excessive) urea and nitrogenous substances in the urine | |
| WR  S(WR) | | |
| 5. hemat/ uria | blood in the urine | |
| WR  S | | |
| 6. ur/ology | study of the male and female urinary systems and the reproductive system of the male | |
| P  S(WR) | | |
| 7. poly/ uria | much (excessive) urine | |
| WR  S | | |
| 8. albumin/uria | albumin in the urine | |
| P  S(WR) | | |
| 9. an/ uria | absence of urine | |
| P WR  S | | |
| 10. di/ ur /esis | condition of urine passing through (increased excretion of urine) | |
| WR  S | | |
| 11. py/uria | pus in the urine | |

WR  S
12. urin/ary      pertaining to urine

WR  S
13. glycos/uria   sugar in the urine

WR  S
14. meat/al       pertaining to the meatus

P  S(WR)
15. dys/ uria     difficult or painful urination

## Exercise 24

| 1. noct/uria | 6. azot/uria | 11. an/uria |
|---|---|---|
| 2. olig/uria | 7. urin/ary | 12. glycos/uria |
| 3. py/uria | 8. hemat/uria | 13. dys/uria |
| 4. ur/ologist | 9. ur/ology | 14. albumin/uria |
| 5. poly/uria | 10. di/ur/esis | 15. meat/al |

## Exercise 25

Spelling exercise; *see* text, p. 174.

## Exercise 26

| 1. urinal | 11. stricture |
|---|---|
| 2. fulguratioin | 12. lithotrite |
| 3. hemodialysis | 13. diuretic |
| 4. distended | 14. resectoscope |
| 5. urinalysis | 15. enuresis |
| 6. catheter | 16. micturate |
| 7. incontinence | 17. specific gravity |
| 8. urinary catheterization | 18. urodynamics |
| 9. peritoneal dialysis | 19. renal transplant |
| 10. evacuate waste material | |

## Exercise 27A

1. e   3. f   5. j   7. c   9. g
2. h   4. a   6. d   8. i

## Exercise 27B

1. c   3. i   5. k   7. d   9. g
2. a   4. f   6. b   8. j   10. e

## Exercise 28

Spelling exercise; *see* text, p. 180.

## Exercise 29

| 1. nephroptosis | 4. polyuria | 7. cystogram |
|---|---|---|
| 2. ureterolithiasis | 5. nephropexy | 8. enuresis |
| 3. pyelogram | 6. urinary suppression | 9. urinary tract infection |

## Exercise 30

| | | | | | |
|---|---|---|---|---|---|
| 1. cystoscopy | | 3. pyelitis | | 5. uremia | |
| 2. anuria | | 4. nephroma | | 6. ureterocele | |

## Exercise 31

1. excessive fat in the blood
2. below-normal amount of glucose in the blood
3. condition of white nail
4. pertaining to the nerves and skin
5. incision of a tumor
6. record of sound
7. pain in the body
8. study of hair

# Answers

```
U R I N O _ _ _ _ T _ H _ _ _ _ _ _
_ _ _ _ _ N _ G L O M E R U L O _ _
_ _ S O N O _ L _ M _ M _ _ _ _ _ _
T _ _ _ C _ Y _ O _ A _ _ _ _ _ U _
R _ _ _ T _ C _ _ _ T _ _ _ _ _ R _
A L B U M I N O _ _ _ O L I G O _ _
C _ R _ _ _ S _ _ H _ I _ _ _ _ _ _
H _ V E S I C O _ C Y S T O _ _ _ _
E _ T _ _ _ A _ D _ H _ _ _ _ _ _ _
L _ H _ N _ Z _ R _ O _ _ _ _ _ _ _
O _ U R E T E R O _ O _ _ V _ _ _ _
_ _ O _ _ P _ T _ _ P _ E _ _ _ _ _
_ _ H _ _ H _ O _ _ Y _ N _ _ _ _ _
_ _ E _ _ R _ _ _ R E N O _ _ _ _ _
_ _ M E A T O _ _ _ L _ _ _ _ _ _ _
_ _ O _ _ _ G L Y C O _ _ _ _ _ _ _
```

# 6

# Male Reproductive System

## Objectives

Upon completion of this chapter you will be able to:

1. Define the anatomical terms of the male reproductive system.

2. Write the definitions of the word parts included in this chapter.

3. Build, analyze, define, pronounce, and spell the diagnostic terms related to the male reproductive system.

4. Define, pronounce, and spell other diagnostic terms related to the male reproductive system.

5. Build, analyze, define, pronounce, and spell the surgical terms related to the male reproductive system.

6. Define, pronounce, and spell other surgical terms related to the male reproductive system.

7. Build, analyze, define, pronounce, and spell additional terms related to the male reproductive system.

8. Define, pronounce, and spell the other additional terms related to the male reproductive system.

## Objective 1    DEFINE THE ANATOMICAL TERMS OF THE MALE REPRODUCTIVE SYSTEM.

## Anatomical Terms

The function of the male reproductive system is to produce sperm, the male reproductive cell, and to secrete the hormone testosterone.

### ORGANS OF THE MALE REPRODUCTIVE SYSTEM (Figure 6-1)

1.  testis, or testicle (*pl.* testes, or testicles). . . . . . . . . . . .  Main male sex organs, oval-shaped and enclosed in a sac called the *scrotum*. The testes produce spermatozoa (sperm cells) and the hormone testosterone.

    a.  seminiferous tubules. . . . . . . . . . .  Coiled tubes within the testes where the sperm have their beginning.

> **Testicle** is derived from the Latin **testis**, meaning **witness**. By Roman law a man could not vote or act as a witness until he could prove that he had testicles.

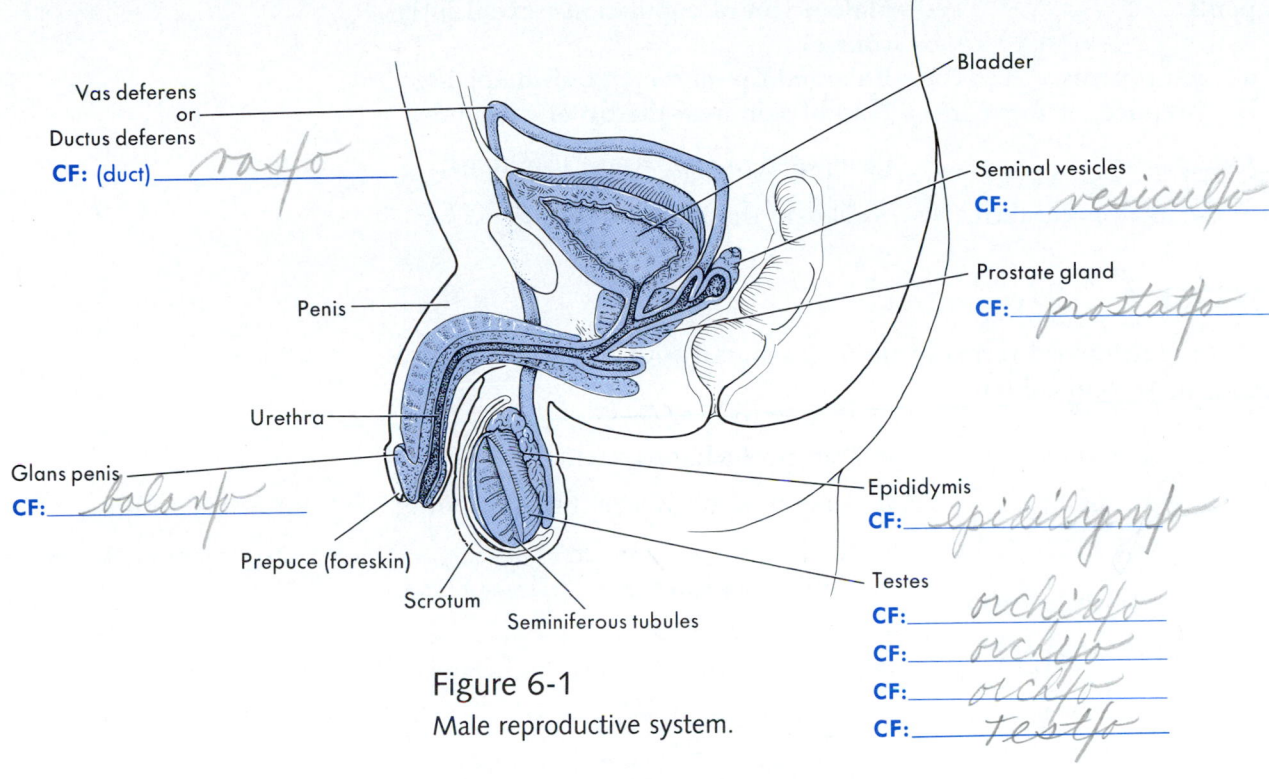

Vas deferens
or
Ductus deferens
**CF:** (duct) _rasfo_

Penis

Urethra

Glans penis
**CF:** _balanfo_

Prepuce (foreskin)

Scrotum

Seminiferous tubules

Bladder

Seminal vesicles
**CF:** _vesiculo_

Prostate gland
**CF:** _prostatfo_

Epididymis
**CF:** _epididymfo_

Testes
**CF:** _orchifo_
**CF:** _orchfo_
**CF:** _orcfo_
**CF:** _testfo_

**Figure 6-1**
Male reproductive system.

b.  epididymis . . . . . . . .    Coiled, 20-foot (6 m) tube atop the testes that carry the mature sperm up to
other tubes, or ducts, called the *vas deferens.*

2.  vas deferens or ductus
deferens . . . . . . . . . . . . .    Duct carrying the sperm into the urethra. (The urethra also connects with the
urinary bladder and carries urine to the
outside of the body.) A circular muscle
constricts during intercourse to prevent
urination.

3.  seminal vesicles . . . . . . .    Glands located at the base of the bladder that open into the vas deferens. The
glands secrete a thick fluid, which forms
a part of the semen.

4.  prostate gland . . . . . . . .    Encircles the upper end of the urethra.
The prostate gland secretes a fluid that
aids in the movement of sperm and ejaculation.

5.  scrotum . . . . . . . . . . . .    Sac suspended on both sides of and just
behind the penis. The testes within are
suspended by the *spermatic cord,* which is
comprised of veins, arteries, nerves, and
the vas deferens.

> **Prostate** is derived from the Greek **pro,** meaning **before,** and **statis,** meaning **standing** or **sitting.** Anatomically it is the gland standing before the bladder.

6.  penis . . . . . . . . . . . . . . . .  Male organ of copulation (sexual intercourse).
    a.   glans penis . . . . . . . .   Enlarged tip on the end of the penis.
    b.   prepuce, or foreskin .   Fold of skin near the tip of the penis.

7.  semen . . . . . . . . . . . . . . . .  Composed of sperm and secretions.

Learn the anatomical terms by completing the following exercises.

## EXERCISE 1

Match the anatomical terms in the first column with the correct definitions in the second column.

_c_   1. epididymis

_i_   2. glans penis

_e_   3. penis

_j_   4. prepuce, or foreskin

_f_   5. prostate gland

_a_   6. scrotum

_k_   7. semen

_g_   8. seminal vesicles

_b_   9. seminiferous tubules

_l_   10. spermatic cord

_h_   11. testes

_d_   12. vas deferens

a. sac in which the testes are suspended

b. area in testes where the sperm originate

c. tube atop testes that carries sperm to the vas deferens

d. duct that carries sperm to urethra

e. male organ of copulation

f. encircles upper end of urethra

g. glands that open into the vas deferens

h. main male sex organs

i. large tip at end of male organ of copulation

j. fold of skin at tip of penis

k. composed of sperm and secretions

l. suspends testes in scrotum

m. engorgement of blood

Place a check mark (√) in the box to indicate that you have completed Objective 1

☐ **DEFINE THE ANATOMICAL TERMS RELATED TO THE MALE REPRODUCTIVE SYSTEM.**

THE DEFINITIONS OF THE WORD PARTS INCLUDED IN THIS CHAPTER.

# Objective 2 WRITE THE DEFINITIONS OF THE WORD PARTS INCLUDED IN THIS CHAPTER.

## Male Reproductive System Word Parts

Study the word parts and their definitions listed as follows. Learning will be made easier by completing the exercises that follow.

| COMBINING FORM | DEFINITION |
|---|---|
| 1. balan/o . . . . . . . . . . . . . . | glans penis |
| 2. epididym/o . . . . . . . . . . . | epididymis |
| 3. orchid/o, orchi/o, orch/o, test/o . . . . . . . . . . . . . . . . | testis, testicle |
| 4. prostat/o . . . . . . . . . . . . . | prostate gland |
| 5. vas/o . . . . . . . . . . . . . . . . | vessel, duct |
| 6. vesicul/o . . . . . . . . . . . . . | seminal vesicles |

Learn the anatomical locations and definitions of the combining forms.

### EXERCISE 2

Write the combining forms in the spaces marked **CF** on the diagram in Figure 6-1, p. 191.

### EXERCISE 3

Write the definitions of the following combining forms.

1. test/o _____ *testis, testicle*
2. vas/o _____ *vessel, duct*
3. balan/o _____ *glans penis*
4. prostat/o _____ *prostate gland*
5. orch/o _____ *testis, testicle*
6. vesicul/o _____ *seminal vesicles*
7. orchi/o _____ *testis, testicle*
8. epididym/o _____ *epididymis*
9. orchid/o _____ *testis, testicle*

## EXERCISE 4

Write the combining form for each of the following.

1. vessel, duct _____vas/o_____

2. prostate gland _____prostat/o_____

3. glans penis _____balan/o_____

4. seminal vesicles _____vesicul/o_____

5. epididymis _____epididym/o_____

6. testicle, or testes

   a. _____test/o_____

   b. _____orchid/o_____

   c. _____orchi/o_____

   d. _____orch/o_____

# Related Word Parts

| COMBINING FORM | DEFINITION |
|---|---|
| 1.  andr/o . . . . . . . . . . . . . . . | male |
| 2.  sperm/o, spermat/o . . . . . . | spermatozoon (*pl.* spermatozoa), or sperm (Figure 6-2) |

Learn the related combining forms by completing the following exercises.

## EXERCISE 5

Write the definitions of the following combining forms.

1. sperm/o _____spermatozoon or sperm_____

2. andr/o _____male_____

3. spermat/o _____spermatozoon or sperm_____

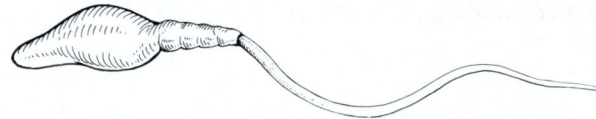

Figure 6-2

Spermatozoon, or sperm. In normal ejaculation there may be as many as 300 million to 500 million sperm.

## EXERCISE 6

Write the combining form for each of the following.

1. sperm      a. _____ *spermo* _____

               b. _____ *spermato* _____

2. male           _____ *andro* _____

# Prefix and Suffix

| PREFIX | DEFINITION |
|---|---|
| trans- . . . . . . . . . . . . . . . . . . | through, across, beyond |

| SUFFIX | DEFINITION |
|---|---|
| -ism . . . . . . . . . . . . . . . . . . . | state of |

## EXERCISE 7

Write the definitions for the prefix and the suffix.

1. -ism _____ *state of* _____

2. trans- _____ *through, across, beyond* _____

Place a check mark (√) in the box to indicate that you have completed Objective 2.

☐   **WRITE THE DEFINITIONS OF THE WORD PARTS INCLUDED IN THIS CHAPTER.**

# Medical Terms

The terms you need to learn to complete this chapter are listed as follows. Now that you know the meaning of the word parts, the exercises found at the end of the list will assist you to learn the definition and the spelling of each word.

# Objective 3   BUILD, ANALYZE, DEFINE, PRONOUNCE, AND SPELL THE DIAGNOSTIC TERMS RELATED TO THE MALE REPRODUCTIVE SYSTEM.

# Diagnostic Terms

| TERM (built from word parts) | DEFINITION |
|---|---|
| 1. anorchism. . . . . . . . . . . (an-OR-kizm) | state of absence of testis (unilaterally or bilaterally) |
| 2. balanitis . . . . . . . . . . . (*bal*-a-NĪ-tis) | inflammation of the glans penis |

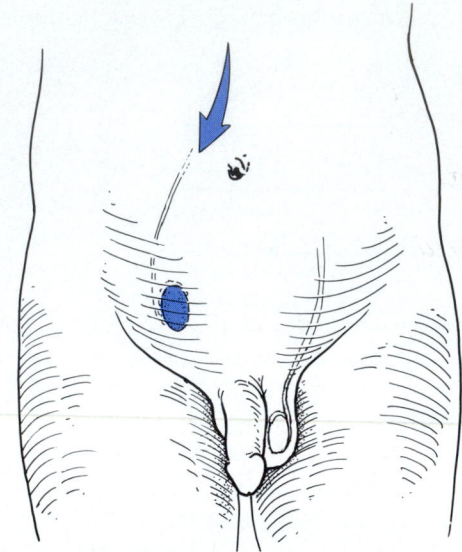

Figure 6-3

Cryptorchidism. Arrow shows path the testis takes in its descent to scrotal sac before birth.

3. balanocele . . . . . . . . . .
(BAL-a-nō-sēl)

protrusion of the glans penis (through the prepuce rupture)

4. balanorrhea . . . . . . . . .
(*bal*-a-nō-RĒ-a)

excessive discharge from the glans penis

5. benign prostatic hypertrophy (BPH) . . . . . . . .
(bē-NĪN) (pros-TAT-ik) (hī-PER-trō-fē)

pertaining to excessive development of the prostate gland

6. cryptorchidism . . . . . . .
(kript-OR-kid-izm)

state of hidden testes (NOTE: During fetal development, testes are located in the abdominal area near the kidneys. Before birth they move down into the scrotal sac. Failure to do so results in cryptorchidism, or undescended testicles.) (Figure 6-3)

7. epididymitis . . . . . . . . .
(*ep*-i-*did*-i-MĪ-tis)

inflammation of the epididymis

8. orchiepididymitis . . . . . .
(*or*-kē-ep-i-did-i-MĪ-tis)

inflammation of the testes and epididymis

9. orchitis, or orchiditis
(or-KĪ-tis) (or-ki-DĪ-tis)
or testitis (tes-TĪ-tis) . . . . .
(NOTE: The *i* from *orchi* is dropped.)

inflammation of the testes or testicles.

10. **prostatitis** . . . . . . . . . . .   inflammation of the prostate gland
    (pros-ta-TĪ-tis)

11. **prostatocystitis** . . . . . . . .   inflammation of the prostate gland and
    (pros-*ta*-tō-sis-TĪ-tis)              **the bladder**

12. **prostatolith** . . . . . . . . . .   stone in the prostate
    (*pros*-TAT-ō-lith)

13. **prostatorrhea** . . . . . . . .      excessive discharge from the prostate
    (pros-*tat*-ōr-RĒ-a)

14. **prostatovesiculitis** . . . . .      inflammation of the prostate gland and
    (*pros*-ta-tō-ves-*ik*-ū-LĪ-tis)       **seminal vesicles**

Practice saying each of these terms aloud. To assist you in pronunciation,
obtain the audiotape designed for use with this text. Learn the definitions
and spellings of the diagnostic terms by completing the following exercises.

## EXERCISE 8

Analyze and define the following medical terms.

1. prostatolith ___stone in the prostate___

2. balanitis ___inflamation of the glans penis___

3. orchitis, orchiditis, or testitis ___inflamatin of the testis or testicles___

4. prostatovesiculitis ___inflamation of the prostate gland + seminal vesicles___

5. prostatocystitis ___inflamation of the prostate gland + the bladder___

6. orchiepididymitis ___inflamatin of the testes + epididymis___

7. prostatorrhea ___excessive discharge from the prostate___

8. epididymitis ___inflamation of the epididymis___

9. benign prostatic hypertrophy ___pertaining to excessive development of the prostate gland___

10. balanocele ___protrusion of the glans penis___

11. cryptorchidism ___state of hidden testes___

12. balanorrhea ___excessive discharge from the glans penis___

13. prostatitis ___inflamation of the prostate gland___

14. anorchism ___state of absence of testis___

## EXERCISE 9

Build medical terms for the following definitions by using the word parts you have learned.

1. inflammation of the prostate gland and urinary
   bladder

   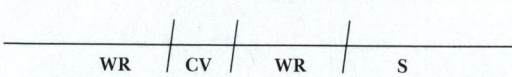
   WR    CV    WR    S

2. stone in the prostate

   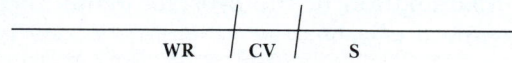
   WR    CV    S

3. inflammation of the testes

   a.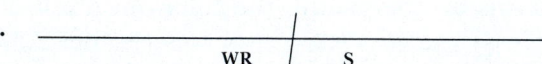
      WR    S

   b.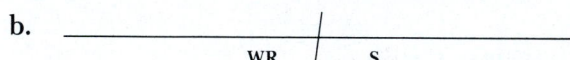
      WR    S

   c.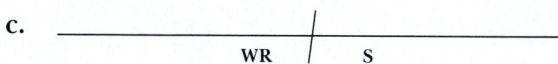
      WR    S

4. pertaining to the non-
   malignant, excessive development of the prostate
   gland

   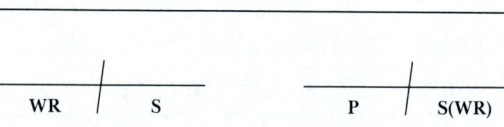
   WR    S         P    S(WR)

5. state of hidden testes

   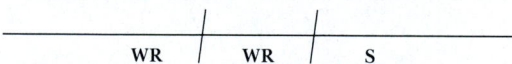
   WR    WR    S

6. inflammation of the prostate and seminal vesicles

   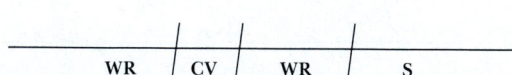
   WR    CV    WR    S

7. state of absence of testis

   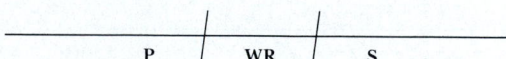
   P    WR    S

8. protrusion of the glans
   penis

   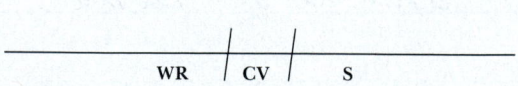
   WR    CV    S

9. inflammation of the prostate gland

_____ / _____
WR          S

10. inflammation of the testes and the epididymis

_____ / _____ / _____
WR          WR          S

11. excessive discharge from the glans penis

_____ / _____
WR          S

12. inflammation of the epididymis

_____ / _____
WR          S

13. inflammation of the glans penis

_____ / _____
WR          S

14. excessive discharge from the prostate

_____ / _____
WR          S

## EXERCISE 10

Spell each of the diagnostic terms. Have someone dictate the terms on pp. 195 to 197 to you or say the words into a tape recorder; then spell the words from your recording as often as necessary. Think about the word parts before attempting to write the word. Study any you have spelled incorrectly.

1. _____        8. _____
2. _____        9. _____
3. _____        10. _____
4. _____        11. _____
5. _____        12. _____
6. _____        13. _____
7. _____        14. _____

Place a check mark (√) in the box to indicate that you have completed Objective 3.

☐ **BUILD, ANALYZE, DEFINE, PRONOUNCE, AND SPELL THE DIAGNOSTIC TERMS RELATED TO THE MALE REPRODUCTIVE SYSTEM.**

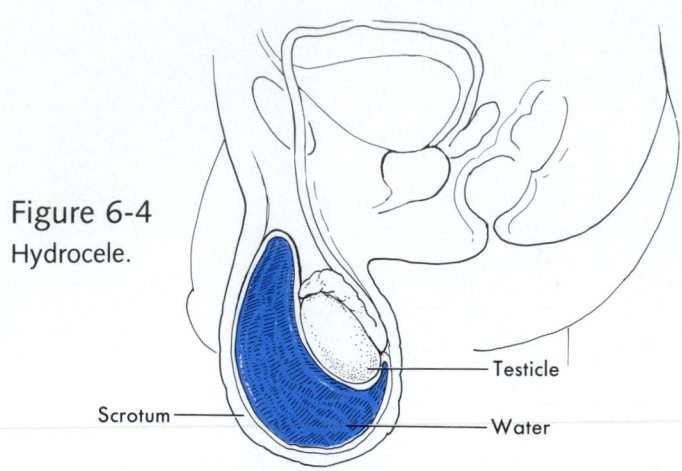

Figure 6-4
Hydrocele.

Testicle

Scrotum

Water

# Objective 4 DEFINE, PRONOUNCE, AND SPELL OTHER DIAGNOSTIC TERMS RELATED TO THE MALE REPRODUCTIVE SYSTEM.

## Other Diagnostic Terms

| TERM | DEFINITION |
|---|---|
| 1. hydrocele . . . . . . . . . . . . . .<br>(HĪ-drō-sēl) | scrotal swelling caused by a collection of fluid along the tubes within the testes (Figure 6-4) |
| 2. impotent. . . . . . . . . . . . .<br>(IM-pō-tent) | lack of power to have an erection or to copulate |

Prostatic cancer is the second most common cause of cancer deaths among American males and typically occurs after the age of 40 (Figure 6-5). Procedures used for detecting prostatic cancer are:

1. **digital rectal exam,** whereby the physician inserts a finger into the rectum and feels for the size and shape of the prostate gland through the rectal wall.

2. **prostatic specific antigen (PSA),** a blood test that measures the level of prostate specific antigen. Elevated test results may indicate the presence of prostatic cancer.

3. **transrectal ultrasound** uses sound waves obtained by placing a probe into the rectum. The sound waves are transformed into an image of the prostate gland on a television screen where it is viewed by the physician.

Treatment includes prostatectomy and/or radiation therapy. For stage C prostatic cancer, hormonal therapy may be used or an orchidectomy may be performed to reduce the production of testosterone, which fuels the prostatic cancer.

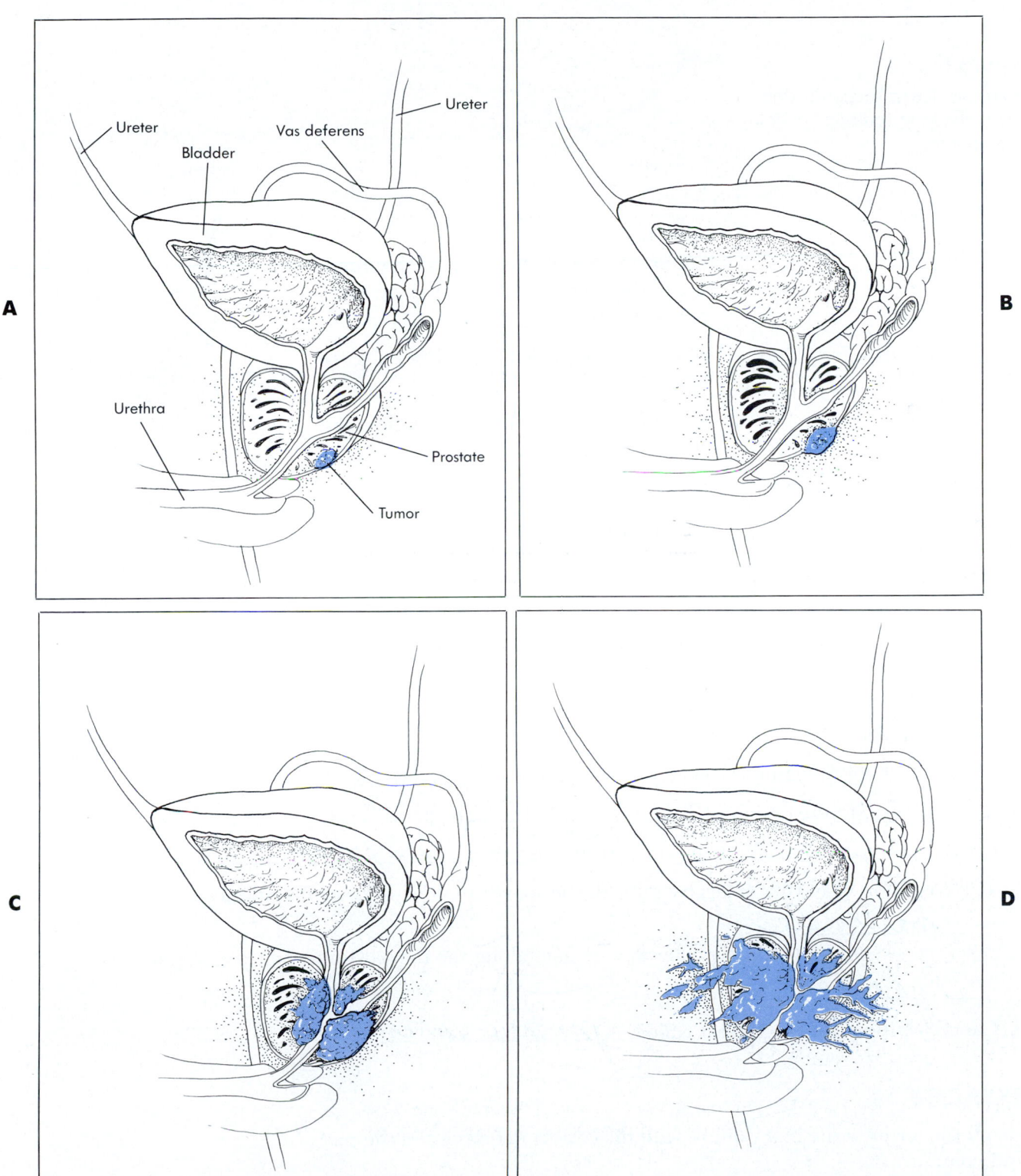

**A**

Ureter
Bladder
Vas deferens
Ureter

Urethra

Prostate

Tumor

**B**

**C**

**D**

Figure 6-5A,B,C,D
Four stages of prostatic cancer.
Courtesy artist May S. Cheney.

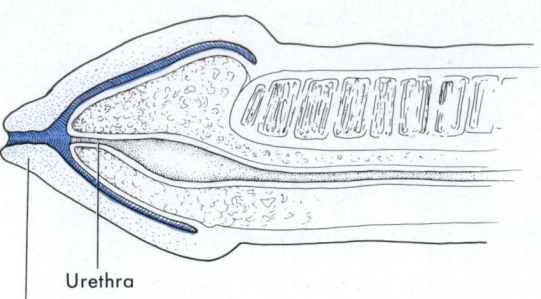

**Figure 6-6**
Phimosis. Cross section of the penis showing foreskin covering the opening.

Urethra

Skin over opening

3.  phimosis . . . . . . . . . . . . .     narrowing, or constriction, of the open-
    (fī-MŌ-sis)                            ing of the prepuce (foreskin) of the glans
                                           penis (Figure 6-6)

4.  prostatic cancer . . . . . . .     cancer of the prostate gland (see Figure
    (prō-STAT-ik)( CAN-ser)            6-5)

5.  varicocele . . . . . . . . . . . .     enlarged veins of the spermatic cord
    (VĂR-i-kō-sēl)                         (Figure 6-7)

6.  testicular carcinoma . . . . .     cancer of the testicles
    (tes-TIK-ū-ler) (*kar*-sin-Ō-ma)

Practice saying each of these terms aloud. To assist you in pronunciation, obtain the audiotape designed for use with this text. Learn the definitions and spellings of the other diagnostic terms by completing the following exercises.

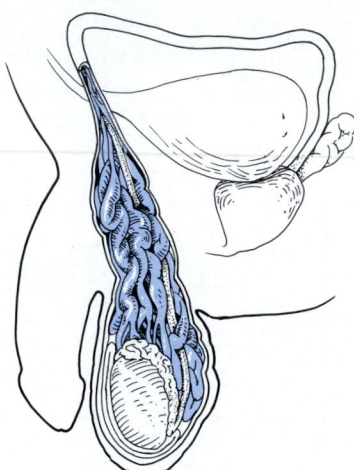

**Figure 6-7**
Varicocele.

## EXERCISE 11

Fill in the blanks with the correct terms.

1.  Another way of referring to cancer of the testicles is ___Testicular carcinoma___

2.  A constriction of the opening of the foreskin of the glans penis is called ___phimosis___ .

3.  Lack of power to copulate or have an erection is called ___impotence___ .

4.  The condition of having enlarged veins of the spermatic cord is known medically as a ___varicocele___ .

5.  A scrotal swelling caused by a collection of fluid along the tubes within the testes is called a ___hydrocele___ .

6.  Cancer of the prostate gland is called ___prostatic cancer___ .

## EXERCISE 12

Match the terms in the first column with the correct definitions in the second column.

___a___ 1. varicocele
___c___ 2. phimosis
___e___ 3. testicular carcinoma

a.  scrotal swelling caused by a collection of fluid along the tubes within the testes

_b_ 4. impotent

_a_ 5. hydrocele

_f_ 6. prostatic cancer

b. lack of power to have an erection or to copulate

c. narrowed opening of the foreskin of the glans penis

d. enlarged veins of the spermatic cord

e. cancer of the testicles

f. cancer of the prostate gland

g. stone in the prostate gland

## EXERCISE 13

Spell each of the other diagnostic terms. Have someone dictate the terms on pp. 200 to 202 to you or say the words into a tape recorder; then spell the words from your recording as often as necessary. Study any you have spelled incorrectly.

1. _____  4. _____

2. _____  5. _____

3. _____  6. _____

Place a check mark (√) in the box to indicate that you have completed Objective 4.

☐ DEFINE, PRONOUNCE, AND SPELL OTHER DIAGNOSTIC TERMS RELATED TO THE MALE REPRODUCTIVE SYSTEM.

# Objective 5  BUILD, ANALYZE, DEFINE, PRONOUNCE, AND SPELL SURGICAL TERMS RELATED TO THE MALE REPRODUCTIVE SYSTEM.

## Surgical Terms

**TERM**
(built from word parts)

**DEFINITION**

1. balanoplasty . . . . . . . . . . (BAL-a-nō-plas-tē) — surgical repair of the glans penis

2. epididymectomy . . . . . . . (ep-i-did-i-MEK-tō-mē) — excision or surgical removal of the epididymis

3. orchioplasty . . . . . . . . . (ŌR-kē-ō-plas-tē) — surgical repair of a testis

4. orchidectomy, orchiectomy . . . . . . . . . . . . . . (ōr-kid-EK-tō-mē) (or-kē-EK-tō-mē) — excision or surgical removal of one or both testes (castration)

5. orchidopexy, or orchiopexy . . . . . . . . . . . . . . (ŌR-kid-ō-pek-sē) (ŌR-kē-ō-pek-sē) — surgical fixation of a testicle (performed to bring undescended testicle[s] into the scrotum)

## Figure 6-8

Transurethral resection. Resecto-scope is inserted through the urethra to the prostate. The end of the instrument is equipped to remove small pieces of enlarged prostate gland.

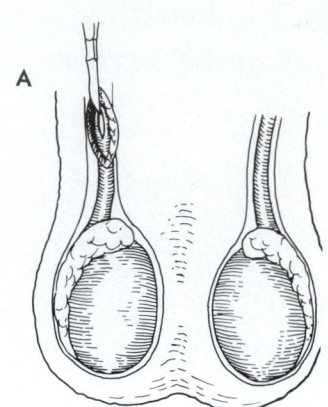

A

6. orchidotomy, or orchiotomy .............. (ōr-kid-OT-ō-mē),   (ōr-kē-OT-ō-mē)      incision into a testis

7. prostatectomy........ (*pros*-ta-TEK-tō-mē)      excision of the prostate gland

8. prostatocystotomy ..... (pros-*tat*-ō-sis-TOT-ō-mē)      incision into the bladder and prostate

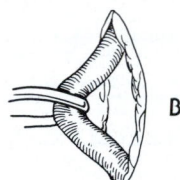

B

9. prostatolithotomy...... (pros-*tat*-ō-li-THOT-ō-mē)      incision into the prostate gland to remove a stone

10. prostatovesiculectomy .. (*pros*-tat-ō-ves-*ik*-ū-LEK-tō-mē)      excision of the prostate gland and seminal vesicles

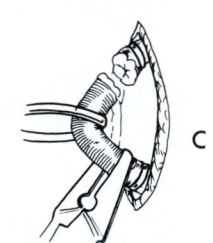

C

11. transurethral   resection (TUR or TURP)....... (*trans*-ū-RĒ-thral)   (re-SEK-shun)      resection (cutting back) through the urethra (performed through the urethra to cut back with a resectoscope the prostate gland when the enlargement of the gland interferes with normal urination) (Figure 6-8)

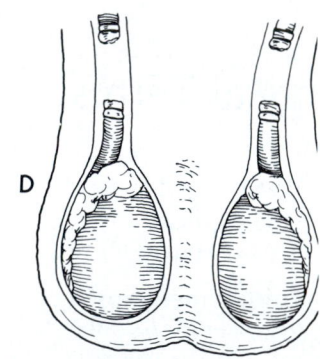

D

12. vasectomy............ (va-SEK-tō-mē)      excision of a duct (actually the surgical removal of a portion of the vas, or ductus deferens; male sterilization) (Figure 6-9)

## Figure 6-9

Vasectomy. **A,** Incision is made into the covering of the vas. **B,** Vas is exposed. **C,** Segment of vas is excised. **D,** Vas is replaced and skin is sutured.

From Phipps WJ, Long BC, and Woods NF: *Shafer's medical-surgical nursing,* ed 7, St. Louis, 1980, Mosby.

13. vasovasostomy ........ (*vas*-ō-va-SOS-tō-mē)      creation of artificial openings between ducts (the severed ends of the vas deferens are reconnected to restore fertility in males who have had a vasectomy)

14. vesiculectomy........ (ve-*sik*-ū-LEK-tō-mē)      excision of the seminal vesicle(s)

## EXERCISE 14

Analyze and define the following surgical terms.

1. vasectomy _____


2. prostatocystotomy _____


3. orchidotomy, or orchiotomy _____


4. epididymectomy _____


5. orchidopexy, or orchiopexy _____


6. prostatovesiculectomy _____


7. orchioplasty _____


8. vesiculectomy _____


9. prostatectomy _____


10. balanoplasty _____


11. transurethral resection _____


12. vasovasostomy _____


13. orchidectomy, or orchiectomy _____


14. prostatolithotomy _____

## EXERCISE 15

Build surgical terms for the following definitions by using the word parts
you have learned.

1. excision of one or both
   testes      a. <u>                        /               </u>
   <br>                                                  WR     S

                          b. <u>                        /               </u>
   <br>                                                  WR     S

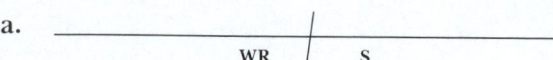

2. surgical repair of the
   glans penis

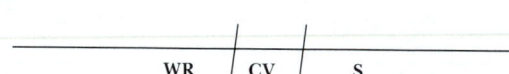

   WR   CV   S

3. incision into the bladder
   and prostate

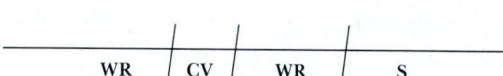

   WR   CV   WR   S

4. excision of the seminal
   vesicle(s)

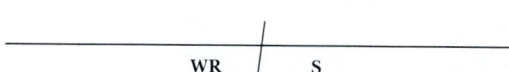

   WR   S

5. incision into the prostate
   gland to remove a stone

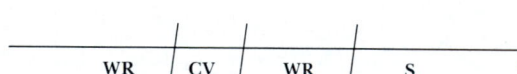

   WR   CV   WR   S

6. incision into a testis    a.

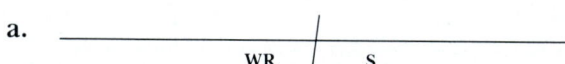

   WR   S

                          b. <u>                        /               </u>
   <br>                                                  WR     S

7. cutting back (the prostate)
   through the urethra

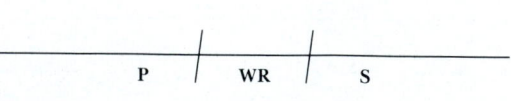

   P   WR   S

8. excision of the epididymis

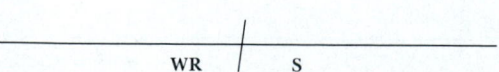

   WR   S

9. surgical repair of a testis

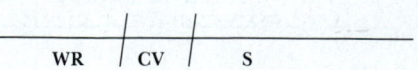

   WR   CV   S

10. excision of the prostate
    gland

    _____ / _____
            WR        S

11. excision of a duct (surgi-
    cal removal of a portion
    of the vas, or ductus def-
    erens)

    _____ / _____
            WR        S

12. excision of the prostate
    gland and seminal vesicles.

    _____ / _____ / _____ / _____
      WR    CV    WR    S

13. surgical fixation of a tes-
    ticle          a.

    _____ / _____ / _____
      WR    CV    S

                   b.

    _____ / _____ / _____
      WR    CV    S

14. creation of artificial
    openings between the
    severed ends of the vas
    deferens

    _____ / _____ / _____ / _____
      WR    CV    WR    S

# EXERCISE 16

Spell each of the surgical terms. Have someone dictate the words on pp.
203 and 204 to you or say the words into a tape recorder; then spell the
words from your recording as often as necessary. Think about the word
parts before attempting to write the word. Study any you have spelled
incorrectly.

1. _____    8. _____

2. _____    9. _____

3. _____    10. _____

4. _____    11. _____

5. _____    12. _____

6. _____    13. _____

7. _____    14. _____

Place a check mark (√) in the box to indicate that you have completed Objective 5.

☐ BUILD, ANALYZE, DEFINE, PRONOUNCE, AND SPELL THE SURGICAL TERMS RELATED TO THE MALE
REPRODUCTIVE SYSTEM.

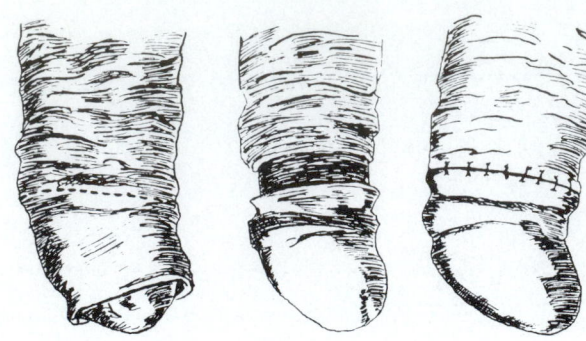

Figure 6-10

Circumcision.

From Meeker MH and Rothrock JC: *Alexander's care of the patient in surgery*, ed 9, St. Louis, 1991, Mosby.

# Objective 6   DEFINE, PRONOUNCE, AND SPELL OTHER SURGICAL TERMS RELATED TO THE MALE REPRODUCTIVE SYSTEM.

## Other Surgical Terms

| TERM | DEFINITION |
| --- | --- |
| 1. circumcision.......... (*ser*-kum-SI-zhun) | surgical removal of the prepuce (foreskin) (Figure 6-10) |
| 2. hydrocelectomy........ (hī-drō-sē-LEK-tō-mē) | surgical removal of a hydrocele |
| 3. penile implant......... (PĒ-nīl) | surgical implantation of a penile prosthesis to correct erectile dysfunction |
| 4. perineal prostatectomy... (*pār*-i-NĒ-al)   (*pros*-ta-TEK-tō-mē) | excision of the prostate gland through an incision in the floor of the pelvis |
| 5. suprapubic prostatectomy (*sū*-pra-PŪ-bik)   (*pros*-ta-TEK-tō-mē) | surgical excision of the prostate gland through an incision made above the pubic bone |

Practice saying each of these terms aloud. To assist you in pronunciation, obtain the audiotape designed for use with this text. Learn the definitions and spellings of the other surgical terms by completing the following exercises.

## EXERCISE 17

Fill in the blanks with the correct terms.

1. Two surgeries performed to remove the prostate gland are the **a.** _perineal prostatectomy_ and the **b.** _suprapubic_ _prostalectomy_.
2. The surgical procedure performed to remove the prepuce is called a(n) _circumcision_.
3. The surgery performed to correct erectile dysfunction of the penis is _penile_ _implant_.
4. Surgical removal of a hydrocele is _hydrocelectomy_

## EXERCISE 18

Spell each of the other surgical terms. Have someone dictate the terms on p. 208 to you or say the words into a tape recorder; then spell the words from your recording as often as necessary. Think about the word parts before attempting to write the words. Study any you have spelled incorrectly.

1. _____     4. _____

2. _____     5. _____

3. _____

Place a check mark (√) in the box to indicate that you have completed Objective 6.

☐ **DEFINE, PRONOUNCE, AND SPELL OTHER SURGICAL TERMS RELATED TO THE MALE REPRODUCTIVE SYSTEM.**

# Objective 7  BUILD, ANALYZE, DEFINE, PRONOUNCE, AND SPELL ADDITIONAL TERMS RELATED TO THE MALE REPRODUCTIVE SYSTEM.

## Additional Terms

| TERM (built from word parts) | DEFINITION |
|---|---|
| 1. andropathy........... (an-DROP-a-thē) | diseases of the male (that is, peculiar to the male, such as testitis) |
| 2. aspermia............. (a-SPER-mē-a) | condition of the absence of sperm |
| 3. oligospermia ......... (ol-i-gō-SPER-mē-a) | condition of scanty sperm (in the semen) |
| 4. spermatolysis ......... (sper-ma-TOL-i-sis) | dissolution (destruction) of sperm |

Practice saying each of these terms aloud. To assist you in pronunciation, obtain the audiotape designed for use with this text. Learn the definitions and spellings of the additional terms by completing the following exercises.

## EXERCISE 19

Analyze and define the following terms.

1. oligospermia _____

2. andropathy _____

3. spermatolysis _____

4. aspermia _____

## EXERCISE 20

Build medical terms for the following definitions by using the word parts you have learned.

1. dissolution (destruction) of
   sperm

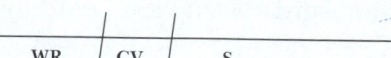

   | WR | CV | S |

2. diseases of the male

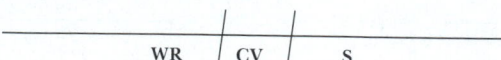

   | WR | CV | S |

3. condition of the absence
   of sperm

   | P | WR | S |

4. condition of scanty sperm

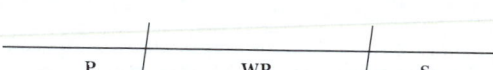

   | WR | CV | WR | S |

## EXERCISE 21

Spell each of the additional terms. Have someone dictate the terms on p. 209 to you or say the words into a tape recorder; then spell the words from your recording as often as necessary. Think about the word parts before attempting to write the word. Study any you have spelled incorrectly.

1. _____    3. _____

2. _____    4. _____

Place a check mark (√) in the box to indicate that you have completed Objective 7.

☐ **BUILD, ANALYZE, DEFINE, PRONOUNCE, AND SPELL ADDITIONAL TERMS RELATED TO THE MALE REPRODUCTIVE SYSTEM.**

# Objective 8    DEFINE, PRONOUNCE, AND SPELL THE OTHER ADDITIONAL TERMS RELATED TO THE MALE REPRODUCTIVE SYSTEM.

# Other Additional Terms

**TERM**

**DEFINITION**

1. acquired immune defi-
   ciency syndrome (AIDS).

   a disease that affects the body's immune system, transmitted by exchange of body fluid during the sexual act, by reuse of

> The sexually transmitted diseases may occur in both the male and female.

contaminated needles, or by using contaminated blood transfusions

2. artificial insemination . . (ar-ti-FISH-al) (in-sem-i-NĀ-shun)
   introduction of semen into vagina by artificial means

3. chlamydia . . . . . . . . . . (klah-MID-ē-a)
   one of the more prevalent sexually transmitted diseases. A bacterium, *Chlamydia trachomatis,* is the causative agent.

4. coitus . . . . . . . . . . . . . (KO-i-tus)
   sexual intercourse between male and female

5. condom . . . . . . . . . . . . (KON-dum)
   cover for the penis worn during coitus

6. ejaculation . . . . . . . . . . (ē-jak-ū-LĀ-shun)
   ejection of semen and fluids (seminal fluids) from the male urethra

7. genitalia (genitals) . . . . . (*jen*-i-TĀ-lē-a)
   reproductive organs (male or female)

8. gonads . . . . . . . . . . . . (GŌ-nads)
   male and female sex glands

9. genital herpes . . . . . . . . (JEN-i-tal) (HER-pēz)
   sexually transmitted disease caused by herpes virus hominis type II

10. gonorrhea . . . . . . . . . . . (gon-or-RĒ-a)
    contagious, inflammatory sexually transmitted disease caused by a bacterial organism that affects the mucous membranes of the genitourinary system

11. heterosexual . . . . . . . . . (*het*-er-ō-SEKS-shū-al)
    person who is attracted to a member of the opposite sex

12. homosexual . . . . . . . . . (*hō*-mō-SEKS-shū-al)
    person who is attracted to a member of the same sex

13. orgasm . . . . . . . . . . . . . (ŌR-gazm)
    climax of sexual stimulation

14. prosthesis . . . . . . . . . . . (PROS-thē-sis)
    an artificial replacement of an absent body part

15. puberty . . . . . . . . . . . . (PU-ber-tē)
    period when secondary sex characteristics develop and the ability to reproduce sexually begins

16. sexually transmitted disease (STD) . . . . . . . . . .
    disease, such as syphilis, gonorrhea, and genital herpes, transmitted during sexual intercourse (also called *venereal disease*)

17. sterilization . . . . . . . . . (*stār*-il-i-ZĀ-shun)
    process that renders an individual unable to produce offspring

**Venereal** is derived from Venus, the goddess of love. In ancient times it was noted that the disease was part of the misfortunes of love.

18.  syphilis . . . . . . . . . . . . .     infectious sexually trasmitted disease
     (SĬF-i-lis)                           having lesions that can affect any organ
                                           or tissue; a syphilitic mother may trans-
                                           mit the disease to her unborn infant,
                                           since the causative organism is able to
                                           pass through the placenta

19.  trichomoniasis . . . . . . .          a sexually transmitted disease caused by
     (trik-ō-mŏ-NĬ-a-sis)                  a one-cell organism, *Trichomonas*. It in-
                                           fects the genitourinary tract. (More com-
                                           mon in females.)

Practice saying each of these terms. To assist you in pronunciation, obtain the audiotape designed for use with this text. Learn the definitions
and spellings of the other additional terms by completing the following
exercises.

## EXERCISE 22

Write the definitions of the following terms.

1.  puberty _____

2.  orgasm _____

3.  gonorrhea _____

4.  homosexual _____

5.  coitus _____

6.  genital herpes _____

7.  heterosexual _____

8.  syphilis _____

9.  ejaculation _____

10. gonads _____

11. STD _____

12. genitalia _____

13. sterilization _____

14. acquired immune deficiency syndrome _____

15. trichomoniasis _____

16. artificial insemination _____

17. chlamydia _____

18. condom _____

19. prosthesis _____

## EXERCISE 23A

Match the terms in the first column with the correct definitions in the second column.

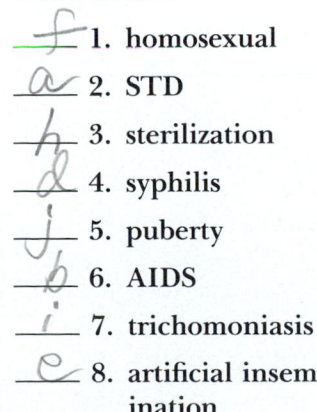

_g_ 1. coitus

_e_ 2. ejaculation

_h_ 3. genitalia

_a_ 4. gonads

_d_ 5. genital herpes

_i_ 6. gonorrhea

_c_ 7. heterosexual

_b_ 8. orgasm

_j_ 9. condom

_f_ 10. prosthesis

a. male and female sex glands

b. climax of sexual stimulation

c. one who is attracted to a member of the opposite sex

d. STD caused by herpes virus hominus type II

e. ejection of semen

f. an artificial replacement of an absent body part

g. sexual intercourse between man and woman

h. reproductive organs

i. contagious and inflammatory STD

j. cover for the penis worn during coitus

k. one who is attracted to a member of the same sex

## EXERCISE 23B

Match the terms in the first column with the correct definitions in the second column.

_f_ 1. homosexual

_a_ 2. STD

_h_ 3. sterilization

_d_ 4. syphilis

_j_ 5. puberty

_b_ 6. AIDS

_i_ 7. trichomoniasis

_e_ 8. artificial insemination

_g_ 9. chlamydia

a. abbreviation for diseases such as syphilis, gonorrhea, and genital herpes,

b. a disease that affects the body's immune system

c. one who is attracted to members of the opposite sex

d. sexually transmitted disease that can affect any organ and that can be transmitted to an unborn infant

e. introduction of semen into vagina by means other than intercourse

   **f.** one who is attracted to members of the same sex

   **g.** a prevalent STD caused by a bacterium, *C. trachomatis*

   **h.** process rendering an individual unable to produce offspring

   **i.** an STD caused by a one-cell organism, *Trichomonas*

   **j.** period when the ability to sexually reproduce begins

## EXERCISE 24

Spell each of the other additional terms. Have someone dictate the terms on pp. 210 to 212 to you or say the words into a tape recorder; then spell the words from your recording as often as necessary. Study any you have spelled incorrectly.

1. _____   11. _____

2. _____   12. _____

3. _____   13. _____

4. _____   14. _____

5. _____   15. _____

6. _____   16. _____

7. _____   17. _____

8. _____   18. _____

9. _____   19. _____

10. _____

Place a check mark (√) in the box to indicate that you have completed Objective 8.

☐ **DEFINE, PRONOUNCE, AND SPELL THE OTHER ADDITIONAL TERMS RELATED TO THE MALE REPRODUCTIVE SYSTEM.**

**Case History:** This male patient is a retired Asian attorney who came into the emergency room at 3 AM complaining that he was in great pain and could not urinate. He had not been seen by a physician for several years but claimed to be in good health otherwise, except for a "little high blood pressure."

**Source of Information:** The patient and his wife, both of whom are reliable historians.

CHIEF COMPLAINT: The patient is a 75-year-old retired gentleman who comes into the emergency room complaining of lower abdominal pain and inability to void for the past 12 hours.

PAST MEDICAL HISTORY: States that several years ago he was told that he had high blood pressure and to decrease his sodium intake and lose fifteen pounds, which he has done. Otherwise unremarkable.

PRESENT ILLNESS: The patient complains of urinary frequency, nocturia × 2, hesitancy, intermittency, diminished force and caliber of the urinary stream, a sensation of not having completely emptied the bladder and postvoid dribbling. Earlier today, he had hematuria at the end of urination. Abdomen shows a suprapubic mass approximately three fingerbreadths below the umbilicus, dull to percussion and slightly tender.

IMPRESSION: Urinary bladder distention secondary to urinary outlet obstruction, probably secondary to benign prostatic hypertrophy.

PLAN:
1. Indwelling Foley catheter for relief of urine obstruction.
2. Urology consult.

# EXERCISE 25

To test your understanding of the terms introduced in this chapter, circle the words that correctly complete the sentences. The italicized words refer to the correct answer.

1. A *discharge from the glans penis* is referred to medically as (balanorrhagia, balanorrhea, balanorrhaphy).
2. The surgical procedure circumcision is the removal of the *foreskin,* or (glans penis, testes, prepuce).
3. *A person who is attracted to a member of the opposite sex* is (heterosexual, homosexual).
4. The patient had a diagnosis of (aspermia, phimosis, impotence), or a *narrowing of the opening of the prepuce.*
5. The *operation for the surgical fixation of the testicle* is (orchidopexy, orchidotomy, orchioplasty).
6. An *artificial replacement* or (condom, prosthesis, artificial insemination) is used to correct erectile dysfunction of the penis.

## EXERCISE 26

Unscramble the following mixed-up terms. The words on the left indicate the word root in each of the following.

1. vas deferens (duct)

    / / / / / / / / /
    t e s y a c v o m

2. glans penis

    / / / / /n/ / /r/ / /
    r a a l b e a r h o n

3. male

    / / / / / /p/ / / / /
    t o d y h a a p r n

4. prostate gland

    / / / / / / / /i/ / /
    a t t i s s t o i p r

5. testes

    / / / / / / / /t/ / /
    m o o c h y d o r i t

## EXERCISE 27

The following words did not appear in this chapter but are composed of word parts studied in this or the previous chapters. Find their definitions by translating the word parts literally.

1. **autophagia** (aw-tō-FĀ-jē-a) _____

2. **bronchadenitis** (bron-kad-e-NĪ-tis) _____

3. **necrospermia** (nek-rō-SPERM-ē-a) _____

4. **paracystitis** (pār-a-sis-TĪ-tis) _____

5. **pathosis** (pa-THŌ-sis) _____

6. **polyhydruria** (pol-ē-hī-DRŪ-rē-a) _____

7. **trachelomyitis** (trā-ke-lō-mī-YĪ-tis) _____

8. **viscerogenic** (vis-er-ō-JEN-ik) _____

# SUFFIXES—CHAPTERS 2 TO 4—CROSSWORD PUZZLE

## Across Clues

2. instrument to measure
4. substance or agent that produces or causes
6. flow, excessive discharge
8. measurement
9. disease
10. plastic or surgical repair
11. sudden involuntary muscle contraction
13. pertaining to sound or voice
14. instrument to cut
15. instrument for visual examination
17. pertaining to
18. cell
19. pertaining to carbon dioxide
22. producing, originating, causing
24. chest
25. cut into or incision
28. abnormal condition
30. rapid flow of blood
32. inflammation
34. creation of an artificial opening
36. one who studies and practices
37. control, stop
38. process of recording

## Down Clues

1. softening
3. a stretching out, dilatation
5. diseased state, abnormal state
7. surgical removal
10. eating, swallowing
11. visual examination
12. breathing
13. surgical fixation, suspension
16. hernia or protrusion
17. blood condition
19. surgical puncture to aspirate fluid
20. pain
21. constriction, narrowing
23. tumor, swelling
26. resembling
27. record, x-ray film
29. pertaining to
31. pertaining to
33. study of
34. pertaining to oxygen
35. to view

# COMBINING FORMS—CHAPTERS 2 TO 4—CROSSWORD PUZZLE

## Across Clues
1. skin
5. dry
8. grapelike clusters
10. cause
11. pus
12. oxygen
14. tissue
17. epithelium
19. life
20. internal organs
22. dust
23. blood
24. flesh, connective tissue
30. wrinkles
32. disease
33. hair
34. fungus

## Down Clues
2. imperfect, incomplete
3. nail
4. straight
5. yellow
6. nose
7. cell
9. lung
13. tumor
15. oil
16. twisted chains
18. breath
21. body
25. hidden
26. horny tissue, hard
27. other
28. self
29. fat
31. muscle

# Summary

Can you build, analyze, define, pronounce, and spell the following terms *built from word parts?*  yes □  no □

## DIAGNOSTIC

anorchism
(an-OR-kizm)

balanitis
(*bal*-a-NĪ-tis)

balanocele
(BAL-a-nō-sēl)

balanorrhea
(*bal*-a-nō-RĒ-a)

benign prostatic
hypertrophy (BPH)
(bē-NĪN) (pros-TAT-ik)
(hī-PER-trō-fē)

cryptorchidism
(kript-OR-kid-izm)

epididymitis
(*ep*-i-*did*-i-MĪ-tis)

orchiepididymitis
(or-kē-ep-i-did-i-MĪ-tis)

orchitis, or orchiditis
(or-KĪ-tis) (or-ki-DĪ-tis)
or testitis (tes-TĪ-tis)

prostatitis
(pros-ta-TĪ-tis)

prostatocystitis
(pros-*ta*-tō-sis-TĪ-tis)

prostatolith
(*pros*-TAT-ō-lith)

prostatorrhea
(pros-*tat*-ōr-RĒ-a)

prostatovesiculitis
(*pros*-ta-tō-ves-*ik*-ū-LĪ-tis)

## SURGICAL

balanoplasty
(BAL-a-nō-plas-tē)

epididymectomy
(*ep*-i-*did*-i-MEK-tō-mē)

orchioplasty
(OR-kē-ō-plas-tē)

orchidectomy,
orchiectomy
(*ōr*-kid-EK-tō-*mē*)
(or-kē-EK-tō-mē)

orchidopexy, or
orchiopexy
(ŌR-kid-ō-pek-sē),
(ŌR-kē-ō-pek-sē)

orchidotomy, or
orchiotomy
(ōr-kid-OT-ō-mē),
(ōr-kē-OT-ō-mē)

prostatectomy
(*pros*-ta-TEK-tō-mē)

prostatocystotomy
(pros-*tat*-ō-sis-TOT-ō-mē)

prostatolithotomy
(pros-*tat*-ō-li-THOT-ō-mē)

prostatovesiculectomy
(*pros*-tat-ō-ves-*ik*-ū-LEK-
tō-mē)

transurethral resection
(*trans*-ū-RĒ-thral)
(re-SEK-shun)

vasectomy
(va-SEK-tō-mē)

vasovasostomy
(*vas*-ō-va-SOS-tō-mē)

vesiculectomy
(ve-*sik*-ū-LEK-tō-mē)

## ADDITIONAL

andropathy
(an-DROP-a-thē)

aspermia
(a-SPER-mē-a)

oligospermia
(*ol*-i-gō-SPER-mē-a)

spermatolysis
(sper-ma-TOL-i-sis)

# Summary

Can you define, pronounce, and spell the following terms *not built from word parts?*   yes ☐   no ☐

| DIAGNOSTIC | SURGICAL | ADDITIONAL | |
|---|---|---|---|
| hydrocele<br>(HĪ-drō-sēl) | circumcision<br>(*ser*-kum-SI-zhun) | acquired immune<br>deficiency syndrome | heterosexual<br>(*het*-er-ō-SEKS-shū-al) |
| impotent<br>(IM-pō-tent) | hydrocelectomy<br>(hī-drō-sē-LEK-tō-mē) | artificial insemination<br>(ar-ti-FISH-al)<br>(in-sem-i-NĀ-shun) | homosexual<br>(*hō*-mō-SEKS-shū-al) |
| phimosis<br>(fī-MŌ-sis) | penile implant<br>(PE-nīl) | chlamydia<br>(klah-MID-ē-a) | orgasm<br>(ŌR-gazm) |
| prostatic cancer<br>(pros-TAT-ik) | perineal prostatectomy<br>(*pār*-i-NĒ-al)<br>(*pros*-ta-TEK-tō-mē) | coitus<br>(KO-i-tus) | prosthesis<br>(PROS-thē-sis) |
| varicocele<br>(VĀR-i-kō-sēl) | suprapubic<br>prostatectomy<br>(*sū*-pra-PŪ-bik)<br>(*pros*-ta-TEK-tō-mē) | condom<br>(KON-dum) | puberty<br>(PU-ber-tē) |
| testicular carcinoma<br>(tes-TIK-ū-ler)<br>(*kar*-sin-Ō-ma) | | ejaculation<br>(ē-jak-ū-LĀ-shun) | sexually transmitted<br>disease |
| | | genitalia<br>(*jen*-i-TĀ-lē-a) | sterilization<br>(*stār*-il-i-ZĀ-shun) |
| | | gonads<br>(GŌ-nads) | syphilis<br>(SĪF-i-lis) |
| | | genital herpes<br>(JEN-i-tal) (HER-pēz) | trichomoniasis<br>(trik-o-mō-NĪ-a-sis) |
| | | gonorrhea<br>(gon-or-RĒ-a) | |

# Answers

## Exercise 1

| | | | |
|---|---|---|---|
| 1. c | 4. j | 7. k | 10. l |
| 2. i | 5. f | 8. g | 11. h |
| 3. e | 6. a | 9. b | 12. d |

## Exercise 4

| | |
|---|---|
| 1. vas/o | 6. a. orchid/o |
| 2. prostat/o | b. orchi/o |
| 3. balan/o | c. orch/o |
| 4. vesicul/o | d. test/o |
| 5. epididym/o | |

## Exercise 2

**Figure 6-1**

Vas, or ductus,
  deferens: vas/o
Glans penis: balan/o
Seminal vesicles: vesicul/o
Prostate gland: prostat/o

Epididymis: epididym/o
Testes: orchid/o, orchi/o,
  orch/o, test/o

## Exercise 5

1. sperm   2. male   3. sperm

## Exercise 6

1. a. sperm/o      2. andr/o
   b. spermat/o

## Exercise 3

| | |
|---|---|
| 1. testes, or testicles | 6. seminal vesicles |
| 2. vessel, duct | 7. testes, or testicles |
| 3. glans penis | 8. epididymis |
| 4. prostate gland | 9. testes, or testicles |
| 5. testes, or testicles | |

## Exercise 7

1. state of   2. through, across, beyond

## Exercise 8

1. prostat/ o /lith
   (WR CV WR / CF)
   stone in the prostate

2. balan/itis
   (WR S)
   inflammation of the glans penis

3. a. orch/itis
      (WR S)
   b. orchid/itis
      (WR S)
   c. test/itis
      (WR S)
   inflammation of the testes

4. prostat/ o /vesicul/itis
   (WR CV WR S / CF)
   inflammation of the prostate gland and seminal vesicles

5. prostat/ o /cyst/itis
   (WR CV WR S / CF)
   inflammation of the prostate gland and bladder

6. orchi/epididym/itis
   (WR WR S)
   inflammation of the testes and epididymis

7. prostat/orrhea
   (WR S)
   excessive discharge from the prostate

8. epididym/itis
   (WR S)
   inflammation of the epididymis

9. benign prostat/ic hyper/trophy
   (WR S P S(WR))
   pertaining to excessive development of the prostate gland

10. balan/ o /cele
    (WR CV S / CF)
    protrusion of the glans penis

11. crypt/orchid/ism
    (WR WR S)
    state of hidden testes

12. balan/orrhea
    (WR S)
    excessive discharge from the glans penis

13. prostat/itis
    (WR S)
    inflammation of the prostate

14. an/orch/ism
    (P WR S)
    state of absence of testis

## Exercise 9

1. prostat/o/cyst/itis
2. prostat/o/lith
3. a. orchid/itis
   b. orch/itis
   c. test/itis
4. benign prostat/ic hyper/trophy
5. crypt/orchid/ism
6. prostat/o/vesicul/itis
7. an/orch/ism
8. balan/o/cele
9. prostat/itis
10. orchi/epididym/itis
11. balan/orrhea
12. epididym/itis
13. balan/itis
14. prostat/orrhea

## Exercise 10

Spelling exercise; *see* text, p. 199.

## Exercise 11

1. testicular carcinoma
2. phimosis
3. impotence
4. varicocele
5. hydrocele
6. prostatic cancer

## Exercise 12

1. d  2. c  3. e  4. b  5. a  6. f

## Exercise 13

Spelling exercise; *see* text, p. 203.

## Exercise 14

1. vas/ectomy
   (WR S)
   excision of a duct

2. prostat/ o /cyst/otomy
   (WR CV WR S / CF)
   incision into the bladder and prostate gland

3. orchid/otomy
   (WR S)
   orchi/otomy
   (WR S)
   incision into a testis

4. epididym/ectomy
   (WR S)
   excision of the epididymis

5. orchid/ o /pexy
   (WR CV S / CF)
   orchi/ o /pexy
   (WR CV S / CF)
   surgical fixation of a testicle

6. prostat/ o /vesicul/ectomy
   (WR CV WR S / CF)
   excision of the prostate gland and seminal vesicles

7. orchi/ o /plasty
   (WR CV S / CF)
   surgical repair of testis

8. vesicul/ectomy
   (WR S)
   excision of the seminal vesicle(s)

9. prostat/ectomy
   (WR S)
   excision of the prostate gland

10. balan/ o /plasty
    (WR CV S / CF)
    surgical repair of the glans penis

11. trans/urethr/al resection
    (P WR S)
    resection (of prostate gland) through the urethra

12. vas/ o /vas/ostomy
    (WR CV WR S / CF)
    creation of artificial opening between ducts

WR    S
13. orchid/ectomy            excision of one or both
                                          testes

WR    S
orchi/ectomy

WR  CV WR    S
14. prostat/ o /lith/otomy      incision into prostate
        CF                                  gland to remove a
                                              stone

## Exercise 15

1. a. orchid/ectomy        8. epididym/ectomy
   b. orchi/ectomy         9. orchi/o/plasty
2. balan/o/plasty         10. prostat/ectomy
3. prostat/o/cyst/otomy   11. vas/ectomy
4. vesicul/ectomy         12. prostat/o/vesicul/
5. prostat/o/lith/otomy       ectomy
6. a. orchid/otomy        13. a. orchid/o/pexy
   b. orchi/otomy             b. orchi/o/pexy
7. trans/urethr/al resec-  14. vas/o/vas/ostomy
   tion

## Exercise 16

Spelling exercise; *see* text, p. 207.

## Exercise 17

1. a. suprapubic prostatectomy, b. perineal
   prostatectomy
2. circumcision
3. penile implant
4. hydrocelectomy

## Exercise 18

Spelling exercise; *see* text, p. 209.

## Exercise 19

WR CV  WR   S
1. olig/ o /sperm/ia     condition of scanty sperm
    CF

WR  CV   S
2. andr/ o /pathy        diseases of the male
    CF

WR    CV  S
3. spermat/ o /lysis     dissolution of sperm
      CF

P  WR   S
4. a/sperm/ia            condition of the absence
                             of sperm

## Exercise 20

1. spermat/o/lysis    3. a/sperm/ia
2. andr/o/pathy       4. olig/o/sperm/ia

## Exercise 21

Spelling exercise; *see* text, p. 210.

## Exercise 22

1. period when secondary sex characteristics develop
   and the ability to sexually reproduce begins
2. climax of sexual stimulation
3. contagious, inflammatory venereal disease
4. person who is attracted to a member of the same sex
5. sexual intercourse between male and female
6. contagious venereal disease caused by the herpes
   hominis type II virus
7. person who is attracted to a member of the opposite
   sex
8. infectious venereal disease having lesions that can
   affect any organ or tissue
9. ejection of semen and fluids from the male urethra
10. male and female sex glands
11. sexually transmitted disease; a disease transmitted
    during sexual intercourse
12. reproductive organs
13. process rendering an individual unable to produce
    offspring
14. a disease transmitted by exchange of body fluids
    during the sexual act, reuse of contaminated needles,
    and contaminated blood transfusions that affect the
    body's immune system
15. sexually transmitted disease caused by a one-cell
    organism, *Trichomonas*. It affects the genitourinary
    system
16. introduction of semen into vagina by artificial means
17. one of the more prevalent STD's. Caused by
    bacterium, *Chlamydia trachomatis*
18. a cover for the penis worn during coitus
19. an artificial replacement of an absent body part

## Exercise 23A

1. g   3. h   5. d   7. c   9. j
2. e   4. a   6. i   8. b   10. f

## Exercise 23B

1. f   3. h   5. j   7. i   9. g
2. a   4. d   6. b   8. e

## Exercise 24

Spelling exercise; *see* text, p. 214.

## Exercise 25

1. balanorrhea   3. heterosexual   5. orchidopexy
2. prepuce       4. phimosis       6. prosthesis

## Exercise 26

1. vasectomy    3. andropathy    5. orchidotomy
2. balanorrhea    4. prostatitis

## Exercise 27

1. eating or biting self
2. inflammation of the bronchial glands
3. pertaining to dead sperm
4. inflammation around the (urinary) bladder
5. abnormal condition of disease
6. excessive amount of water in the urine
7. inflammation of the muscles of the neck
8. originating in the internal organs

# Answers: Suffixes—Chapters 2 to 4

| M |   |   | M | E | T | E | R |   | G | E | N |   |   |   |   |   | I |
|---|---|---|---|---|---|---|---|---|---|---|---|---|---|---|---|---|---|
| A |   |   |   | C |   |   |   |   |   |   |   | O | R | R | H | E | A |
| L |   | M | E | T | R | Y |   | P | A | T | H | Y |   |   |   | C |   |
| A |   |   |   | A |   |   |   |   |   |   | P | L | A | S | T | Y |
| C |   | S | P | A | S | M |   |   |   | P |   | H |   |   |   | O |
| I |   | C |   | I |   |   | P | H | O | N | I | A |   | T | O | M | E |
| A |   | O |   | S | C | O | P | E |   | E |   | G |   |   |   | Y |
|   |   | P |   | E |   |   | E |   | X |   | A |   | I |   |   |   |
|   |   | Y |   | E | A | L |   | C | Y | T | E |   | C | A | P | N | I | A |
|   |   |   | M |   | E |   |   |   |   |   | E |   |   |   | L |
| S |   |   | I |   |   | G | E | N | I | C |   | N |   | O |   | G |
| T | H | O | R | A | X |   |   |   |   | O | T | O | M | Y |   | I |
| E |   |   |   |   |   |   |   |   |   | E |   | A |   | A |
| N | O |   |   |   | G |   |   |   |   | S |   |   |   |   |
| O | S | I | S |   | O |   | O | R | R | H | A | G | I | A |   | I | T | I | S |
| S |   | D |   |   | U |   | A |   |   | R |   | S |   | O |
| I |   |   |   | O | S | T | O | M | Y |   |   |   | L |
| S |   |   | X |   | P |   |   |   |   | O | L | O | G | I | S | T |
|   |   |   | I |   | S | T | A | S | I | S |   | G |
|   | G | R | A | P | H | Y |   |   |   |   |   | Y |

# Answers: Combining Forms—Chapters 2 to 4

| C | U | T | A | N | E | O |   | O |   |   | X | E | R | O |   |   | N |
|---|---|---|---|---|---|---|---|---|---|---|---|---|---|---|---|---|---|
|   |   | T |   | N |   | R |   | A |   |   |   |   |   |   |   | A |
|   |   | E |   | Y |   | T |   | N |   |   |   | C |   | S |
|   |   | L |   | C |   | H | S | T | A | P | H | Y | L | O |
| E | T | I | O |   | H |   | O |   | H | U |   | T |
|   |   | O |   |   |   | P | Y | O |   | L |   | O | X | O |
| H | I | S | T | O |   |   | S |   |   |   | M |   | N |
|   | E |   |   | E | P | I | T | H | E | L | I | O |   | S |   | C |
|   | B |   |   |   | R |   |   |   | N |   | P |   | O |
| B | I | O | V | I | S | C | E | R | O | C | O | N | I | O |
|   |   | O |   | P |   |   |   |   | R |
|   |   | H | E | M | A | T | O | S | A | R | C | O |
| K |   | H |   | A | O |   |   |   | R |   | A |
| E |   | E |   | T |   |   | L |   | Y |   | U |
| R | H | Y | T | I | D | O |   | I |   | P |   | T |
| A |   | E |   |   | M | P | A | T | H | O |
| T | T | R | I | C | H | O | M | Y | C | O | O |
| O |   | O |   |   |   | O |

# 7
# Female Reproductive System

## Objectives

Upon completion of this chapter you will be able to:

1. Define the anatomical terms of the female reproductive system.

2. Write the definitions of the word parts included in this chapter.

3. Build, analyze, define, pronounce, and spell the diagnostic terms related to the female reproductive system.

4. Define, pronounce, and spell other diagnostic terms related to the female reproductive system.

5. Build, analyze, define, pronounce, and spell the surgical terms related to the female reproductive system.

6. Define, pronounce, and spell other surgical terms related to the female reproductive system.

7. Build, analyze, define, pronounce, and spell the diagnostic procedural terms related to the female reproductive system.

8. Build, analyze, define, pronounce, and spell additional terms related to the female reproductive system.

9. Define, pronounce, and spell the other additional terms related to the female reproductive system.

## Objective 1   DEFINE THE ANATOMICAL TERMS OF THE FEMALE REPRODUCTIVE SYSTEM.

## Anatomical Terms

The female reproductive system produces the female sex cells and hormones and also provides for conception and pregnancy.

### INTERNAL ORGANS OF THE FEMALE REPRODUCTIVE SYSTEM

1. ovaries . . . . . . . . . . . . . . .   Pair of almond-shaped organs located in the pelvic cavity. Sex cells are formed in the ovaries (Figure 7-1).

    a.  ovum (*pl.* ova) . . . . . .   female sex cell.

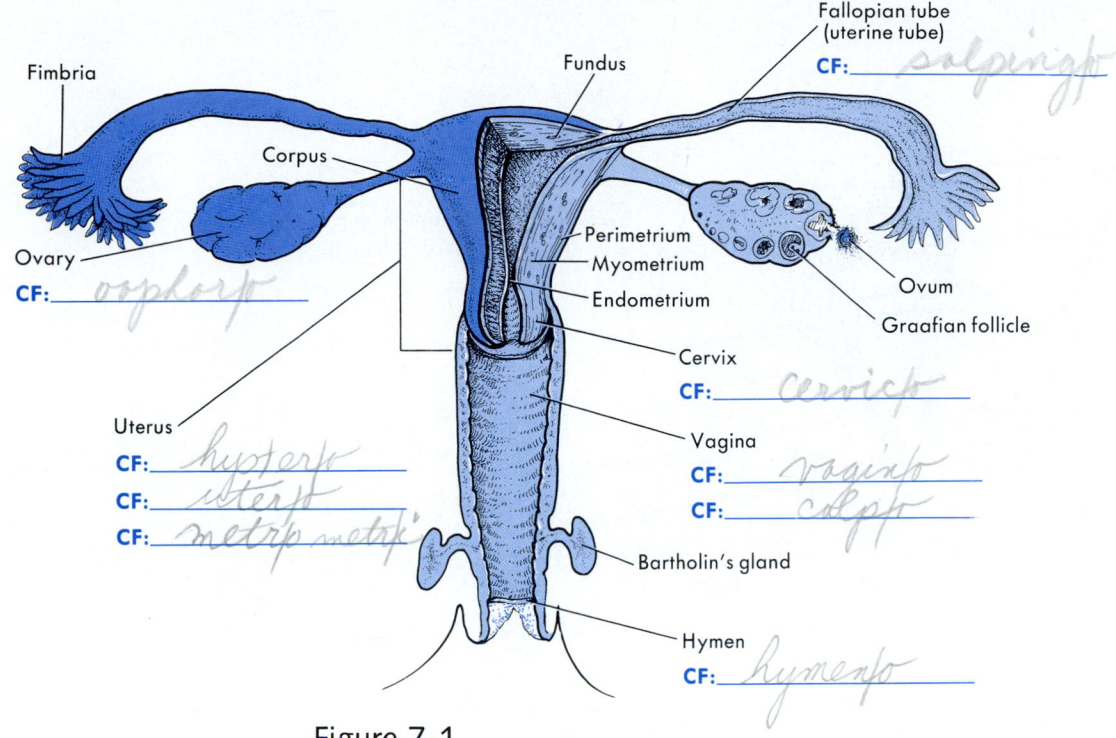

Fimbria

Fundus

Fallopian tube (uterine tube)
**CF:** _salpingo_

Corpus

Ovary
**CF:** _oophoro_

Perimetrium
Myometrium
Endometrium

Ovum

Graafian follicle

Uterus
**CF:** _hystero_
**CF:** _utero_
**CF:** _metro metrio_

Cervix
**CF:** _cervico_

Vagina
**CF:** _vagino_
**CF:** _colpo_

Bartholin's gland

Hymen
**CF:** _hymeno_

**Figure 7-1**

Frontal view of female reproductive system.

|   |   |   |
|---|---|---|
| b. | graafian follicles . . . . | Several thousand microscopic sacs that make up a large portion of the ovaries. Each follicle contains an immature ovum. |
| 2. | fallopian tube or uterine tube . . . . . . . . . . . . . . . | Pair of 5-inch (12 cm) tubes, attached to the uterus, that provide a passageway for the ovum to move from the ovary to the uterus. |
| a. | fimbria (*pl.* fimbriae) . | Fingerlike ends of the fallopian tubes. |
| 3. | uterus . . . . . . . . . . . . . . | Pear-sized and pear-shaped muscular organ that lies in the pelvic cavity except during pregnancy. Its functions are menstruation, pregnancy, and labor (Figure 7-1). |
| a. | endometrium . . . . . . . | Lining of the uterus. |
| b. | myometrium . . . . . . . | Muscular middle layer of the uterus. |
| c. | perimetrium . . . . . . . | Outer thin layer that covers the surface of the uterus. |
| d. | corpus or body . . . . . | Large central portion of the uterus. |
| e. | fundus . . . . . . . . . . . | Rounded upper portion of the uterus. |
| f. | cervix . . . . . . . . . . . . | Narrow lower portion of the uterus. |

The **graafian follicle** is named for a Dutch anatomist named Regnier de Graaf, who discovered the sac in 1672.

The **fallopian tube** was named in honor of Gabriele Fallopius because he described it in his works. Fallopius also gave the **vagina** and the **placenta** their present names.

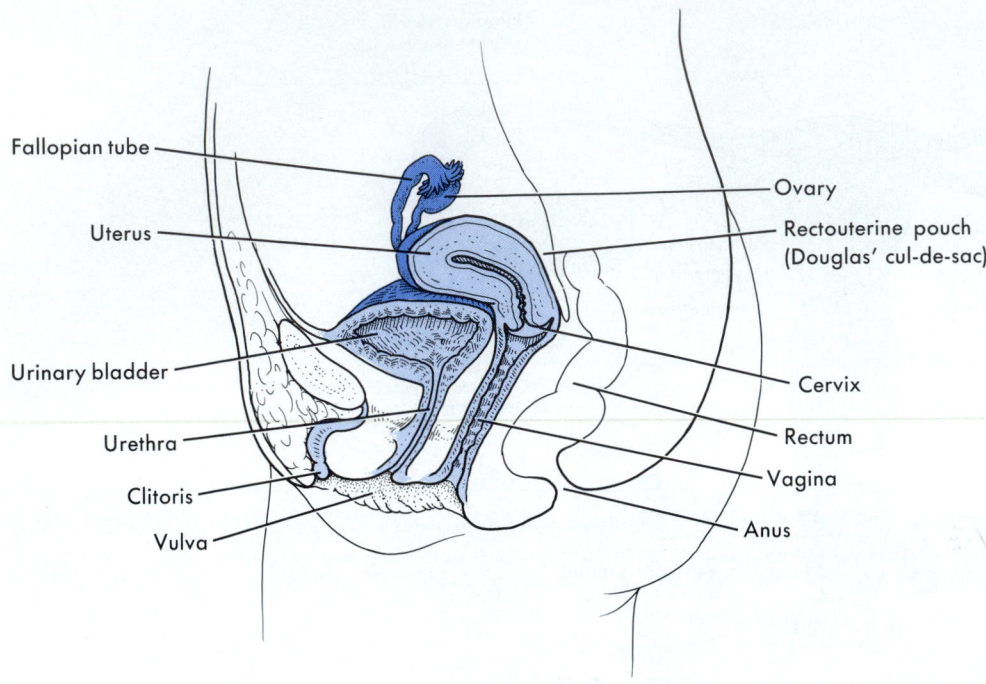

**Figure 7-2**
Side view of female reproductive system.

| | |
|---|---|
| 4. vagina . . . . . . . . . . . . . . | A 3-inch (7-8 cm) tube that connects the uterus to the outside of the body. |
| a. hymen . . . . . . . . . . . | Fold of membrane found near the opening of the vagina. |
| 5. rectouterine pouch (also called Douglas' cul-de-sac) . . . . . . . . . . . . . . . . | Pouch between the posterior wall of the uterus and the anterior wall of the rectum (Figure 7-2). |

## GLANDS OF THE FEMALE REPRODUCTIVE SYSTEM

| | |
|---|---|
| 1. Bartholin's glands . . . . . . | Pair of mucus-producing glands located on each side just above the vaginal opening. |
| 2. mammary glands, or breasts . . . . . . . . . . . . . | Milk-producing glands of the female. Each breast consists of 15 to 20 divisions, or lobes. |
| a. mammary papilla . . . | Breast nipple. |
| b. areola . . . . . . . . . . . | Dark area around the breast nipple. |

**Bartholin's glands** were described by Thomas Bartholinus, a Danish anatomist, in 1675.

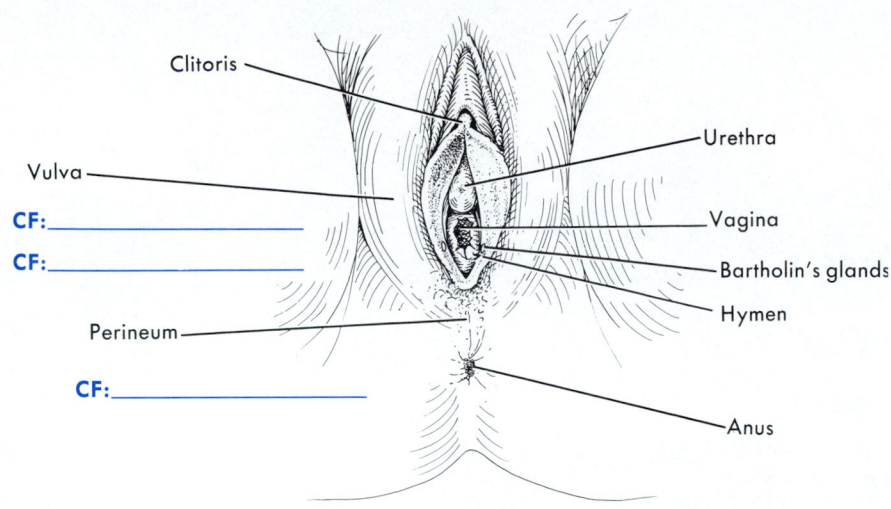

**Figure 7-3**
External female reproductive organs.

## EXTERNAL FEMALE REPRODUCTIVE STRUCTURES

1.  vulva, or external genitals.    Two pairs of lips that surround the va-
                                     gina (Figure 7-3).

    a.  clitoris . . . . . . . . . . .    Highly erogenous erectile body located
                                     anterior to the urethra.

2.  perineum . . . . . . . . . . . .    Pelvic floor in both the male and female.
                                     In women it usually refers to the area be-
                                     tween the vaginal opening and the anus.

Learn the anatomical terms by completing the following exercises.

## EXERCISE 1

Match the terms in the first column with the correct definitions in the second column.

_c_ 1. organ in which sex
         cells are formed

_f_ 2. lower portion of the
         uterus

_g_ 3. lining of the uterus

_b_ 4. upper portion of the
         uterus

_d_ 5. pelvic floor

_e_ 6. ends of fallopian
         tubes

_h_ 7. large central portion
         of the uterus

a.  perimetrium

b.  fundus

c.  ovaries

d.  perineum

e.  fimbriae

f.  cervix

g.  endometrium

h.  corpus

i.  myometrium

j.  ovum

_a_ 8. layer that covers the uterus

_i_ 9. muscle layer of the uterus

## EXERCISE 2

Match the terms in the first column with the correct definitions in the second column.

_b_ 1. connects the uterus to the outside of the body

_c_ 2. located above the vaginal opening

_d_ 3. breast

_k_ 4. female sex cells

_e_ 5. external genitals

_f_ 6. passageway for ovum

_g_ 7. colored area around the nipple

_l_ 8. microscopic sacs in the ovaries

_i_ 9. muscular organ

_j_ 10. nipples

_h_ 11. rectouterine pouch

a. ovary

b. vagina

c. Bartholin's glands

d. mammary gland

e. vulva

f. fallopian tube

g. areola

h. Douglas' cul-de-sac

i. uterus

j. mammary papillae

k. ova

l. graafian follicles

Place a check mark (√) in the box to indicate that you have completed Objective 1.

☐ **DEFINE THE ANATOMICAL TERMS OF THE FEMALE REPRODUCTIVE SYSTEM.**

# Objective 2    WRITE THE DEFINITIONS OF THE WORD PARTS INCLUDED IN THIS CHAPTER.

# Female Reproductive System Word Parts

Study the word parts and their definitions listed as follows. Learning will be made easier by completing the exercises that follow.

| COMBINING FORM | DEFINITION |
|---|---|
| 1. arche/o . . . . . . . . . . . . . | first, beginning |
| 2. cervic/o . . . . . . . . . . . . . | cervix |
| 3. colp/o<br>vagin/o . . . . . . . . . . . . | vagina |

4.  culd/o . . . . . . . . . . . . . .    cul-de-sac

5.  episi/o
    vulv/o . . . . . . . . . . . . . .    vulva

6.  gynec/o
    gyn/o . . . . . . . . . . . . . .    woman

7.  hymen/o . . . . . . . . . . . .    hymen

8.  hyster/o
    metr/o, metr/i
    uter/o . . . . . . . . . . . . . .    uterus
    (NOTE: The combining vowel *i*
    or *o* may be used with metr/.)

9.  mamm/o
    mast/o . . . . . . . . . . . . . .    breast

10. men/o . . . . . . . . . . . . . .    menstruation

11. oophor/o . . . . . . . . . . . .    ovary

12. perine/o . . . . . . . . . . . .    perineum

13. salping/o . . . . . . . . . . . .    fallopian tube (uterine tube)

Learn the anatomical locations and definitions of the combining forms by completing the following exercises.

## EXERCISE 3

Write the combining forms in the spaces provided on the diagrams in Figures 7-1, 7-2, and 7-3, pp. 255 to 257.

## EXERCISE 4

Write the definitions of the following combining forms.

1.  vagin/o _____ *vagina* _____

2.  oophor/o _____ *ovary* _____

3.  metr/o
    metr/i _____ *uterus* _____

4.  uter/o _____ *uterus* _____

5.  hymen/o _____ *hymen* _____

6.  hyster/o _____ *uterus* _____

7.  men/o _____ *menstration* _____

8.  episi/o _____ *vulva* _____

9.  cervic/o _____ *cervix* _____

10. colp/o _____ *vagina* _____

11. gynec/o _____ *woman* _____

12. mamm/o _____ *breast* _____

13. perine/o _____ *perineum* _____

14. salping/o _____ *fallopian tube* _____

15. vulv/o _____ *vulva* _____

16. mast/o _____ *breast* _____

17. arche/o _____ *first, beginning* _____

18. culd/o _____ *culde-sac* _____

19. gyn/o _____ *woman* _____

## EXERCISE 5

Write the combining form for each of the following.

1. vulva        a. _____

            b. _____

2. breast       a. _____

            b. _____

3. menstruation    _____

4. ovary        _____

5. fallopian tube   _____

6. perineum      _____

7. vagina       a. _____

            b. _____

8. uterus       a. _____

            b. _____

            c. _____

9. woman        a. _____

            b. _____

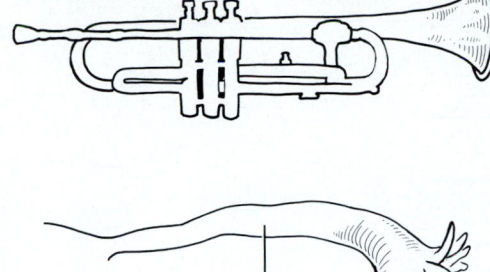

**Figure 7-4**
*Salpinx* is derived from *salpingx*, the Greek term for trumpet. The term was used for the fallopian tubes because of their trumpet-like shape.

Fallopian tube

10. hymen _____

11. cul-de-sac _____

12. cervix _____

13. beginning _____

# Prefix and Suffixes

**PREFIX** **DEFINITION**
1. peri- . . . . . . . . . . . . . . . surrounding (outer)

**SUFFIXES** **DEFINITION**
2. -atresia . . . . . . . . . . . . . absence of a normal body opening; occlusion; closure

3. -ial . . . . . . . . . . . . . . . . pertaining to

4. -salpinx. . . . . . . . . . . . . . fallopian tube (Figure 7-4)
(NOTE: For learning purposes *salpinx* and *atresia* are presented as suffixes.)

**Atresia** literally means no perforation or hole. It is composed of the Greek words **a**, meaning **without**, and **tresis**, meaning **perforation**. The term may be used alone as in "atresia of vagina" or combined with other word parts as in "gynatresia" meaning closure of a part of the female genital tract, usually the vagina.

Learn the suffixes and prefix by completing the following exercises.

## EXERCISE 6

Write the word part for each of the following.

1. fallopian tube _____salpinx_____

2. pertaining to _____ial_____

3. surrounding _____peri_____

4. absence of a normal body opening _____atresia_____

## EXERCISE 7

Write the definitions of the following word parts.

1. -salpinx _____ *fallopian tube* _____

2. peri- _____ *surrounding, outer* _____

3. -ial _____ *pertaining to* _____

4. -atresia _____ *absence of normal body opening* _____

Place a check mark (√) in the box to indicate that you have completed Objective 2.

☐ WRITE THE DEFINITIONS OF THE WORD PARTS INCLUDED IN THIS CHAPTER.

# Medical Terms

The terms you need to complete this chapter are listed as follows. Now that you know the meaning of the word parts, the exercises found at the end of the list will assist you to learn the definition and the spelling of each word.

# Objective 3    BUILD, ANALYZE, DEFINE, PRONOUNCE, AND SPELL THE DIAGNOSTIC TERMS RELATED TO THE FEMALE REPRODUCTIVE SYSTEM.

# Diagnostic Terms

| TERM (built from word parts) | DEFINITION |
|---|---|
| 1. amenorrhea . . . . . . . . . (ā-*men*-ō-RĒ-a) | absence of menstrual discharge (menostasis) |
| 2. Bartholin's adenitis . . . . (BAR-tō-lins) (*ad*-e-NĪ-tis) | inflammation of Bartholin's gland |
| 3. cervicitis . . . . . . . . . . . . (*ser*-vi-SĪ-tis) | inflammation of the cervix |
| 4. colpitis . . . . . . . . . . . . . (kol-PĪ-tis) | inflammation of the vagina |
| 5. dysmenorrhea . . . . . . . . (*dis*-men-ō-RĒ-a) | painful menstrual discharge |
| 6. endocervicitis . . . . . . . . (en-dō-*ser*-vi-SĪ-tis) | inflammation of the inner lining of the cervix |
| 7. endometritis . . . . . . . . . (en-dō-mē-TRĪ-tis) | inflammation of the inner lining of the uterus (endometrium) |
| 8. hematosalpinx . . . . . . . . (*hem*-a-tō-SAL-pinks) | blood in the fallopian tube |

9.  hydrosalpinx . . . . . . . . .    water in the fallopian tube
    (hī-drō-SAL-pinks)

10. hysteratresia . . . . . . . . . .    closure of the uterus (uterine cavity)
    (his-ter-a-TRĒ-zē-a)

11. mastitis . . . . . . . . . . . . .    inflammation of the breast
    (*mas*-TĪ-tis)

12. menometrorrhagia . . . . .    rapid flow of bleeding from the uterus
    (*men*-ō-*met*-rō-RĀ-jē-a)      at and between menstruation

13. metrorrhea . . . . . . . . . . .    excessive discharge from the uterus
    (me-trō-RĒ-a)

14. myometritis . . . . . . . . .    inflammation of the uterine muscle
    (*mī*-o-mē-TRĪ-tis)              (myometrium)

15. oophoritis . . . . . . . . . . .    inflammation of the ovary
    (ō-of-ō-RĪ-tis)

16. perimetritis . . . . . . . . . .    inflammation surrounding (outer layer)
    (*per*-i-mē-TRĪ-tis)            of the uterus (perimetrium)

17. pyosalpinx . . . . . . . . . . .    pus in the fallopian tube
    (pī-o-SAL-pinks)

18. salpingitis . . . . . . . . . . .    inflammation of the fallopian tube (Fig-
    (*sal*-pin-JĪ-tis)              ure 7-5)

19. salpingocele . . . . . . . . .    hernia of the fallopian tube
    (sal-PING-gō-sēl)

20. vulvovaginitis . . . . . . . .    inflammation of the vulva and vagina
    (*vul*-vō-VAJ-i-nī-tis)

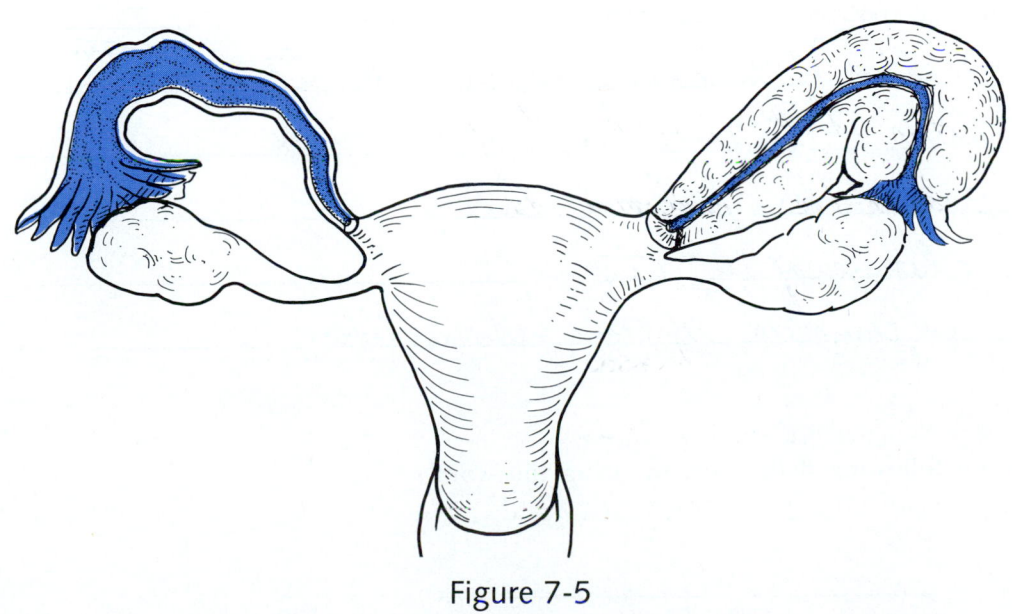

Figure 7-5
Salpingitis.

## EXERCISE 8

Analyze and define the following medical terms.

1. colpitis _inflamation of the vagina_
2. cervicitis _inflamation of the cervix_
3. hydrosalpinx _water in the fallopian tube_
4. hematosalpinx _blood in the fallopian tube_
5. metrorrhea _excessive discharge from the uterus_
6. oophoritis _inflamation of the ovary_
7. (Bartholin's) adenitis _inflamation of Bartholin's glands_
8. vulvovaginitis _inflamation of the vagina + the vulva_
9. salpingocele _hernia of the fallopian tube_
10. menometrorrhagia _rapid flow of bleeding from the uterus at + between menstruation_
11. amenorrhea _absence of menstrual discharge_
12. dysmenorrhea _painful menstrual discharge_
13. mastitis _inflamation of the breast_
14. perimetritis _inflamation surrounding outer layer of the uterus (perimetrum)_
15. myometritis _inflamation of the uterine muscle_
16. endometritis _inflamation of the inner layer of the uterus (endometrium)_
17. endocervicitis _inflamation of the inner lining of the cervix_
18. pyosalpinx _pus in the fallopian tube_
19. hysteratresia _closure of the uterus_
20. salpingitis _inflamation of the fallopian tube_

## EXERCISE 9

Build diagnostic terms for the following definitions by using the word parts you have learned.

1. inflammation of the breast

```
_____ / _____
       WR              S
```

2. excessive discharge from the uterus

    WR   |   S

3. inflammation of the fallopian tube

    WR   |   S

4. inflammation of the vulva and vagina

    WR  |  CV  |  WR  |  S

5. absence of menstrual discharge

    P  |  WR  |  S

6. inflammation of the cervix

    WR   |   S

7. inflammation of (Bartholin's) gland

    WR   |   S

8. water in the fallopian tube

    WR  |  CV  |  S

9. painful menstrual discharge

    P  |  WR  |  S

10. blood in the fallopian tube

    WR  |  CV  |  S

11. inflammation of the vagina

    WR   |   S

12. rapid flow of blood at or between menstruation

    WR  |  CV  |  WR  |  S

13. inflammation of the
    ovary

    _____
                        WR  |  S

14. hernia of the fallopian
    tube

    _____
                  WR  |  CV  |  S

15. inflammation surround-
    ing the uterus

    _____
              P  |  WR  |  S

16. inflammation of the in-
    ner lining of the uterus

    _____
              P  |  WR  |  S

17. inflammation of the in-
    ner lining of the cervix

    _____
              P  |  WR  |  S

18. inflammation of the uter-
    ine muscle

    _____
            WR  |  CV  |  WR  |  S

19. pus in the fallopian tube

    _____
                  WR  |  CV  |  S

20. closure of the uterus

    _____
                        WR  |  S

## EXERCISE 10

Spell each of the diagnostic terms. Have someone dicate the terms on pp. 232 and 233 to you or say the words into a tape recorder; then spell the words from your recording as often as necessary. Think about the word parts before attempting to write the word. Study any you have spelled incorrectly.

1. _____     7. _____

2. _____     8. _____

3. _____     9. _____

4. _____     10. _____

5. _____     11. _____

6. _____     12. _____

13. _____          17. _____
14. _____          18. _____
15. _____          19. _____
16. _____          20. _____

Place a check mark (√) in the box to indicate that you have completed Objective 3.

☐ BUILD, ANALYZE, DEFINE, PRONOUNCE, AND SPELL THE DIAGNOSTIC TERMS RELATED TO THE FEMALE REPRODUCTIVE SYSTEM.

## Objective 4   DEFINE, PRONOUNCE, AND SPELL OTHER DIAGNOSTIC TERMS RELATED TO THE FEMALE REPRODUCTIVE SYSTEM.

## Other Diagnostic Terms

| TERM | DEFINITION |
|------|------------|
| 1. adenomyosis.......... <br>(ad-e-nō-mī-Ō-sis) | growth of endometrium into the muscular portion of the uterus |
| 2. endometriosis......... <br>(*en*-dō-*mē*-trē-Ō-sis) | abnormal condition in which endometrial tissue occurs in various areas in the pelvic cavity (Figure 7-6) |
| 3. fibroid tumor.......... <br>(FĪ-broyd) | benign fibroid tumor of the uterine muscle (also called *myoma of the uterus*) (Figure 7-7) |
| 4. pelvic inflammatory disease (PID)............ | inflammation of the female pelvic organs |
| 5. prolapsed uterus ....... | downward displacement of the uterus in the vagina (also called *hysteroptosis*) (Figure 7-8) |

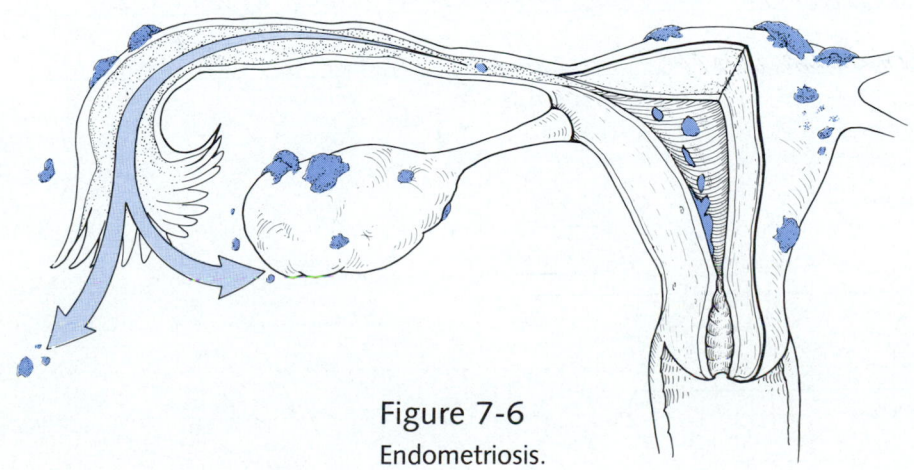

Figure 7-6
Endometriosis.

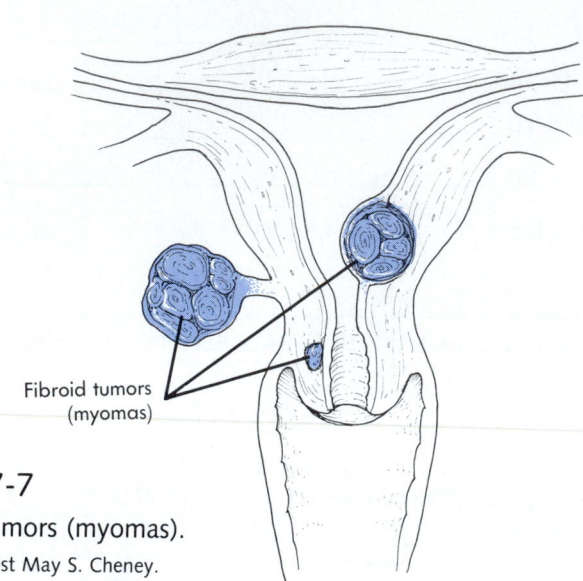

**Figure 7-7**
Fibroid tumors (myomas).
Courtesy artist May S. Cheney.

Fibroid tumors
(myomas)

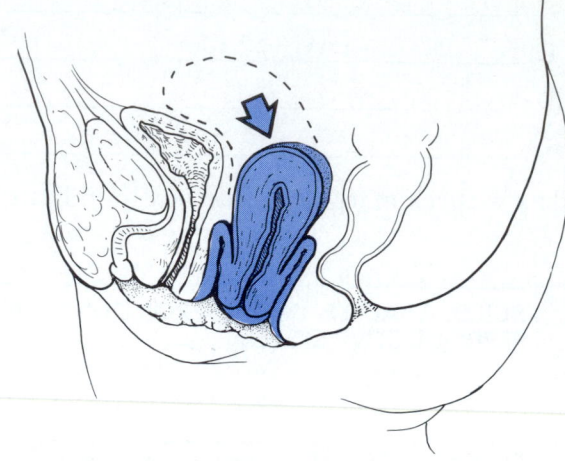

**Figure 7-8**
Prolapsed uterus, or hysteroptosis.

6.   **vesicovaginal fistula** . . . . .    **opening between the bladder and the va-**
     (*ves*-i-kō-VAJ-i-nal) (FIS-tū-la)    **gina (Figure 7-15, see p. 254)**

Practice saying each of these terms aloud. To assist you in pronunciation, obtain the audiotape designed for use with this text. Learn the definitions and spellings of the other diagnostic terms by completing the following exercises.

## EXERCISE 11

Write the definition of the following terms.

1. prolapsed uterus ___*downward displacement of the uterus in the vagina*___

2. pelvic inflammatory disease ___*inflamation of the female pelvic organs*___

3. vesicovaginal fistula ___*opening between the bladder + the vagina*___

4. fibroid tumor ___*benign fibroid tumor of the uterine muscle*___

5. endometriosis ___*abnormal condition in which the endometrial tissue appears in pelvic cavity*___

6. adenomyosis ___*growth of endometrium into the muscular portion of the uterus*___

## EXERCISE 12

Write the term for each of the following.

1. opening between the bladder and the vagina _____  _____

2. benign fibroid tumor of the
   uterine wall _____

3. inflammation of the female
   pelvic organs _____  _____  _____

4. downward displacement of
   the uterus in the vagina _____  _____

5. endometrial tissue in the pelvic cavity _____  _____

6. growth of endometrium into
   the muscular portion of the uterus _____

## EXERCISE 13

Spell each of the other diagnostic terms. Have someone dictate the terms
on pp. 237 and 238 to you or say the words into a tape recorder; then
spell the words from your recording as often as necessary. Study any you
have spelled incorrectly.

1. _____     4. _____

2. _____     5. _____

3. _____     6. _____

Place a check mark (√) in the box to indicate that you have completed Objective 4.

☐ **DEFINE, PRONOUNCE, AND SPELL OTHER DIAGNOSTIC TERMS RELATED TO THE FEMALE
REPRODUCTIVE SYSTEM.**

# Objective 5   BUILD, ANALYZE, DEFINE, PRONOUNCE, AND SPELL THE SURGICAL TERMS RELATED
TO THE FEMALE REPRODUCTIVE SYSTEM.

## Surgical Terms

| TERM (built from word parts) | DEFINITION |
|---|---|
| 1. cervicectomy <br> (*ser*-vi-SEK-tō-mē) | excision of the cervix |
| 2. colpoperineorrhaphy <br> (*kōl*-pō-*pār*-i-nē-OR-a-fē) | suture of the vagina and perineum (per-formed to mend perineal vaginal tears) |
| 3. colpoplasty <br> (KOL-pō-*plas*-tē) | plastic repair of the vagina |
| 4. colporrhaphy <br> (*kōl*-PŌR-a-fē) | suture of the vagina |
| 5. episioperineoplasty <br> (e-*piz*-ē-ō-pār-i-nē-o-PLAST-ē) | plastic repair of the vulva and perineum |
| 6. episiorrhaphy <br> (ē-*piz*-ē-ŌR-a-fē) | suture of (a tear in) the vulva |
| 7. hymenectomy <br> (*hī*-men-EK-tō-mē) | excision of the hymen |
| 8. hymenotomy <br> (*hī*-men-OT-ō-mē) | incision of the hymen |
| 9. hysterectomy <br> (*his*-te-REK-tō-mē) | excision of the uterus (Figure 7-9) |

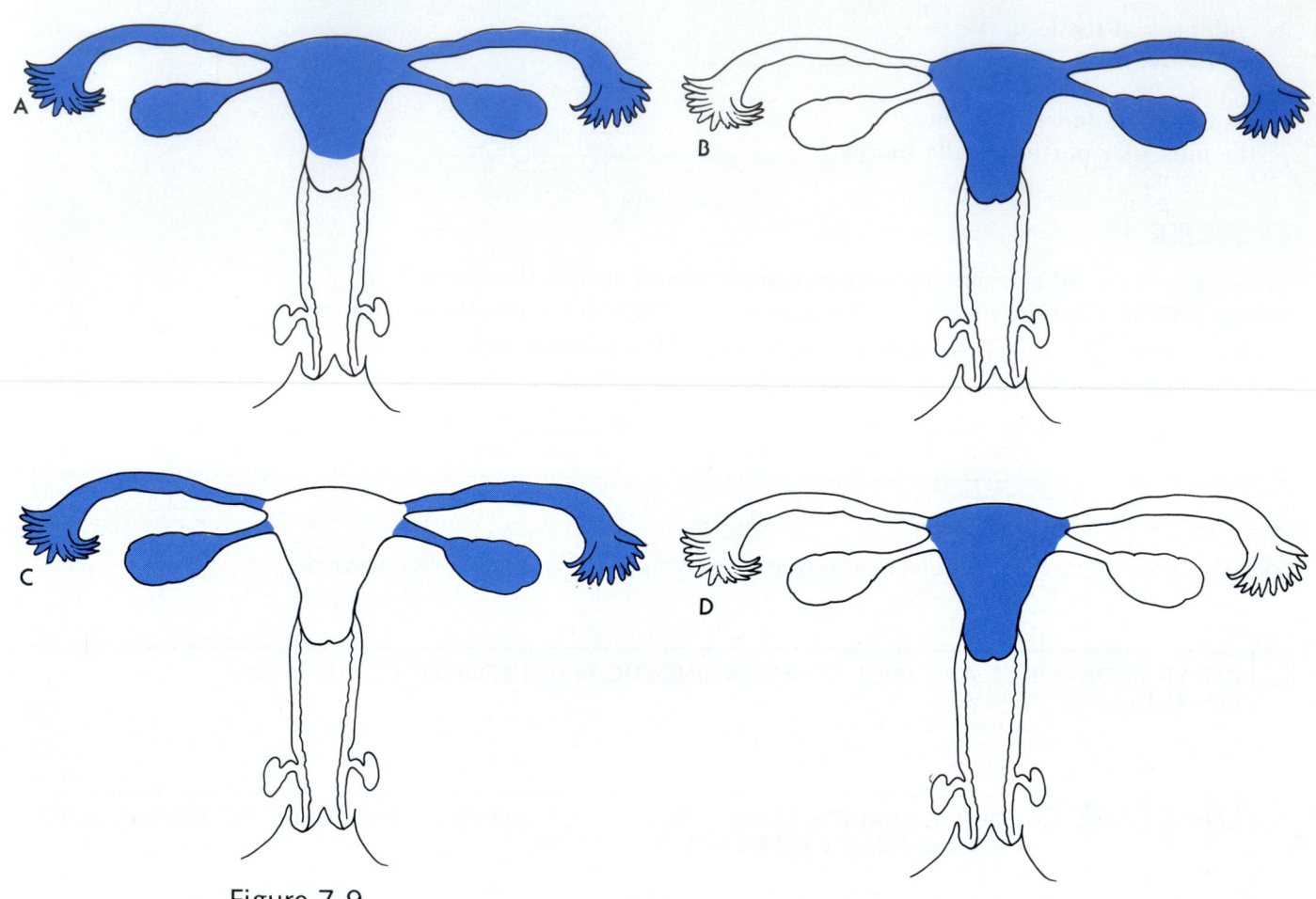

**Figure 7-9**

Types of surgeries. **A,** Hysterectomy, bilateral salpingo-oophorectomy. **B,** Hysterosalpingo-oophorectomy. **C,** Bilateral oophorosalpingectomy. **D,** Hysterectomy.

| | | |
|---|---|---|
| 10. | **hysteropexy** . . . . . . . . .<br>(HIS-ter-ō-*pek*-sē) | surgical fixation of the uterus |
| 11. | **hysterosalpingo-**<br>**oophorectomy** . . . . . . .<br>(*his*-ter-ō-sal-*ping*-gō-ō-of-ō-<br>REK-tō-mē) | excision of the uterus, fallopian tubes,<br>and ovaries (Figure 7-9) |
| 12. | **mammoplasty** . . . . . . . .<br>(MAM-ō-*plas*-tē) | plastic repair of the breasts (performed<br>to enlarge or reduce in size, to lift, or to<br>reconstruct after removal of a tumor) |
| 13. | **mastectomy** . . . . . . . . .<br>(mas-TEK-tō-mē) | surgical removal of a breast |
| 14. | **oophorectomy** . . . . . . .<br>(ō-of-ō-REK-tō-mē) | excision of an ovary |
| 15. | **oophorosalpingectomy** . .<br>(ō-*of*-ō-rō-sal-pin-JEK-tō-mē) | excision of the ovary and fallopian tube<br>(Figure 7-9) |

16. **perineorrhaphy** . . . . . . .    suture of (a tear in) the perineum
    (*pār*-i-nē-ŌR-a-fē)

17. **salpingectomy** . . . . . . . .    excision of a fallopian tube
    (*sal*-pin-JEK-tō-mē)

18. **salpingostomy** . . . . . . . .    creation of an artificial opening in a fal-
    (*sal*-ping-GOS-tō-mē)                lopian tube (performed to restore pa-
                                          tency)

19. **vulvectomy** . . . . . . . . . .    excision of the vulva
    (vul-VEK-tō-mē)

Practice saying each of these terms aloud. To assist you in pronunciation, obtain the audiotape designed for use with this text. Learn the definitions and spellings of the surgical terms by completing the following exercises.

---

### ENDOSCOPIC SURGERY

There has been a remarkable advance in endoscopic surgery since the first laparoscopic cholecystectomy was performed in 1989 to remove a diseased gallbladder. Endoscopic surgery includes the use of a slender flexible fiberoptic endoscope that is inserted into a natural body cavity such as the mouth or into other body areas through a small incision. Three or four other tiny incisions may be made to accommodate laser or electrosurgery units used to destroy or remove tissue, to accommodate visualization equipment that projects the patient's internal organs to a TV screen, and to accommodate other instruments and devices needed to complete the surgery (Figure 7-10).

Because the surgeon performs endoscopic surgery, sometimes referred to as videoscope surgery, by viewing a TV screen, the surgeon must master a new set of skills. Although it is thought that endoscopic surgery will not replace large incision surgery, its use is in demand because of the reduced trauma and medical cost to the patient. Continued advances in technology will improve and expand its use.

### TYPES OF ENDOSCOPIC SURGERY

| INSTRUMENT | PROCEDURE | TYPE OF SURGERY |
|---|---|---|
| arthroscope | arthroscopy or arthroscopic surgery | biopsy<br>meniscus repair<br>synovectomy<br>ligament repair |
| colonoscope | colonoscopy | polypectomy |
| hysteroscope | hysteroscopy | myomectomy<br>polypectomy |
| laparoscope | laparoscopy or laparoscopic surgery | tubal sterilization<br>ovary biopsy<br>adhesiolysis<br>cholesystectomy<br>appendectomy<br>herniorrhaphy<br>hysterectomy |
| pelviscope | pelviscopy | oophorectomy<br>adhesiolysis<br>myomectomy<br>ovarian cystectomy |
| thoracoscope | thoracoscopy | biopsy<br>wedge resection of the lung |

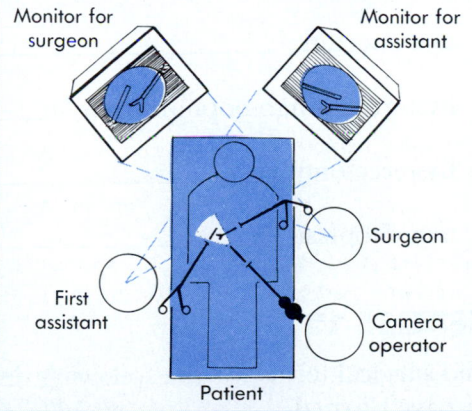

**Figure 7-10**

Operative setup for laparoscopic hysterectomy.

Courtesy artist May S. Cheney.

## EXERCISE 14

Analyze and define the following surgical terms.

1. colporrhaphy _____

2. colpoplasty _____

3. episiorrhaphy _____

4. hymenotomy _____

5. hysteropexy _____

6. vulvectomy _____

7. perineorrhaphy _____

8. salpingostomy _____

9. oophorosalpingectomy _____

10. oophorectomy _____

11. mastectomy _____

12. salpingectomy _____

13. cervicectomy _____

14. colpoperineorrhaphy _____

15. episioperineoplasty _____

16. hymenectomy _____

17. hysterosalpingo-oophorectomy _____

18. hysterectomy _____

19. mammoplasty _____

## EXERCISE 15

Build surgical terms for the following definitions by using the word parts
you have learned.

1. suture of the vagina    _____ colp / orrhaphy _____
                                     WR    S

2. excision of the cervix    _____ cervic / ectomy _____
                                        WR     S

3. suture of the vulva

episi / orrhaphy
WR / S

4. plastic repair of the vulva and perineum

episi o perine o plasty
WR CV WR CV S

5. plastic repair of the vagina

colp o plasty
WR CV S

6. suture of the vagina and perineum

colp o perine orrhaphy
WR CV WR S

7. excision of the uterus, ovaries, and fallopian tubes

hyster o salping o oophor ectomy
WR CV WR CV WR S

8. surgical fixation of the uterus

hyster o pexy
WR CV S

9. excision of the hymen

hymen ectomy
WR S

10. incision of the hymen

hymen otomy
WR S

11. excision of the uterus

hyster ectomy
WR S

12. excision of the ovary

oophor ectomy
WR S

13. surgical removal of a breast

mast ectomy
WR S

14. excision of a fallopian tube

salping ectomy
WR S

15. suture of the perineum      _perine / orrphy_
                                       WR      S

16. excision of the ovary and
    fallopian tube              _ooplor / o / salping / ectomy_
                                    WR      CV     WR       S

17. creation of an artificial
    opening in the fallopian
    tube                        _salping / ostomy_
                                    WR        S

18. excision of the vulva       _vulv / ectomy_
                                   WR       S

19. plastic repair of the
    breasts                     _mammo / mast / o / plasty_
                                      WR      CV    S

## EXERCISE 16

Spell each of the surgical terms. Have someone dictate the terms on pp.
239 to 241 to you or say the words into a tape recorder; then spell the
words from your recording as often as necessary. Think about the word
parts before attempting to write the word. Study any you have spelled
incorrectly.

1. _____        11. _____
2. _____        12. _____
3. _____        13. _____
4. _____        14. _____
5. _____        15. _____
6. _____        16. _____
7. _____        17. _____
8. _____        18. _____
9. _____        19. _____
10. _____

Place a check mark (√) in the box to indicate that you have completed Objective 5.

☐ **BUILD, ANALYZE, DEFINE, PRONOUNCE, AND SPELL THE SURGICAL TERMS RELATED TO THE FEMALE REPRODUCTIVE SYSTEM.**

# Objective 6  DEFINE, PRONOUNCE, AND SPELL OTHER SURGICAL TERMS RELATED TO THE FEMALE REPRODUCTIVE SYSTEM.

## Other Surgical Terms

| TERM | DEFINITION |
|---|---|
| 1. anterior and posterior colporrhaphy (A & P repair) | when a weakened vaginal wall results in a cystocele (protrusion of the bladder against the anterior wall of the vagina) and a rectocele (protrusion of the rectum against the posterior wall of the vagina), an A & P repair corrects the condition (Figure 7-11) |
| 2. dilatation and curettage (D & C) . . . . . . . . . . . . . (*dil*-a-TĀ-shun and kū-re-TAHZH) | dilation of the cervix and scraping of the endometrium with an instrument called a *curette*. It is performed to diagnose disease, to correct bleeding, and to empty uterine contents. |
| 3. laparoscopy or laparoscopic surgery . . . . . . . . (*lap*-a-ROS-kō-pē) | visual examination of the abdominal cavity, accomplished by insertion of a laparoscope through a tiny incision near |

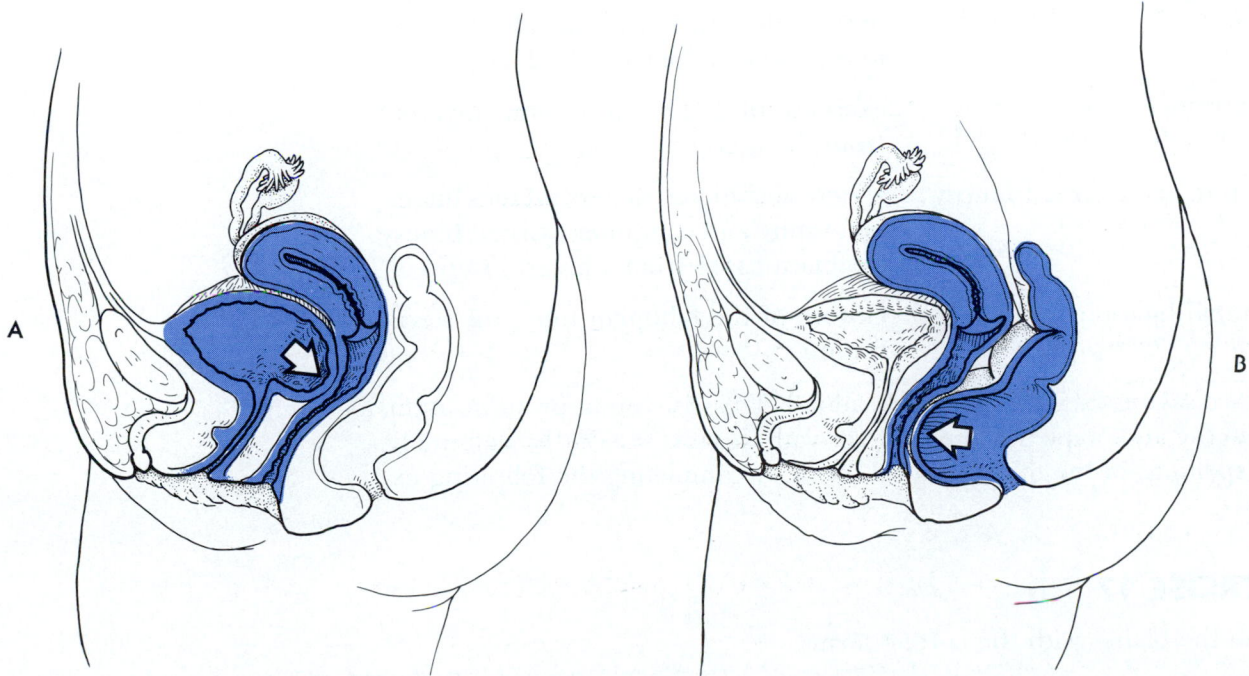

## Figure 7-11

**A,** Cystocele. **B,** Rectocele. Anterior and posterior colporrhaphies correct this condition.

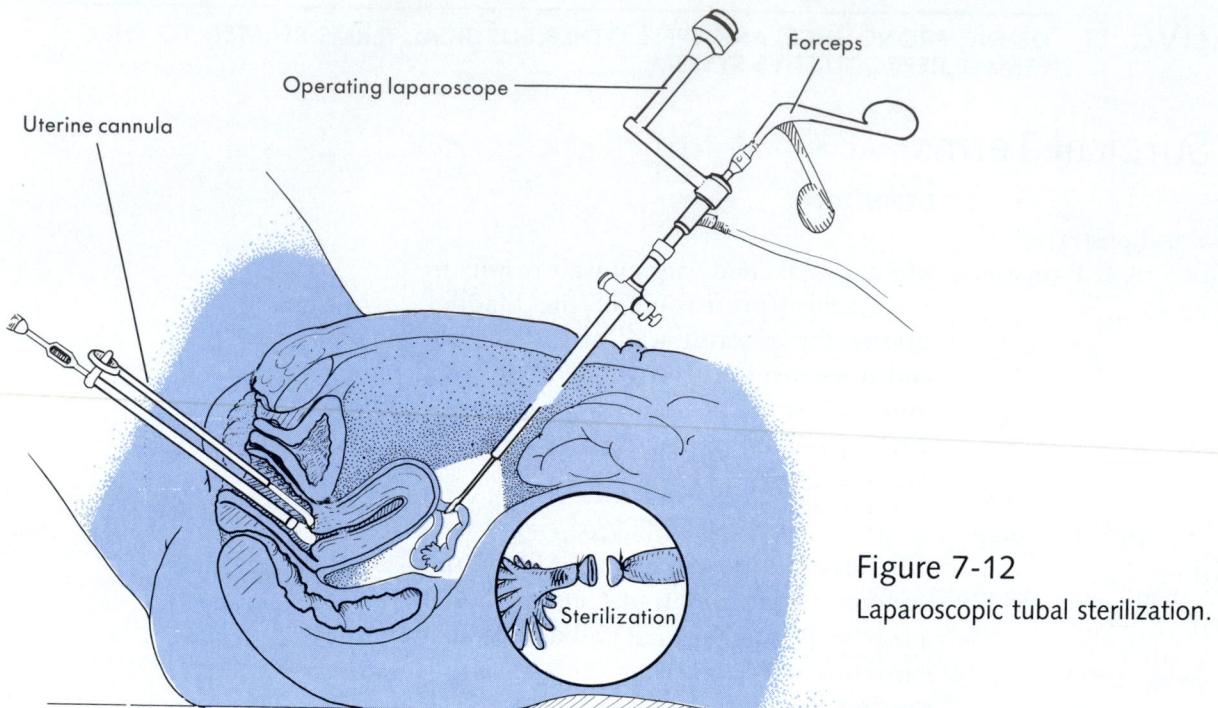

Uterine cannula

Operating laparoscope

Forceps

Sterilization

**Figure 7-12**
Laparoscopic tubal sterilization.

the umbilicus. It is used for surgical procedures such as tubal sterilization (blocking of the fallopian tubes) or biopsy of the ovaries. It may also be used to diagnose endometriosis (Figure 7-12)

4.  myomectomy . . . . . . . . . .    excision of a fibroid tumor (myoma) from the uterus
    (mī-ō-MEK-tō-mē)

5.  stereotactic breast biopsy .    a new technique that combines mammography and computer assisted biopsy to obtain tissue from a breast lump
    (ster-ē-ō-TAC-tic)

6.  tubal ligation . . . . . . . . . .    closure of the fallopian tubes for sterilization
    (lī-GĀ-shun)

Practice saying each of these terms aloud. To assist you in pronunciation, obtain the audiotape designed for use with this text. Learn the definitions and spellings of the other surgical terms by completing the following exercises.

## EXERCISE 17

Fill in the blanks with the correct terms.

1.  Two procedures used for sterilization of the female are _tubal ligation_ and _laparoscopy_ .

2.  The surgery used to repair a cystocele and rectocele is a(n) _anterior & posterior colporrhaphy_

3. D & C is the abbreviation for _____dilatation_____ and _____curettage_____

4. _____stereotactic_____breast_____biopsy_____ is used to obtain tissue
   from a breast lump.

5. Excision of a fibroid tumor from the uterus is called _____myomectomy_____

## EXERCISE 18

Match the surgical procedures in the first column with the corresponding
organs in the second column. You may use the answers in the second column more than once.

_C_ 1. dilatation and curet-
tage

_a_ 2. laparoscopy sterilization

_a_ 3. tubal ligation

_b_ 4. A & P repair

_c_ 5. myomectomy

_f_ 6. stereotactic breast biopsy

a. fallopian tubes

b. vagina

c. uterus

d. ovaries

e. vulva

f. mammary glands

## EXERCISE 19

Spell each of the other surgical terms. Have someone dictate the terms
on pp. 245 and 246 to you or say the words into a tape recorder; then
spell the words from your recording as often as necessary. Study any you
have spelled incorrectly.

1. _____  4. _____

2. _____  5. _____

3. _____  6. _____

Place a check mark (√) in the box to indicate that you have completed Objective 6.

☐ **DEFINE, PRONOUNCE, AND SPELL OTHER SURGICAL TERMS RELATED
TO THE FEMALE REPRODUCTIVE SYSTEM.**

# Objective 7 BUILD, ANALYZE, DEFINE, PRONOUNCE, AND SPELL THE DIAGNOSTIC PROCEDURAL TERMS RELATED TO THE FEMALE REPRODUCTIVE SYSTEM.

## Diagnostic Procedural Terms

| TERM | DEFINITION |
|---|---|
| 1. colposcope ........... <br>(KOL-pō-skōp) | instrument used for visual examination of the vagina (and cervix) |

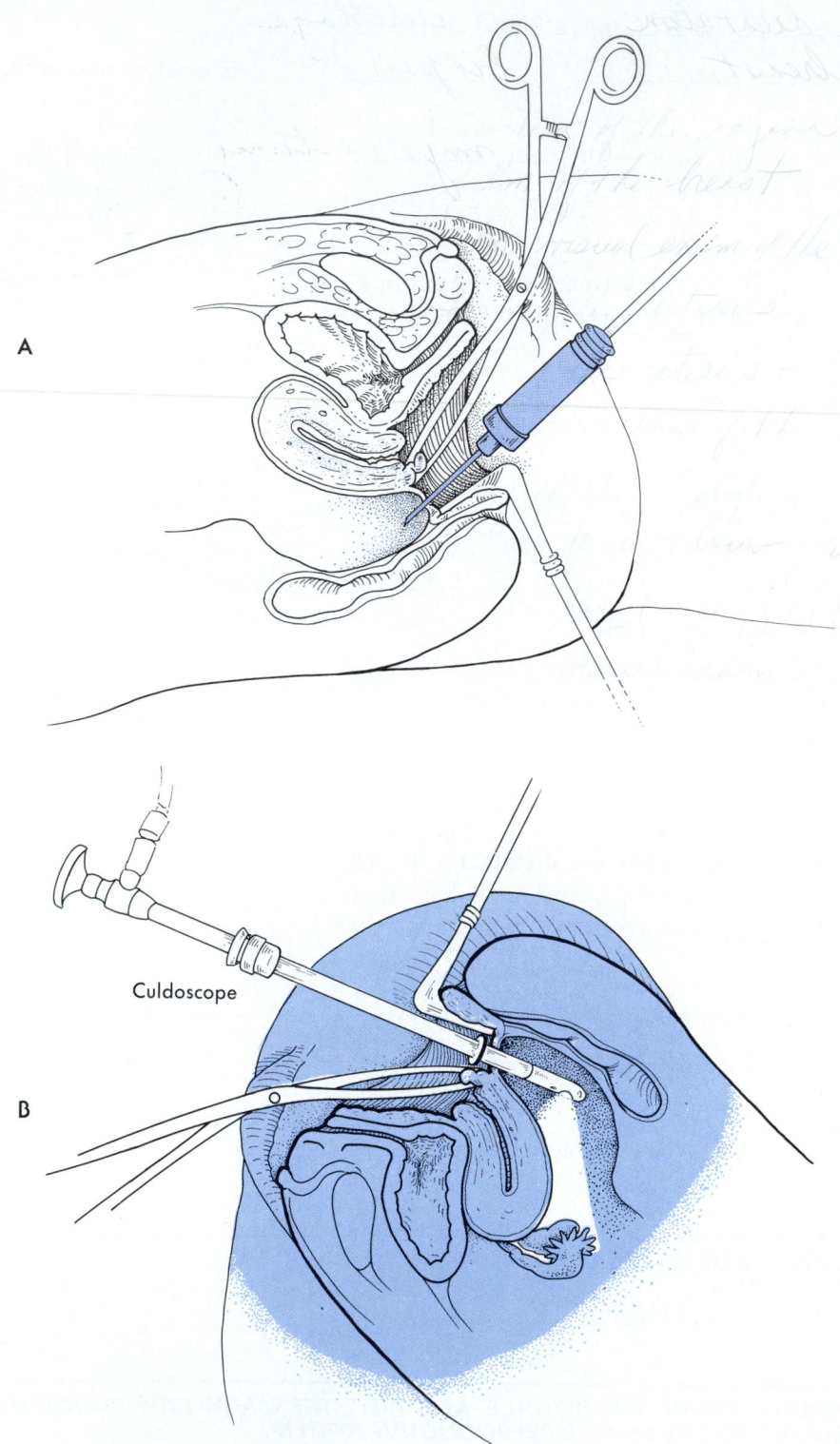

A

B

Culdoscope

## Figure 7-13

**A,** Culdocentesis performed to remove pus or other fluid from the rectouterine pouch. **B,** Culdoscopy performed to view the pelvic cavity and organs; it may be used to diagnose ectopic pregnancy.

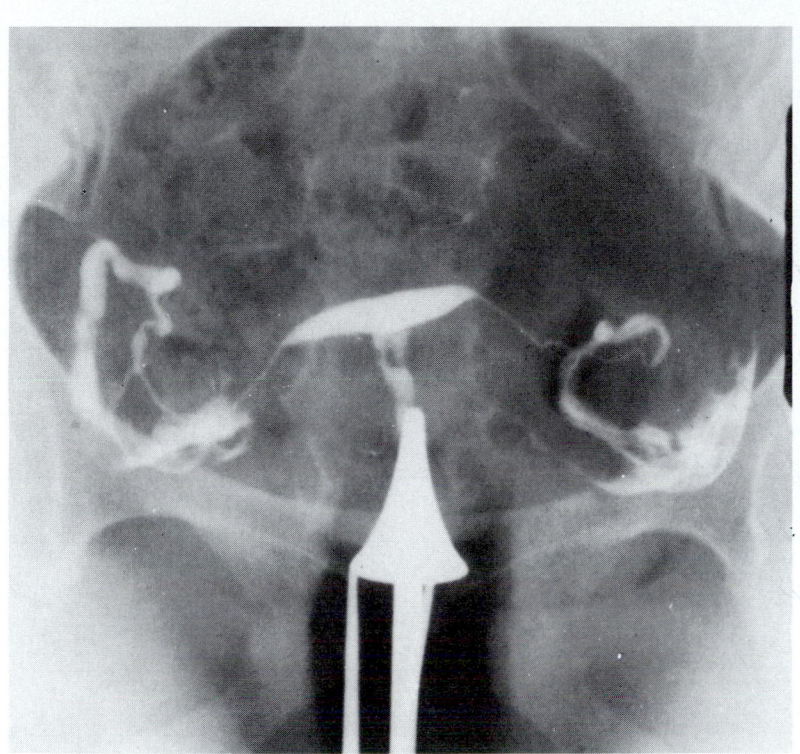

## Figure 7-14
Hysterosalpingogram. Liquid contrast material is used to outline the uterus and fallopian tubes before the x-ray film is made. This procedure is usually performed to determine whether an obstruction exists in the fallopian tubes that may cause sterility.

From Jensen MD, Benson RC, and Bobak IM: *Maternity care: the nurse and the family*, ed 2, St. Louis, 1981, Mosby.

2. **colposcopy** . . . . . . . . . . visual examination (with a magnified
   (kol-POS-kō-pē)                 view) of the vagina (and cervix)

3. **culdocentesis** . . . . . . . . surgical puncture to remove fluid from
   (*kul*-dō-sen-TĒ-sis)            the Douglas' cul-de-sac (Figure 7-13)

4. **culdoscope** . . . . . . . . . . . instrument used for visual examination
   (KUL-dō-skōp)                    of the Douglas' cul-de-sac (Figure 7-13)

5. **culdoscopy** . . . . . . . . . . visual examination of the Douglas' cul-
   (kul-DOS-kō-pē)                  de-sac (Figure 7-13)

6. **hysterosalpingogram** . . . x-ray film of the uterus and the fallopian
   (*his*-ter-ō-*sal*-PING-go-gram) tubes (Figure 7-14)

7. **hysteroscope** . . . . . . . . . instrument used for visual examination
   (HIS-ter-o-skōp)                 of the uterus

8. **hysteroscopy** . . . . . . . . . visual examination of the uterus
   (*his*-ter-OS-kō-pē)

9. **mammography** . . . . . . . . process of recording (x-ray) of the breast
   (ma-MOG-ra-fē)

10. **mammogram** . . . . . . . . x-ray film of the breast
    (MAM-ō-gram)

Practice saying each of these terms aloud. To assist you in pronunciation, obtain the audiotape designed for use with this text. Learn the definitions and spellings of the diagnostic procedural terms by completing the following exercises.

## EXERCISE 20

Analyze and define the following diagnostic procedural terms.

1. colposcopy      *visual examination of the vagina*
   WR CV S

2. mammogram      *x-ray film of the breast*
   WR CV S

3. colposcope      *instrument for visual exam of the vagina*
   WR CV S

4. hysteroscopy      *visual exam of the uterus*
   WR CV S

5. hysterosalpingogram      *x-ray film of the uterus + fallopian tubes*
   WR CV WR CV S

6. culdoscope      *instrument for visual exam of the Douglas cul-de-sac*
   WR CV S

7. culdoscopy      *visual exam of the Douglas cul-de-sac*
   WR CV S

8. culdocentesis      *surgical puncture to withdraw fluid from the Douglas cul-de-sac*
   WR CV S

9. mammography      *process of recording (x-ray) of the breast*
   WR CV S

10. hysteroscope      *instrument for visual exam of the uterus*
    WR CV S

---

**Endoscopy** dates back to the time of Hippocrates II (460-375 BC) who mentions using a speculum to look into a rectum to see where it was affected. By the end of the nineteenth century cystoscopy, proctoscopy, laryngoscopy, and esophagoscopy were well established. Use of the endoscope for surgery was not widely used in the United States until the 1970s when gynecologists started performing laparoscopic tubal sterilization. The first ectopic pregnancy was removed by laparoscopic surgery in 1973, the first laparoscopic appendectomy occurred in 1983, and the first laparoscopic cholecystectomy in 1989.

---

## EXERCISE 21

Build diagnostic procedural terms for the following definitions by using the word parts you have learned.

1. x-ray film of the uterus
   and fallopian tubes

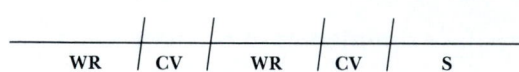

   WR / CV / WR / CV / S

2. visual examination of the
   vagina (and cervix)

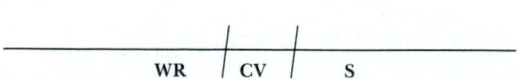

   WR / CV / S

3. instrument used for visual examination of the
   vagina (and cervix)

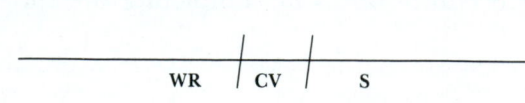

   WR / CV / S

4. visual examination of the uterus

　　　　　　　　_____ / _____ / _____
　　　　　　　　　　WR　　　CV　　　 S

5. x-ray film of the breast

　　　　　　　　_____ / _____ / _____
　　　　　　　　　　WR　　　CV　　　 S

6. instrument used for visual examination of the Douglas' cul-de-sac

　　　　　　　　_____ / _____ / _____
　　　　　　　　　　WR　　　CV　　　 S

7. visual examination of the Douglas' cul-de-sac

　　　　　　　　_____ / _____ / _____
　　　　　　　　　　WR　　　CV　　　 S

8. surgical puncture to remove fluid from the Douglas' cul-de-sac

　　　　　　　　_____ / _____ / _____
　　　　　　　　　　WR　　　CV　　　 S

9. instrument used for visual examination of the uterus

　　　　　　　　_____ / _____ / _____
　　　　　　　　　　WR　　　CV　　　 S

10. process of recording the breast

　　　　　　　　_____ / _____ / _____
　　　　　　　　　　WR　　　CV　　　 S

## EXERCISE 22

Spell each of the diagnostic procedural terms. Have someone dictate the terms on pp. 247 to 249 to you or say the words into a tape recorder; then spell the words from your recording as often as necessary. Think about the word parts before attempting to write the word. Study any you have spelled incorrectly.

1. _____    6. _____

2. _____    7. _____

3. _____    8. _____

4. _____    9. _____

5. _____   10. _____

Place a check mark (√) in the box to indicate that you have completed Objective 7.

☐ **BUILD, ANALYZE, DEFINE, PRONOUNCE, AND SPELL THE DIAGNOSTIC PROCEDURAL TERMS RELATED TO THE FEMALE REPRODUCTIVE SYSTEM.**

# Objective 8

**BUILD, ANALYZE, DEFINE, PRONOUNCE, AND SPELL ADDITIONAL TERMS RELATED TO THE FEMALE REPRODUCTIVE SYSTEM.**

## Additional Terms

| TERM | DEFINITION |
|---|---|
| (built from word parts) | |
| 1. colpalgia (kol-PAL-jē-a) | pain in the vagina |
| 2. gynecologist (gīn-e-KOL-ō-jist) | physician who specializes in gynecology |
| 3. gynecology (gīn-e-KOL-ō-jē) | branch of medicine dealing with diseases of the female reproductive system |
| 4. gynopathic (gīn-ō-PATH-ic) | pertaining to disease of women |
| 5. leukorrhea (lū-kō-RĒ-a) | white discharge (from the vagina) |
| 6. mastalgia (mas-TAL-jē-a) | pain in the breast |
| 7. mastoptosis (mas-tō-TŌ-sis) | sagging breast |
| 8. menarche (me-NAR-kē) | beginning of menstruation |
| 9. oligomenorrhea (ol-i-gō-men-ō-RĒ-a) | scanty menstrual flow |
| 10. vulvovaginal (vul-vō-VAJ-i-nal) | pertaining to the vulva and the vagina |

Practice saying these terms aloud. To assist you in pronunciation, obtain the audiotape designed for use with this text. Learn the definitions and spellings of the additional terms by completing the following exercises.

## EXERCISE 23

Analyze and define the following additional terms.

1. gynecologist _____ physician who specializes in gynecology
2. gynecology _____ branch of medicine dealing with diseases of the female reproductive system
3. colpalgia _____ pain in the vagina
4. vulvovaginal _____ pertaining to the vulva + vagina
5. mastalgia _____ pain in the breast
6. menarche _____ beginning of menstruation
7. leukorrhea _____ white discharge (from the vagina)

8. oligomenorrhea  *scanty menstrual flow*
   <small>WR CV WR S</small>
9. gynopathic  *pertaining to disease of woman*
   <small>WR CV WR S</small>
10. mastoptosis  *sagging breast*
    <small>WR CV S</small>

## EXERCISE 24

Build medical terms for the following definitions by using the word parts you have learned.

1. scanty menstrual flow

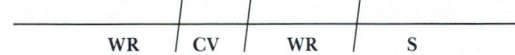

     WR    CV    WR    S

2. white discharge (from the vagina)

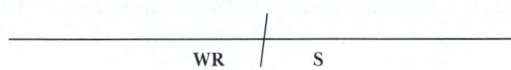

     WR    S

3. beginning of menstruation

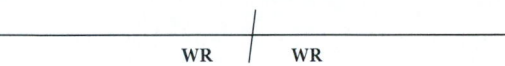

     WR    WR

4. pain in the breast

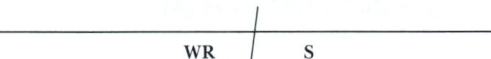

     WR    S

5. pertaining to the vulva and vagina

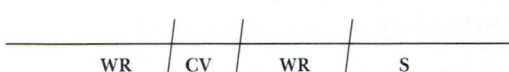

     WR    CV    WR    S

6. pain in the vagina

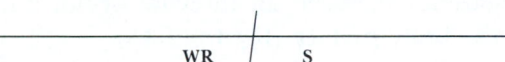

     WR    S

7. physician who specializes in gynecology

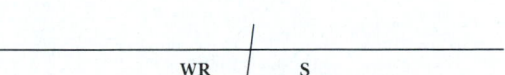

     WR    S

8. branch of medicine dealing with diseases of the female reproductive system

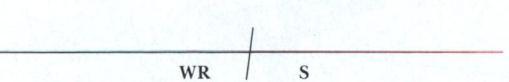

     WR    S

9. sagging breast

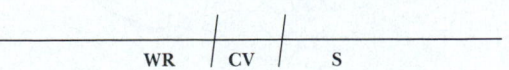

     WR    CV    S

10. pertaining to disease of women

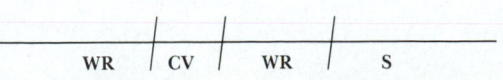

     WR    CV    WR    S

## EXERCISE 25

Spell each of the additional terms. Have someone dictate the terms on p. 252 to you or say the words into a tape recorder; then spell the words from your recording as often as necessary. Think about the word parts before attempting to write the word. Study any you have spelled incorrectly.

1. _____     6. _____
2. _____     7. _____
3. _____     8. _____
4. _____     9. _____
5. _____     10. _____

Place a check mark (√) in the box to indicate that you have completed Objective 8.

☐ BUILD, ANALYZE, DEFINE, PRONOUNCE, AND SPELL ADDITIONAL TERMS RELATED TO THE FEMALE REPRODUCTIVE SYSTEM.

# Objective 9
### DEFINE, PRONOUNCE, AND SPELL THE OTHER ADDITIONAL TERMS RELATED TO THE FEMALE REPRODUCTIVE SYSTEM.

# Other Additional Terms

| TERM | DEFINITION |
| --- | --- |
| 1. dyspareunia . . . . . . . . . . (*dis*-pa-RŪ-nē-a) | difficult or painful intercourse |
| 2. fistula . . . . . . . . . . . . . . . . (FIS-tū-la) | abnormal passageway between two organs or between an internal organ and the body surface (Figure 7-15) |

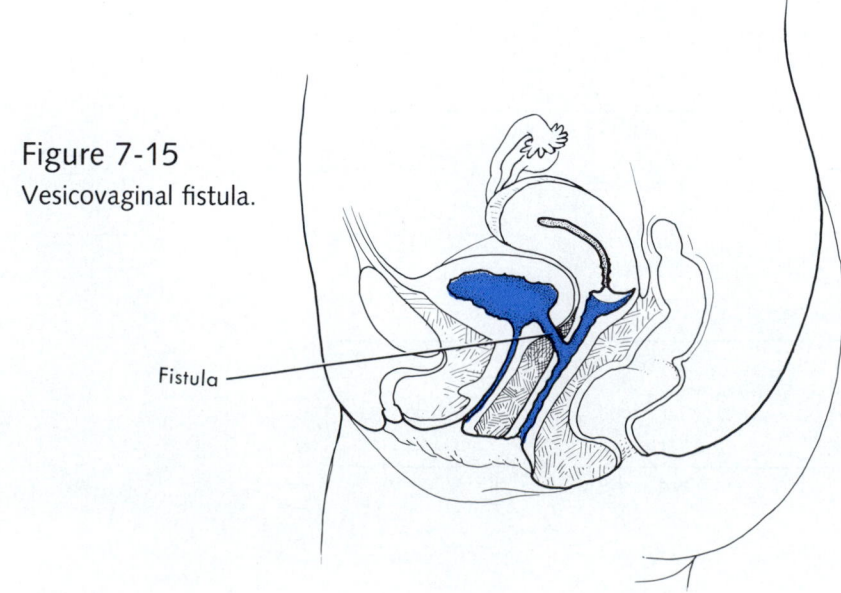

Figure 7-15
Vesicovaginal fistula.

Fistula

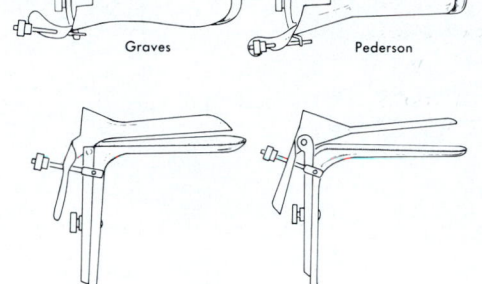

Graves       Pederson

Speculums

### Figure 7-16
Speculums.

From Mosby's medical, nursing, and allied health dictionary, ed 3, St. Louis, 1990, Mosby.

3. menopause . . . . . . . . . . . .    cessation of menstruation, usually
   (MEN-o-pawz)                        around the ages of 48 and 50

4. premenstrual
   syndrome (PMS) . . . . . . . .   a syndrome involving physical and emo-
                                    tional symptoms occurring in the ten
                                    days before menstruation. Symptoms in-
                                    clude nervous tension, irritability, mas-
                                    talgia, edema, and headache. Cause is
                                    not fully understood.

5. speculum . . . . . . . . . . . .    instrument for opening a body cavity to
   (SPEK-ū-lum)                        allow visual inspection (Figure 7-16)

Practice saying each of these terms. To assist you in pronunciation, obtain the audiotape designed for use with this text. Learn the definitions
and spellings of the other additional terms by completing the following
exercises.

## EXERCISE 26

Write the definitions of the following terms.

1. menopause _cessation of menstration usually around age 48 + 50_

2. dyspareunia _difficult or painful intercourse_

3. fistula _abnormal passageway_

4. premenstrual syndrome _syndrome involving physical + emotin symptoms_

5. speculum _instrument for opening a body canity to allow visual inspection_

## EXERCISE 27

Write the term for each of the following.

1. abnormal passageway _____

2. painful intercourse _____

3. cessation of menstrua-
   tion _____

4. syndrome involving physical and emotional symptoms

    _____

5. instrument for opening a body cavity

    _____

## EXERCISE 28

Spell each of the other additional terms. Have someone dictate the terms on pp. 254 and 255 to you or say the words into a tape recorder; then spell the words from your recording as often as necessary. Study any you have spelled incorrectly.

1. _____     4. _____

2. _____     5. _____

3. _____

Place a check mark (√) in the box to indicate that you have completed Objective 9.

☐ **DEFINE, PRONOUNCE, AND SPELL THE OTHER ADDITIONAL TERMS RELATED TO THE FEMALE REPRODUCTIVE SYSTEM.**

---

**Case History:** A 48-year-old Puerto Rican female is referred for follow-up after a suspicious mass in the left breast was discovered in routine mammography. She has a positive family history (mother's sister) of carcinoma of the breast. She also has had a hysterectomy for adenomyosis and endometriosis. She elects to have the biopsy in the outpatient surgery department.

---

**Pathology Report:** <u>GROSS DESCRIPTION</u>: Received labeled "breast biopsy" is an ovoid mass of predominantly adipose breast tissue measuring 4.5 × 3.0 × 1.3 cm. Sectioning reveals a focal area of suspicious induration. Frozen section reveals fat necrosis and evidence of invasive malignancy in an area measuring 0.25 cm in the center of the specimen. The surgeon is so informed. <u>MICROSCOPIC DESCRIPTION</u>: Microscopic examination of the frozen section specimen confirms the presence of fat necrosis. There is a focal duct epithelial hyperplasia exhibiting a papillomatous pattern. In this area is found a well-differentiated adenocarcinoma. Occasional breast parenchymal fragments are also identified and show fibrocystic changes. These are predominantly nonproliferative, although in slide D a small radial scar containing ducts showing proliferative fibrocystic changes with significant atypia and adjacent sclerosis adenosis is identified.

<u>DIAGNOSIS</u>:  Left breast biopsy:
1. radial scar
2. nonproliferative and proliferative fibrocystic changes with significant atypia
3. papillary duct adenocarcinoma
4. focal sclerosing adenosis

## EXERCISE 29

To test your understanding of the terms introduced in this chapter, circle the words that correctly complete the sentences. The italicized words refer to the correct answer.

1. The patient was diagnosed as having *painful menstruation,* or (oligomenorrhea, dysmenorrhea, amenorrhea).
2. *Inflammation of the inner lining of the uterus* is (endocervicitis, endometritis, endometriosis).
3. The patient is scheduled in surgery for a *salpingectomy,* which is the *excision* of the (fallopian tube, ovary, uterus).
4. An *episiorrhaphy* is a (suture of the vulva, discharge from the vulva, rapid discharge from the vulva).
5. A surgical procedure to *reduce breast size* is called (mammogram, mammography, mammoplasty).
6. A *hysterosalpingo-oophorectomy* is the excision of the (uterus, fallopian tubes, and ovaries; uterus, ovaries, and cervix; uterus, fallopian tubes, and vagina).
7. *Blood in the fallopian tube* is called (hematosalpinx, hydrosalpinx, pyosalpinx).
8. *Endometrial tissue occurring in various areas of the pelvic cavity* is called (adenomyosis, endometriosis, hysteratresia).
9. The doctor requested a (hysteroscope, colposcope, speculum) *to open the vagina for visual examination.*

## EXERCISE 30

Unscramble the following mixed-up terms. The word on the left indicates the word root in each of the following.

1. uterus

/ / / s / / / / / / / / /
x e p r o y e t h s y

2. white

/ / e / / / / / / / e / /
e e k u l r r o h a

3. woman

/ / / / / / / l / / / /
y o g o g y c e n l

4. breast

/ / / / / a / / / / /
g l a a s t m a i

5. menstruation

/ / / / / r / / / /
h e r n a c m e

## EXERCISE 31

The following exercise includes words and word parts introduced in previous chapters. Circle the letter of the correct answer in each of the following.

1. The term that means *excision of the nail* is
   a. onychectomy
   b. rhytidectomy
   c. pneumonectomy
   d. nephrectomy
   e. vesiculoectomy

2. The patient was admitted to the hospital with the diagnosis of a *kidney stone*, or
   a. nephroma
   b. nephrohypertrophy
   c. nephromegaly
   d. nephroptosis
   e. nephrolithiasis

3. The patient was admitted to the hospital with possible lung cancer. To assist in confirming the diagnosis the physician ordered an *x-ray film of the bronchi*, or
   a. bronchography
   b. bronchogram
   c. bronchoscopy
   d. bronchoplasty
   e. bronchiectasis

4. The medical term for *pinpoint hemorrhages* is
   a. papule
   b. purpura
   c. pustules
   d. petechiae
   e. pallor

5. The word root for the color *blue* is
   a. erythr
   b. leuk
   c. melan
   d. xanth
   e. cyan

6. A *tumor composed of connective tissue* is called a(n)
   a. neuroma
   b. sarcoma
   c. epithelioma
   d. carcinoma
   e. lipoma

# COMBINING FORMS—CHAPTERS 6 AND 7—CROSSWORD PUZZLE

## Across Clues

1. vagina
2. prostate
5. vulva
8. cervix
9. fallopian tube
11. male
14. epididymis
17. uterus
18. ovary
22. sperm
23. abdomen
24. abbreviation for occupational medicine
26. vulva
27. glans penis
28. uterus

## Down Clues

3. sperm
4. cul-de-sac
6. vessel, duct
7. menstruation
10. perineum
12. woman
13. seminal vesicles
15. testis
16. first, beginning
19. testis, testicle
20. uterus
21. testis
25. breast

# Summary

Can you build, analyze, define, pronounce, and spell the following terms *built from word parts?* yes ☐ no ☐

| DIAGNOSTIC | SURGICAL | PROCEDURAL | ADDITIONAL |
|---|---|---|---|
| amenorrhea (ā-*men*-ō-RĒ-a) | cervicectomy (*ser*-vi-SEK-tō-mē) | colposcope (KŌL-pō-skōp) | colpalgia (kol-PAL-jē-a) |
| Bartholin's adenitis (BAR-tō-lins) (*ad*-e-NĪ-tis) | colpoperineorrhaphy (*kōl*-pō-*pār*-i-nē-ŌR-a-fē) | colposcopy (kol-POS-kō-pē) | gynecologist (*gīn*-e-KOL-ō-jist) |
| cervicitis (*ser*-vi-SĪ-tis) | colpoplasty (KŌL-pō-*plas*-tē) | culdocentesis (*kul*-dō-sen-TĒ-sis) | gynecology (*gīn*-e-KOL-ō-jē) |
| colpitis (kol-PĪ-tis) | colporrhaphy (kōl-PŌR-a-fē) | culdoscope (KUL-dō-skōp) | gynopathic (*gīn*-ō-PATH-ic) |
| dysmenorrhea (*dis*-men-ō-RĒ-a) | episioperineoplasty (e-*piz*-ē-ō-*pār*-i-nē-o-PLAST-ē) | culdoscopy (kul-DOS-kō-pē) | leukorrhea (*lū*-kō-RĒ-a) |
| endocervicitis (*en*-dō-*ser*-vi-SĪ-tis) | episiorrhaphy (ē-*piz*-ē-ŌR-a-fē) | hysterosalpingogram (*his*-ter-ō-*sal*-ping-GŌ-gram) | mastalgia (mas-TAL-jē-a) |
| endometritis (*en*-dō-mē-TRĪ-tis) | hymenectomy (*hī*-men-EK-tō-mē) | hysteroscope (HIS-ter-ō-scōpe) | mastoptosis (mas-tō-TŌ-sis) |
| hematosalpinx (*hem*-a-tō-SAL-pinks) | hymenotomy (*hī*-men-OT-ō-mē) | hysteroscopy (*his*-ter-OS-kō-pē) | menarche (me-NAR-kē) |
| hydrosalpinx (hī-drō-SAL-pinks) | hysterectomy (*his*-te-REK-tō-mē) | mammography (ma-MOG-ra-fē) | oligomenorrhea (*ol*-i-gō-men-ō-RĒ-a) |
| hysteratresia (his-ter-a-TRĒ-zē-a) | hysteropexy (HIS-ter-ō-*pek*-sē) | mammogram (MAM-ō-gram) | vulvovaginal (*vul*-vō-VAJ-i-nal) |
| mastitis (*mas*-TĪ-tis) | hysterosalpingo-oophorectomy (*his*-ter-ō-sal-*ping*-gō-ō-of-ō-REK-tō-mē) | | |
| menometrorrhagia (men-ō-*met*-rō-RĀ-jē-a) | mammoplasty (MAM-ō-*plas*-tē) | | |
| metrorrhea (me-trō-RĒ-a) | mastectomy (mas-TEK-tō-mē) | | |
| myometritis (*mī*-o-mē-TRĪ-tis) | oophorectomy (ō-of-ō-REK-tō-mē) | | |
| oophoritis (ō-of-ō-RĪ-tis) | oophorosalpingectomy (ō-*of*-ō-rō-sal-pin-JEK-tō-mē) | | |
| perimetritis (*per*-i-mē-TRĪ-tis) | perineorrhaphy (*pār*-i-nē-ŌR-a-fē) | | |
| pyosalpinx (pī-ō-SAL-pinks) | salpingectomy (*sal*-pin-JEK-tō-mē) | | |
| salpingitis (*sal*-pin-JĪ-tis) | salpingostomy (*sal*-ping-GOS-tō-mē) | | |
| salpingocele (sal-PING-gō-sēl) | vulvectomy (vul-VEK-tō-mē) | | |
| vulvovaginitis (*vul*-vō-VAJ-i-nī-tis) | | | |

# Summary

Can you define, pronounce, and spell the following terms *not built from word parts?*  yes ☐  no ☐

| DIAGNOSTIC | SURGICAL | ADDITIONAL |
|---|---|---|
| adenomyosis (ad-e-nō-mī-Ō-sis) | anterior and posterior colporrhaphy | dyspareunia (*dis*-pa-RŪ-nē-a) |
| endometriosis (*en*-dō-*mē*-trē-Ō-sis) | dilatation and curettage (*dil*-a-TĀ-shun and kū-re-TAHZH) | fistula (FIS-tū-la) |
| fibroid tumor (FĪ-broyd) | laparoscopy (*lap*-a-ROS-kō-pē) | menopause (MEN-o-pawz) |
| pelvic inflammatory disease | myomectomy (mi-ō-MEK-tō-mē) | premenstrual syndrome |
| prolapsed uterus | stereotactic breast biopsy (ster-ē-ō-TAC-tic) | speculum (SPEK-ū-lum) |
| vesicovaginal fistula (*ves*-i-kō-VAJ-i-nal) (FIS-tū-la) | tubal ligation (lī-GĀ-shun) | |

# Answers

**Exercise 1**

1. c  3. g  5. d  7. h  9. i
2. f  4. b  6. e  8. a

**Exercise 2**

1. b  4. k  7. g  10. j
2. c  5. e  8. l  11. h
3. d  6. f  9. i

**Exercise 3**

**Figure 7-1**
Ovary: oophor/o    Cervix: cervic/o
Uterus: hyster/o, metr/o    Vagina: colp/o, vagin/o
  (metr/i), uter/o    Hymen: hymen/o
Fallopian, or uterine,
  tube: salping/o

**Figure 7-2**    **Figure 7-3**
Rectouterine pouch    Vulva: episi/o, vulv/o
(Douglas' cul-de-sac)    Perineum: perine/o
culd/o

**Exercise 4**

1. vagina  8. vulva  15. vulva
2. ovary  9. cervix  16. breast
3. uterus  10. vagina  17. beginning, first
4. uterus  11. woman  18. cul-de-sac
5. hymen  12. breast  19. woman
6. uterus  13. perineum
7. menstruation  14. fallopian tube

**Exercise 5**

1. a. episi/o  6. perine/o  9. a. gynec/o
   b. vulv/o  7. a. vagin/o     b. gyn/o
2. a. mamm/o     b. colp/o  10. hymen/o
   b. mast/o  8. a. **uter/o**  11. culd/o
3. men/o     b. metr/i, metr/o  12. cervic/o
4. oophor/o     c. hyster/o  13. arche/o
5. salping/o

**Exercise 6**

1. -salpinx  2. -ial  3. peri-  4. -atresia

**Exercise 7**

1. fallopian tube
2. around
3. pertaining to
4. absence of a normal body opening

**Exercise 8**

       WR  S
1. colp/itis    inflammation of the vagina

       WR  S
2. cervic/itis    inflammation of the cervix

     WR  CV  S
3. hydr/ o /salpinx    water in the fallopian tube
     CF

     WR  CV  S
4. hemat/ o /salpinx    blood in the fallopian tube
     CF

5. metr/orrhea         WR  S      excessive discharge from the uterus

6. oophor/itis     WR   S      inflammation of the ovary

7. (Bartholin's) aden/itis     WR  S      inflammation of Bartholin's gland

8. vulv/ o /vagin/itis   WR CV WR S   CF      inflammation of the vulva and vagina

9. salping/ o /cele   WR CV S   CF      hernia of the fallopian tube

10. men/ o /metr/orrhagia   WR CV WR S   CF      rapid flow of blood from the uterus at or between menstruation

11. a/men/orrhea   P WR S      absence of menstrual discharge

12. dys/men/orrhea   P WR S      painful menstrual discharge

13. mast/itis   WR S      inflammation of the breast

14. peri/metr/itis   P WR S      inflammation surrounding the uterus

15. my/ o /metr/itis   WR CV WR S   CF      inflammation of the uterine muscle

16. endo/metr/itis   P WR S      inflammation of the inner lining of the uterus

17. endo/cervic/itis   P WR S      inflammation of the inner lining of the cervix

18. py/ o /salpinx   WR CV S   CF      pus in the fallopian tube

19. hyster/atresia   WR S      closure of the uterus

20. salping/itis   WR S      inflammation of the fallopian tube

## Exercise 9

1. mast/itis
2. metr/orrhea
3. salping/itis
4. vulv/o/vagin/itis
5. a/men/orrhea
6. cervic/itis
7. Bartholin's aden/itis
8. hydr/o/salpinx
9. dys/men/orrhea
10. hemat/o/salpinx
11. colp/itis
12. men/o/metr/orrhagia
13. oophor/itis
14. salping/o/cele
15. peri/metr/itis
16. endo/metr/itis

17. endo/cervic/itis
18. my/o/metr/itis
19. py/o/salpinx
20. hyster/atresia

## Exercise 10

Spelling exercise; *see* text, pp. 236, 237.

## Exercise 11

1. downward placement of the uterus in the vagina
2. inflammation of the female pelvic organs
3. opening between the bladder and vagina
4. benign fibroid tumor of the uterine wall
5. abnormal condition in which endometrial tissue occurs in various areas of the pelvic cavity
6. growth of endometrium into the muscular portion of the uterus

## Exercise 12

1. vesicovaginal fistula
2. fibroid tumor
3. pelvic inflammatory disease
4. prolapsed uterus
5. endometriosis
6. adenomyosis

## Exercise 13

Spelling exercise; *see* text, p. 239.

## Exercise 14

1. colp/orrhaphy   WR S      suture of the vagina

2. colp/ o /plasty   WR CV S   CF      plastic repair of the vagina

3. episi/orrhaphy   WR S      suture of the vulva (tear)

4. hymen/otomy   WR S      incision of the hymen

5. hyster/ o /pexy   WR CV S   CF      surgical fixation of the uterus

6. vulv/ectomy   WR S      excision of the vulva

7. perine/orrhaphy   WR S      suture of the perineum (tear)

8. salping/ostomy   WR S      creation of an artificial opening in the fallopian tube

9. oophor/ o /salping/ectomy   WR CV WR S   CF      excision of the ovary and fallopian tube

        WR     S
10. oophor/ectomy              excision of the ovary

        WR     S
11. mast/ectomy              surgical removal of a
                                       breast

        WR     S
12. salping/ectomy            excision of a fallopian
                                       tube

        WR     S
13. cervic/ectomy            excision of the cervix

      WR CV   WR     S
14. colp/ o /perine/orrhaphy     suture of the vagina and
          CF                                 perineum

      WR CV   WR CV   S
15. episi/ o /perine/ o /plasty     plastic repair of the
         CF       CF                           vulva and perineum

        WR     S
16. hymen/ectomy          excision of the hymen

     WR   CV   WR   CV   WR     S
17. hyster/ o /salping/ o /-oophor/ectomy
         CF        CF

                              excision of the uterus,
                              fallopian tubes, and
                              ovaries

        WR     S
18. hyster/ectomy          excision of the uterus

      WR CV   S
19. mamm o /plasty         plastic repair of the
         CF                               breast

## Exercise 15

| | |
|---|---|
| 1. colp/orrhaphy | 11. hyster/ectomy |
| 2. cervic/ectomy | 12. oophor/ectomy |
| 3. episi/orrhaphy | 13. mast/ectomy |
| 4. episi/o/perine/o/plasty | 14. salping/ectomy |
| 5. colp/o/plasty | 15. perine/orrhaphy |
| 6. colp/o/perine/ orrhaphy | 16. oophor/o/salping/ ectomy |
| 7. hyster/o/salping/o/- oophor/ectomy | 17. salping/ostomy |
| 8. hyster/o/pexy | 18. vulv/ectomy |
| 9. hymen/ectomy | 19. mamm/o/plasty |
| 10. hymen/otomy | |

## Exercise 16

Spelling exercise; *see* text, p. 244.

## Exercise 17

1. laparoscopy (steriliza-tion); tubal ligation
2. A & P repair
3. dilatation and curet-tage
4. stereotactic breast bi-opsy
5. myomectomy

## Exercise 18

1. c   2. a   3. a   4. b   5. c   6. f

## Exercise 19

Spelling exercise; *see* text, p. 247.

## Exercise 20

      WR CV   S
1. colp/ o /scopy          visual examination of the
         CF                              vagina

      WR   CV   S
2. mamm/ o /gram        x-ray film of the breast
         CF

      WR CV   S
3. colp/ o /scope          instrument used for visual
         CF                              examination of the va-
                              gina

      WR   CV   S
4. hyster/ o /scopy       visual examination of the
         CF                              uterus

      WR   CV   WR   CV   S
5. hyster/ o /salping/ o /gram    x-ray film of the uterus
         CF         CF                 and fallopian tube

      WR CV   S
6. culd/ o /scope          instrument used for visual
         CF                              examination of the
                              Douglas' cul-de-sac

      WR CV   S
7. culd/ o /scopy          visual examination of the
         CF                              Douglas' cul-de-sac

      WR CV     S
8. culd/ o /centesis       surgical puncture to re-
         CF                              move fluid from the
                              Douglas' cul-de-sac

      WR   CV   S
9. mamm/ o /graphy      process of recording (x-
         CF                              ray) the breast

     WR   CV   S
10. hyster/ o /scope       instrument used for visual
         CF                              examination of the
                              uterus

## Exercise 21

| | |
|---|---|
| 1. hyster/o/salping/o/ gram | 6. culd/o/scope |
| 2. colp/o/scopy | 7. culd/o/scopy |
| 3. colp/o/scope | 8. culd/o/centesis |
| 4. hyster/o/scopy | 9. hyster/o/scope |
| 5. mamm/o/gram | 10. mamm/o/graph |

## Exercise 22

Spelling exercise; *see* text, p. 251.

## Exercise 23

1. WR S
   gynec/ologist — physician who specializes in gynecology

2. WR S
   gynec/ology — branch of medicine dealing with diseases of the female reproductive system

3. WR S
   colp/algia — pain in the vagina

4. WR CV WR S
   vulv/ o /vagin/al — pertaining to the vulva and vagina
   CF

5. WR S
   mast/algia — pain in the breast

6. WR WR
   men/arche — beginning of menstruation

7. WR S
   leuk/orrhea — white discharge (from the vagina)

8. WR CV WR S
   olig/ o /men/orrhea — scanty menstrual flow
   CF

9. WR CV WR S
   gyn/ o /path/ic — pertaining to disease of women
   CF

10. WR CV S
    mast/ o /ptosis — sagging breast
    CF

## Exercise 24

1. olig/o/men/orrhea
2. leuk/orrhea
3. men/arche
4. mast/algia
5. vulv/o/vagin/al
6. colp/algia
7. gynec/ologist
8. gynec/ology
9. mast/o/ptosis
10. gyn/o/path/ic

## Exercise 25

Spelling exercise; *see* text, p. 252.

## Exercise 26

1. cessation of menstruation
2. painful intercourse
3. abnormal passageway between two organs or between an internal organ and the body surface
4. a syndrome involving physical and emotional symptoms occurring during the 10 days prior to menstruation
5. instrument for opening a body cavity to allow for visual inspection

## Exercise 27

1. fistula
2. dyspareunia
3. menopause
4. premenstrual syndrome
5. speculum

## Exercise 28

Spelling exercise; *see* text, p. 256.

## Exercise 29

1. dysmenorrhea
2. endometritis
3. fallopian tube
4. suture of the vulva
5. mammoplasty
6. uterus, fallopian tubes and ovaries
7. hematosalpinx
8. endometriosis
9. speculum

## Exercise 30

1. hysteropexy
2. leukorrhea
3. gynecology
4. mastalgia
5. menarche

## Exercise 31

1. a
2. e
3. b
4. d
5. e
6. b

# Answers: Combining Forms—Chapters 6 and 7

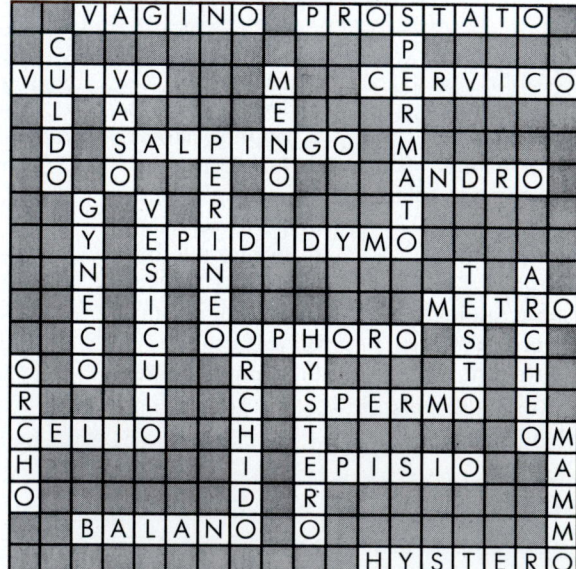

# 8

# Obstetrics and Neonatology

## Objectives

**Upon completion of this chapter you will be able to:**

1. Define the anatomical terms relating to pregnancy.

2. Write the definitions of the word parts included in this chapter.

3. Build, analyze, define, pronounce, and spell the diagnostic terms related to obstetrics.

4. Define, pronounce, and spell other diagnostic terms related to obstetrics.

5. Build, analyze, define, pronounce, and spell the diagnostic terms related to neonatology.

6. Define, pronounce, and spell other diagnostic terms related to neonatology.

7. Build, analyze, define, pronounce, and spell the surgical and diagnostic procedural terms related to obstetrics.

8. Build, analyze, define, pronounce, and spell additional terms related to obstetrics and neonatology.

9. Define, pronounce, and spell the other additional terms related to obstetrics and neonatology.

## Objective 1   DEFINE THE ANATOMICAL TERMS RELATING TO PREGNANCY.

## Anatomical Terms

Human life or pregnancy begins with the union of a mature female sex cell with a mature male sex cell. The duration of pregnancy in a human is 280 days: 9 calendar months, or 10 lunar months (a lunar month is 4 weeks, or 28 days).

### TERMS RELATING TO PREGNANCY

1. gamete . . . . . . . . . . . . . Mature sex cell: sperm (male) or ovum (female).

2. ovulation . . . . . . . . . . . Expulsion of an ovum from an ovary. (Figure 8-1).

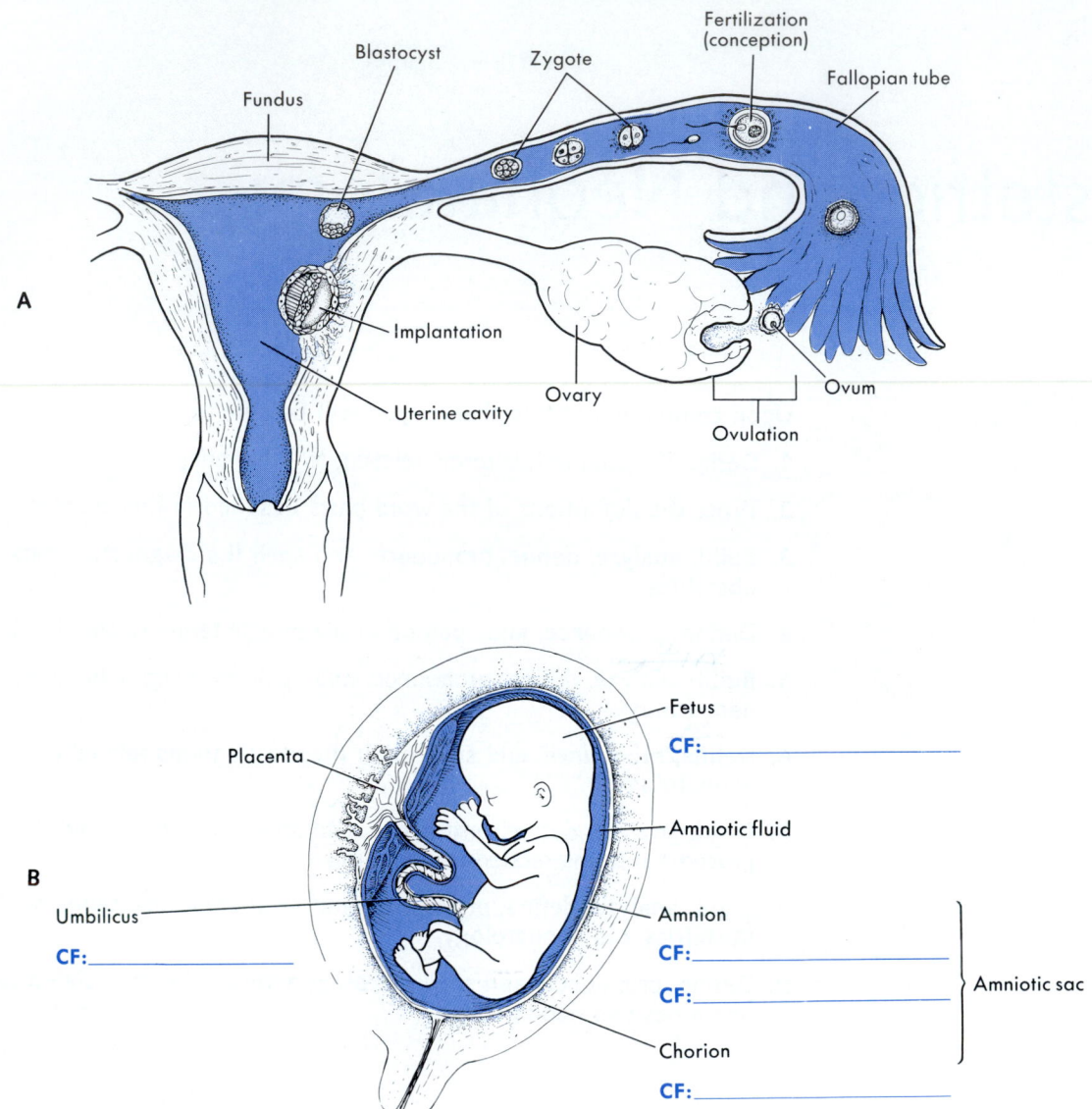

Figure 8-1

**A,** Ovulation, fertilization, and implantation. **B,** Development of the fetus.

3. conception, or fertiliza-
   tion................ Beginning of pregnancy, when the
   sperm enters the ovum. Fertilization
   normally occurs in the fallopian tubes
   (Figure 8-1).

4. zygote.............. Cell formed by the union of the sperm
   and the ovum (Figure 8-2).

5. gestation, or pregnancy. Development of a new individual from
   conception to birth.

   a. gestation period.... Duration of pregnancy.

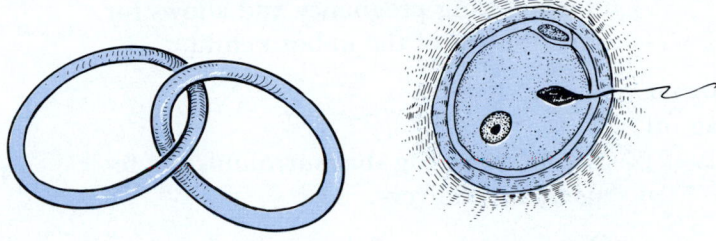

Figure 8-2

*Zygote* is derived from the Greek *zygosis*, which means *yoking* or *joining together.*

Em  +  bruo  =  Embryo

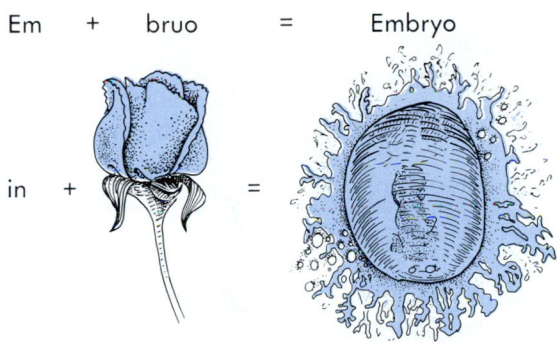

in  +  =

Figure 8-3

*Embryo* comes from the Greek *em* meaning *in*, plus *bruo*, meaning *to bud* or *shoot*.

6. implantation, or nidation................. Embedding of the zygote in the uterine lining. The process normally begins about 7 days after fertilization and continues to occur for several days (Figure 8-1).

7. embryo.............. Unborn offspring in the stage of development from implantation of the zygote to the second month of pregnancy. This period is characterized by rapid growth of the embryo. (Figure 8-3).

8. fetus............... Unborn offspring from the second month of pregnancy until birth.

9.   placenta, or afterbirth . .   Substance that grows on the wall of the uterus during pregnancy and allows for nourishment of the unborn child.

10.   amniotic or amnionic sac (also known as bag of waters) . . . . . . . . . . . .   Membranous bag that surrounds the fetus before delivery.

    a.   chorion . . . . . . . . .   Outermost layer of the fetal membrane.

    b.   amnion . . . . . . . . .   Innermost layer of the fetal membrane.

    c.   amniotic fluid . . . . .   Fluid within the amniotic sac that surrounds the fetus.

Learn the anatomical terms by completing the following exercises.

## EXERCISE 1

Fill in the blanks with the correct terms.

1.  The expulsion of a mature ovum, or ___*ovulation*___ *(gamete)*, from an ovary is called ___*ovulation*___. When the male gamete enters the female gamete, ___*conception*___ occurs, and a(n) ___*zygote*___ is formed. This marks the beginning of the ___*gestation*___ period.

2.  Once the zygote is implanted, it becomes a(n) ___*embryo*___ until the second month of gestation. The unborn offspring from the second month until birth is called a(n) ___*fetus*___.

3.  The fetus is surrounded by a(n) ___*amniotic*___ sac, which has an outermost layer, called the ___*chorion*___, and an innermost layer, called the ___*amnion*___. This sac contains the ___*amniotic*___ fluid that surrounds the fetus.

Place a check mark (√) in the box to indicate that you have completed Objective 1.

☐ **DEFINE THE ANATOMICAL TERMS RELATING TO PREGNANCY.**

# Objective 2   WRITE THE DEFINITIONS OF THE WORD PARTS INCLUDED IN THIS CHAPTER.

# Obstetrical and Neonatological Word Parts

Study the word parts and their definitions listed as follows. Learning will be made easier by completing the exercises that follow.

| COMBINING FORM | DEFINITION |
| --- | --- |
| 1.   amni/o, amnion/o . . . . . . | amnion |
| 2.   chori/o . . . . . . . . . . . . . | chorion |

3. embry/o . . . . . . . . . . . .  embryo, to be full

4. fet/o, fet/i . . . . . . . . . . .  fetus, unborn child
   (NOTE: Both *i* and *o* may be used as combining vowels with *fet.*)

5. gravid/o
   cyes/o, cyes/i . . . . . . . . .  pregnancy
   (NOTE: Both *o* and *i* may be used as combining vowels with *cyes.*)

6. lact/o . . . . . . . . . . . . . .  milk

7. nat/o . . . . . . . . . . . . . .  birth

8. omphal/o . . . . . . . . . . .  umbilicus, navel

9. par/o, part/o . . . . . . . . .  bear, give birth to; labor

10. puerper/o . . . . . . . . . . .  childbirth

> **Puerper** is made up of two Latin word roots: **puer**, meaning **child**, and **per**, meaning **through.**

Learn the anatomical locations and definitions of the combining forms by completing the following exercises.

## EXERCISE 2

Write the combining forms in the spaces marked **CF** on the diagram in Figure 8-1, p. 266.

## EXERCISE 3

Write the definitions of the following combining forms.

1. fet/o, fet/i _____ *fetus unborn child* _____

2. lact/o _____ *milk* _____

3. par/o, part/o _____ *bear, give birth to* _____

4. omphal/o _____ *umbilicus, navel* _____

5. amni/o, amnion/o _____ *amnion* _____

6. puerper/o _____ *childbirth* _____

7. gravid/o
   cyes/o, cyes/i _____ *pregnancy* _____

8. nat/o _____ *birth* _____

9. chori/o _____ *chorion* _____

10. embry/o _____ *embryo, to be full* _____

## EXERCISE 4

Write the combining form for each of the following.

1. milk                    _____

2. fetus                   _____

3. chorion                 _____

4. amnion          a.   _____

                   b.   _____

5. childbirth              _____

6. give birth to   a.   _____

                   b.   _____

7. pregnancy       a.   _____

                   b.   _____

8. embryo                  _____

9. birth                   _____

10. umbilicus, or navel    _____

# Related Word Parts

| COMBINING FORM | DEFINITION |
| --- | --- |
| 1. cephal/o . . . . . . . . . . . . . | head |
| 2. esophag/o . . . . . . . . . . . | esophagus (tube leading from the throat to the stomach) (see Figure 10-1, p. 364) |
| 3. pelvi/i, pelv/o . . . . . . . . . (NOTE: Both *i* and *o* may be used as the combining vowel with *pelv*.) | pelvic bone, pelvis (see Figures 13-2 and 13-5, pp. 478 and 480) |
| 4. prim/i . . . . . . . . . . . . . . . (NOTE: The combining vowel is *i*.) | first |
| 5. pseud/o . . . . . . . . . . . . . | false |
| 6. pylor/o . . . . . . . . . . . . . | pylorus (pyloric sphincter) (see Figure 10-2, p. 366) |

## EXERCISE 5

Write the definitions of the following combining forms.

1. prim/i _____ *first* _____

2. pylor/o _____ *pylorus* _____

3. cephal/o ___ *head* ___

4. esophag/o ___ *esophagus* ___

5. pseud/o ___ *false* ___

6. pelv/o, pelv/i ___ *pelvic bone, pelvis* ___

## EXERCISE 6

Write the combining form for each of the following.

1. head _____

2. pylorus _____

3. false _____

4. esophagus _____

5. first _____

6. pelvic bone, pelvis _____

# Prefixes

| PREFIX | DEFINITION |
|---|---|
| 1. ante- . . . . . . . . . . . . . . . . | before |
| 2. micro- . . . . . . . . . . . . . . | small |
| 3. multi- . . . . . . . . . . . . . . | many |
| 4. nulli- . . . . . . . . . . . . . . | none |
| 5. post- . . . . . . . . . . . . . . | after |

## EXERCISE 7

Write the definitions of the following prefixes.

1. post- ___ *after* ___

2. multi- ___ *many* ___

3. nulli- ___ *none* ___

4. micro- ___ *small* ___

5. ante- ___ *before* ___

## EXERCISE 8

Write the prefix for each of the following definitions.

1. none _____

2. small    _____

3. many    _____

4. before    _____

5. after    _____

## Suffixes

| SUFFIX | DEFINITION |
|---|---|
| 1. -orrhexis.............. | rupture |
| 2. -tocia ............... | birth, labor |

> Several terms introduced in this chapter end with the noun suffixes **-a, -e, -is,** and **-us.** The suffixes have no special meaning but should be analyzed as suffixes.

Orrhexis is the last of the four **-orrh-** suffixes to be learned. The other three introduced in earlier chapters are **-orrhea** (excessive flow or discharge), **-orrhagia** (rapid flow [of blood]), and **-orrhaphy** (suturing, repair).

Place a check mark (√) in the box to indicate that you have completed Objective 2.

☐ **WRITE THE DEFINITIONS OF THE WORD PARTS INCLUDED IN THIS CHAPTER.**

## Medical Terms

The terms you need to learn to complete this chapter are listed as follows. Now that you know the meaning of the word parts, the exercises found at the end of the list will assist you to learn the definition and spelling of each word.

## Objective 3   BUILD, ANALYZE, DEFINE, PRONOUNCE, AND SPELL THE DIAGNOSTIC TERMS RELATED TO OBSTETRICS.

## Diagnostic Terms

**TERM**
(built from word parts) — **DEFINITION**

1. amnionitis ............
(am-nē-ō-NĪ-tis) — inflammation of the amnion

2. chorioamnionitis .......
(kō-rē-ō-am-nē-ō-NĪ-tis) — inflammation of the amnion and chorion

3. choriocarcinoma .......
(kō-rē-ō-kar-si-NŌ-ma) — cancerous tumor of the chorion

4. dystocia ............
(dis-TŌ-sē-a) — difficult labor

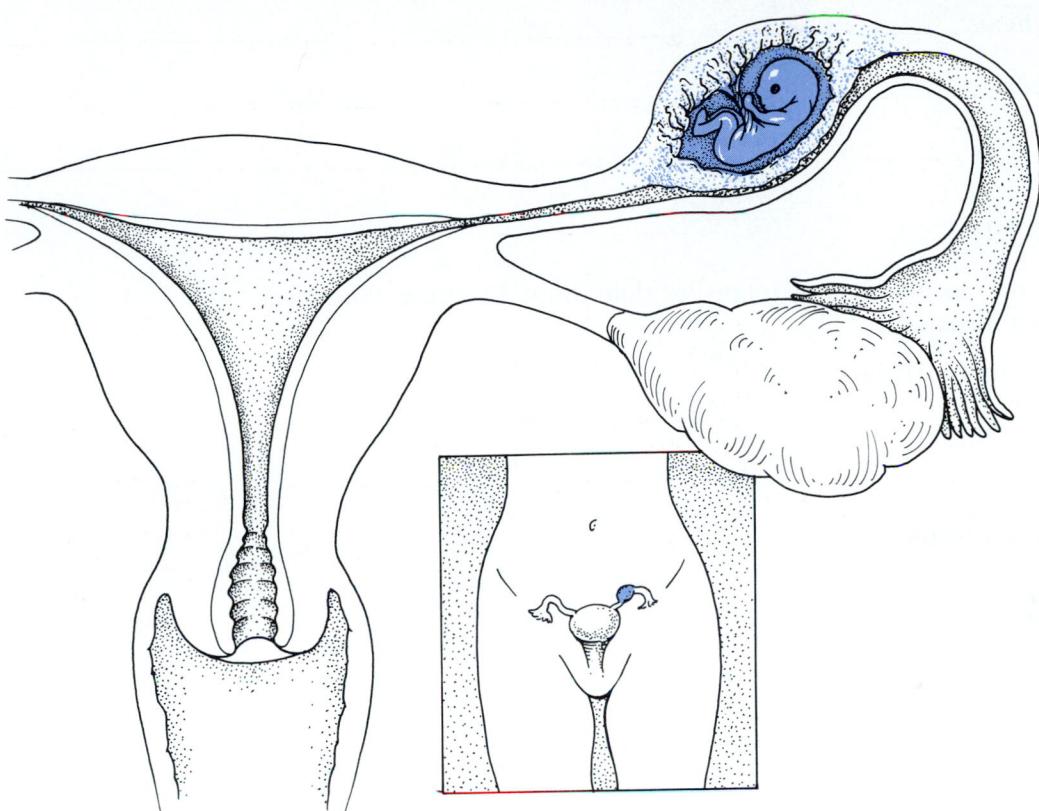

Figure 8-4
Ectopic pregnancy (in the fallopian tubes) or salpingocyesis.

5. **embryotocia** . . . . . . . . . . .    **birth of an embryo (abortion)**
   (*em*-brē-ō-TŌ-sē-a)

6. **hysterorrhexis** . . . . . . . . .    **rupture of the uterus**
   (his-ter-ō-REK-sis)

7. **salpingocyesis** . . . . . . . . .    **pregnancy occurring in the fallopian**
   (sal-PING-gō-sī-ē-sis)    **tube (an ectopic pregnancy) (Figure 8-4)**

Practice saying each of these terms aloud. To assist you in pronunciation, obatin the audiotape designed for use with this text. Learn the definitions and spellings of the diagnostic terms by completing the following exercises.

## EXERCISE 9

Analyze and define the following diagnostic terms.

1. chorioamnionitis _____ *inflamation of the amnion + the chorion* _____

2. choriocarcinoma _____ *cancerous tumor of the chorion* _____

3. dystocia _____ *painful labor* _____

4. amnionitis _____ *inflamation of the amnion* _____

5. hysterorrhexis _____ rupture of the uterus

6. embryotocia _____ birth of an embryo

7. salpingocyesis _____ pregnancy in the fallopian tubes

## EXERCISE 10

Build diagnostic terms for the following definitions by using the word parts you have learned.

1. cancerous tumor of the chorion

$$\frac{\quad\quad}{WR} / \frac{\quad}{CV} / \frac{\quad\quad}{WR} / \frac{\quad\quad}{S}$$

2. inflammation of the amnion

$$\frac{\quad\quad}{WR} / \frac{\quad\quad}{S}$$

3. inflammation of the amnion and chorion

$$\frac{\quad\quad}{WR} / \frac{\quad}{CV} / \frac{\quad\quad}{WR} / \frac{\quad\quad}{S}$$

4. birth of an embryo (abortion)

$$\frac{\quad\quad}{WR} / \frac{\quad}{CV} / \frac{\quad\quad}{S}$$

5. difficult labor

$$\frac{\quad\quad}{P} / \frac{\quad\quad}{S(WR)}$$

6. rupture of the uterus

$$\frac{\quad\quad}{WR} / \frac{\quad\quad}{S}$$

7. pregnancy occurring in the fallopian tube

$$\frac{\quad\quad}{WR} / \frac{\quad}{CV} / \frac{\quad\quad}{WR} / \frac{\quad\quad}{S}$$

## EXERCISE 11

Spell each of the diagnostic terms. Have someone dictate the terms on pp. 272 and 273 to you or say the words into a tape recorder; then spell the words from your recording as often as necessary. Think about the word parts before attempting to write the word. Study any you have spelled incorrectly.

1. _____    3. _____

2. _____    4. _____

5. _____    7. _____

6. _____

Place a check mark (√) in the box to indicate that you have completed Objective 3.

☐ BUILD, ANALYZE, DEFINE, PRONOUNCE, AND SPELL THE DIAGNOSTIC TERMS RELATED TO OBSTETRICS.

# Objective 4 DEFINE, PRONOUNCE, AND SPELL OTHER DIAGNOSTIC TERMS RELATED TO OBSTETRICS.

## Other Diagnostic Terms

| TERM | DEFINITION |
|---|---|
| 1. abortion . . . . . . . . . . . . .<br>(ab-ŌR-shun) | termination of pregnancy by the expulsion from the uterus of an embryo or a nonviable fetus |
| 2. abruptio placentae . . . . . .<br>(ab-RŬP-shē-ō) (pla-SEN-tē) | premature separation of the placenta from the uterine wall (Figure 8-5) |

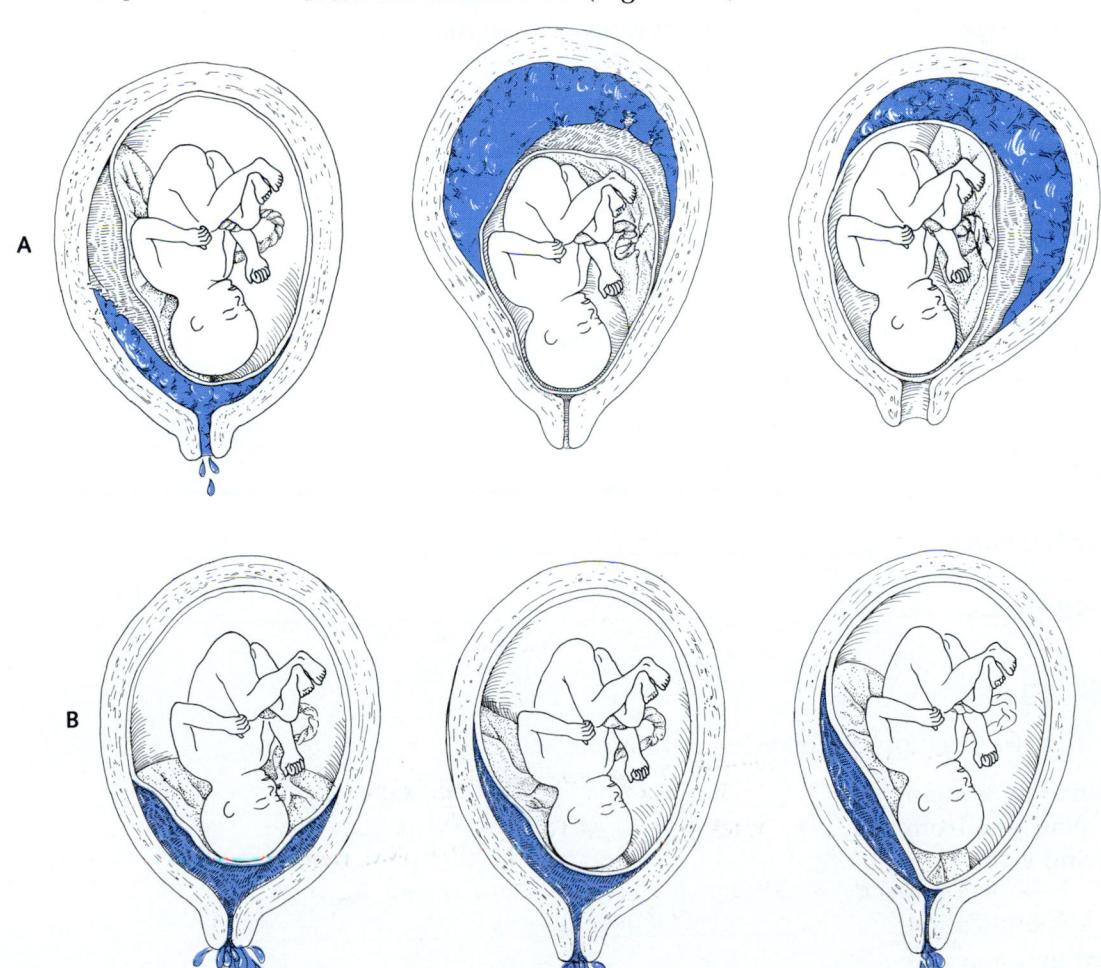

Figure 8-5

**A,** Various stages of abruptio placentae. **B,** Placenta previa.

3. eclampsia . . . . . . . . . . . .    severe complication and progression of
   (ē-KLAMP-sē-a)    preeclampsia characterized by convul-
   sion and coma (see *preeclampsia* below)

4. ectopic pregnancy . . . . . .    pregnancy occurring outside the uterus,
   (ek-TOP-ik)    commonly in the fallopian tube

5. placenta previa. . . . . . . .    abnormally low implantation of the pla-
   (pla-SEN-ta) (PREV-ē-a)    centa on the uterine wall. (Dilatation of
   the cervix can cause separation of the
   placenta from the uterine wall, resulting
   in bleeding. With severe hemorrhage, a
   cesarean section may be necessary to
   save the mother's life.) (Figure 8-5)

6. preeclampsia . . . . . . . . .    abnormal condition encountered during
   (prē-ē-KLAMP-sē-a)    pregnancy or shortly after delivery,
   characterized by high blood pressure,
   edema, and proteinuria, and with no
   convulsions or coma

**Cesarean section** (C section) is the birth of a baby through an incision in the mother's abdomen and uterus. The origin of the term has no relation to the birth of Julius Caesar, as is commonly believed. One suggested etymology is that from 715 to 672 BC it was Roman law that the operation be performed on dying women in the last few months of pregnancy in the hope of saving the child. At that time the operation was called **a caeso matris utero**, which means **the cutting of the mother's uterus.**

Practice saying each of these terms aloud. To assist you in pronunciation, obtain the audiotape designed for use with this text. Learn the definitions and spellings of the other diagnostic terms by completing the following exercises.

## EXERCISE 12

Write the definitions of the following terms.

1. abruptio placentae _____

2. abortion _____

3. placenta previa _____

4. eclampsia _____

5. ectopic pregnancy _____

6. preeclampsia _____

## EXERCISE 13

Write the term for each of the following definitions.

1. premature separation      *abruptio placentae*
   of the placenta from
   the uterine wall

2. severe complication      *eclampsia*
   and progression of
   preeclampsia

3. termination of pregnancy by the expulsion from the uterus of an embryo or nonviable fetus

*abortion*

4. pregnancy occurring outside the uterus

*ectopic pregnancy*

5. abnormally low implantation of the placenta on the uterine wall

*placenta previa*

6. abnormal condition encountered during pregnancy or shortly after delivery

*preeclampsia*

## EXERCISE 14

Spell the other diagnostic terms. Have someone dictate the terms on pp. 275 and 276 to you or say the words into a tape recorder; then spell the words from your recording as often as necessary. Study any you have spelled incorrectly.

1. _____    4. _____

2. _____    5. _____

3. _____    6. _____

Place a check mark (√) in the box to indicate that you have completed Objective 4.

☐ **DEFINE, PRONOUNCE, AND SPELL OTHER DIAGNOSTIC TERMS RELATED TO OBSTETRICS.**

# Objective 5  **BUILD, ANALYZE, DEFINE, PRONOUNCE, AND SPELL THE DIAGNOSTIC TERMS RELATED TO NEONATOLOGY.**

## Diagnostic Terms

| TERM (built from word parts) | DEFINITION |
|---|---|
| 1. microcephalus . . . . . . . . . (mī-krō-SEF-a-lus) | (fetus with a very) small head |
| 2. omphalitis . . . . . . . . . . . (om-fa-LĪ-tis) | inflammation of the umbilicus |

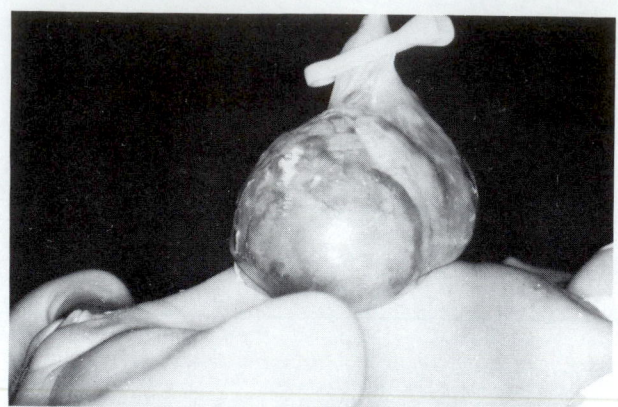

## Figure 8-6
Omphalocele containing liver.

From Bobak IM, Jensen MD, and Zalar MK: *Maternity care: the nurse and the family*, ed 4, St. Louis, 1989, Mosby.

3. omphalocele . . . . . . . . . . (congenital) herniation (of part of the in-
   (OM-fal-ō-*sēl*)        testine through the abdominal wall) at
                            the umbilicus (Figure 8-6)

4. pyloric stenosis . . . . . . . . narrowing of the pyloric sphincter. Con-
   (pī-LŌR-ik) (ste-NŌ-sis)  genital pyloric stenosis occurs in 1 of ev-
                            ery 200 newborns.

5. tracheoesophageal fistula . abnormal   passageway   between   the
   (TRĀ-kē-ō-ē-*sof*-a-*jē*-al)   (FIS-  esophagus and the trachea
   tū-la)

Practice saying each of these terms aloud. To assist you in pronunciation,
obtain the audiotape designed for this text. Learn the definitions and spellings of the diagnostic terms by completing the following exercises.

## EXERCISE 15

Analyze and define the following diagnostic terms.

1. pyloric stenosis _____ narrowing of the pyloric sphincter
2. omphalocele _____ herniation at the umbilicus
3. omphalitis _____ inflamation of the umbilicus
4. microcephalus _____ small head (fetus)
5. tracheoesophageal fistula _____ abnormal passageway between esophagus trachea

## EXERCISE 16

Build diagnostic terms for the following by using the word parts you have learned.

1. hernia (of part of the intestine through the abdominal wall) at the umbilicus

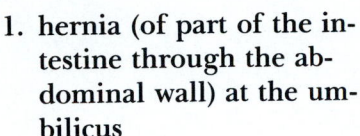

_____
WR / CV / S

2. (fetus with a very) small head

_____
P / WR / S

3. narrowing of the pyloric sphincter

_____ stenosis
WR / S

4. abnormal passageway between the esophagus and the trachea

_____ fistula
WR / CV / WR / S

5. inflammation of the umbilicus

_____
WR / S

## EXERCISE 17

Spell each of the diagnostic terms. Have someone dictate the terms on pp. 277 and 278 to you or say the words into a tape recorder; then spell the words from your recording as often as necessary. Think about the word parts before attempting to write the word. Study any you have spelled incorrectly.

1. _____      4. _____

2. _____      5. _____

3. _____

Place a check mark (√) in the box to indicate that you have completed Objective 5.

☐ **BUILD, ANALYZE, DEFINE, PRONOUNCE, AND SPELL THE DIAGNOSTIC TERMS RELATED TO NEONATOLOGY.**

# Objective 6   DEFINE, PRONOUNCE, AND SPELL OTHER DIAGNOSTIC TERMS RELATED TO NEONATOLOGY.

## Other Diagnostic Terms

| TERM | DEFINITION |
|---|---|
| 1.  cleft lip and palate...... | congenital split of the lip and roof of the mouth (*cleft* indicates a fissure) |
| 2.  Down's syndrome....... | Congenital condition characterized by varying degrees of mental retardation and multiple defects (formerly called *mongolism*) |
| 3.  erythroblastosis fetalis ...<br>(e-*rith*-rō-blas-TŌ-sis)<br>(fet-A-lis) | condition of the newborn characterized by hemolysis of the erythrocytes. The condition is usually caused by the incompatibility of the infant's and mother's blood, occurring when the mother's blood is Rh negative and the infant's blood is Rh positive. |
| 4.  esophageal atresia ......<br>(ē-sof-a-JE-al) (a-TRĒ-zē-a) | congenital absence of part of the esophagus. Food cannot pass from the baby's mouth to the stomach (Figure 8-7) |

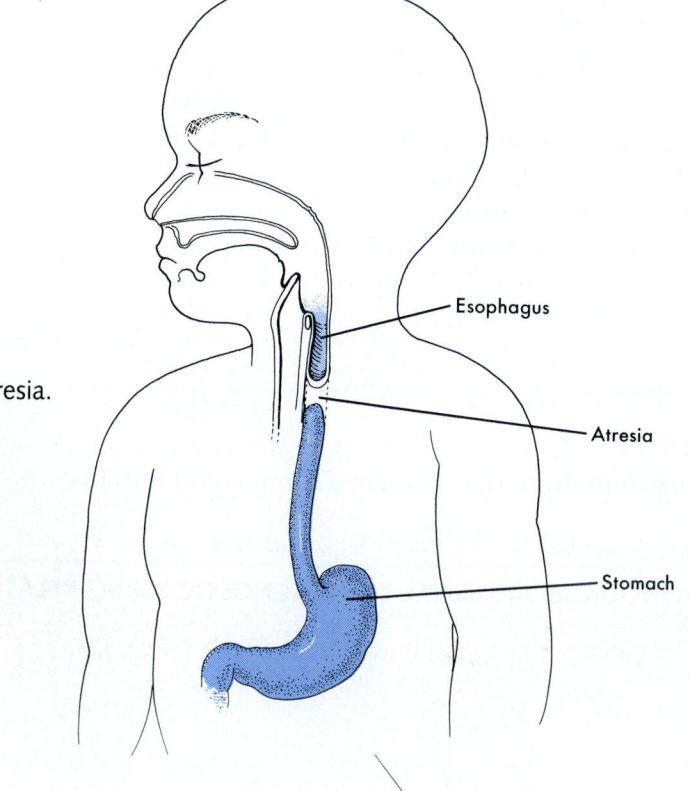

Figure 8-7
Esophageal atresia.

Esophagus

Atresia

Stomach

5. spina    bifida    (divided spine) . . . . . . . . . . . . . .
   (SPĪ-na) (BIF-i-da)

   congenital defect in the vertebral column caused by the failure of the vertebral arch to fuse (see Figure 14-5, p. 543)

6. hyaline membrane disease (HMD) . . . . . . . . . . . . . .
   (HĪ-a-lĭn)

   respiratory complication found especially in premature infants (also known as *respiratory distress syndrome—RDS*)

Practice saying each of these terms aloud. To assist you in pronunciation, obtain the audiotape designed for use with this text. Learn the definitions and spellings of the other diagnostic terms by completing the following exercises.

## EXERCISE 18

Match the terms in the first column with the correct definitions in the second column.

____f___ 1. Down's syndrome

____c___ 2. cleft lip and palate

____a___ 3. spina bifida

____d___ 4. erythroblastosis fetalis

____b___ 5. hyaline    membrane disease

____e___ 6. esophageal atresia

a. defect of the vertebral column

b. respiratory complication

c. split of the lip and roof of the mouth

d. caused by incompatibility of the infant's and the mother's blood

e. congenital absence of part of the esophagus

f. congenital condition characterized by mental retardation

g. pregnancy occurring outside the uterus

## EXERCISE 19

Spell the other diagnostic terms. Have someone dictate the terms on pp. 280 and 281 to you or say the words into a tape recorder; then spell the words from your recording as often as necessary. Study any you have spelled incorrectly.

1. _____    4. _____

2. _____    5. _____

3. _____    6. _____

Place a check mark (√) in the box to indicate that you have completed Objective 6.

☐ DEFINE, PRONOUNCE, AND SPELL OTHER DIAGNOSTIC TERMS RELATED TO NEONATOLOGY.

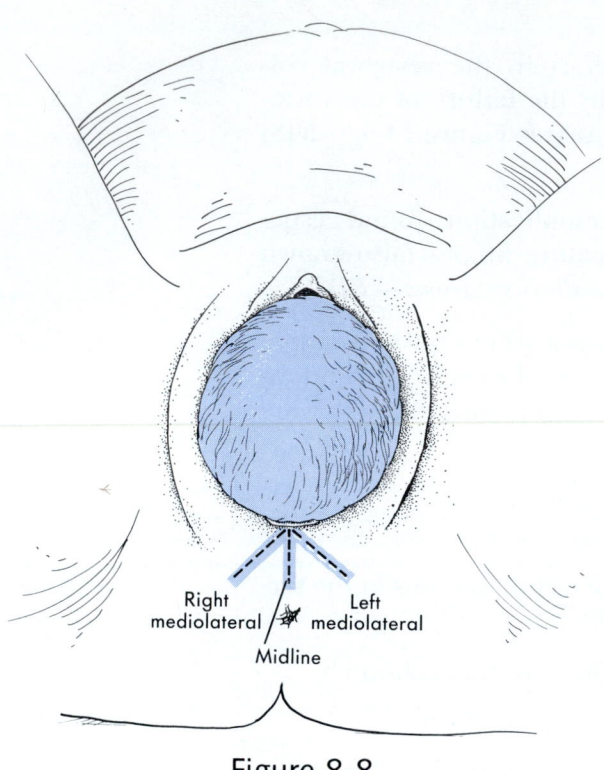

Right mediolateral    Left mediolateral

Midline

Figure 8-8
Episiotomies.

# Objective 7 | BUILD, ANALYZE, DEFINE, PRONOUNCE, AND SPELL THE SURGICAL AND DIAGNOSTIC PROCEDURAL TERMS RELATED TO OBSTETRICS.

## Surgical Terms

| **TERM** (built from word parts) | **DEFINITION** |
| --- | --- |
| 1. amniotomy . . . . . . . . . . . (am-nē-OT-ō-mē) | incision into the fetal membranes (performed to induce labor) |
| 2. episiotomy . . . . . . . . . . . (e-*piz*-ē-OT-ō-mē) | incision of the vulva (perineum) usually done during delivery to prevent tearing of the perineum (also called *perineotomy*) (Figure 8-8) |

## Diagnostic Procedural Terms

| **TERM** (built from word parts) | **DEFINITION** |
| --- | --- |
| 1. amniocentesis . . . . . . . . . (am-nē-ō-sen-TĒ-sis) | surgical puncture to remove amniotic fluid (the needle is inserted through the abdominal and uterine walls, utilizing ultrasound to guide the needle. The fluid is used for the assessment of fetal |

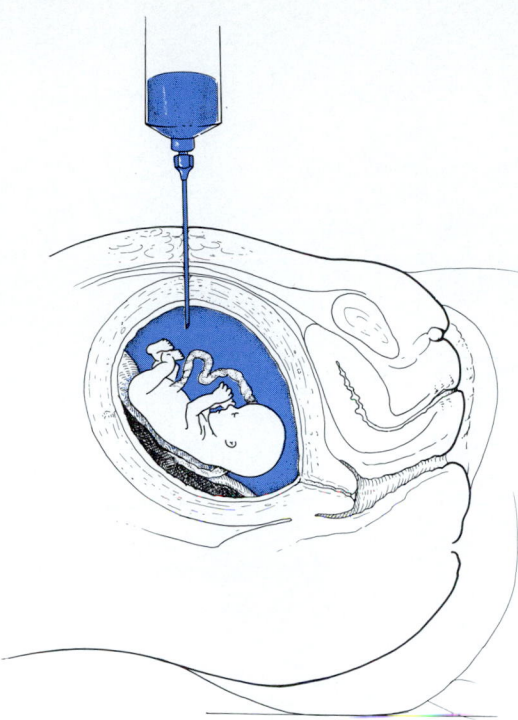

Figure 8-9
Amniocentesis.

health and maturity to aid in diagnosing fetal abnormalities) (Figure 8-9)

2. **amniography** . . . . . . . . . .
   (*am*-nē-OG-ra-fē)
   process of x-ray filming of the uterus (after the injection of contrast medium into the amniotic fluid, which outlines the amniotic cavity and fetus)

3. **amnioscope** . . . . . . . . . . .
   (AM-nē-ō-skōp)
   instrument (inserted through the cervix and used) for visual examination of the fetus and amniotic fluid

4. **amnioscopy** . . . . . . . . . .
   (*am*-nē-OS-kō-pē)
   visual examination of the fetus and amniotic fluid

5. **fetography** . . . . . . . . . . .
   (fē-TOG-ra-fē)
   process of x-ray filming the fetus

6. **fetometry** . . . . . . . . . . . .
   (fē-TOM-e-trē)
   measurement of the size of the fetus

7. **fetoscope** . . . . . . . . . . . .
   (FĒ-tō-scōp)
   instrument used for examining fetal heart tones (Figure 8-10)

8. **pelvimetry** . . . . . . . . . . .
   (pel-VIM-e-trē)
   measurement of the mother's pelvis (to determine ability of the fetus to pass through)

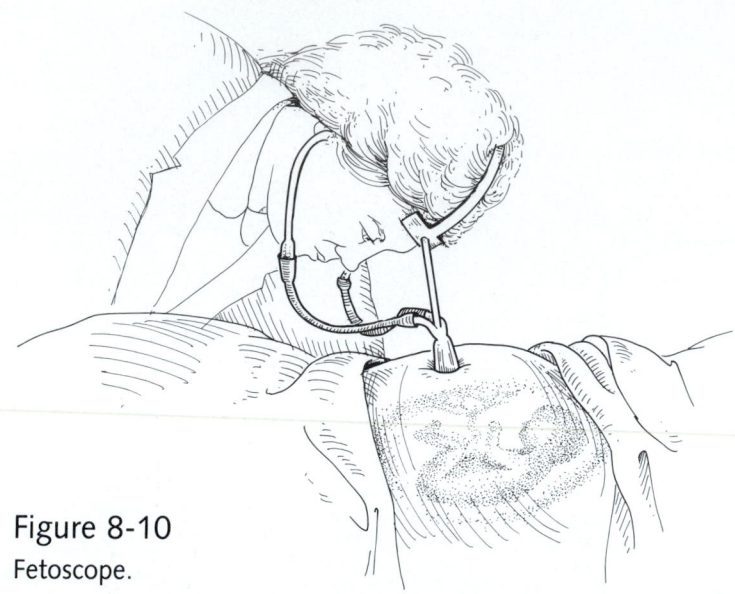

**Figure 8-10**
Fetoscope.

Practice saying these terms aloud. To assist you in pronunciation, obtain the audiotape designed for use with this text. Learn the definitions and spellings of the surgical and diagnostic procedural terms by completing the following exercises. (Since there are few terms in the surgical and procedural diagnostic categories, the exercises are combined.)

## EXERCISE 20

Analyze and define the following terms.

1. episiotomy _____

2. amniotomy _____

3. amnioscope _____

4. amniography _____

5. fetography _____

6. amniocentesis _____

7. amnioscopy _____

8. pelvimetry _____

9. fetoscope _____

10. fetometry _____

## EXERCISE 21

Build terms for the following definitions by using the word parts you have learned.

1. incision into the fetal membranes

_amni_ | _otomy_
WR | S

2. incision of the vulva

_episi_ | _otomy_
WR | S

3. process of x-ray filming the uterus to outline the amniotic cavity and fetus

_amnio_ | _o_ | _graphy_
WR | CV | S

4. visual examination of the fetus and amniotic fluid

_amni_ | _o_ | _scopy_
WR | CV | S

5. surgical puncture to remove amniotic fluid

_amni_ | _o_ | _centesis_
WR | CV | S

6. instrument used for visual examination of the fetus and amniotic fluid

_amni_ | _o_ | _scope_
WR | CV | S

7. process of x-ray filming the fetus

_fet_ | _o_ | _graphy_
WR | CV | S

8. instrument used for examining fetal heart tones

_fet_ | _o_ | _scope_
WR | CV | S

9. measurement of the mother's pelvis

_pelvi_ | _i_ | _metry_
WR | CV | S

10. measurement of the size of the fetus

_fet_ | _o_ | _metry_
WR | CV | S

## EXERCISE 22

Spell each of the surgical and diagnostic procedural terms. Have someone dictate the terms on pp. 282 and 283 to you or say the words into a tape recorder; then spell the words from your recording as often as necessary. Think about the word parts before attempting to spell the word. Study any you have spelled incorrectly.

1. _____      6. _____
2. _____      7. _____
3. _____      8. _____
4. _____      9. _____
5. _____      10. _____

Place a check mark (√) in the box to indicate that you have completed Objective 7.

☐ **BUILD, ANALYZE, DEFINE, PRONOUNCE, AND SPELL THE SURGICAL AND DIAGNOSTIC PROCEDURAL TERMS RELATED TO OBSTETRICS AND NEONATOLOGY.**

## Objective 8   BUILD, ANALYZE, DEFINE, PRONOUNCE, AND SPELL ADDITIONAL TERMS RELATED TO OBSTETRICS AND NEONATOLOGY.

## Additional Terms

| TERM (built from word parts) | DEFINITION |
|---|---|
| 1. amniochorial (am-nē-ō-KŌ-rē-al) | pertaining to the amnion and chorion |
| 2. amniorrhea (am-nē-ō-RĒ-a) | discharge (escape) of amniotic fluid |
| 3. amniorrhexis (am-nē-ō-REK-sis) | rupture of the amnion |
| 4. antepartum (an-tē-PAR-tum) | occurring before childbirth |
| 5. cyesiology (sī-ē-sē-OL-ō-jē) | study of pregnancy |
| 6. cyesis (sī-Ē-sis) | pregnancy |
| 7. embryogenic (em-brē-ō-JEN-ik) | producing an embryo |
| 8. embryoid (EM-brē-oyd) | resembling an embryo |
| 9. embryologist (em-brē-OL-ō-jist) | one who specializes in embryology |
| 10. embryology (em-brē-OL-ō-jē) | study or science of the development of the embryo |

11. fetal . . . . . . . . . . . . . . . pertaining to the fetus
    (FĒ-tal)

12. gravida . . . . . . . . . . . . . pregnant woman
    (GRAV-i-da)

13. gravidopuerperal . . . . . pertaining to pregnancy and the puerperium
    (grav-i-dō-pū-ER-per-al)

14. intrapartum . . . . . . . . . occurring during labor and childbirth
    (in-tra-PAR-tum)

15. lactic . . . . . . . . . . . . . . pertaining to milk
    (LAK-tik)

16. lactogenic . . . . . . . . . . . (stimulating) the production of milk
    (lak-tō-JEN-ik)

17. lactorrhea . . . . . . . . . . . (spontaneous) discharge of milk
    (lak-tō-RĒ-a)

18. multigravida . . . . . . . . . woman who has been pregnant two or more times
    (mul-tī-GRAV-i-da)

19. multipara . . . . . . . . . . . woman who has given birth to two or more (viable) offspring
    (mul-TIP-a-ra)

20. natal . . . . . . . . . . . . . . . pertaining to birth
    (NĀ-tal)

21. neonate . . . . . . . . . . . . . an infant from birth to four weeks of age
    (NĒ-ō-nāt)

22. neonatology . . . . . . . . . branch of medicine that deals with diagnosis and treatment of disorders in newborn infants
    (nē-ō-nā-TOL-ō-jē)

23. nulligravida . . . . . . . . . woman who has never been pregnant
    (nul-li-GRAV-i-da)

24. nullipara . . . . . . . . . . . . woman who has not given birth to a viable offspring
    (nu-LIP-a-ra)

25. para . . . . . . . . . . . . . . . woman who has given birth to a viable offspring
    (PAR-a)

26. postpartum . . . . . . . . . . occurring after childbirth
    (pōst-PAR-tum)

27. primigravida . . . . . . . . woman in her first pregnancy
    (prī-mi-GRAV-i-da)

28. primipara . . . . . . . . . . . woman who has borne one viable offspring
    (prī-MIP-a-ra)

29. pseudocyesis . . . . . . . . . false pregnancy
    (sū-dō-sī-Ē-sis)

30. puerpera . . . . . . . . . . . . woman who has just given birth
    (pū-ER-per-a)

31. puerperal . . . . . . . . . . . pertaining to (immediately after) childbirth
    (pū-ER-per-al)

Practice saying each of these terms aloud. To assist you in pronunciation, obtain the audiotape designed for use with this text. Learn the definitions and spellings of the additional terms by completing the following exercises.

## EXERCISE 23

Analyze and define the following terms.

1. puerpera _____

2. amniorrhexis _____

3. antepartum _____

4. cyesiology _____

5. pseudocyesis _____

6. cyesis _____

7. lactic _____

8. lactorrhea _____

9. amniorrhea _____

10. embryologist _____

11. multipara _____

12. embryogenic _____

13. embryoid _____

14. fetal _____

15. gravida _____

16. embryology _____

17. amniochorial _____

18. multigravida _____

19. lactogenic _____

20. natal _____

21. gravidopuerperal _____

22. neonatology _____

23. nullipara _____

24. para _____

25. primigravida _____

26. postpartum _____

27. neonate _____

28. primipara _____

29. puerperal _____

30. nulligravida _____

31. intrapartum _____

## EXERCISE 24

Build the word for each of the following definitions.

1. pertaining to the amnion and chorion

   _amni / o / chor / ial_
   WR   CV   WR   S

2. before childbirth

   _ante / o / partum_
   P   WR   S

3. producing an embryo

   _ebryo / gen / ic_
   WR   CV   S

4. study of pregnancy

   _cyes / i / ology_
   WR   CV   S

5. pertaining to the fetus

   _fet / al_
   WR   S

6. pregnancy

   _cyesis_
   WR   S

7. pertaining to milk

   _lact / ic_
   WR   S

8. (spontaneous) discharge of milk

   _lact / orrhea_
   WR   S

9. discharge (escape) of amniotic fluid

_amni_ / _orrhea_
WR / S

10. false pregnancy

_pseud_ / _o_ / _cyes_ / _is_
P / CV / WR / S

11. one who specializes in embryology

_embry_ / _ologist_
WR / S

12. (stimulating) the production of milk

_lact_ / _o_ / _genic_
WR / CV / S

13. study or science of the development of embryos

_embryo_ / _ology_
WR / S

14. rupture of the amnion

_amni_ / _orrhexis_
WR / S

15. resembling an embryo

_embry_ / _oid_
WR / S

16. pregnant woman

_gravid_ / _a_
WR / S

17. pertaining to pregnancy and the puerperium

_gravid_ / _o_ / _puerper_ / _al_
WR / CV / WR / S

18. woman who has given birth to two or more viable offspring

_multi_ / _par_ / _a_
P / WR / S

19. pertaining to birth

_nat_ / _al_
WR / S

20. an infant from birth to 4 weeks of age

_neo_ / _nat_ / _e_
P / WR / S

21. branch of medicine that deals with the newborn infant

neo | nat | ology
P | WR | S

22. woman who has not given birth to a viable offspring

nulli | par | para
P | WR | S

23. woman who has given birth to a viable offspring

par | a
WR | S

24. woman in her first pregnancy

prim | i | gravid | a
WR | CV | WR | S

25. after childbirth

post | part | um
P | WR | S

26. woman who has borne one viable offspring

prim | i | par | a
WR | CV | WR | S

27. woman who has been pregnant two or more times

multi | gravid | a
P | WR | S

28. pertaining to (immediately after) childbirth

puerper | al
WR | S

29. woman who has never been pregnant

nulli | gravid | a
P | WR | S

30. woman who has just given birth

puerper | a
WR | S

31. during labor and childbirth

intra | part | um
P | WR | S

## EXERCISE 25

Spell each of the additional terms. Have someone dictate the terms on pp. 286 and 287 to you or say the words into a tape recorder; then spell the words from your recording as often as necessary. Think about the word parts before attempting to write the word. Study any you have spelled incorrectly.

1. _____          17. _____
2. _____          18. _____
3. _____          19. _____
4. _____          20. _____
5. _____          21. _____
6. _____          22. _____
7. _____          23. _____
8. _____          24. _____
9. _____          25. _____
10. _____         26. _____
11. _____         27. _____
12. _____         28. _____
13. _____         29. _____
14. _____         30. _____
15. _____         31. _____
16. _____

Place a check mark (√) in the box to indicate that you have completed Objective 8.

☐ **BUILD, ANALYZE, DEFINE, PRONOUNCE, AND SPELL ADDITIONAL TERMS RELATED TO OBSTETRICS AND NEONATOLOGY.**

# Objective 9    DEFINE, PRONOUNCE, AND SPELL THE OTHER ADDITIONAL TERMS RELATED TO OBSTETRICS AND NEONATOLOGY.

# Other Additional Terms

| TERM | DEFINITION |
|---|---|
| 1. breech birth . . . . . . . . . . . <br> (brēch) | parturition in which the buttocks, feet, or knees emerge first |
| 2. congenital anomaly . . . . . <br> (kon-JEN-i-tal) (a-NOM-a-lē) | abnormality present at birth |
| 3. lochia . . . . . . . . . . . . . . . <br> (LŌ-kē-a) | vaginal discharge following childbirth |

4. meconium . . . . . . . . . . . first stool of the newborn (greenish-
   (me-KŌ-nē-um)                black in color)

5. obstetrician . . . . . . . . . . . physician who specializes in obstetrics
   (ob-ste-TRISH-an)

6. obstetrics . . . . . . . . . . . . medical specialty dealing with preg-
   (ob-STET-riks)               nancy, childbirth, and puerperium

7. parturition . . . . . . . . . . . act of giving birth
   (par-tū-RISH-un)

8. premature infant . . . . . . . infant born before completing 37 weeks
                                 of gestation

9. puerperium . . . . . . . . . . period from delivery until the reproduc-
   (pū-er-PĒ-rē-um)             tive organs return to normal (about 6
                                 weeks)

Practice saying each of these terms aloud. To assist in pronunciation, obtain the audiotape designed for use with this text. Learn the definitions and spellings of the other additional terms by completing the following exercises.

## EXERCISE 26

Match the definitions in the first column with the correct terms in the second column.

_a_ 1. vaginal discharge
_e_ 2. medical specialty
_i_ 3. abnormality that is present at birth
_g_ 4. period after delivery
_f_ 5. giving birth
_b_ 6. physician-specialist
_j_ 7. buttocks, feet, or knees first
_d_ 8. first stool
_c_ 9. born before completing 37 weeks of gestation

a. lochia
b. obstetrician
c. premature infant
d. meconium
e. obstetrics
f. parturition
g. puerperium
h. lactorrhea
i. congenital anomaly
j. breech birth

## EXERCISE 27

Write the definitions of the following terms.

1. meconium _____

2. obstetrics _____

3. premature infant _____

4. lochia _____

5. puerperium _____

6. parturition _____

7. obstetrician _____

8. congenital anomaly _____

9. breech _____

## EXERCISE 28

Spell each of the other additional terms. Have someone dictate the terms on pp. 292 and 293 to you or say the words into a tape recorder; then spell the words from your recording as often as necessary. Study any you have spelled incorrectly.

1. _____    6. _____
2. _____    7. _____
3. _____    8. _____
4. _____    9. _____
5. _____

Place a check mark (√) in the box to indicate that you have completed Objective 9.

☐ DEFINE, PRONOUNCE, AND SPELL THE OTHER ADDITIONAL TERMS RELATED TO OBSTETRICS AND NEONATOLOGY.

**Case History:** The patient is a 24-year-old married Hispanic female, Gravida III Para II, whose EDC is 1 week from today. She has received prenatal care since the second month of pregnancy. This gestation has been uncomplicated with no spotting, albuminuria, hypertension, edema, or glycosuria. She has gained 25 pounds. Routine ultrasonography revealed a single fetus. Pelvimetry indicates adequate pelvis for normal sized fetus. When examined at the obstetrician's office this week, it was noted that fetus' presentation was cephalic. Patient has attended Lamaze classes with her husband.

> **Nurse's Admitting Notes:**
> **Date:** 4/23/93 **Time:** 2330
> 24-year-old GIII PII Hispanic female admitted to room 271. History of two 12-14 hour uncomplicated labors. Uterine contractions began at 2100. Contractions every 5 minutes at 2200. Current uterine contractions every 3 minutes frequency with duration of 40-60 seconds and moderate intensity. Contractions originate in lower back and spread to lower abdomen. FHT 140, regular, good variability. Refuses continuous electronic fetal monitoring after full explanation of procedure's advantages from nurse. Last ate small sandwich and glass of milk 6 hours ago. Offered ice chips and advised not to eat or drink while in active labor. 1000 cc 5% D/W started IV in left hand at keep open rate. Vaginal exam reveals cervix 4 cm dilated and 100% effaced, station +1, head engaged, BOW intact, LOA position, fetal head flexed. BP 118/80, radial pulse 86, R 18. Wt. 150 lb. Urinated qs. Negative for protein and glucose. Small BM without enema. Husband present. Participating together with Lamaze breathing and relaxation techniques. Coping apparently well with uterine contractions.

## EXERCISE 29

To test your understanding of the terms introduced in this chapter, circle the words that correctly complete the sentences. The italicized words refer to the correct answer.

1. The premature infant was diagnosed as having *hyaline membrane disease,* a disease of the (umbilicus, erythrocytes, lungs).
2. Because of the inadequate uterine contractions the patient was experiencing *difficult labor,* or (dysphasia, dystocia, dysuria).
3. Down's syndrome was diagnosed prenatally by laboratory analysis of *amniotic fluid removed by surgical puncture,* or (amniocentesis, amniography, amnioscope).
4. The word that means *before childbirth* is (intrapartum, antepartum, antipartum).
5. *Nulligravida* is a woman who (has never been pregnant, has not given birth).
6. *Multipara* is a woman who has (borne two or more viable offspring, been pregnant two or more times).
7. *Primigravida* is a woman (in her first pregnancy, who has borne one child).
8. The word that means the *act of giving birth* is (parturition, puerperium, gravidopuerperal).
9. *Rupture of the uterus* is called (hysterorrhaphy, hysterorrhexis, hysteroptosis).

## EXERCISE 30

Unscramble the following mixed-up terms. The word on the left indicates the word root in each of the following.

1. vulva

/ / / / s / / / t / / / /
t  e  y  m  p  o  s  i  i  o

2. umbilicus

/ / / p / / / / / c / / / /
e  e  l  l  o  o  m  a  h  p  c

3. fetus

/ / / t / / / / / / /
c  e  p  o  o  t  e  f  s

4. amnion

/ / / / / o / / / /
m  a  n  t  i  o  i  c

5. pregnancy

/ / / / t / / / / a / / / / /
d  a  v  i  m  t  i  g  r  a  u  l

## EXERCISE 31

The following are words studied in previous chapters. Write the definitions of the italicized word parts.

1. *cyto*genic _____ cell
2. *leuko*cyte _____ white
3. dermato*plasty* _____ plastic repair
4. *laryng*itis _____ larynx
5. *pneumon*ectomy _____ lung
6. uretero*cele* _____ hernia
7. *nephr*osis _____ ~~death~~ kidney
8. *cervic*itis _____ cervix
9. rhino*rrhagia* _____ rapid flow of blood
10. prostato*rrhea* _____ excessive discharge
11. colpo*rrhaphy* _____ suture

## COMBINING FORMS CROSSWORD PUZZLE

### Across Clues

1. pregnancy
4. childbirth
5. pregnancy
6. first
8. amnion
11. umbilicus
12. bear, give birth
13. head

### Down Clues

2. amnion
3. fetus, unborn child
4. pelvis
5. chorion
6. false
7. milk
9. embryo
10. birth

# Summary

Can you build, analyze, define, spell, and pronounce the following terms *built from word parts?*   yes ☐   no ☐

| DIAGNOSTIC (OBSTETRICS) | SURGICAL (OBSTETRICS) | PROCEDURAL (OBSTETRICS) | ADDITIONAL (OBSTETRICS AND NEONATOLOGY) |
|---|---|---|---|
| amnionitis (*am*-nē-ō-NĪ-tis) | amniotomy (*am*-nē-OT-ō-mē) | amniocentesis (*am*-nē-ō-sen-TĒ-sis) | amniochorial (*am*-nē-ō-KŌ-rē-al) |
| chorioamnionitis (*kō*-rē-ō-*am*-nē-ō-NĪ-tis) | episiotomy (e-*piz*-ē-OT-ō-mē) | amniography (*am*-nē-OG-ra-fē) | amniorrhea (*am*-nē-ō-RĒ-a) |
| choriocarcinoma (*kō*-rē-ō-*kar*-si-NŌ-ma) | | amnioscope (AM-nē-ō-skōp) | amniorrhexis (*am*-nē-ō-REK-sis) |
| dystocia (dis-TŌ-sē-a) | | amnioscopy (*am*-nē-OS-kō-pē) | antepartum (*an*-tē-PAR-tum) |

| DIAGNOSTIC (OBSTETRICS) | SURGICAL (OBSTETRICS) | PROCEDURAL (OBSTETRICS) | ADDITIONAL (OBSTETRICS AND NEONATIOLOGY) |
|---|---|---|---|

embryotocia
(*em*-brē-ō-TŌ-sē-a)

hysterorrhexis
(his-ter-ō-REK-sis)

salpingocyesis
(sal-PING-gō-sī-ē-sis)

## NEONATOLOGY

microcephalus
(*mī*-krō-SEF-a-lus)

omphalitis
(*om*-fa-LĪ-tis)

omphalocele
(OM-fal-ō-*sēl*)

pyloric stenosis
(pī-LŌR-ik) (ste-NŌ-sis)

tracheoesophageal
fistula
(TRĀ-kē-ō-ē-*sof*-a-jē-al)
(FIS-tū-la)

fetography
(fē-TOG-ra-fē)

fetometry
(fē-TOM-e-trē)

fetoscope
(FĒ-tō-scōp)

pelvimetry
(pel-VIM-e-trē)

cyesiology
(sī-*ē*-sē-OL-ō-jē)

cyesis
(sī-Ē-sis)

embryogenic
(*em*-brē-ō-JEN-ik)

embryoid
(EM-brē-oyd)

embryologist
(*em*-brē-OL-ō-jist)

embryology
(*em*-brē-OL-ō-jē)

fetal
(FĒ-tal)

gravida
(GRAV-i-da)

gravidopuerperal
(*grav*-i-dō-pū-ER-per-al)

intrapartum
(*in*-tra-PAR-tum)

lactic
(LAK-tik)

lactogenic
(*lak*-tō-JEN-ik)

lactorrhea
(*lak*-tō-RĒ-a)

multigravida
(*mul*-tī-GRAV-i-da)

multipara
(mul-TIP-a-ra)

natal
(NĀ-tal)

neonate
(NĒ-ō-nāt)

neonatology
(*nē*-ō-nā-TOL-ō-jē)

nulligravida
(*nul*-li-GRAV-i-da)

nullipara
(nu-LIP-a-ra)

para
(PAR-a)

## ADDITIONAL (OBSTETRICS AND NEONATIOLOGY)

postpartum
(pōst-PAR-tum)

primigravida
(prī-mi-GRAV-i-da)

primipara
(prī-MIP-a-ra)

pseudocyesis
(*sū*-dō-sī-Ē-sis)

puerpera
(pū-ER-per-a)

puerperal
(pū-ER-per-al)

# Summary

Can you define, pronounce, and spell the following terms *not built from word parts?*   yes □   no □

## DIAGNOSTIC (OBSTETRICS)

abortion
(ab-ŌR-shun)

abruptio placentae
(ab-RUP-shē-o)
(pla-SEN-tē)

eclampsia
(ē-KLAMP-sē-a)

ectopic pregnancy
(ek-TOP-ik)

placenta previa
(pla-SEN-ta) (PREV-ē-a)

preeclampsia
(prē-ē-KLAMP-sē-a)

## NEONATOLOGY

cleft lip and palate
Down's syndrome
erythroblastosis fetalis
(e-*rith*-rō-blas-TŌ-sis)
(fet-A-lis)

esophageal atresia
(ē-sof-a-JĒ-al) (a-TRĒ-zē-a)

spina bifida
(SPĪ-na) (BIF-i-da)

hyaline membrane
disease
(HĪ-a-lin)

## ADDITIONAL (OBSTETRICS AND NEONATOLOGY)

breech birth
(brēch)

congenital anomaly
(kon-JEN-i-tal)
(a-NOM-a-lē)

lochia
(LŌ-kē-a)

meconium
(me-KŌ-nē-um)

obstetrician
(*ob*-ste-TRISH-an)

obstetrics
(ob-STET-riks)

parturition
(*par*-tū-RISH-un)

premature infant
puerperium
(*pū*-er-PĒ-rē-um)

# Answers

## Exercise 1

1. gamete; ovulation; fertilization; zygote; gestation
2. embryo; fetus
3. amniotic; chorion; amnion; amniotic

## Exercise 2

**Figure 8-1**

Umbilicus: omphal/o     Amnion: amni/o, amnion/o

Fetus: fet/o (fet/i)     Chorion: chori/o

## Exercise 3

1. fetus
2. milk
3. give birth to, bear, labor
4. umbilicus, navel
5. amnion
6. childbirth
7. pregnancy
8. birth
9. chorion
10. embryo

## Exercise 4

1. lact/o
2. fet/o, fet/i
3. chori/o
4. a. amni/o
   b. amnion/o
5. puerper/o
6. a. par/o
   b. part/o
7. a. gravid/o
   b. cyes/o, cyes/i
8. embry/o
9. nat/o
10. omphal/o

## Exercise 5

1. first
2. pylorus
3. head
4. esophagus
5. false
6. pelvic bone, pelvis

## Exercise 6

1. cephal/o
2. pylor/o
3. pseud/o
4. esophag/o
5. prim/i
6. pelv/i, pelv/o

## Exercise 7

1. after
2. many
3. none
4. small
5. before

## Exercise 8

1. nulli-
2. micro-
3. multi-
4. ante-
5. post-

## Exercise 9

```
      WR  CV   WR    S
1. chori/ o /amnion/itis        inflammation of the am-
         ‾‾‾‾                   nion and chorion
          CF
```

```
      WR  CV   WR    S
2. chori/ o /carcin/oma         cancerous tumor of the
         ‾‾‾‾                   chorion
          CF
```

```
       P   S(WR)
3. dys/tocia                    difficult labor
```

```
      WR      S
4. amnion/itis                  inflammation of the am-
                                nion
```

```
      WR      S
5. hyster/orrhexis              rupture of the uterus
```

```
      WR  CV  S
6. embry/ o /tocia              birth of any embryo;
         ‾‾‾‾                   abortion
          CF
```

```
      WR   CV WR  S
7. salping/ o /cyes/is          pregnancy in a fallopian
          ‾‾‾‾                  tube (ectopic preg-
           CF                   nancy)
```

## Exercise 10

1. chori/o/carcin/oma
2. amnion/itis
3. chori/o/amnion/itis
4. embry/o/tocia
5. dys/tocia
6. hyster/orrhexis
7. salping/o/cyes/is

## Exercise 11

Spelling exercise; *see* text, pp. 274 and 275.

## Exercise 12

1. premature separation of the placenta from the uterine wall
2. termination of pregnancy by the expulsion from the uterus of an embryo or nonviable fetus
3. abnormally low implantation of the placenta on the uterine wall
4. severe complication and progression of preeclampsia
5. pregnancy occurring outside the uterus
6. abnormal condition, encountered during pregnancy or shortly after delivery, of high blood pressure, edema, and proteinuria

## Exercise 13

1. abruptio placentae
2. eclampsia
3. abortion
4. ectopic pregnancy
5. placenta previa
6. preeclampsia

## Exercise 14

Spelling exercise; *see* text, p. 277.

## Exercise 15

```
      WR   S
1. pylor/ic stenosis            congenital narrowing of
                                the pyloric sphincter
```

```
     WR   CV  S
2. omphal/ o /cele                    hernia at the umbilicus
        CF

     WR     S
3. omphal/itis                        inflammation of the
                                         umbilicus

      P    WR   S
4. micro/cephal/us                    fetus with a very small
                                         head

     WR  CV   WR    S
5. trache/ o /esophag/eal fistula     abnormal passageway
        CF                               between the esopha-
                                         gus and the trachea
```

```
     WR  CV   S
8. pelv/ i /metry                     measurement of the
        CF                               mother's pelvis to de-
                                         termine the ability of
                                         the fetus to pass
                                         through

     WR  CV   S
9. fet/ o /scope                      instrument used for ex-
        CF                               amining fetal heart
                                         tones

     WR  CV   S
10. fet/ o /metry                     measurement of the size
        CF                               of the fetus
```

## Exercise 16

1. omphal/o/cele
2. micro/cephal/us
3. pylor/ic stenosis
4. trache/o/esophag/eal fistula
5. omphal/itis

## Exercise 17

Spelling exercise; *see* text, p. 279.

## Exercise 18

1. f  2. c  3. a  4. d  5. b  6. e

## Exercise 19

Spelling exercise; *see* text, p. 281.

## Exercise 20

```
     WR      S
1. episi/otomy                incision of the vulva (per-
                                 ineum)

     WR    S
2. amni/otomy                 incision into the fetal
                                 membrane

     WR  CV   S
3. amni/ o /scope             instrument used for visual
        CF                       examination of the fe-
                                 tus and amniotic fluid

     WR  CV   S
4. amni/ o /graphy            process of x-ray filming
        CF                       the amniotic fluid (after
                                 injection of dye)

     WR  CV  S
5. fet/ o /graphy             process of x-ray filming
        CF                       the fetus in the uterus

     WR  CV   S
6. amni/ o /centesis          surgical puncture to re-
        CF                       move amniotic fluid

     WR  CV   S
7. amni/ o /scopy             visual examination of the
        CF                       uterus outlining the
                                 fetus and amniotic cav-
                                 ity
```

## Exercise 21

1. amni/otomy
2. episi/otomy
3. amni/o/graphy
4. amni/o/scopy
5. amni/o/centesis
6. amni/o/scope
7. fet/o/graphy
8. fet/o/scope
9. pelv/i/metry
10. fet/o/metry

## Exercise 22

Spelling exercise; *see* text, p. 286.

## Exercise 23

```
       WR    S
1. puerper/a                 woman who has just
                               given birth

       WR       S
2. amni/orrhexis             rupture of the amnion

      P    WR   S
3. ante/part/um              occurring before child-
                               birth

     WR  CV   S
4. cyes/ i /ology            study of pregnancy
        CF

     WR  CV   WR  S
5. pseud/ o /cyes/is         false pregnancy
        CF

      WR   S
6. cyes/is                   pregnancy

      WR  S
7. lact/ic                   pertaining to milk

      WR      S
8. lact/orrhea               spontaneous discharge of
                               milk

       WR      S
9. amni/orrhea              discharge of amniotic
                               fluid

       WR      S
10. embry/ologist            one who specializes in
                               embryology

       P    WR  S
11. multi/par/a              woman who has given
                               birth to two or more
                               viable offspring
```

WR CV S
12. embry/ o /genic        producing an embryo
     CF

WR S
13. embry/oid              resembling an embryo

WR S
14. fet/al                 pertaining to the fetus

WR S
15. gravid/a               pregnant woman

WR S
16. embry/ology            study or science of the
                           development of the em-
                           bryo

WR CV WR S
17. amni/ o /chori/al      pertaining to the amnion
   CF                        and chorion

P WR S
18. multi/gravid/a         woman who has been
                           pregnant two or more
                           times

WR CV S
19. lact/ o /genic         (stimulating) the produc-
   CF                        tion of milk

WR S
20. nat/al                 pertaining to birth

WR CV WR S
21. gravid/ o /puerper/al  pertaining to pregnancy
    CF

P WR S
22. neo/nat/ology          branch of medicine that
                           deals with diagnosis
                           and treatment of the
                           newborn infant

P WR S
23. nulli/par/a            woman who has not given
                           birth to a viable off-
                           spring

WR S
24. par/a                  woman who has given
                           birth to a viable off-
                           spring

WR CV WR S
25. prim/ i /gravid/a      woman in her first preg-
   CF                        nancy

P WR S
26. post/part/um           occurring after childbirth

P WR S
27. neo/nat/e              an infant from birth to 4
                           weeks of age

WR CV WR S
28. prim/ i /par/a         woman who has borne
   CF                        one viable offspring

WR S
29. puerper/al             pertaining to (immedi-
                           ately after) childbirth

P WR S
30. nulli/gravid/a         woman who has never
                           been pregnant

P WR S
31. intra/part/um          occurring during labor
                           and childbirth

## Exercise 24

| | |
|---|---|
| 1. amni/o/chori/al | 17. gravid/o/puerper/al |
| 2. ante/part/um | 18. multi/par/a |
| 3. embry/o/genic | 19. nat/al |
| 4. cyes/i/ology | 20. neo/nat/e |
| 5. fet/al | 21. neo/nat/ology |
| 6. cyes/is | 22. nulli/par/a |
| 7. lact/ic | 23. par/a |
| 8. lact/orrhea | 24. prim/i/gravid/a |
| 9. amni/orrhea | 25. post/part/um |
| 10. pseud/o/cyes/is | 26. prim/i/par/a |
| 11. embry/ologist | 27. multi/gravid/a |
| 12. lact/o/genic | 28. puerper/al |
| 13. embry/ology | 29. nulli/gravid/a |
| 14. amni/orrhexis | 30. puerper/a |
| 15. embry/oid | 31. intra/part/um |
| 16. gravid/a | |

## Exercise 25

Spelling exercise; *see* text, p. 292.

## Exercise 26

| | | | | |
|---|---|---|---|---|
| 1. a | 3. i | 5. f | 7. j | 9. c |
| 2. e | 4. g | 6. b | 8. d | |

## Exercise 27

1. first stool of the newborn
2. medical specialty dealing with pregnancy, childbirth, and puerperium
3. infant born before completing 37 weeks of gestation
4. vaginal discharge following childbirth
5. period after delivery until the reproductive organs return to normal
6. act of giving birth
7. physician who specializes in obstetrics
8. abnormality present at birth
9. parturition in which the buttocks, feet, or knees emerge first

## Exercise 28

Spelling exercise; *see* text, p. 294.

## Exercise 29

1. lungs
2. dystocia
3. amniocentesis
4. antepartum
5. has never been pregnant
6. borne two or more viable offspring
7. first pregnancy
8. parturition
9. hysterorrhexis

## Exercise 30

1. episiotomy
2. omphalocele
3. fetoscope
4. amniotic
5. multigravida

## Exercise 31

1. cell
2. white
3. surgical repair
4. larynx
5. lung
6. hernia, or protrusion
7. kidney
8. cervix
9. rapid flow (of blood)
10. excessive discharge
11. suture

# Answers

```
            G R A V I D O       A
        F                       M
      P U E R P E R O           N
      E   T           C Y E S O I
      L   O           H         O
      V   H           N
P R I M I             O         O
S           L         R
E           A M N I O           E
U           C         O         M
D         N T                   B
O M P H A L O                   R
          T                     Y
P A R T O         C E P H A L O
```

# 9

# Cardiovascular and Lymphatic Systems

## Objectives

Upon completion of this chapter you will be able to:

1. Define the anatomical terms of the cardiovascular and lymphatic systems.

2. Write the definitions of the word parts included in this chapter.

3. Build, analyze, define, pronounce, and spell the diagnostic terms related to the cardiovascular and lymphatic systems.

4. Define, pronounce, and spell other diagnostic terms related to the cardiovascular and lymphatic systems.

5. Build, analyze, define, pronounce, an spell the surgical terms related to the cardiovascular and lymphatic systems.

6. Define, pronounce, and spell other surgical and treatment terms related to the cardiovascular and lymphatic systems.

7. Build, analyze, define, pronounce, and spell the diagnostic procedural terms related to the cardiovascular and lymphatic systems.

8. Define, pronounce, and spell other diagnostic procedural terms related to the cardiovascular and lymphatic systems.

9. Build, analyze, define, pronounce, and spell additional terms related to the cardiovascular and lymphatic systems.

10. Define, pronounce, and spell the other additional terms related to the cardiovascular and lymphatic systems.

## Objective 1    DEFINE THE ANATOMICAL TERMS OF THE CARDIOVASCULAR AND LYMPHATIC SYSTEMS.

## Anatomical Terms

The cardiovascular system is composed of the heart, blood vessels, and blood. The function of the system is to nourish the body by transporting nutrients and oxygen to the cells and removing carbon dioxide and other waste products.

### PARTS OF THE CARDIOVASCULAR SYSTEM (FIGURE 9-1)

1. heart . . . . . . . . . . . . . . . . .   Muscular organ the size of a closed fist located behind the breast bone between the lungs. The pumping action of the

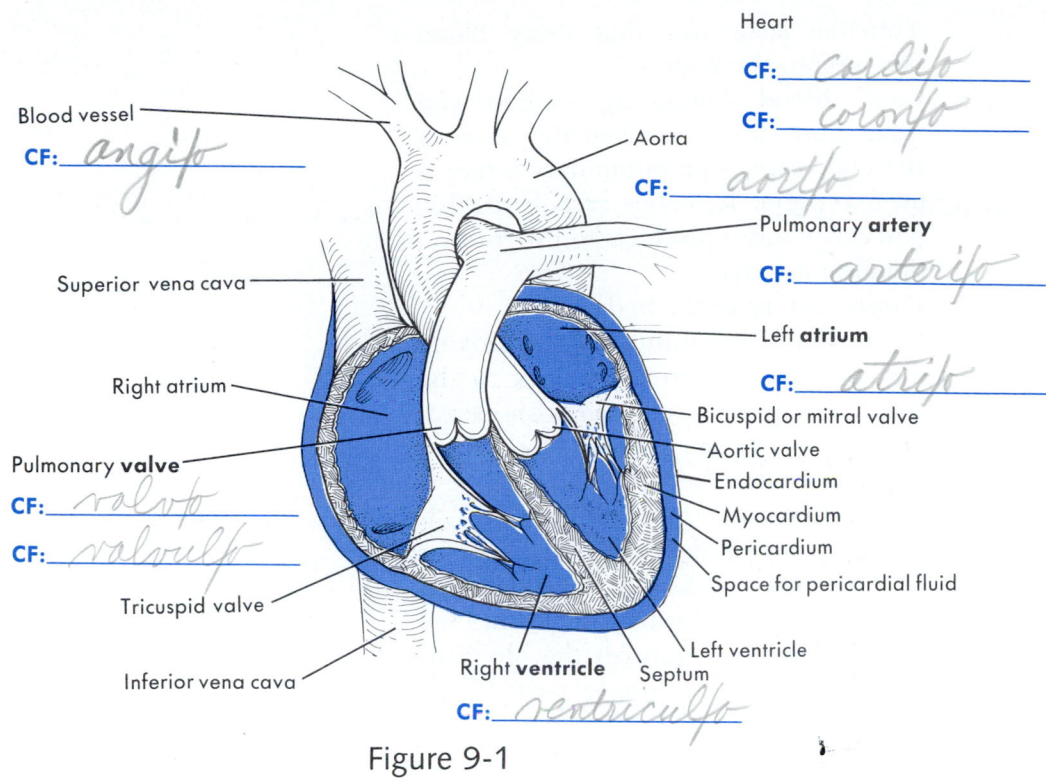

Heart
CF: _cardio_
CF: _coronio_
CF: _aorto_

Blood vessel
CF: _angio_

Aorta
CF: _aorto_

Pulmonary **artery**
CF: _arterio_

Superior vena cava

Left **atrium**
CF: _atrio_

Right atrium

Bicuspid or mitral valve
Aortic valve
Endocardium
Myocardium
Pericardium
Space for pericardial fluid

Pulmonary **valve**
CF: _valvo_
CF: _valvulo_

Tricuspid valve

Inferior vena cava

Right **ventricle**    Left ventricle
Septum
CF: _ventriculo_

**Figure 9-1**
Cutaway section of the heart.

heart circulates blood throughout the body. The heart consists of two upper chambers, the *right atrium (pl. atria)* and the *left atrium*, and two lower chambers, the *right ventricle* and the *left ventricle*. Valves of the heart keep the blood flowing in one direction. The *cardiac septum* separates the right and left sides of the heart.

a. tricuspid valve . . . . . .    Located between the right atrium and right ventricle.

b. bicuspid valve . . . . . .    Located between the left atrium and left ventricle.

c. semilunar valves . . . .    Located between the right ventricle and the pulmonary artery and between the left ventricle and the aorta.

2. three layers of the heart
   a. pericardium. . . . . . . .    Two-layer sac (*pericardial sac*) covering the heart (*pericardial fluid* allows the layers to move without friction)

   (1) visceral layer . . .    Lies closest to the myocardium.
   (2) parietal layer . . .    Lines the pericardium.
   b. myocardium . . . . . . .    Middle, thick, muscular layer.
   c. endocardium . . . . . .    Inner lining of the heart.

3. blood vessels............. Tubelike structures that carry blood throughout the body.

   a.  arteries........... Carry blood containing oxygen and other nutrients away from the heart to the body cells. The pulmonary artery is an exception: it carries carbon dioxide and other waste products to the lungs.

      (1)  arterioles ...... Smallest arteries.

      (2)  aorta......... Largest artery in the body.

   b.  veins ............ Carry blood containing carbon dioxide and other waste products back to the heart. The pulmonary vein is an exception: it carries oxygenated blood from the lungs to the heart.

      (1)  venules........ Smallest veins.

      (2)  vena cava ...... Largest vein in the body. The *inferior vena cava* carries blood to the heart from body parts below the diaphragm, and the *superior vena cava* returns the blood to the heart from the upper part of the body.

   c.  capillaries ........ Connect arterioles with venules.

4. blood ............... Composed of *plasma* and *formed elements*, such as *cells*.

   a.  plasma........... Liquid portion of blood in which cells float.

   b.  cells

      (1)  erythrocytes .... Red blood cells.

      (2)  leukocytes...... White blood cells.

      (3)  platelets (thrombocytes) ....... Necessary for the coagulation process.

## PARTS OF THE LYMPHATIC SYSTEM

The lymphatic system has as its major function the removal of excessive tissue fluid, which develops from increased metabolic activity. Lymphatics, or lymph vessels, are found throughout the body.

1. lymph................ Transparent, usually colorless, tissue fluid.

2. lymph nodes.......... Small, spherical bodies made up of lymphoid tissue. They are found singularly or may be grouped together. The nodes act as filters in keeping substances such as bacteria from the blood.

3. spleen............... Located in the left side of the abdominal cavity between the stomach and the diaphragm. The spleen is the largest lymphatic organ in the body.

4.  thymus gland . . . . . . . . .  Located behind the breast bone between the lungs. It plays an important role in the development of the body's immune system.

Learn the anatomical terms by completing the following exercises.

# EXERCISE 1

Match the terms in the first column with the correct definitions in the second column.

_g_  1. aorta
_j_  2. artery
_e_  3. arterioles
_m_  4. atria
_b_  5. bicuspid valve
_k_  6. blood
_i_  7. capillaries
_f_  8. endocardium
_l_  9. visceral layer
_h_ 10. erythrocyte
_d_ 11. heart
_a_ 12. leukocyte
_n_ 13. lymph

a.  white blood cell
b.  lies between the left atrium and left ventricle
c.  outer layer of the pericardial sac
d.  pumps blood throughout the body
e.  smallest arteries
f.  inner lining of the heart
g.  largest artery in the body
h.  red blood cell
i.  connects arterioles and venules
j.  carries blood away from the heart
k.  composed of plasma and cells
l.  layer of the pericardial sac that lies closest to the myocardium
m.  upper chambers of the heart
n.  colorless tissue fluid

# EXERCISE 2

Match the terms in the first column with the correct definitions in the second column.

_f_  1. lymph node
_b_  2. myocardium
_h_  3. parietal layer
_b_  4. pericardium
_k_  5. pericardial fluid
_m_  6. plasma
_c_  7. platelet
_l_  8. semilunar valves
_g_  9. cardiac septum

a.  carries blood back to the heart
b.  two-layer sac covering the heart
c.  thrombocyte
d.  largest lymphatic organ in the body
e.  smallest veins
f.  acts as a filter to keep bacteria from the blood
g.  plays an important role in the body's immune system

_d_ 10. spleen                     h.  lines the pericardial sac

_o_ 11. tricuspid valves           i.  lower chambers of the heart

_a_ 12. vein                       j.  largest vein in the body

_i_ 13. ventricles                 k.  allows the double layer of the cover-
                                       ing of the heart to move without fric-
_e_ 14. venules                        tion

_j_ 15. vena cava                  l.  between the right ventricle and the
                                       pulmonary artery and between the
_g_ 16. thymus gland                   left ventricle and the aorta

                                   m.  liquid portion of the blood

                                   n.  carries oxygenated blood away from
                                       the heart

                                   o.  between the right atrium and the
                                       right ventricle

                                   p.  muscular layer of the heart

                                   q.  separates heart into right and left
                                       sides

Place a check mark (√) in the box to indicate that you have completed Objective 1.

☐ DEFINE THE ANATOMICAL TERMS OF THE CARDIOVASCULAR AND LYMPHATIC SYSTEMS.

# Objective 2   WRITE THE DEFINITIONS OF THE WORD PARTS INCLUDED IN THIS CHAPTER.

# Cardiovascular and Lymphatic System Word Parts

Study the word parts and their definitions as follows. Learning will be made easier by completing the exercises that follow.

**COMBINING FORM**

1. angi/o . . . . . . . . . . . . . .   **DEFINITION**
                                        vessel (usually refers to blood vessel)

2. aort/o . . . . . . . . . . . . .     aorta

3. arteri/o . . . . . . . . . . . . .   artery

4. atri/o . . . . . . . . . . . . . .   atrium

5. cardi/o
   coron/o . . . . . . . . . . . . .    heart
   (NOTE: *coron/o* is used for blood
   vessels of the heart, such as the
   coronary artery.)

6. lymph/o . . . . . . . . . . . . .    lymph

7. phleb/o . . . . . . . . . . . . .    vein (another word root for vein is ven/o,
                                        covered in Chapter 5)

It was believed in ancient times that arteries carried air. Vital air, or **pneuma**, did not allow blood in the arteries. A cut in an artery allowed vital air to escape and blood to replace it. The Greek **arteria**, meaning **windpipe**, was given for this reason.

**Coronary** is derived from the Latin **coronalis**, meaning **crown** or **wreath**. It describes the arteries encircling the heart.

8. plasm/o . . . . . . . . . . . . plasma
9. splen/o . . . . . . . . . . . . spleen
10. thym/o . . . . . . . . . . . . thymus gland
11. valv/o, valvul/o . . . . . . . valve
12. ventricul/o . . . . . . . . . . ventricle

Learn the anatomical locations and definitions of the combining forms by completing the following exercises.

## EXERCISE 3

Write the combining forms in the spaces marked **CF** on the diagram in Fig. 9-1, p. 305.

## EXERCISE 4

Write the definitions of the following combining forms.

1. cardi/o _____ heart _____
2. atri/o _____ atrium _____
3. plasm/o _____ plasma _____
4. angi/o _____ vessel _____
5. coron/o _____ heart _____
6. aort/o _____ aorta _____
7. valv/o _____ valve _____
8. splen/o _____ spleen _____
9. thym/o _____ thymus gland _____
10. phleb/o _____ vein _____
11. ventricul/o _____ ventricle _____
12. arteri/o _____ artery _____
13. valvul/o _____ valve _____
14. lymph/o _____ lymph _____

## EXERCISE 5

Write the combining form for each of the following.

1. artery _____

2. vein _____

3. heart    a. _____

   b. _____

4. atrium _____

5. ventricle _____

6. lymph _____

7. aorta _____

8. vessel
   (usually blood vessel) _____

9. valve    a. _____

   b. _____

10. spleen _____

11. plasma _____

12. thymus gland _____

# Related Word Parts

| COMBINING FORM | DEFINITIONS |
| --- | --- |
| 1. ather/o . . . . . . . . . . . . . . | yellowish, fatty plaque |
| 2. bacteri/o . . . . . . . . . . . . . | bacteria |
| 3. ech/o. . . . . . . . . . . . . . . | sound |
| 4. electr/o . . . . . . . . . . . . . | electricity, electrical activity |
| 5. isch/o . . . . . . . . . . . . . . | deficiency, blockage |
| 6. sphygm/o . . . . . . . . . . . | pulse |
| 7. steth/o. . . . . . . . . . . . . | chest |
| 8. therm/o. . . . . . . . . . . . | heat |
| 9. thromb/o . . . . . . . . . . . | clot |

Learn the other combining forms by completing the following exercises.

## EXERCISE 6

Write the definitions of the following combining forms.

1. ech/o _____ *sound* _____

2. steth/o _____ *chest* _____

3. thromb/o _____ *clot* _____

4. isch/o _____ *deficiency, blockage* _____

5. therm/o _____ *heat* _____

6. sphygm/o _____ *pulse* _____

7. ather/o _____ *yellowish fatty plaque* _____

8. electr/o _____ *electricity* _____

9. bacteri/o _____ *bacteria* _____

## EXERCISE 7

Write the combining form for each of the following.

1. clot _____

2. chest _____

3. sound _____

4. deficiency, blockage _____

5. yellowish, fatty plaque _____

6. heat _____

7. bacteria _____

8. electricity, electrical _____

9. pulse _____

## Prefixes

| PREFIX | DEFINITION |
| --- | --- |
| 1.  brady- . . . . . . . . . . . . . . . | slow |
| 2.  tachy- . . . . . . . . . . . . . . . | fast, rapid |

Learn the prefixes by completing the exercises that follow.

## EXERCISE 8

Write the definitions of the following prefixes.

1. tachy- _____ *fast, rapid* _____
2. brady- _____ *slow* _____

## EXERCISE 9

Write the prefix for each of the following.

1. fast, rapid _____ *tachy* _____

2. slow _____ *brady* _____

# Suffixes

| SUFFIX | DEFINITIONS |
| --- | --- |
| 1. -ac................. | pertaining to |
| 2. -apheresis............ | removal |
| 3. -crit................ | to separate |
| 4. -graph.............. | instrument used to record (see Chapter 4 for suffixes -*gram* and -*graphy*) |
| 5. -odynia............. | pain |
| 6. -penia.............. | abnormal reduction in number |
| 7. -poiesis............. | formation |
| 8. -sclerosis............ | hardening |

Learn the suffixes by completing the following exercises.

## EXERCISE 10

Write the definitions of the following suffixes.

1. -crit _____ *to separate* _____
2. -graph _____ *instrument used to record* _____
3. -penia _____ *abnormal reduction in number* _____
4. -sclerosis _____ *hardening* _____
5. -odynia _____ *pain* _____
6. -apheresis _____ *removal* _____
7. -poiesis _____ *formation* _____
8. -ac _____ *pertaining to* _____

## EXERCISE 11

Write the suffix for each of the following.

1. formation _____

2. pertaining to _____

3. hardening _____

4. instrument used to record _____

5. abnormal reduction in numbers _____

6. pain _____

7. separate _____

8. removal _____

Place a check mark (√) in the box to indicate that you have completed Objective 2.

☐ **WRITE THE DEFINITIONS OF THE WORD PARTS INCLUDED IN THIS CHAPTER.**

# Medical Terms

The terms you need to learn to complete this chapter are listed as follows. Now that you know the meaning of the word parts, the exercises found at the end of the list will assist you to learn the definition and the spelling of each word.

# Objective 3  BUILD, ANALYZE, DEFINE, PRONOUNCE, AND SPELL THE DIAGNOSTIC TERMS RELATED TO THE CARDIOVASCULAR AND LYMPHATIC SYSTEMS.

# Diagnostic Terms

**TERM**
(built from word parts)

**DEFINITION**

**HEART AND BLOOD VESSELS**

1. angiocarditis. . . . . . . . .
   (*an*-jē-ō-kar-DĪ-tis)
   (NOTE: the *i* in card/i is dropped because the suffix begins with an *i*.)

   inflammation of the blood vessels and heart

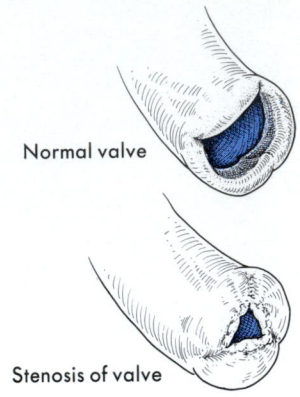
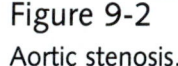

Normal valve

Stenosis of valve

**Figure 9-2**
Aortic stenosis.

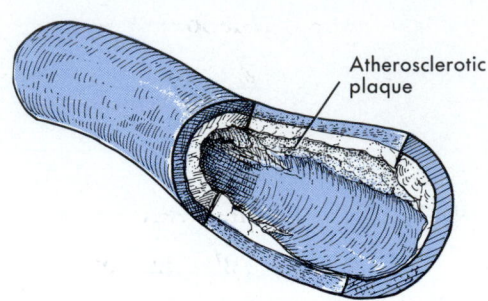

Atherosclerotic plaque

**Figure 9-3**
Atherosclerosis.

2. angioma . . . . . . . . . . . .    tumor composed of blood vessels
   (an-jē-Ō-ma)

3. angiospasm. . . . . . . . . .    spasm (contraction) of the blood vessels
   (AN-jē-ō-spazm)

4. angiostenosis . . . . . . . .    narrowing of a blood vessel
   (an-jē-o-ste-NŌ-sis)

5. aortic stenosis. . . . . . . .    narrowing of the aorta (Figure 9-2)
   (ā-OR-tik) (ste-NŌ-sis)

6. arteriorrhexis . . . . . . . .    rupture of an artery
   (ar-*tē*-rē-ō-REK-sis)

7. arteriosclerosis . . . . . . .    hardening of the arteries
   (ar-*tē*-rē-ō-skle-*RŌ-sis*)

8. atherosclerosis . . . . . . .    hardening of the arteries (in which yel-
   (*ath*-er-ō-skle-RŌ-sis)           lowish, fatty plaque is deposited on the
                                      arterial wall) (Figure 9-3)

9. atrioventricular defect . .    defect pertaining to an atrium and ven-
   (*ā*-trē-ō-ven-TRIK-ū-lar)        tricle

10. bacterial endocarditis. . .    inflammation of the inner lining within
    (bak-TĒ-rē-al) (en-dō-kar-DĪ-    the heart caused by bacteria
    tis)

11. bradycardia . . . . . . . . .    abnormal state of a slow heart rate
    (brād-ē-KAR-dē-a)
    (NOTE: The *i* in card/i has been
    dropped.)

12. cardiodynia . . . . . . . . .    pain in the heart
    (*kar*-dē-ō-DĪN-ē-a)

13. cardiomegaly . . . . . . . .    enlargement of the heart
    (*kar*-dē-ō-MEG-a-lē)

14. cardiomyopathy . . . . . . .    disease of the heart muscle
    (kar-dē-ō-mī-OP-a-thē)

15. cardiovalvulitis . . . . . . .     inflammation of the valves of the heart
    (kar-dē-ō-val-vū-LĪ-tis)

16. coronary ischemia . . . . .     deficient supply of blood to the heart's
    (KŌR-ō-nā-rē) (is-KĒ-mē-a)     blood vessels

17. coronary thrombosis . . .     abnormal condition of a clot in a blood
    (KŌR-ō-nā-rē)   (throm-BŌ-     vessel of the heart
    sis)

18. endocarditis . . . . . . . . .     inflammation of the inner lining within
    (en-dō-kar-DĪ-tis)     the heart

19. myocarditis . . . . . . . . . .     inflammation of the muscle of the heart
    (mī-ō-kar-DĪ-tis)

20. pericarditis . . . . . . . . . .     inflammation of the outer (double layer
    (pār-i-kar-DĪ-tis)     of the) heart

21. polyarteritis . . . . . . . . .     inflammation of many (sites) in the ar-
    (pol-ē-ar-te-RĪ-tis)     teries
    (NOTE: The *i* in arteri/o has
    been dropped.)

22. tachycardia . . . . . . . . . .     abnormally rapid heart rate (of over 100
    (*tak*-i-KAR-dē-a)     beats per minute, which may be caused
    (NOTE: The *i* in cardi/o has     by illness or exercise)
    been dropped.)

## BLOOD AND LYMPHATIC SYSTEMS

1. hematocytopenia . . . . . . .     deficiency of blood cells
   (*hem*-a-tō-sī-tō-PĒ-nē-a)

2. hematoma . . . . . . . . . . .     tumor of blood (swelling caused by an
   (*hem*-a-TŌ-ma)     accumulation of clotted blood in the tis-
       sues)

3. lymphadenitis . . . . . . . .     inflammation of the lymph glands
   (*limf*-ad-en-Ī-tis)

4. lymphadenopathy . . . . . .     disease of the lymph glands. Lymphad-
   (lim-*fad*-e-NOP-a-thē)     enopathy syndrome (LAS) is a persistent
       generalized swelling of the lymph nodes
       often preceding the development of
       AIDS.

5. lymphoma . . . . . . . . . . .     tumor of lymphatic tissue
   (limf-Ō-ma)

6. splenomegaly . . . . . . . . .     enlargement of the spleen
   (*sple*-nō-MEG-a-lē)

7. thymoma . . . . . . . . . . . .     tumor of the thymus gland
   (thī-MŌ-ma)

Practice saying each of these terms aloud. To assist you in pronunciation, obtain the audiotape designed for use with this text. Learn the definitions and spellings of the diagnostic terms by completing the following exercises.

## EXERCISE 12

Analyze and define the following terms.

1. endocarditis _____

2. bradycardia _____

3. cardiomegaly _____

4. arteriosclerosis _____

5. cardiovalvulitis _____

6. angiocarditis _____

7. arteriorrhexis _____

8. tachycardia _____

9. angiostenosis _____

10. atrioventricular defect _____

11. coronary ischemia _____

12. pericarditis _____

13. cardiodynia _____

14. aortic stenosis _____

15. coronary thrombosis _____

16. atherosclerosis _____

17. myocarditis _____

18. angioma _____

19. thymoma _____

20. hematocytopenia _____

21. lymphoma _____

22. lymphadenitis _____

23. splenomegaly _____

24. hematoma _____

25. polyarteritis _____

26. cardiomyopathy _____

27. bacterial endocarditis _____

28. angiospasm _____

29. lymphadenopathy _____

## EXERCISE 13

Build diagnostic terms for the following definitions by using the word parts you have learned.

1. rupture of an artery

   _arteri_ / _orrhexis_
   WR / S

2. enlargement of the heart

   _cardi_ / _o_ / _megaly_
   WR / CV / S

3. deficient supply of blood to the heart's blood vessels

   _coron_ / _ary_
   WR / S

   _isch_ / _emia_
   WR / S

4. inflammation of the blood vessels and the heart

   _angi_ / _o_ / _card_ / _itis_
   WR / CV / WR / S

5. inflammation of the inner layer of the heart

   _endo_ / _card_ / _itis_
   P / WR / S

6. abnormal state of slow heart rate

   _brady_ / _card_ / _ia_
   P / WR / S

7. hardening of the arteries

   _arteri_ / _o_ / _sclerosis_
   WR / CV / S

8. abnormal condition of a clot in the blood vessel of the heart

   _coron_ / _ary_
   WR / S

   _thromb_ / _osis_
   WR / S

9. pain in the heart

_cardiodynia_
WR | S

10. inflammation of the muscle of the heart

_myo o card itis_
WR | CV | WR | S

11. narrowing of blood vessels

_angi o stenosis_
WR | CV | S

12. abnormal state of a rapid heart rate

_tachy cardia_
P | WR | S

13. hardening of the arteries (yellowish, fatty plaque is deposited on the arterial wall)

_arther o sclerosis_
WR | CV | S

14. tumor composed of blood vessels

_angi oma_
WR | S

15. inflammation of the valves of the heart

_card i valvul itis_
WR | CV | WR | S

16. narrowing of the aorta

_aort ic_
WR | S

_stenosis_

17. inflammation of the outer double layer of the heart

_peri card itis_
P | WR | S

18. abnormality concerning the atrium and ventricle of the heart

_atri o ventricul ar_
WR | CV | WR | S

_defect_

19. deficiency in the cells of the blood

_hemato o cyt o penia_
WR | CV | WR | CV | S

20. tumor of lymphatic tissue

lymph / oma
WR / S

21. tumor of the thymus gland

thym / oma
WR / S

22. enlargement of the spleen

splen / o / megaly
WR / CV / S

23. tumor of blood (swelling caused by an accumulation of clotted blood in the tissues)

hemat / oma
WR / S

24. inflammation of lymph glands

lymphaden / itis
WR / WR / S

25. disease of the heart muscle

cardi / o / my / o / pathy
WR / CV / WR / CV / S

26. inflammation of many (sites) in the arteries

poly / arter / itis
P / WR / S

27. spasm of the blood vessels

angi / o / spasm
WR / CV / S

28. inflammation of the inner lining within the heart caused by bacteria

bacterial          endo / card / itis
WR / S              P / WR / S

29. disease of the lymph glands

lymph aden / o / pathy
WR / WR / CV / S

## EXERCISE 14

Spell each of the diagnostic terms. Have someone dictate the terms on pp. 313 to 315 to you or say the words into a tape recorder; then spell the words from your recording as often as necessary. Think about the word parts before attempting to write the word. Study any you have spelled incorrectly.

1. _____        16. _____
2. _____        17. _____
3. _____        18. _____
4. _____        19. _____
5. _____        20. _____
6. _____        21. _____
7. _____        22. _____
8. _____        23. _____
9. _____        24. _____
10. _____        25. _____
11. _____        26. _____
12. _____        27. _____
13. _____        28. _____
14. _____        29. _____
15. _____

Place a check mark (√) in the box to indicate that you have completed Objective 3.

☐ BUILD, ANALYZE, DEFINE, PRONOUNCE, AND SPELL THE DIAGNOSTIC TERMS RELATED TO THE CARDIOVASCULAR AND LYMPHATIC SYSTEMS.

# Objective 4 DEFINE, PRONOUNCE, AND SPELL OTHER DIAGNOSTIC TERMS RELATED TO THE CARDIOVASCULAR AND LYMPHATIC SYSTEMS.

# Other Diagnostic Terms

| TERM | DEFINITION |
| --- | --- |
| 1. anemia . . . . . . . . . . . . . . <br> (a-NĒ-mē-a) | reduction in the amount of hemoglobin in the blood |
| 2. aneurysm . . . . . . . . . . . <br> (AN-ū-rizm) | ballooning of a weakened portion of an arterial wall (Figure 9-4) |
| 3. angina pectoris. . . . . . . . <br> (an-JĪ-na) (PEK-to-ris) | chest pain, which may radiate to the left arm and jaw, that occurs when there is an insufficient supply of blood to the heart muscle |

Ancients believed angina pectoris to be a disorder of the breast. The Latin **angere,** meaning **to throttle,** was used to represent the sudden pain, and was added to **pectus** for **breast.**

4.  arrhythmia . . . . . . . . . .
    (a-RITH-mē-a)
    any variation from the normal heart rhythm

5.  cardiac arrest . . . . . . . .
    (KAR-dē-ak)    (a-REST)
    sudden cessation of cardiac output and effective circulation which requires cardiopulmonary resuscitation (CPR)

6.  cardiac tamponade . . . . .
    (KAR-dē-ak) (tam-pō-NĀD)
    acute compression of the heart caused by fluid accumulation in the pericardial cavity

7.  coarctation of the aorta .
    (kō-ark-TĀ-shun)
    congenital cardiac condition characterized by a narrowing of the aorta (Figure 9-5)

8.  congenital heart disease .
    (kon-JEN-i-tal)
    heart abnormality present at birth

9.  congestive heart failure (CHF) . . . . . . . . . . . . . .
    (kon-JES-tiv)
    inability of the heart to pump enough blood through the body to supply the tissues and organs

10. coronary occlusion . . . . .
    (KŌR-ō-nā-rē) (o-KLŪ-zhun)
    obstruction of an artery of the heart, usually from atherosclerosis (also called *heart attack*)

11. deep vein thrombosis (DVT) . . . . . . . . . . . . . .
    a condition of thrombus in a deep vein of the body. Iliac and femoral veins are commonly affected.

12. embolus, *pl.* emboli . . . .
    (EM-bō-lus) (EM-bō-lī)
    clot or foreign material, such as air or fat, which enters the bloodstream and moves until it lodges at another point in the circulation

13. fibrillation . . . . . . . . . . .
    (fi-bril-Ā-shun)
    rapid, quivering, noncoordinated contractions of the atria or ventricles

14. hemophilia . . . . . . . . . . .
    (hē-mō-FIL-ē-a)
    inherited bleeding disease caused by a deficiency of the coagulation factor VIII

15. hemorrhoid . . . . . . . . .
    (HEM-ō-royd)
    varicose vein in the rectal area which may be internal or external

16. Hodgkin's disease . . . . .
    (HOJ-kins)
    malignant disorder of the lymphatic tissue characterized by progressive enlargement of the lymph nodes, usually beginning in the cervical nodes

17. hypertensive heart disease (HHD) . . . . . . . . .
    (hī-per-TEN-siv)
    disorder of the heart brought about by persistent high blood pressure

18. intermittent claudication . . . . . . . . . . . . . . . .
    (klaw-di-KĀ-shun)
    pain and discomfort in calf muscles while walking. A condition seen in occlusive artery disease.

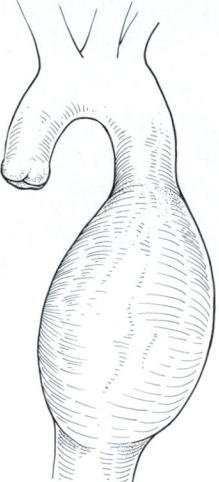

**Figure 9-4**
Aneurysm.

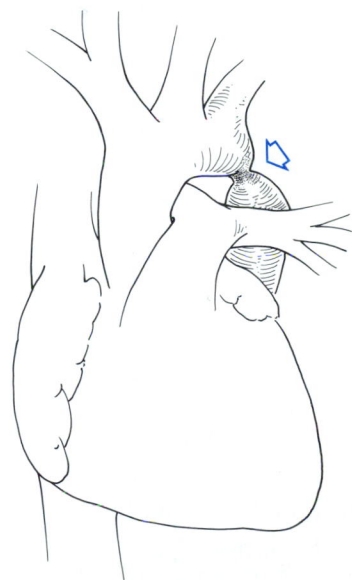

**Figure 9-5**
Coarctation of the aorta.

Thomas Hodgkin, a pathologist at Guy's Hospital in London, described the condition in 1832. In 1865 the name **Hodgkin's disease** was given to the condition by another English physician, Sir Samuel Wilks.

19. **leukemia**. . . . . . . . . . . .
    (lū-KĒ-mē-a)

    disease characterized by excessive increase in white blood cells formed in the bone marrow

20. **mitral valve stenosis**. . . .
    (MĪ-tral)

    a narrowing of the mitral valves from scarring, usually caused by episodes of rheumatic fever.

21. **myocardial infarction (MI)** . . . . . . . . . . . . . . .
    (mī-ō-KAR-dē-al) (in-FARK-shun)

    death of a portion of the myocardial muscle caused by an interrupted blood supply (also called *heart attack*)

22. **rheumatic fever** . . . . . . .
    (rū-MAT-ik)

    an inflammatory disease usually occurring in children and often following an upper respiratory streptococcal infection.

23. **rheumatic heart disease**.
    (rū-MAT-ik)

    damage to the heart muscle or heart valves caused by one or more episodes of rheumatic fever

24. **sickle cell anemia**. . . . . .
    (SIK-el) (sel) (a-NE-mē-a)

    a hereditary, chronic hemolytic disease characterized by crescent or sickle-shaped red blood cells

25. **thromboangiitis obliterans** . . . . . . . . . . . . . . . .
    (*throm*-bō-*an*-jē-Ī-tis) (ob-LIT-er-anz)

    vascular inflammatory disorder usually affecting the lower extremities (also called *Buerger's disease*)

26. **varicose veins (varicosities)** . . . . . . . . . . . . . .
    (VĀR-i-kōs)

    distended or tortuous veins usually found in the lower extremities (Figure 9-6)

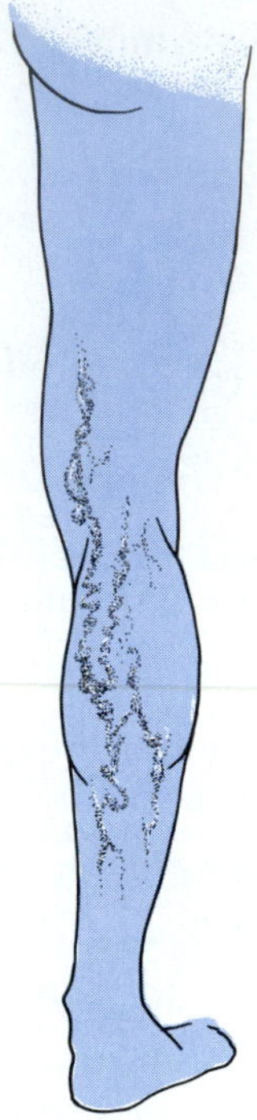

**Figure 9-6**
Varicose veins in the leg.

**Thromboangiitis obliterans** still bears the name of Dr. Leo Buerger, a New York physician who differentiated the disease from another condition, called **obliterating endarteritis.**

Practice saying each of these terms aloud. To assist you in pronunciation, obtain the audiotape designed for use with this text. Learn the definitions and spellings of the other diagnostic terms by completing the exercises that follow.

## EXERCISE 15

Fill in the blanks with the correct terms.

1. A congenital cardiac condition characterized by a narrowing of the aorta is called *Coarctation* of the aorta.
2. A clot or foreign material that enters the bloodstream and moves until it lodges at another point in the circulation is called a(n) *embolus* .
3. Sudden cessation of cardiac output and effective circulation is referred to as a(n) *cardiac* *arrest* .
4. *Congenital* heart disease is the name given to a heart abnormality present at birth.

5. Veins that are distended or tortuous are called ___varicose___ _____.

6. Obstruction of an artery of the heart usually from atherosclerosis is called a(n) ___coronary___ ___occlusion___.

7. ___Aneurysm___ is the name given to the ballooning of a weakened portion of an artery wall.

8. ___Hodgkin's___ disease is the name given to a malignant disorder of lymphatic tissue characterized by enlarged lymph nodes.

9. Varicose veins in the rectal area are called ___hemorroids___.

10. ___angina___ ___pectoris___ is a cardiac condition characterized by center chest pain caused by an insufficient blood supply to the cardiac muscle.

11. Death of a portion of myocardial muscle caused by an interrupted blood supply is called a(n) ___myocardial___ ___infarction___.

12. The condition in which the atria or ventricles have rapid, quivering, noncoordinated contractions is called ___fibrillation___.

13. Any variation from the normal heart rhythm is called a(n) ___arrhythmia___.

14. A disorder of the heart brought about by a persistently elevated blood pressure is called ___hypertensive___ heart disease.

15. ___Congestive___ ___heart___ ___failure___ is the inability of the heart to pump enough blood through the body to supply tissues and organs.

16. ___thromboangitis___ ___obliterans___ is the name given to an inflammatory vascular disorder affecting the lower extremities.

17. ___hemophilia___ is an inherited bleeding disease caused by a deficiency of the coagulation factor VIII.

18. ___Leukemia___ is a disease in which the number of white blood cells in the bone marrow is excessively increased.

19. A reduction in the amount of hemoglobin in the blood results in a condition known as ___anemia___.

20. A hereditary, chronic hemolytic disease in which the red blood cells are crescent-shaped is called ___sickle___ ___cell___ ___anemia___.

21. ___Intermittent___ ___claudication___ is a condition in which a patient suffers pain and discomfort in calf muscles while walking.

22. Acute compression of the heart caused by fluid accumulation in the pericardial cavity is known as ___cardiac___ ___tamponade___.

23. Episodes of rheumatic fever may/can cause ___rheumatic___ ___heart___ ___disease___ and ___mitral___ ___valve___ ___stenosis___.

24. ___Deep___ ___vein___ ___thrombosis___ usually affects the iliac and femoral veins.

25. An inflammatory disease usually occurring in children is ___rheumatic___ ___fever___.

## EXERCISE 16A

Match the terms in the first column with the correct definitions in the second column.

d  1. anemia
c  2. aneurysm
f  3. angina pectoris
e  4. arrhythmia
a  5. cardiac arrest
j  6. cardiac tamponade
i  7. coarctation of the aorta
k  8. congenital heart disease
g  9. congestive heart failure
b  10. coronary occlusion
h  11. intermittent claudication
l  12. deep vein thrombosis

a. sudden cessation of cardiac output and effective circulation

b. obstruction of an artery of the heart, usually from atherosclerosis

c. ballooning or weakening of an artery wall

d. reduction of the amount of hemoglobin in the blood

e. any variation from normal heart rhythm

f. center chest pain occurring because of insufficient blood supply to the heart muscle

g. inability of heart to pump enough blood through the body to supply tissues or organs

h. pain in calf muscles while walking

i. congenital cardiac condition with narrowing of the aorta

j. acute compression of heart caused by fluid in the pericardial cavity

k. heart abnormality present at birth

l. commonly affects the iliac and femoral veins

m. rapid, quivering, noncoordinated contractions of the atria or ventricles

## EXERCISE 16B

Match the terms in the first column with the correct definitions in the second column.

i  1. embolus
e  2. fibrillation
a  3. hemophilia
h  4. hemorrhoids
j  5. Hodgkin's disease
b  6. hypertensive heart disease

a. inherited bleeding disease caused by a deficiency of the coagulation factor VIII

b. heart disorder brought on by persistent high blood pressure

c. distended or tortuous veins

d. excessive increase of white blood cells in the bone marrow

_d_ 7. leukemia

_k_ 8. myocardial infarction

_l_ 9. sickle cell anemia

_g_ 10. thromboangiitis obliterans

_c_ 11. varicose veins

_f_ 12. mitral valve stenosis and rheumatic heart disease

_m_ 13. rheumatic fever

e. rapid, quivering, noncoordinated contractions of the atria or ventricles

f. caused by episodes of rheumatic fever

g. vascular inflammatory disorder usually affecting the lower extremities

h. varicose veins in the rectal area

i. clot or foreign material that enters bloodstream and moves until it lodges at another point

j. malignant disorder of lymphatic tissue with enlargement of lymph nodes

k. death of a portion of myocardial muscle caused by an interrupted blood supply

l. chronic, hemolytic disease having crescent-shaped blood cells

m. often follows an upper respiratory streptococcal infection

## EXERCISE 17

Spell each of the other diagnostic terms. Have someone dictate the terms on pp. 320 to 322 to you or say the words into a tape recorder; then spell the words from your recording as often as necessary. Study any you have spelled incorrectly.

1. _____
2. _____
3. _____
4. _____
5. _____
6. _____
7. _____
8. _____
9. _____
10. _____
11. _____
12. _____
13. _____

14. _____
15. _____
16. _____
17. _____
18. _____
19. _____
20. _____
21. _____
22. _____
23. _____
24. _____
25. _____
26. _____

Place a check mark (√) in the box to indicate that you have completed Objective 4.

☐ **DEFINE, PRONOUNCE, AND SPELL OTHER DIAGNOSTIC TERMS RELATED TO THE CARDIOVASCULAR AND LYMPHATIC SYSTEMS.**

## Objective 5 | BUILD, ANALYZE, DEFINE, PRONOUNCE, AND SPELL THE SURGICAL TERMS RELATED TO THE CARDIOVASCULAR AND LYMPHATIC SYSTEMS.

## Surgical Terms

| **TERMS** (built from word parts) | **DEFINITIONS** |
|---|---|
| 1. **angioplasty** . . . . . . . . . . . (AN-jē-ō-plas-tē) | surgical repair of a blood vessel |
| 2. **angiorrhaphy** . . . . . . . . . . (an-jē-OR-a-fē) | suturing of a blood vessel |
| 3. **endarterectomy** . . . . . . . (*end*-ar-ter-EK-tō-mē) (NOTE: The *o* from *endo-* is dropped for easier pronunciation.) | excision of the thickened interior (intima) of an artery (usually named for the artery to be cleaned out such as *carotid endarterectomy*) (Figure 9-7) |
| 4. **pericardiostomy** . . . . . . . (*par*-i-kar-dē-OS-tō-mē) | creation of an artificial opening in the outer (double) layer of the heart |
| 5. **phlebectomy** . . . . . . . . . . (fle-BEK-tō-mē) | excision of a vein |
| 6. **phlebotomy** . . . . . . . . . . (fle-BOT-ō-mē) | incision into a vein to remove blood or to give blood or intravenous fluids, also called venipuncture |
| 7. **splenectomy** . . . . . . . . . . (sple-NEK-tō-mē) | excision of the spleen |

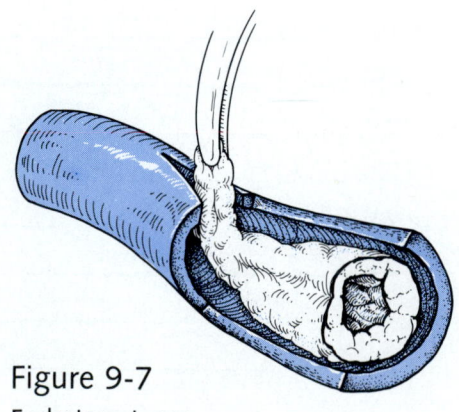

**Figure 9-7**
Endarterectomy.

8. splenopexy . . . . . . . . . . .    surgical fixation of the spleen
   (SPLE-nō-peks-ē)

9. thymectomy . . . . . . . . . .    excision of the thymus gland
   (thī-MEK-tō-mē)

Practice saying each of these terms aloud. To assist you in pronunciation, obtain the audiotape designed for use wth this text. Learn definitions and spellings of the surgical terms by completing the following exercises.

## EXERCISE 18

Analyze and define the following surgical terms.

1. pericardiostomy  _creation of an artifical opening in the outer layer of the heart_
2. thymectomy  _excision of the thymus gland_
3. angioplasty  _surgical repair of a blood vessel_
4. splenopexy  _surgical fixation of the spleen_
5. angiorrhaphy  _suturing of a blood vessel_
6. endarterectomy  _excision of the interior of an artery_
7. phlebotomy  _incision into a vein_
8. splenectomy  _excision of the spleen_
9. phlebectomy  _excision of a vein_

## EXERCISE 19

Build surgical terms for the following definitions by using the word parts you have learned.

1. excision of the thickened interior of an artery
   _____ / _____ / _____
       P     WR     S

2. surgical fixation of the spleen
   _____ / _____ / _____
       WR    CV    S

3. suturing of a blood vessel
   _____ / _____
       WR    S

4. incision into a vein
   _____ / _____
       WR    S

5. excision of the thymus
   gland

   _____ / _____
          WR         S

6. creation of an artificial
   opening in the outer layer
   of the heart

   _____ / _____ / _____
     P        WR       S

7. surgical repair of a blood
   vessel

   _____ / _____ / _____
     WR      CV      S

8. excision of a spleen

   _____ / _____
          WR         S

9. excision of a vein

   _____ / _____
          WR         S

Place a check mark (√) in the box to indicate that you have completed Objective 5.

☐ **BUILD, ANALYZE, DEFINE, PRONOUNCE, AND SPELL THE SURGICAL TERMS RELATED TO THE CARDIOVASCULAR AND LYMPHATIC SYSTEMS.**

## Objective 6   DEFINE, PRONOUNCE, AND SPELL OTHER SURGICAL TERMS RELATED TO THE CARDIOVASCULAR AND LYMPHATIC SYSTEMS.

# Other Surgical and Treatment Terms

| TERM | DEFINITION |
|---|---|
| 1. aneurysmectomy . . . . . .<br>(an-ū-riz-MEK-tō-mē) | surgical excision of an aneurysm (the ballooning of a weakened blood vessel wall) |
| 2. bone marrow transplant. | infusion of normal bone marrow cells from a donor with matching cells and tissue to a recipient with a certain type of leukemia or anemia |
| 3. cardiac pacemaker . . . . . | battery-powered or nuclear-powered apparatus implanted under the skin to regulate heart rate (Figure 9-8) |
| 4. coronary artery bypass graft (CABG) . . . . . . . . | surgical technique to bring a new blood supply to heart muscles by detouring around blocked arteries (Figure 9-9) |

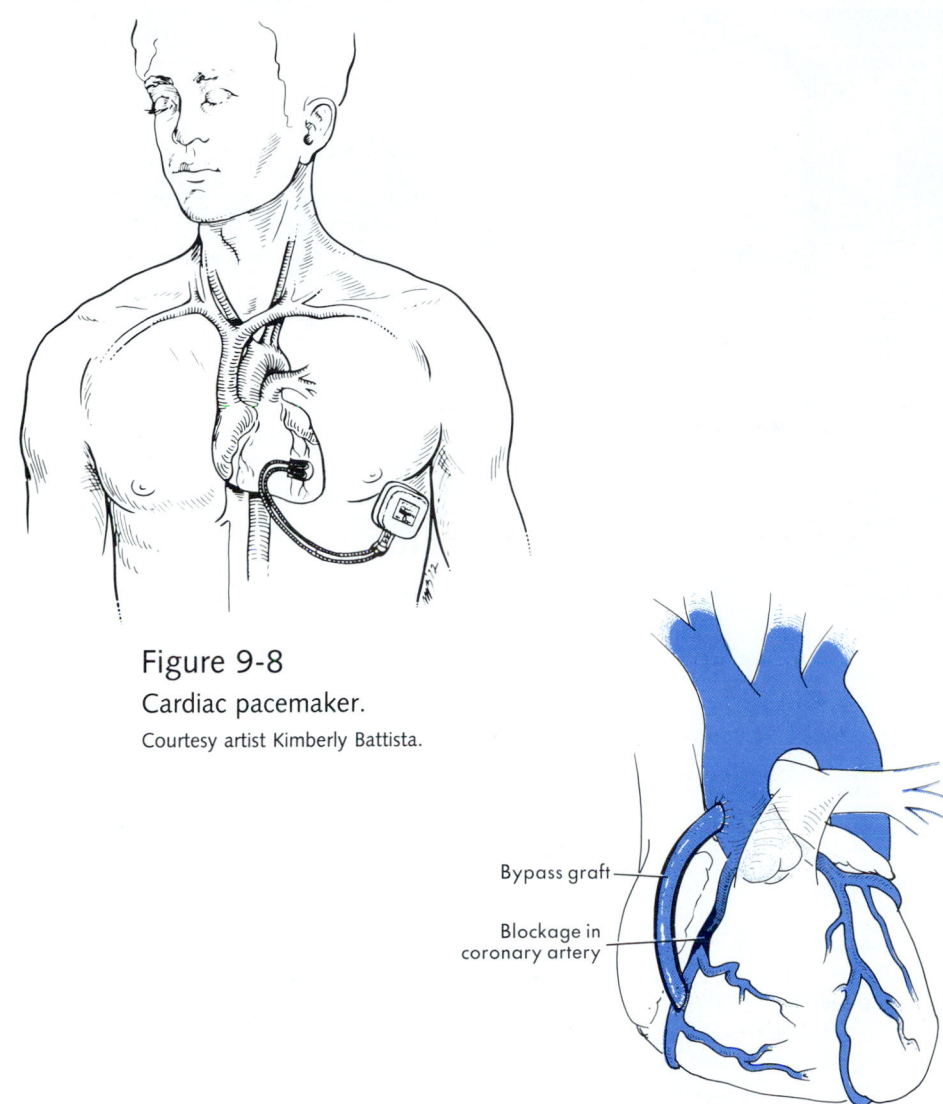

Figure 9-8
Cardiac pacemaker.
Courtesy artist Kimberly Battista.

Bypass graft

Blockage in
coronary artery

Figure 9-9
Coronary artery bypass graft.

5.  **defibrillation** . . . . . . . .    application of an electric shock to the
    (dē-fib-ri-LĀ-shun)                   myocardium through the chest wall to
                                          restore normal cardiac rhythm (Figure
                                          9-10)

6.  **embolectomy** . . . . . . . . .    surgical removal of an embolus or clot
    (*em*-bō-LEK-tō-mē)

7.  **femoropopliteal bypass** .    surgery to establish an alternate route
    (FEM-or-ō-pop-li-TĒ-al)             from femoral artery to popliteal artery to
                                        bypass obstructive portion (Figure 9-11)

8.  **hemorrhoidectomy**. . . . .    excision of hemorrhoids, the varicosed
    (hem-ō-royd-EK-tō-mē)              veins in the rectal region

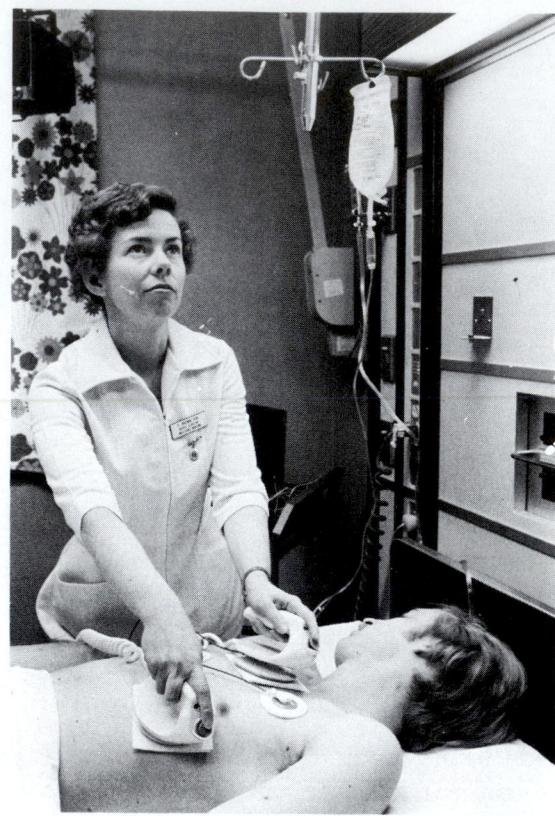

**Figure 9-10**
Defibrillation being performed on patient.
From Phipps WJ, Long BC, Woods NF and others: *Medical-surgical nursing*, ed 4, St. Louis, 1991, Mosby.

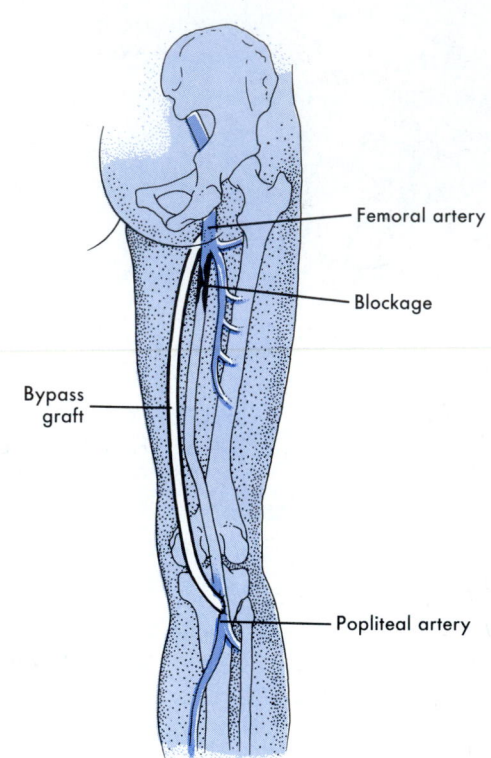

Femoral artery

Blockage

Bypass graft

Popliteal artery

**Figure 9-11**
Femoropopliteal bypass.

9.  intracoronary thrombo-
    lytic therapy..........
    (in-tra-KOR-ō-na-rē) (throm-
    bol-LI-tik)

an injection of a medication in a blocked coronary vessel to dissolve blood clots

10. laser angioplasty ......
    (LĀ-zer) (AN-jē-ō-*plas*-tē)

the use of *l*ight *a*mplification by *s*imulated *e*mission of *r*adiation or laser beam to open blocked arteries especially in lower extremities

11. mitral commissurotomy.
    (MI-tral)    (*kom*-i-shūr-OT-
    ō-mē)

surgical procedure to repair a stenosed mitral valve by breaking apart the leaves (commissures) of the valve (Figure 9-12)

12. percutaneous translumi-
    nal coronary angioplasty
    (PTCA)..............
    (*per*-kū-TĀ-nē-us)
    (trans-LŪM-in-al)
    (KOR-ō-na-rē)
    (AN-jē-ō-*plas*-tē)

procedure in which a balloon is passed through a blood vessel to the area in which plaque is formed. Inflation of the balloon then flattens the plaque against the vessel wall and allows the blood to circulate more freely.

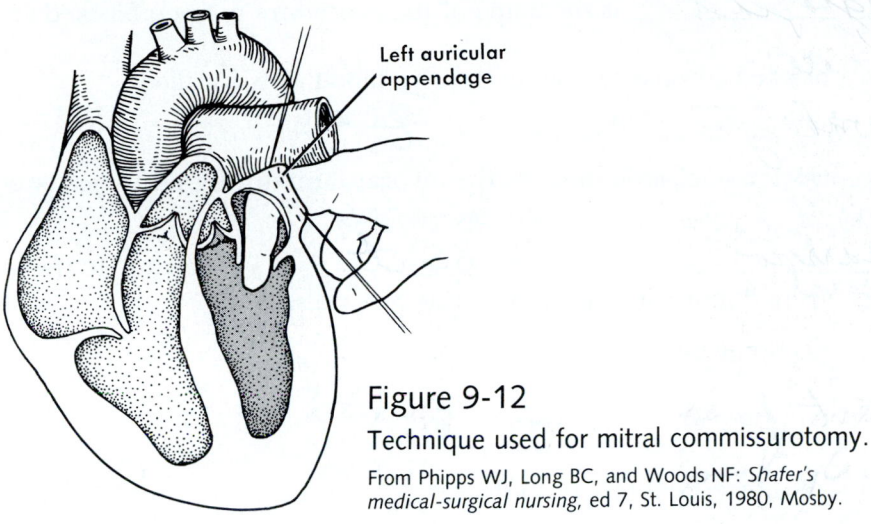

Left auricular appendage

Figure 9-12

Technique used for mitral commissurotomy.

From Phipps WJ, Long BC, and Woods NF: *Shafer's medical-surgical nursing*, ed 7, St. Louis, 1980, Mosby.

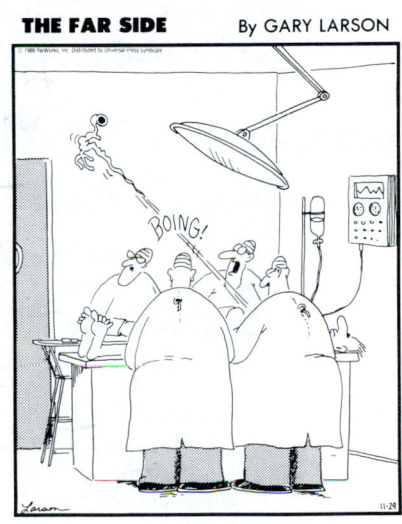

THE FAR SIDE    By GARY LARSON

"Whoa! Watch where that thing lands — we'll probably need it."

13. vein ligation and stripping . . . . . . . . . . . . . . .
(lī-GA-shun)

surgical method of tying off a varicose vein and removing it

Practice saying each of these terms aloud. To assist you in pronunciation, obtain the audiotape designed for use with this text. Learn the definitions and spellings of the other surgical terms by completing the following exercises.

## EXERCISE 20

Fill in the blanks with the correct terms.

1. Surgical excision of hemorrhoids is called a(n) _hemorrhoidectomy_.

2. The surgical method of tying off a varicosed vein and removing it is called _vein_ _ligation_ _and_ _stripping_.

3. The procedure in which a balloon is passed through a blood vessel to flatten plaque against the vessel wall when the balloon is inflated is called _percutaneous_ _transluminal_ _coronary_ _angioplasty_.

4. To regulate the heart rate, the physician may insert a(n) _pacemaker_ under the patient's skin.

5. A mitral _commissurotomy_ is the name of the surgery performed to repair a stenosed mitral valve.

6. The surgery performed to detour blood around a blocked artery so that a new blood supply can be given to heart muscles is called _coronary_ _artery_ _bypass_ _graft_.

7. The surgical excision of an aneurysm is called a(n) _aneurysmectomy_.

8. A(n) _femoropopliteal_ _bypass_ is the name of the surgery performed to establish an alternate route from femoral artery to popliteal artery to bypass obstructive portion.

9. _Laser_ _angioplasty_ is the name of the procedure to open blocked arteries with a laser beam.

10. An injection of a medication into a blocked coronary vessel to dissolve blood clots is called _intracoronary_ _thrombolytic_ therapy.

11. _defibrillation_ is the application of electric shock to the myocardium through the chest wall to restore cardiac rhythm.

12. _Bone_ _marrow_ _transplant_ is a procedure to transfuse bone marrow cells to recipient from donor with matching tissue and cells.

13. _embolectomy_ is the surgical removal of embolus or clot.

## EXERCISE 21

Match the terms in the first column with the correct definitions in the second column.

_h_ 1. aneurysmectomy

_f_ 2. coronary artery by-pass graft

_k_ 3. femoropopliteal by-pass

_l_ 4. hemorrhoidectomy

_d_ 5. cardiac pacemaker

_m_ 6. mitral commissurotomy

_a_ 7. percutaneous trans-luminal coronary angioplasty

_b_ 8. vein ligation and stripping

_c_ 9. defibrillation

_e_ 10. laser angioplasty

_i_ 11. bone marrow transplant

_g_ 12. intracoronary thrombolytic therapy

_j_ 13. embolectomy

a. pressing plaque against a blood vessel wall by inflating a balloon passed through the blood vessel

b. tying off and removal of a varicose vein

c. application of electric shock to myocardium through chest wall to restore cardiac rhythm

d. apparatus implanted under the skin to regulate heart beat

e. procedure performed to open blocked arteries using a laser beam

f. diverts blood past a blocked artery in the heart

g. use of a medication to dissolve blood clots in blocked coronary vessel

h. excision of a weakened ballooning blood vessel wall

i. normal bone marrow cells infused from donor with matching tissues and cells into recipient with leukemia

j. surgical removal of an embolus

k. surgical procedure to establish an alternate route from femoral artery to popliteal artery to bypass obstructive portion

l. surgical excision of varicose veins in the rectal area

   **m.** surgical procedure to break apart the leaves of the mitral valve

   **n.** surgical removal of a thickened artery

## EXERCISE 22

Spell each of the surgical terms. Have someone dictate the terms on pp. 328 to 331 to you or say the words into a tape recorder; then spell the words from your recording as often as necessary. Study any you have spelled incorrectly.

1. _____  8. _____

2. _____  9. _____

3. _____  10. _____

4. _____  11. _____

5. _____  12. _____

6. _____  13. _____

7. _____

Place a check mark (√) in the box to indicate that you have completed Objective 6.

☐ **DEFINE, PRONOUNCE, AND SPELL OTHER SURGICAL TERMS RELATED TO THE CARDIOVASCULAR AND LYMPHATIC SYSTEMS.**

## Objective 7   BUILD, ANALYZE, DEFINE, PRONOUNCE, AND SPELL THE DIAGNOSTIC PROCEDURAL TERMS RELATED TO THE CARDIOVASCULAR AND LYMPHATIC SYSTEMS.

## Diagnostic Procedural Terms

**TERM**       **DEFINITION**
(built from word parts)

**HEART AND BLOOD VESSELS**

1. angiography . . . . . . . . .  process of x-ray filming a blood vessel
   (an-jē-OG-ra-fē)     (after an injection of contrast medium; the procedure named for the vessel to be studied, such as a *femoral angiography*)

2. angioscope . . . . . . . . . .  instrument used to visualize a blood vessel.
   (AN-jē-ō-skōp)

3. angioscopy . . . . . . . . . .  visual examination of a blood vessel
   (an-jē-OS-kō-pē)

4. aortogram. . . . . . . . . . .  x-ray film of the aorta (made after an injection of contrast medium)
   (ā-OR-tō-gram)

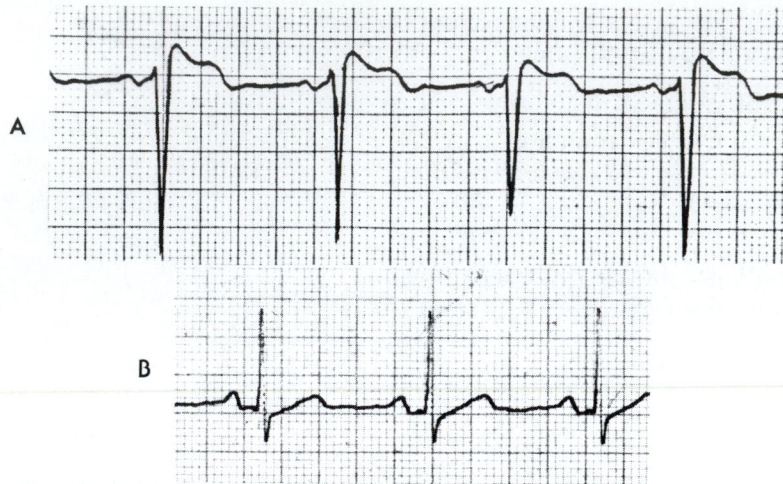

## Figure 9-13

Electrocardiogram tracings. Normal ECGs in lead V **(A)** and lead II (B).

From Phipps WJ, Long BC, and Woods NF: *Shafer's medical-surgical nursing*, ed 7, St. Louis, 1980, Mosby.

5.  arteriogram . . . . . . . . . . 
    (ar-TE-rē-ō-gram)
    x-ray film of an artery (taken after an injection of contrast medium)

6.  echocardiogram . . . . . . . 
    (ek-ō-KAR-dē-ō-gram)
    record made of the structure and motion of the heart using sound waves

7.  electrocardiogram (EKG) . . . . . . . . . . . . . . 
    (e-*lek*-trō-KAR-dē-ō-gram)
    record of the electrical activity of the heart (Figure 9-13)

8.  electrocardiograph . . . . . 
    (e-*lek*-trō-KAR-dē-ō-graf)
    instrument used to record the electrical activity of the heart

9.  electrocardiography . . . . 
    (e-*lek*-trō-*kar*-dē-OG-ra-fē)
    process of recording the electrical activity of the heart

10. phlebography . . . . . . . . 
    (fle-BOG-ra-fē)
    process of x-ray filming a vein (filled with contrast medium)

11. phonocardiogram . . . . . . 
    (*fō*-nō-KAR-dē-ō-gram)
    graphic record of heart sound

12. sphygmocardiograph . . . 
    (*sfig*-mō-KAR-dē-ō-graf)
    instrument used to measure pulse waves and heart beat

13. stethoscope . . . . . . . . . . 
    (STETH-ō-skōp)
    instrument used to listen to chest sounds produced by heart and lungs

14. venogram . . . . . . . . . . . 
    (VĒ-nō-gram)
    x-ray film of the veins (taken after an injection of dye)

### BLOOD AND LYMPHATIC SYSTEMS

1.  erythrocyte count (RBC) . 
    (e-RITH-rō-sīt)
    red blood cell count (number of red blood cells per cubic millimeter of blood)

> The stethoscope was first called a **baton** or **cylinder**. Its name is derived from the Greek **stethos** meaning **chest** and **scopeo**, meaning **to view** or **examine**. The term means **"to see"** what is in the body by listening to the body sounds.

2. hematocrit (HCT) . . . . . .
   (he-MAT-ō-krit)

   separated blood (volume percentage of erythrocytes in whole blood after separation by centrifuge)

3. leukocyte count (WBC) . .
   (LŪ-kō-sīt)

   white blood cell count (number of white blood cells per cubic millimeter of blood)

4. lymphadenography . . . . .
   (lim-*fad*-e-NOG-ra-fē)

   process of x-ray filming the lymph nodes and glands (after an injection of contrast medium)

5. lymphangiogram . . . . . . .
   (lim-FAN-jē-ō-gram)

   x-ray film of the lymphatic vessels

6. lymphangiography. . . . . .
   (lim-*fan*-jē-OG-ra-fē)

   process of x-ray filming the lymphatic vessels (after an injection of contrast medium)

Practice saying each of these terms aloud. To assist you in pronunciation, obtain the audiotape designed for use with this text. Learn the definitions and spellings of the diagnostic procedural terms by completing the following exercises.

## EXERCISE 23

Analyze and define the following diagnostic procedural terms.

1. electrocardiograph *instrument used to record the electrical activity of the heart*

2. sphygmocardiograph *instrument used to measure pulse waves + heart beat*

3. venogram *x-ray film of the veins*

4. angiography *process of x-ray filming a blood vessel*

5. echocardiogram *record made of the structure + motion of the heart using sound waves*

6. stethoscope *instrument used to listen to chest sounds*

7. aortogram *x-ray film of the aorta*

8. electrocardiogram *record of the electrical activity of the heart*

9. phonocardiogram *graphic record of heart sounds*

10. arteriogram *x-ray film of an artery*

11. electrocardiography *process of recording the electrical activity of the heart*

12. erythrocyte count *red blood cell count*

13. lymphangiogram *x-ray film of lymphatic vessels*

14. hematocrit  *WR CV S*  — _separated blood_

15. lymphadenography  *WR F WR CV S*  — _process of x-ray filming the lymph nodes + gland_

16. leukocyte count  *WR CV S*  — _white blood cell count_

17. lymphangiography  *WR F WR CV*  — _process of x-ray filming the lymphatic vessels_

18. angioscopy  *WR CV S*  — _visual exam of a blood vessel_

19. phlebography  *WR CV S*  — _process of x-ray filming a vein_

20. angioscope  *WR CV S*  — _instrument for visual exam of a vessel_

## EXERCISE 24

Build diagnostic procedural terms for the following definitions by using the word parts you have learned.

1. instrument used to record
   the electrical activity of
   the heart

   _____ / _____ / _____ / _____ / _____
      WR    CV    WR    CV    S

2. instrument used to listen
   to chest sounds

   _____ / _____ / _____
      WR    CV    S

3. x-ray film of an artery
   (taken after an injection
   of contrast medium)

   _____ / _____ / _____
      WR    CV    S

4. x-ray film of the veins
   (taken after an injection
   of contrast medium)

   _____ / _____ / _____
      WR    CV    S

5. process of making an
   x-ray film of a blood vessel

   _____ / _____ / _____
      WR    CV    S

6. record of the electrical
   activity of the heart

   _____ / _____ / _____ / _____ / _____
      WR    CV    WR    CV    S

7. record made of the structure and motion of the heart using sound waves

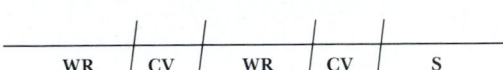

WR / CV / WR / CV / S

8. graphic record of heart sounds

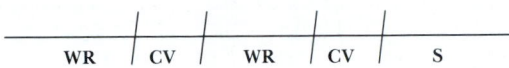

WR / CV / WR / CV / S

9. instrument used to measure pulse waves and heart beat

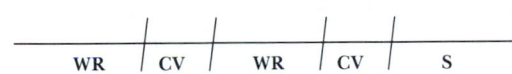

WR / CV / WR / CV / S

10. x-ray film of the aorta (taken after an injection of contrast medium)

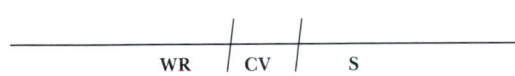

WR / CV / S

11. process of recording the electrical activity of the heart

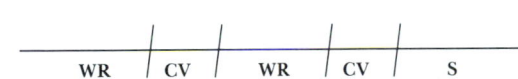

WR / CV / WR / CV / S

12. separated blood (volume percentage of erythrocytes in whole blood after separation by centrifuge)

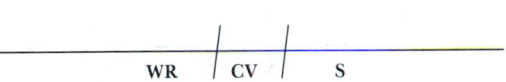

WR / CV / S

13. x-ray film of lymphatic vessels

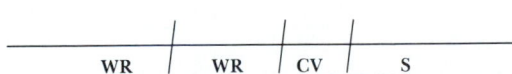

WR / WR / CV / S

14. white blood cell count (number of white blood cells per cubic millimeter of blood)

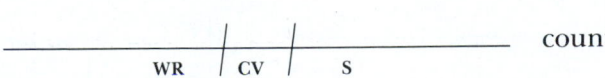 count

WR / CV / S

15. process of x-ray filming the lymph nodes and glands

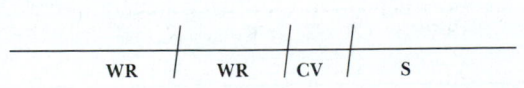

WR / WR / CV / S

16. red blood cell count (number of red blood cells per cubic millimeter of blood) _____\|_____\|_____ count
    WR   CV   S

17. process of x-ray filming the lymphatic vessels _____\|_____\|_____\|_____
    WR   WR   CV   S

18. instrument used to visually examine a blood vessel _____\|_____\|_____
    WR   CV   S

19. process of x-ray filming a vein _____\|_____\|_____
    WR   CV   S

20. instrument used for visual examination of a blood vessel _____\|_____\|_____
    WR   CV   S

## EXERCISE 25

Spell each of the diagnostic procedural terms. Have someone dictate the terms on pp. 333 to 335 to you or say the words into a tape recorder; then spell the words from your recording as often as necessary. Think about the word parts before attempting to write the word. Study any you have spelled incorrectly.

1. _____    11. _____
2. _____    12. _____
3. _____    13. _____
4. _____    14. _____
5. _____    15. _____
6. _____    16. _____
7. _____    17. _____
8. _____    18. _____
9. _____    19. _____
10. _____    20. _____

☐ **BUILD, ANALYZE, DEFINE, PRONOUNCE, AND SPELL THE DIAGNOSTIC PROCEDURAL TERMS RELATED TO THE CARDIOVASCULAR AND LYMPHATIC SYSTEMS.**

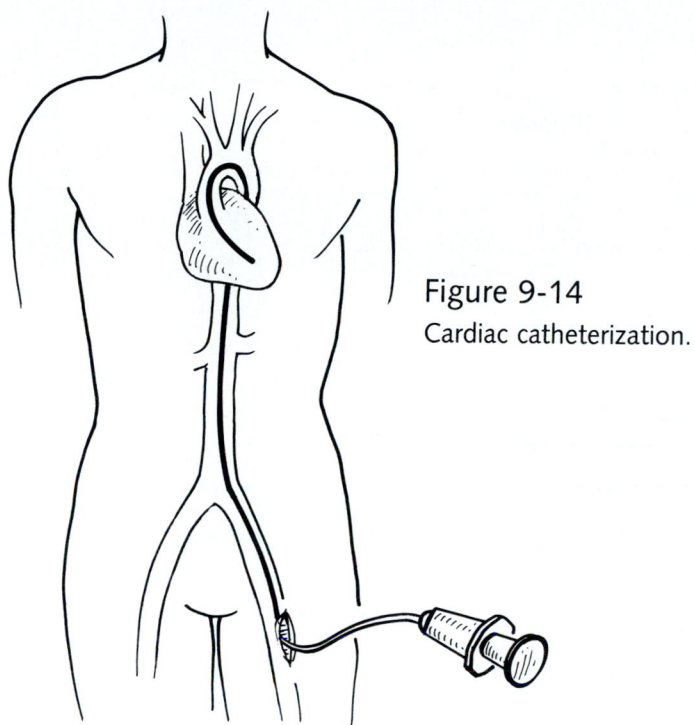

Figure 9-14
Cardiac catheterization.

## Objective 8 DEFINE, PRONOUNCE, AND SPELL OTHER DIAGNOSTIC PROCEDURAL TERMS RELATING TO THE CARDIOVASCULAR AND LYMPHATIC SYSTEMS.

# Other Diagnostic Procedural Terms

| TERM | DEFINITION |
| --- | --- |
| **HEART AND BLOOD VESSELS** | |
| 1. cardiac catheterization... (KAR-dē-ak) (*kath*-e-ter-ī-ZĀ-shun) | introduction of a catheter into the heart by way of a blood vessel for the purpose of determining cardiac disease (Figure 9-14) |
| 2. cardiac scan . . . . . . . . . . | two-dimensional photographic representation of the heart taken after the introduction of radioactive material into the body |
| 3. Doppler flow studies . . . . (DOP-ler) | study that uses ultrasound to determine the velocity of the flow of blood within the vessels (Figure 9-15) |
| 4. impedance plethysmography . . . . . . . . . . . . . . . . . (im-PĒD-dans) (pleth-iz-MOG-ra-fē) | measures venous flow to the limbs using a plethysmograph, which records electrical resistance (impedance) caused by venous occlusion. Used to detect deep vein thrombosis |

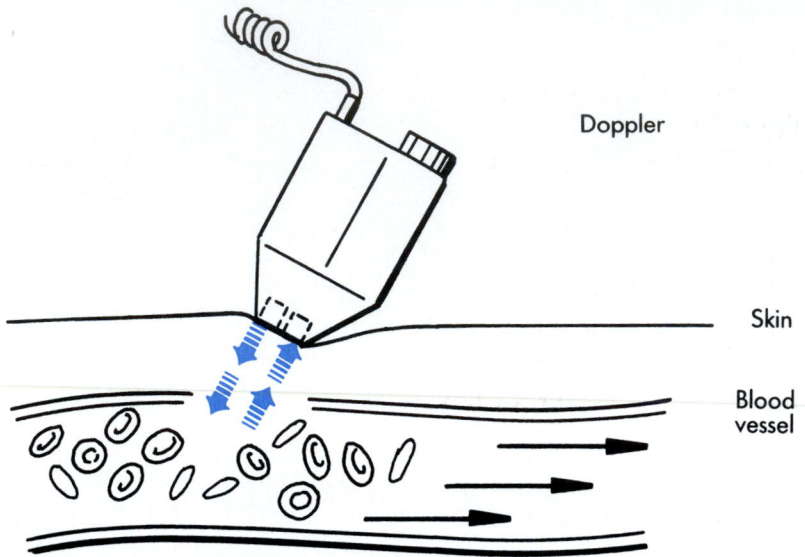

## Figure 9-15

Doppler flow effect showing the red blood cells reflecting sound.

From Phipps WJ, Long BC, Woods NF and others: *Medical-surgical nursing,* ed 4, St. Louis, 1991, Mosby.

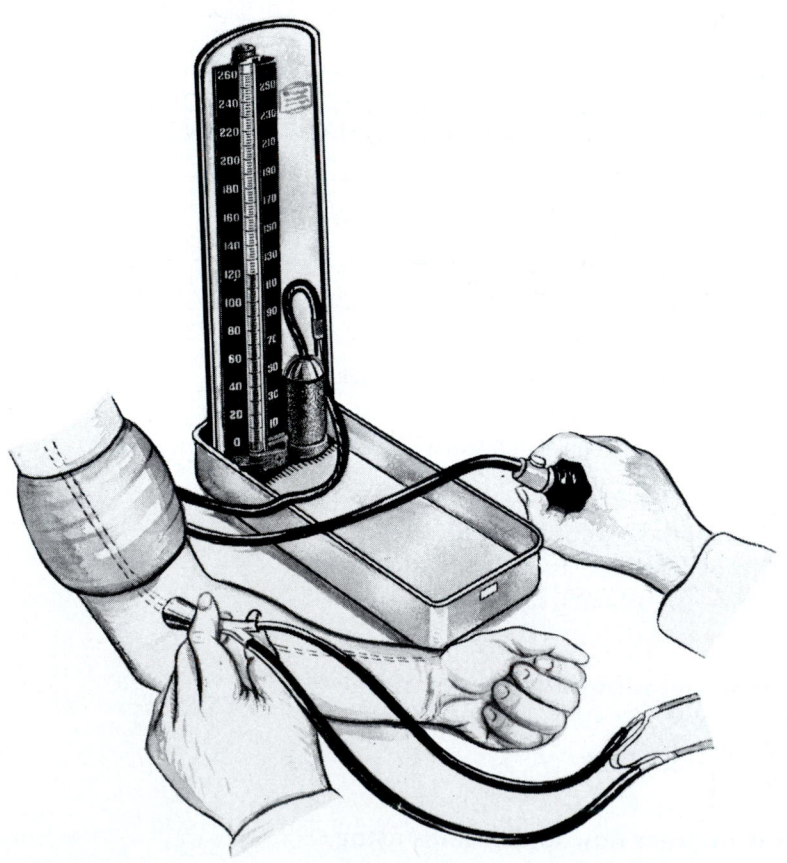

## Figure 9-16

Sphygmomanometer.

From Schottelius BA and Schottelius DD: *Textbook of physiology,* ed 17, St. Louis, 1973, Mosby.

5.  sphygmomanometer . . . . .     device used for measuring arterial blood
    (*sfig*-mō-ma-NOM-e-ter)        pressure (Figure 9-16)

6.  treadmill stress test . . . . .     test to assess the ability of the coronary
                                    circulation to handle the increased load
                                    placed on the heart by exercise

### BLOOD AND LYMPHATIC SYSTEM

1.  complete     blood     count
    (CBC) . . . . . . . . . . . . . .     basic blood screening that includes tests
                                    on hemoglobin, hematocrit, red blood
                                    cell morphology (size and shape), leuko-
                                    cyte count, and white blood cell differ-
                                    ential (types of WBCs)

2.  coagulation time . . . . . . .     blood test to determine the time it takes
    (kō-ag-ū-LĀ-shun)              for blood to form a clot

3.  hemoglobin (Hgb) . . . . . .     oxygen-carrying components in red
    (HĒ-mō-glō-bin)                blood cells, responsible for giving blood
                                    its color

4.  prothrombin time (PT) . .     test to determine certain coagulation ac-
    (prō-THROM-bin)                tivity defects; also used to monitor anti-
                                    coagulation therapy

5.  bone marrow biopsy . . . . .     needle puncture to remove bone marrow
                                    for study, usually from the sternum or
                                    ilium, to determine certain blood cell
                                    diseases, such as leukemia and anemia
                                    (Figure 9-17)

Practice saying each of these terms aloud. To assist you in pronunciation, obtain the audiotape designed for use with this text. Learn the definitions and spellings of the other diagnostic procedural terms by completing the following exercises.

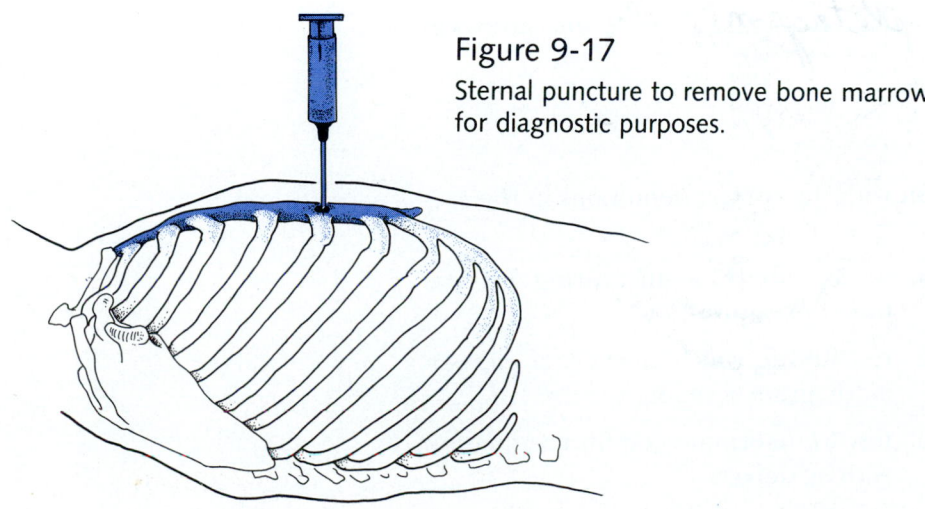

Figure 9-17
Sternal puncture to remove bone marrow for diagnostic purposes.

## EXERCISE 26

Fill in the blanks with the correct terms.

1. A device for measuring blood pressure is called a(n) _sphygmomanometer_.

2. _coagulation_ _time_ is the name of the blood test that determines the time it takes for blood to form a clot.

3. A test, performed to diagnose coronary artery disease, in which the patient walks while an exercise cardiogram is recorded is a(n) _treadmill_ _stress_ test.

4. _Complete_ _blood_ _count_ is the name of a basic blood-screening test.

5. The name of the study in which ultrasound is used to determine the velocity of flow of blood within vessels is called _Doppler_ _flow_ _studies_.

6. Two-dimensional photographic representation of the heart taken after the introduction of radioactive material is called a(n) _cardiac_ _scan_.

7. _Bone_ _marrow_ _biopsy_ is the name given to a procedure performed to determine certain blood diseases, such as leukemia.

8. A blood test performed to determine certain coagulation defects and to monitor anticoagulation therapy is called _Prothrombin_ _time_.

9. _cardiac_ _catheterization_ is the name given to a procedure in which a catheter is introduced into the heart to determine pathology in the heart or its vessels.

10. The oxygen-carrying component in the red blood cells is called _Hemoglobin_.

11. A _impedance_ _plethysmography_ measures venous flow to the limbs.

## EXERCISE 27

Match the terms in the first column with the correct definitions in the second column.

_d_ 1. cardiac catheterization

_e_ 2. cardiac scan

_h_ 3. complete blood count

_i_ 4. coagulation time

a. device used for measuring arterial blood pressure

b. test during which an exercise electrocardiogram is made

c. test to determine certain coagulation activity defects

_g_ 5. hemoglobin

_j_ 6. Doppler flow studies

_c_ 7. prothrombin time

_a_ 8. sphygmomanometer

_k_ 9. bone marrow biopsy

_b_ 10. treadmill stress test

_f_ 11. impedance plethysmography

d. passage of a tube into the heart to determine disease within the heart

e. two-dimensional photograph of heart

f. measures venous flow to the limbs

g. responsible for the red color of blood

h. basic blood screening test

i. determines the time it takes for blood to form a clot

j. study in which ultrasound is used to determine the velocity of the flow of blood within vessels

k. performed to determine certain blood cell diseases, such as leukemia

l. test to determine the number of red blood cells

## EXERCISE 28

Spell each of the other diagnostic procedural terms. Have someone dictate the terms on pp. 333 to 335 to you or say the words into a tape recorder; then spell the words from your recording as often as necessary. Study any you have spelled incorrectly.

1. _____

2. _____

3. _____

4. _____

5. _____

6. _____

7. _____

8. _____

9. _____

10. _____

11. _____

Place a check mark (√) in the box to indicate that you have completed Objective 8.

☐ DEFINE, PRONOUNCE, AND SPELL THE DIAGNOSTIC PROCEDURAL TERMS RELATING TO THE CARDIOVASCULAR AND LYMPHATIC SYSTEMS.

# Objective 9 — BUILD, ANALYZE, DEFINE, PRONOUNCE, AND SPELL ADDITIONAL TERMS RELATED TO THE CARDIOVASCULAR AND LYMPHATIC SYSTEMS.

# Additional Terms

| TERM (Built from word parts) | DEFINITION |
|---|---|
| 1. cardiac .............. (KAR-dē-ak) | pertaining to the heart |

2.  cardiogenic. . . . . . . . .     originating in the heart
    (*kar*-dē-ō-JEN-ik)

3.  cardiologist. . . . . . . . .     physician who studies and treats diseases
    (*kar*-dē-OL-ō-jist)                of the heart

4.  cardiology . . . . . . . . .     study of the heart
    (*kar*-dē-OL-ō-jē)

5.  hematologist. . . . . . . .     physician who studies and treats diseases
    (*hē*-ma-TOL-ō-jist)                of the blood

6.  hematology. . . . . . . . .     study of the blood
    (*hē*-ma-TOL-ō-jē)

7.  hematopoiesis. . . . . . . .     formation of blood cells
    (*hē*-ma-tō-poy-Ē-sis)

8.  hemolysis . . . . . . . . . .     destruction of (red) blood cells
    (hē-MOL-i-sis)

9.  hemostasis . . . . . . . . .     stoppage of bleeding
    (*hē*-mō-STĀ-sis)

10. hypothermia. . . . . . . .     condition of body temperature that is be-
    (*hī*-pō-THER-mē-a)               low normal (sometimes induced for var-
                                     ious surgical procedures, such as bypass
                                     surgery)

11. plasmapheresis. . . . . . .     removal of plasma (from withdrawn
    (plaz-ma-fe-RĒ-sis)               blood)

12. tachypnea. . . . . . . . . .     rapid breathing
    (tak-ip-NĒ-a)

Practice saying each of these terms aloud. To assist you in pronunciation,
obtain the audiotape designed for use with this text. Learn the terms by
completing the following exercises.

## EXERCISE 29

Analyze and define the following additional terms.

1. hypothermia _____

2. hematopoiesis _____

3. cardiology _____

4. cardiologist _____

5. hemolysis _____

6. hematologist _____

7. cardiac _____

8. hematology _____

9. plasmapheresis _____

10. hemostasis _____

11. cardiogenic _____

12. tachypnea _____

## EXERCISE 30

Build terms for the following definitions by using the word parts you have learned.

1. study of the heart

   _____ cardi | ology _____
         WR     S

2. formation of red blood cells

   _____ hemat | o | poiesis _____
         WR   CV   S

3. body temperature that is below normal

   _____ hyp | o | thermia _____
         P   WR   S

4. destruction of red blood cells

   _____ hem | o | lysis _____
         WR   CV   S

5. removal of plasma from withdrawn blood

   _____ plasm | apheresis _____
         WR   S

6. physician who studies and treats diseases of the blood

   _____ hemat | ologist _____
         WR   S

7. pertaining to the heart

   _____ cardi | ac _____
         WR   S

8. physician who studies and treats diseases of the heart

   _____ cardi | ologist _____
         WR   S

9. study of the blood

   _____ hemat | ology _____
         WR   S

10. stoppage of bleeding     *hemo o stasis*

                                                  WR    CV    S

11. rapid breathing     *tachy pnea*

                                                  P     S(WR)

12. originating in the heart     *cardi o genic*

                                                  WR    CV    S

## EXERCISE 31

Spell each of the additional terms. Have someone dictate the terms on pp. 343-344 to you or say the words into a tape recorder; then spell the words from your recording as often as necessary. Think about the word parts before attempting to write the word. Study any you have spelled incorrectly.

1. _____
2. _____
3. _____
4. _____
5. _____
6. _____

7. _____
8. _____
9. _____
10. _____
11. _____
12. _____

Place a check mark (√) in the box to indicate that you have completed Objective 9.

☐ **BUILD, ANALYZE, DEFINE, PRONOUNCE, AND SPELL ADDITIONAL TERMS RELATED TO THE CARDIOVASCULAR AND LYMPHATIC SYSTEMS.**

# Objective 10   DEFINE, PRONOUNCE, AND SPELL THE OTHER ADDITIONAL TERMS RELATED TO THE CARDIOVASCULAR AND LYMPHATIC SYSTEMS.

# Other Additional Terms

**TERM**              **DEFINITION**

**HEART AND BLOOD VESSELS**

1. auscultation . . . . . . . . . .   the hearing of sounds within the body through a stethoscope
   (*aws*-kul-TĀ-shun)

2. blood pressure (BP) . . . .   pressure exerted by the blood against the blood vessel walls

3. cardiopulmonary resuscitation (CPR) . . . . . . . .   emergency procedure consisting of artificial ventilation and external cardiac massage
   (*kar*-dē-ō-PUL-mō-năr-ē) (rē-*sus*-i-TĀ-shun)

4. diastole.............. phase in the cardiac cycle in which the
   (dī-AS-tō-lē) ventricles relax between contractions

5. extracorporeal ........ occurring outside the body (during open
   (*ek*-stra-kōr-PŌ-rē-al) heart surgery extracorporeal circulation
   occurs when blood is diverted outside
   the body to a heart-lung machine)

6. extravasation ......... escape of blood from the blood vessel
   (eks-trav-a-SĀ-shun) into the tissue

7. heart murmur ........ a short duration humming sound of car-
   (MER-mer) diac or vascular origin

8. hypertension ......... blood pressure that is above normal
   (*hī*-per-TEN-shun)

9. hypotension ......... blood pressure that is below normal
   (*hī*-pō-TEN-shun)

10. lumen............... space within a tubular part or organ,
    (LŪ-men) such as the space within a blood vessel

11. occlude.............. to close tightly
    (o-KLŪD)

12. percussion .......... tapping of a body surface with the fin-
    (per-KUSH-un) gers to determine the density of the part
    beneath (Figure 9-18)

13. peripheral vascular .... referring to the blood vessels outside the
    (per-IF-er-al) (VAS-kū-lar) heart and the lymphatic vessels

14. systole.............. phase in the cardiac cycle in which the
    (SIS-tō-lē) ventricles contract

15. vasoconstrictor........ agent or nerve that narrows the lumen
    (vas-ō-kon-STRIK-tor) of blood vessels

16. vasodilator .......... agent or nerve that enlarges the lumen
    (vas-ō-dī-LĀ-tor) of blood vessels

17. venipuncture ........ puncture of a vein to remove blood, in-
    (VEN-i-*punk*-chūr) still a medication, or start an intravenous
    infusion

## BLOOD AND LYMPHATIC SYSTEM

1. anticoagulant.......... agent that slows down the clotting pro-
   (*an*-tē-kō-AG-ū-lant) cess

2. dyscrasia.............. abnormal or pathological condition of
   (dis-KRĀ-zhē-a) the blood

3. hemorrhage .......... rapid flow of blood
   (HEM-or-ij)

4. manometer............ instrument used to measure the pressure
   (ma-NOM-e-ter) of fluids

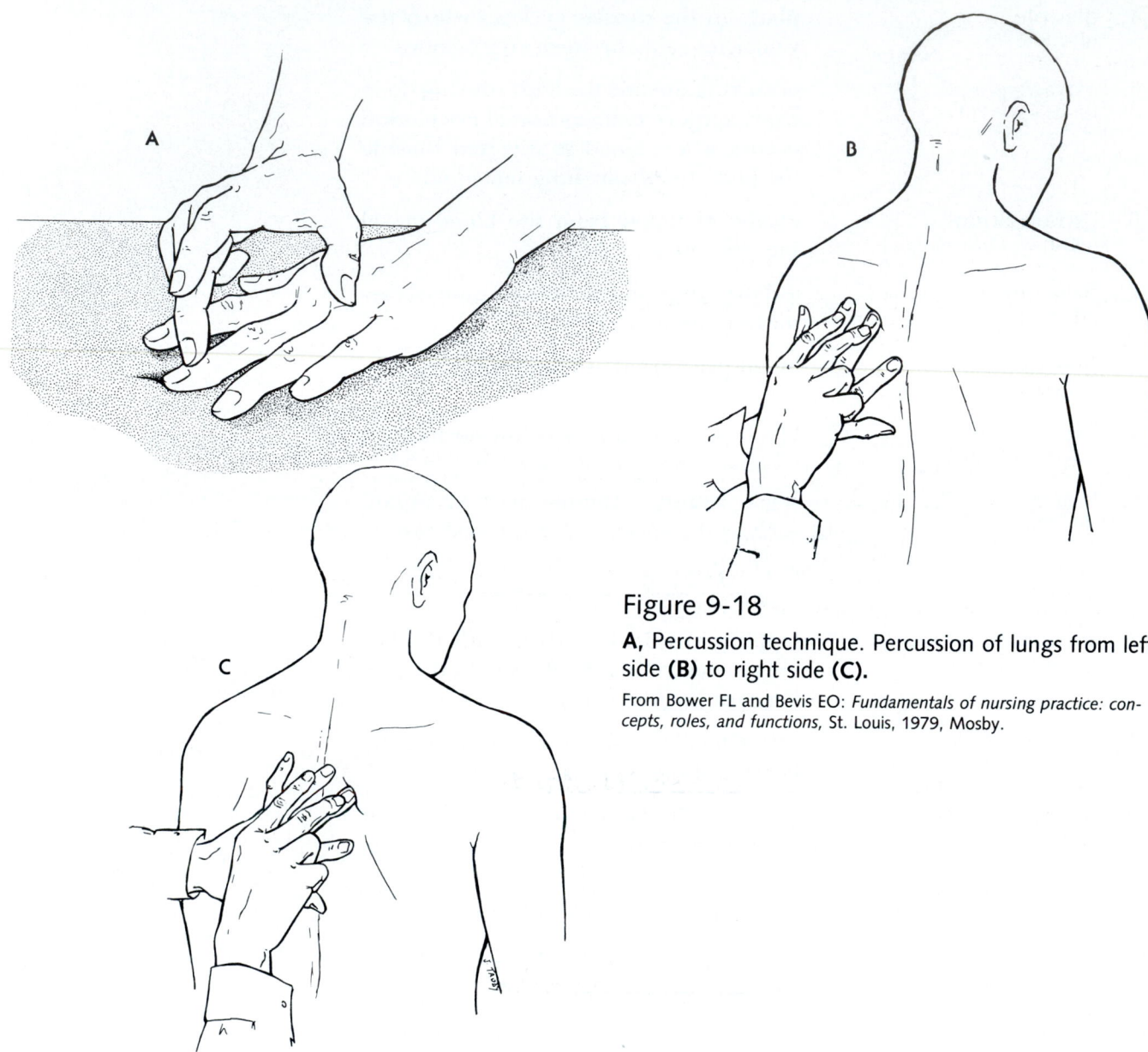

A

B

C

**Figure 9-18**

**A,** Percussion technique. Percussion of lungs from left side **(B)** to right side **(C).**

From Bower FL and Bevis EO: *Fundamentals of nursing practice: concepts, roles, and functions,* St. Louis, 1979, Mosby.

5.  plasma . . . . . . . . . . . . . .     liquid portion of the blood in which the
    (PLAZ-ma)                             elements or cells are suspended, and
                                          which also contains some of the clotting
                                          factors

6.  serum . . . . . . . . . . . . . .     liquid portion of the blood without the
    (SĒR-um)                              clotting factors

Practice saying each of these terms aloud. To assist you in pronunciation, obtain the audiotape designed for use with this text. Learn the definitions and spellings of the other additional terms by completing the following exercises.

## EXERCISE 32

Write the term for each of the following definitions.

1. agent that narrows the lumen of a blood vessel

_vasoconstrictor_

2. space within a tube-like structure

_lumen_

3. emergency procedure consisting of artificial ventilation and external cardiac massage

_cardiopulmonary resuscitation_

4. phase in the cardiac cycle in which the ventricles relax

_diastole_

5. pressure exerted by blood against artery walls

_blood pressure_

6. blood pressure that is below normal

_hypotension_

7. escape of blood from the blood vessel into the tissue

_extravasation_

8. puncture of a vein to remove blood

_venipuncture_

9. phase in the cardiac cycle in which the ventricles contract

_systole_

10. agent that enlarges the lumen of a blood vessel

_vasodilator_

11. blood pressure that is above normal

_hypertension_

12. referring to the blood vessels outside the heart and the lymphatic vessels

_peripheral vascular_

13. to close tightly

_occlude_

14. tapping of a body surface with the fingers to determine the density of the part beneath

_percussion_

15. hearing of sounds within the body through a stethoscope

_auscultation_

16. liquid portion of the blood that contains clotting factors

_plasma_

17. instrument used to measure the pressure of fluids

_manometer_

18. rapid flow of blood

_hemorrhage_

19. agent that slows down the clotting process

_anticoagulant_

20. liquid portion of the blood without the clotting factors

_serum_

21. pathological condition of the blood

_dyscrasia_

22. A humming sound of cardiac or vascular origin is a

_heart murmur_

23. Occurring outside the body

_extracorporeal_

# EXERCISE 33

Write the definitions of the following other additional terms.

1. lumen _____

2. extravasation _____

3. blood pressure _____

4. venipuncture _____

5. peripheral vascular _____

6. vasodilator _____

7. hypertension _____

8. cardiopulmonary resuscitation _____

9. systole _____

10. hypotension _____

11. vasoconstrictor _____

12. diastole _____

13. auscultation _____

14. occlude _____

15. percussion _____

16. serum _____

17. dyscrasia _____

18. manometer _____

19. plasma _____

20. hemorrhage _____

21. anticoagulant _____

22. extracorporeal _____

23. heart murmur _____

## EXERCISE 34

Spell each of the other additional terms. Have someone dictate the terms on pp. 346 to 348 to you or say the words into a tape recorder; then spell the words from your recording as often as necessary. Study any you have spelled incorrectly.

1. _____    10. _____
2. _____    11. _____
3. _____    12. _____
4. _____    13. _____
5. _____    14. _____
6. _____    15. _____
7. _____    16. _____
8. _____    17. _____
9. _____    18. _____

19. _____     22. _____

20. _____     23. _____

21. _____

Place a check mark (√) in the box to indicate that you have completed Objective 9.

☐ **DEFINE, PRONOUNCE, AND SPELL THE OTHER ADDITIONAL TERMS RELATED TO THE CARDIOVASCULAR AND LYMPHATIC SYSTEMS.**

---

**Case History:** This is the third hospitalization for this 76-year-old widowed Filipino female who was admitted for recurrent angina.

**History of Present Illness:** The patient has a long history of stable angina pectoris and had a positive treadmill test in 1988. A thallium treadmill test in 1991 showed reversible apical ischemia. In May of 1992 she underwent cataract surgery. She developed severe chest pain postoperatively. The EKG at that time showed ischemic ST changes in the anterior leads. A subsequent coronary angiography revealed a 90% focal left anterior descending stenosis. The patient then underwent angioplasty of this lesion. The 90% stenosis was dilated to a 20% stenosis. The patient had an uncomplicated course and was discharged home.

Over the last 10 days the patient has had at least five episodes of chest pain, all relieved by rest or a single nitroglycerin tablet. She had an episode yesterday while gardening, which lasted almost 20 minutes before subsiding after a second nitroglycerin. She came to her cardiologist's office today. An electrocardiogram was done which showed marked anterior T wave inversion in the anterior leads and she was immediately sent to this hospital for an evaluation.

Atherogenic risk factors include hypercholesterolemia for which she is now taking lovastatin. She is also hypertensive and smokes one pack per day. She is not diabetic. Current medications are lovastatin 20 mg daily, enalapril 20 mg bid, nifedipine 10 mg tid, nitroglycerin prn.

**Recommendations:** Patient is being admitted on an urgent basis for emergency cardiac catheterization and redilatation if necessary. Serial EKGs and enzymes will be obtained to rule out a myocardial infarction.

---

## EXERCISE 35

To test your understanding of the terms introduced in this chapter, circle the words that correctly complete the sentences. The italicized words refer to the correct answer.

1. *Yellowish, fatty plaque within the arteries* is (arteriosclerosis, atherosclerosis, aortosclerosis).
2. *Enlargement of the spleen* is (splenatrophy, spleniasis, splenomegaly).
3. *Inflammation of the middle muscular layer of the heart* is (endocarditis, myocarditis, pericarditis).
4. Another name for a *heart attack* is (myocardial infarction, coronary fibrillation, angina pectoris).
5. The *surgical excision of a thickened artery interior* is an (arteriorrhaphy, angioplasty, endarterectomy).
6. *Varicose veins in the rectal area* are (plasma, thrombi, hemorrhoids).

7. A *graphic record of heart sounds* is called a(n) (electrocardiogram, pho-nocardiogram, vectorcardiogram).
8. *Reduction of body temperature to a level below normal* results in a condi-tion called (hypothermia, hypertension, hyperthermia).
9. (Impedance plethysmography, cardiac scan, aortogram) is used *to de-termine if the patient had a blood clot in her femoral vein.*
10. *A humming sound* or (hemorrhage, murmur, auscultation) *originating in the heart* was the result of many episodes of rheumatic fever, *an in-flammatory disease occurring in children.*
11. The doctor used an (echocardiograph, electrocardiogram, angio-scope) *to visualize the blood vessel* and guide the laser beam to open blocked arteries; this procedure is called (echocardiography, angios-copy).

## EXERCISE 36

Unscramble the following mixed-up terms. The word(s) on the left indi-cate the word root in each of the following.

1. spleen

    / / / l / / / / c / / / / /
    c o m t e l e n v p s

2. vein

    / / / / / / / t / / / /
    b e t h o y p l m o

3. heart

    / / / o / / / / / i / / / /
    t i c y o m i r d a s

4. thymus

    / / / / / / / /
    h o m m a t y

5. blood vessel

    / / / / i / / / t / / / / / / /
    g e s i n o s i s t a n o

6. blood

    / / / / / / l / / / /
    t a e g h o o m y l

## EXERCISE 37

The following words did not appear in this chapter but are composed of word parts studied in this or the previous chapters. Find their definitions by translating the word parts literally.

1. **cytoscopy** (si-TOS-kō-pē) _____

2. **dysphonia** (dis-FŌ-nē-a) _____

3. **electrotome** (ē-LEK-trō-tōm) _____

4. **lipemia** (li-PĒ-mē-a) _____

5. **nephropyosis** (*nef*-rō-pī-Ō-sis) _____

6. **oligomenorrhea** (*ol*-i-gō-*men*-ō-RĒ-a) _____

7. **oophoropexy** (ō-OF-ō-rō-pek-sē) _____

8. **pleurodynia** (*plŭr*-ō-DĪN-nē-a) _____

9. **pyelectasis** (pī-e-LEK-ta-sis) _____

10. **subungual** (sub-UNG-gwal) _____

## COMBINING FORMS CROSSWORD PUZZLE

**Across Clues**
1. heart
7. ventricle
15. clot
16. heart (refers to blood vessels)
20. blockage, deficiency
21. spleen
22. aorta

**Down Clues**
2. vessel
3. valve
4. artery
5. yellowish, fatty plaque
6. chest
8. electricity, electrical activity
10. plasma
12. pulse
17. valve
18. atrium
19. sound

# Summary

Can you build, analyze, define, spell, and pronounce the following terms *built from word parts?*   yes □   no □

## DIAGNOSTIC

**Heart and Blood Vessels**

angiocarditis
(*an*-jē-ō-kar-DĪ-tis)

angioma
(an-jē-Ō-ma)

angiospasm
(AN-jē-ō-spazm)

angiostenosis
(an-jē-o-ste-NŌ-sis)

aortic stenosis
(ā-ŌR-tik) (ste-NŌ-sis)

arteriorrhexis
(ar-*tē*-rē-ō-REK-sis)

arteriosclerosis
(ar-*tē*-rē-ō-skle-RŌ-sis)

atherosclerosis
(*ath*-er-ō-skle-RŌ-sis)

atrioventricular defect
(ā-trē-ō-ven-TRIK-ū-lar)

bacterial endocarditis
(bak-TE-rē-al)
(en-dō-kar-DĪ-tis)

bradycardia
(brād-ē-KAR-dē-a)

cardiodynia
(*kar*-dē-ō-DĪN-ē-a)

cardiomegaly
(*kar*-dē-ō-MEG-a-lē)

cardiomyopathy
(kar-dē-ō-mī-OP-a-thē)

cardiovalvulitis
(kar-dē-ō-val-vū-LĪ-tis)

coronary ischemia
(KŌR-ō-nā-rē) (is-KĒ-mē-a)

coronary thrombosis
(KŌR-ō-nā-rē)
(throm-BŌ-sis)

endocarditis
(*en*-dō-kar-DĪ-tis)

## SURGICAL

angioplasty
(AN-jē-ō-plas-tē)

angiorrhaphy
(an-jē-ŌR-a-fē)

endarterectomy
(*end*-ar-ter-EK-tō-mē)

pericardiostomy
(*par*-i-kar-dē-OS-tō-mē)

phlebectomy
(fle-BEK-tō-mē)

phlebotomy
(fle-BOT-ō-mē)

splenectomy
(sple-NEK-tō-mē)

splenopexy
(SPLE-nō-peks-ē)

thymectomy
(thī-MEK-tō-mē)

## PROCEDURAL

**Heart and Blood Vessels**

angiography
(an-jē-OG-ra-fē)

angioscope
(AN-jē-ō-skōp)

angioscopy
(an-jē-OS-kō-pē)

aortogram
(ā-ŌR-tō-gram)

arteriogram
(ar-TE-rē-ō-gram)

echocardiogram
(ek-ō-KAR-dē-ō-gram)

electrocardiogram
(e-*lek*-trō-KAR-dē-ō-gram)

electrocardiograph
(e-*lek*-trō-KAR-dē-ō-graf)

electrocardiography
(e-*lek*-trō-kar-dē-OG-ra-fē)

phlebography
(fle-BOG-ra-fē)

phonocardiogram
(*fō*-nō-KAR-dē-ō-gram)

sphygmocardiograph
(*sfig*-mō-KAR-dē-ō-graf)

stethoscope
(STETH-ō-skōp)

venogram
(VE-nō-gram)

**Blood and Lymphatic System**

erythrocyte count
(e-RITH-rō-sīt)

hematocrit
(he-MAT-ō-krit)

leukocyte count
(LŪ-kō-sīt)

## ADDITIONAL

cardiac
(KAR-dē-ak)

cardiogenic
(kar-dē-ō-JEN-ik)

cardiologist
(*kar*-dē-OL-ō-jist)

cardiology
(*kar*-dē-OL-ō-jē)

hematologist
(*hē*-ma-TOL-ō-jist)

hematology
(*hē*-ma-TOL-ō-jē)

hematopoiesis
(*hē*-ma-to-poy-Ē-sis)

hemolysis
(hē-MOL-i-sis)

hemostasis
(*hē*-mō-STĀ-sis)

hypothermia
(*hī*-pō-THER-mē-a)

plasmapheresis
(plaz-ma-fe-RĒ-sis)

tachypnea
(tak-ip-NĒ-a)

**DIAGNOSTIC—cont'd**

myocarditis
(mī-ō-kar-DĪ-tis)

pericarditis
(pār-i-kar-DĪ-tis)

polyarteritis
(pol-ē-ar-te-RĪ-tis)

tachycardia
(tak-i-KAR-dē-a)

**Blood and Lymphatic System**

hematocytopenia
(hem-a-tō-sī-tō-PĒ-nē-a)

hematoma
(hem-a-TŌ-ma)

lymphadenitis
(limf-ad-en-Ī-tis)

lymphadenopathy
(lim-fad-e-NOP-a-thě)

lymphoma
(limf-Ō-ma)

splenomegaly
(sple-nō-MEG-a-lē)

thymoma
(thī-MŌ-ma)

**PROCEDURAL—cont'd**

lymphadenography
(lim-fad-e-NOG-ra-fē)

lymphangiogram
(lim-FAN-jē-ō-gram)

lymphangiography
(lim-fan-jē-OG-ra-fē)

# Summary

Can you define, pronounce, and spell the following terms *not built from word parts?*   yes ☐   no ☐

| **DIAGNOSTIC** | **SURGICAL** | **PROCEDURAL** | **ADDITIONAL** |
|---|---|---|---|
| anemia<br>(a-Nē-mē-a) | aneurysmectomy<br>(an-ū-riz-MEK-tō-mē) | **Heart and Blood Vessels** | **Heart and Blood Vessels** |
| aneurysm<br>(AN-ū-rizm) | bone marrow transplant<br>cardiac pacemaker<br>coronary artery bypass<br>defibrillation<br>(dē-fib-ri-LĀ-shun) | cardiac catheterization<br>(KAR-dē-ak)<br>(kath-e-ter-ī-ZA-shun) | auscultation<br>(aws-kul-TĀ-shun) |
| angina pectoris<br>(an-JĪ-na) (PEK-to-ris) | | cardiac scan<br>Doppler flow studies<br>(DOP-ler) | blood pressure<br>cardiopulmonary resuscitation<br>(kar-dē-ō-PUL-mō-nār-ē)<br>(rē-sus-i-TĀ-shun) |
| arrhythmia<br>(a-RITH-mē-a) | embolectomy<br>(em-bō-LEK-tō-mē) | impedance plethysmography<br>(im-PĒD-dans)<br>(pleth-iz-MOG-ra-fē) | diastole<br>(dī-AS-tō-lē) |
| cardiac arrest<br>(KAR-dē-ak) (a-REST) | femoropopliteal bypass<br>(FEM-or-ō-pop-LIT-ē-al) | | extracorporeal<br>(ek-stra-kōr-pō-rē-al) |
| cardiac tamponade<br>(KAR-dē-ak) (tam-pō-NĀD) | | sphygmomanometer<br>(sfig-mō-ma-NOM-e-ter) | |

## DIAGNOSTIC—cont'd

coarctation of the aorta
(kō-ark-TĀ-shun)

congenital heart disease
(kon-JEN-i-tal)

congestive heart failure
coronary occlusion
(KŌR-ō-nā-rē)     (o-KLŪ-zhun)

deep vein thrombosis
embolus, *pl.* emboli
(EM-bō-lus) EM-bō-lī)

fibrillation
(fi-bril-Ā-shun)

hemophilia
(hē-mō-FIL-ē-a)

hemorrhoid
(HEM-ō-royd)

Hodgkin's disease
(HOJ-kins)

hypertensive heart disease
(hī-per-TEN-siv)

intermittent claudication
(klaw-di-KĀ-shun)

leukemia
(lū-KĒ-mē-a)

mitral valve stenosis
(MĪ-tral)

myocardial infarction
(mī-ō-KAR-dē-al) (in-FARK-shun)

rheumatic fever
(rū-MAT-ic)

rheumatic heart disease
sickle cell anemia
(SIK-el) (sel)

thromboangiitis obliterans
(*throm*-bō-*an*-jē-Ī-tis) (ob-LIT-er-anz)

varicose veins
(VĀR-i-kōs)

## SURGICAL—cont'd

hemorrhoidectomy
(hem-ō-royd-EK-tō-mē)

intracoronary
thrombolytic therapy
(in-tra-KŌR-ō-na-rē)
(throm-bol-LI-tik)

laser angioplasty
(LĀ-zer) (AN-jē-ō-plas-tē)

mitral commissurotomy
(mī-tral) (kom-i-shūr-OT-ō-mē)

percutaneous
transluminal coronary
angioplasty
(*per*-kū-TĀ-nē-us)
(trans-LŪM-in-al)
(KOR-ō-na-rē)
(AN-jē-ō-*plas*-tē)

vein ligation and
stripping
(lī-GĀ-shun)

## PROCEDURAL—cont'd

treadmill stress test

### Blood and Lymphatic System
complete blood count
coagulation time
(kō-ag-ū-LĀ-shun)

hemoglobin
(HĒ-mo-glō-bin)

prothrombin time
(prō-THROM-bin)

bone marrow biopsy

## ADDITIONAL—cont'd

extravasation
(eks-trav-a-SĀ-shun)

heart murmur
(MER-mer)

hypertension
(hī-per-TEN-shun)

hypotension
(hī-pō-TEN-shun)

lumen
(LŪ-men)

occlude
(o-KLŪD)

percussion
(per-KUSH-un)

peripheral vascular
(per-IF-er-al) (VAS-kū-lar)

systole
(SIS-tō-lē)

vasoconstrictor
(vas-ō-kon-STRIK-tor)

vasodilator
(vas-ō-dī-LĀ-tor)

venipuncture
(VEN-i-*punk*-chūr)

### Blood and Lymphatic System

anticoagulant
(*an*-tē-kō-AG-ū-lant)

dyscrasia
(dis-KRĀ-zhē-a)

hemorrhage
(HEM-or-ij)

manometer
(ma-NOM-e-ter)

plasma
(PLAZ-ma)

serum
(SĒR-um)

# Answers

## Exercise 1
1. g    4. m    7. i    10. h    12. a
2. j    5. b    8. f    11. d    13. n
3. e    6. k    9. l

## Exercise 2
1. f    5. k    9. q    13. i
2. p    6. m    10. d    14. e
3. h    7. c    11. o    15. j
4. b    8. l    12. a    16. g

## Exercise 3
**Figure 9-1**
blood vessel: angi/o    Artery: arteri/o
Valve: valv/o, valvul/o    Atrium: atri/o
Heart: cardi/o, coron/o    Ventricle: ventricul/o
Aorta: aort/o

## Exercise 4
1. heart    6. aorta    11. ventricle
2. atrium    7. valve    12. artery
3. plasma    8. spleen    13. valve
4. vessel    9. thymus gland    14. lymph
5. heart    10. vein

## Exercise 5
1. arteri/o    6. lymph/o    11. plasm/o
2. phleb/o    7. aort/o    12. thym/o
3. a. cardi/o    8. angi/o
   b. coron/o    9. a. valv/o
4. atri/o       b. valvul/o
5. ventricul/o    10. splen/o

## Exercise 6
1. sound    6. pulse
2. chest    7. yellowish, fatty plaque
3. clot    8. electricity, electrical
4. deficiency, blockage    activity
5. heat    9. bacteria

## Exercise 7
1. thromb/o    4. isch/o    7. bacteri/o
2. steth/o    5. ather/o    8. electr/o
3. ech/o    6. therm/o    9. sphygm/o

## Exercise 8
1. fast, rapid    2. slow

## Exercise 9
1. tachy-    2. brady-

## Exercise 10
1. to separate    5. pain
2. instrument used to    6. removal
   record    7. formation
3. abnormal reduction in    8. pertaining to
   numbers
4. hardening

## Exercise 11
1. -poiesis    4. -graph    7. -crit
2. -ac    5. -penia    8. -apheresis
3. -sclerosis    6. -odynia

## Exercise 12
1. endo/card/itis — inflammation of the inner layer of the heart
2. brady/card/ia — abnormal state of slow heart rate
3. cardi/o/megaly — enlargement of the heart
4. arteri/o/sclerosis — hardening of the arteries
5. cardi/o/valvul/itis — inflammation of the valves of the heart
6. angi/o/card/itis — inflammation of the heart and blood vessels
7. arteri/orrhexis — rupture of an artery
8. tachy/card/ia — abnormally rapid heart rate
9. angi/o/stenosis — narrowing of blood vessels
10. atri/o/ventricul/ar defect — defect pertaining to the atrium and ventricles
11. coron/ary isch/emia — deficient supply of blood to the heart's blood vessels
12. peri/card/itis — inflammation of outer layer of heart

WR     S
13. cardi/odynia                     pain in the heart

WR      CV
14. aort/ ic stenosis                narrowing of the aorta

WR     S     WR     S
15. coron/ary thromb/osis            abnormal condition of a
                                     clot in a blood vessel of
                                     the heart

WR   CV    S
16. ather/ o /sclerosis              hardening of the arteries.
    CF

WR CV WR  S
17. my/ o /card/itis                 inflammation of the mus-
    CF                               cle of the heart

WR    S
18. angi/oma                         tumor composed of blood
                                     vessels

WR    S
19. thym/oma                         tumor of the thymus
                                     gland

WR   CV WR CV   S
20. hemat/ o /cyt/ o /penia          deficiency of blood cells
         CF      CF

WR    S
21. lymph/oma                        tumor of lymphatic tissue

WR    WR   S
22. lymph/aden/itis                  inflammation of lymph
                                     glands (nodes)

WR  CV    S
23. splen/ o /megaly                 enlargement of the
        CF                           spleen

WR    S
24. hemat/oma                        tumor of blood (swelling
                                     caused by an accumula-
                                     tion of clotted blood in
                                     the tissues)

P    WR    S
25. poly/arter/itis                  inflammation of many
                                     (sites) in the arteries

WR   CV WR CV    S
26. cardi/ o /my/ o /pathy           disease of the heart mus-
        CF      CF                   cles

WR   S  P    WR   S
27. bacteri/al endo/card/itis        inflammation within the
                                     heart caused by bacte-
                                     ria

WR   CV    S
28. angi/ o /spasm                   spasm of the blood ves-
        CF                           sels

WR    WR  CV   S
29. lymph/aden/ o /pathy             disease of the lymph
             CF                      glands

## Exercise 13

| | |
|---|---|
| 1. arteri/orrhexis | 17. peri/card/itis |
| 2. cardi/o/megaly | 18. atri/o/ventricul/ar de- |
| 3. coron/ary isch/emia | fect |
| 4. angi/o/card/itis | 19. hemat/o/cyt/o/penia |
| 5. endo/card/itis | 20. lymph/oma |
| 6. brady/card/ia | 21. thym/oma |
| 7. arteri/o/sclerosis | 22. splen/o/megaly |
| 8. coron/ary thromb/osis | 23. hemat/oma |
| 9. cardi/odynia | 24. lymph/aden/itis |
| 10. my/o/card/itis | 25. cardi/o/my/o/pathy |
| 11. angi/o/stenosis | 26. poly/arter/itis |
| 12. tachy/card/ia | 27. angi/o/spasm |
| 13. ather/o/sclerosis | 28. bacteri/al endo/card/ |
| 14. angi/oma | itis |
| 15. cardi/o/valvul/itis | 29. lymph/aden/o/pathy |
| 16. aort/ic stenosis | |

## Exercise 14

Spelling exercise; *see* pp. 313-315.

## Exercise 15

| | |
|---|---|
| 1. coarctation | 16. thromboangiitis oblit- |
| 2. embolus | erans (Buerger's dis- |
| 3. cardiac arrest | ease) |
| 4. congenital | 17. hemophilia |
| 5. varicose veins | 18. leukemia |
| 6. coronary occlusion | 19. anemia |
| 7. aneurysm | 20. sickle cell anemia |
| 8. Hodgkin's | 21. intermittent claudica- |
| 9. hemorrhoids | tion |
| 10. angina pectoris | 22. cardiac tamponade |
| 11. myocardial infarction | 23. mitral valve stenosis |
| 12. fibrillation | and rheumatic heart |
| 13. arrhythmia | disease |
| 14. hypertensive | 24. deep vein thrombosis |
| 15. congestive heart dis- | 25. rheumatic fever |
| ease | |

## Exercise 16A

| | | | | | |
|---|---|---|---|---|---|
| 1. d | 3. f | 5. a | 7. i | 9. g | 11. h |
| 2. c | 4. e | 6. j | 8. k | 10. b | 12. l |

## Exercise 16B

| | | | | | | |
|---|---|---|---|---|---|---|
| 1. i | 3. a | 5. j | 7. d | 9. l | 11. c | 13. m |
| 2. e | 4. h | 6. b | 8. k | 10. g | 12. f | |

## Exercise 17

Spelling exercise; *see* text, p. 325.

## Exercise 18

      P   WR    S
1. peri/cardi/ostomy      creation of an artificial opening in the outer (double) layer of the heart

      WR    S
2. thym/ectomy      excision of the thymus gland

      WR  CV   S
3. angi/ o /plasty      surgical repair of a blood vessel
         CF

      WR  CV  S
4. splen/ o /pexy      surgical fixation of the spleen
         CF

      WR    S
5. angi/orrhaphy      suturing of a blood vessel

      P   WR    S
6. end/arter/ectomy      excision of the thickened interior of an artery

      WR    S
7. phleb/otomy      incision into a vein

      WR    S
8. splen/ectomy      excision of the spleen

      WR    S
9. phleb/ectomy      excision of a vein

## Exercise 19

1. end/arter/ectomy
2. splen/o/pexy
3. angi/orrhaphy
4. phleb/otomy
5. thym/ectomy
6. peri/cardi/ostomy
7. angi/o/plasty
8. splen/ectomy
9. phleb/ectomy

## Exercise 20

1. hemorrhoidectomy
2. vein ligation and stripping
3. percutaneous transluminal coronary angioplasty
4. pacemaker
5. commissurotomy
6. coronary artery bypass graft
7. aneurysmectomy
8. femoropopliteal bypass
9. laser angioplasty
10. intracoronary thrombolytic
11. defibrillation
12. bone marrow transplant
13. embolectomy

## Exercise 21

1. h   3. k   5. d   7. a   9. c   11. i   13. j
2. f   4. l   6. m   8. b   10. e   12. g

## Exercise 22

Spelling exercise; *see* text, pp. 328 to 331.

## Exercise 23

    WR CV WR CV  S
1. electr/ o /cardi/ o /graph      instrument used to record the electrical activity of the heart
       CF     CF

    WR  CV WR CV  S
2. sphygm/ o /cardi/ o /graph      instrument used to measure pulse waves and heart beat
        CF     CF

    WR CV  S
3. ven/ o /gram      x-ray film of the veins (taken after an injection of contrast medium)
      CF

    WR CV   S
4. angi/ o /graphy      process of x-ray filming a blood vessel
      CF

    WR CV WR CV  S
5. ech/ o /cardi/ o /gram      record made of the structure and motion of the heart using sound waves
      CF     CF

    WR CV   S
6. steth/ o /scope      instrument used to examine sounds in the chest
      CF

    WR CV  S
7. aort/ o /gram      x-ray film of the aorta (taken after an injection of contrast medium)
      CF

    WR CV WR CV  S
8. electr/ o /cardi/ o /gram      record of the electrical activity of the heart
      CF     CF

    WR CV WR CV  S
9. phon/ o /cardi/ o /gram      graphic record of heart sounds
      CF     CF

     WR CV  S
10. arteri/ o /gram      x-ray film of an artery (after an injection of contrast medium)
       CF

```
       WR CV WR CV  S
11. electr/ o /cardi/ o /graphy
         CF        CF
```
process of recording the electrical activity of the heart

```
     WR  CV S
12. erythr/ o /cyte count
         CF
```
red blood cell count (number of red blood cells per cubic millimeter of blood)

```
     WR   WR CV  S
13. lymph/angi/ o /gram
             CF
```
x-ray record of lymphatic vessels

```
     WR  CV S
14. hemat/ o /crit
         CF
```
separated blood (volume percentage of erythrocytes in whole blood)

```
     WR    WR CV   S
15. lymph/aden/ o /graphy
               CF
```
process of recording an x-ray film of the lymph nodes and glands after an injection of contrast medium

```
     WR CV S
16. leuk/ o /cyte count
        CF
```
white blood cell count (number of white blood cells per cubic millimeter of blood)

```
     WR   WR CV    S
17. lymph/angi/ o /graphy
              CF
```
process of recording an x-ray film of the lymphatic vessels (after an injection of the contrast medium)

```
     WR CV  S
18. angi/ o /scopy
        CF
```
visual examination of a blood vessel

```
     WR CV  S
19. phleb/ o /graphy
         CF
```
process of x-ray filming a vein

```
     WR CV  S
20. angi/ o /scope
        CF
```
instrument used for visual examination of a blood vessel

## Exercise 24

1. electr/o/cardi/o/graph
2. steth/o/scope
3. arteri/o/gram
4. ven/o/gram
5. angi/o/graphy
6. electr/o/cardi/o/gram
7. ech/o/cardi/o/gram
8. phon/o/cardi/o/gram
9. sphygm/o/cardi/o/graph
10. aort/o/gram
11. electr/o/cardi/o/graphy
12. hemat/o/crit
13. lymph/angi/o/gram
14. leuk/o/cyte
15. lymph/aden/o/graphy
16. erythr/o/cyte
17. lymph/angi/o/graphy
18. angi/o/scope
19. angi/o/graphy
20. phleb/o/scope

## Exercise 25
Spelling exercise; *see* text, pp. 333-335.

## Exercise 26
1. sphygmomanometer
2. coagulation time
3. treadmill stress
4. complete blood count
5. Doppler flow studies
6. cardiac scan
7. bone marrow biopsy
8. prothrombin time
9. cardiac catheterization
10. hemoglobin
11. impedance plethysmography

## Exercise 27
1. d  3. h  5. g  7. c  9. k  11. f
2. e  4. i  6. j  8. a  10. b

## Exercise 28
Spelling exercise; *see* text, pp. 333 to 335.

## Exercise 29

```
      P    WR  S
1. hypo/therm/ia
```
condition of body temperature that is below normal

```
     WR  CV  S
2. hemat/ o /poiesis
         CF
```
formation of red blood cells

```
    WR    S
3. cardi/ology
```
study of the heart

```
    WR     S
4. cardi/ologist
```
physician who studies and treats diseases of the heart

```
    WR CV  S
5. hem/ o /lysis
       CF
```
destruction of (red) blood cells

```
     WR     S
6. hemat/ologist
```
physician who studies and treats diseases of the blood

```
    WR  S
7. cardi/ac
```
pertaining to the heart

```
     WR    S
8. hemat/ology
```
study of the blood

```
    WR      S
9. plasm/apheresis
```
removal of plasma from withdrawn blood

```
    WR CV  S
10. hem/ o /stasis
       CF
```
stoppage of bleeding

11. $\underset{\text{CF}}{\underbrace{\overset{\text{WR}\ \text{CV}}{\text{cardi/ o}}\ /\overset{\text{S}}{\text{genic}}}}$     originating in the heart

12. $\overset{\text{P}}{\text{tachy}}/\overset{\text{S(WR)}}{\text{pnea}}$     rapid breathing

## Exercise 30

1. cardi/ology
2. hemat/o/poiesis
3. hypo/therm/ia
4. hem/o/lysis
5. plasm/apheresis
6. hemat/ologist
7. cardi/ac
8. cardi/ologist
9. hemat/ology
10. hem/o/stasis
11. tachy/pnea
12. cardi/o/genic

## Exercise 31

Spelling exercise; *see* p. ●●●

## Exercise 32

1. vasoconstrictor
2. lumen
3. cardiopulmonary resuscitation
4. diastole
5. blood pressure
6. hypotension
7. extravasation
8. venipuncture
9. systole
10. vasodilator
11. hypertension
12. peripheral vascular
13. occlude
14. percussion
15. auscultation
16. plasma
17. manometer
18. hemorrhage
19. anticoagulant
20. serum
21. dyscrasia
22. heart murmur
23. extracorporeal

## Exercise 33

1. space within a tubelike structure
2. escape of blood from the blood vessel into the tissues
3. pressure exerted by the blood against the vessel walls
4. puncture of a vein to remove blood, start an intravenous infusion, or instill a medication
5. referring to blood vessels outside the heart and lymphatic vessels
6. agent or nerve that enlarges the lumen of blood vessels
7. blood pressure that is above normal
8. emergency procedure consisting of artificial ventilation and external cardiac massage
9. phase in the cardiac cycle in which ventricles contract
10. blood pressure that is below normal
11. agent or nerve that narrows the lumen of blood vessels
12. cardiac cycle phase in which ventricles relax
13. hearing of sounds within the body through a stethoscope
14. to close tightly
15. tapping of a body surface with fingers to determine the density of parts beneath

16. liquid portion of the blood without clotting factors
17. abnormal or pathological condition of the blood
18. instrument used to measure the pressure of fluids
19. liquid portion of the blood in which the elements or cells are suspended and which contains the clotting factors
20. rapid flow of blood
21. agent that slows down the clotting process
22. occurring outside the body
23. humming sound of cardiac or vascular origin

## Exercise 34

Spelling exercise; *see* text, pp. 351 and 352.

## Exercise 35

1. atherosclerosis
2. splenomegaly
3. myocarditis
4. myocardial infarction
5. endarterectomy
6. hemorrhoids
7. phonocardiogram
8. hypothermia
9. impedance plethysmography
10. murmur
11. angioscope, angioscopy

## Exercise 36

1. splenectomy
2. phlebotomy
3. myocarditis
4. thymoma
5. angiostenosis
6. hematology

## Exercise 37

1. visual examination of a cell
2. difficulty in speaking
3. electrical cutting instrument
4. blood containing fat
5. abnormal condition of pus in the kidney
6. scanty menstrual discharge
7. surgical fixation of an ovary
8. pain in the pleura
9. dilatation of the renal pelvis
10. pertaining to under the nail

| C | A | R | D | I | O |   | A |   |   | V |   | A |
|   |   |   |   |   | N |   | G |   | V | A |   | R |
| A |   |   | S |   | G |   | A |   |   |   |   | T |
| T | V | E | N | T | R | I | C | U | L | O |   | E |
| H | P |   | L |   | E |   | O |   | V |   |   | R |
| E | L |   | E |   | T |   | S |   | U |   |   | I |
| R | A |   | C |   | H |   | P |   | L |   |   | I |
| O | S |   | T |   | O | T | H | R | O | M | B | O |
|   | M |   | R |   |   |   | Y |   |   |   |   |   |
| C | O | R | O | N | O |   | G |   | V |   |   | A |
|   |   |   |   | E |   | M |   | A |   |   | T |
|   |   | I | S | C | H | O |   | L |   |   | R |
|   |   |   |   | H |   |   |   | V |   |   | I |
| S | P | L | E | N | O |   | A | O | R | T | O |

# 10

# Digestive System

## Objectives

**Upon completion of this chapter you will be able to:**

1. Define the anatomical terms of the digestive system.

2. Write the definitions of the word parts included in this chapter.

3. Build, analyze, define, pronounce, and spell the diagnostic terms related to the digestive system.

4. Define, pronounce, and spell other diagnostic terms related to the digestive system.

5. Build, analyze, define, pronounce, and spell the surgical terms related to the digestive system.

6. Define, pronounce, and spell other surgical terms related to the digestive system.

7. Build, analyze, define, pronounce, and spell the diagnostic procedural terms related to the digestive system.

8. Define, pronounce, and spell other diagnostic procedural terms related to the digestive system.

9. Build, analyze, define, pronounce, and spell additional terms related to the digestive system.

10. Define, pronounce, and spell the other additional terms related to the digestive system.

## Objective 1    DEFINE THE ANATOMICAL TERMS OF THE DIGESTIVE SYSTEM.

## Anatomical Terms

The digestive tract, also known as the *alimentary canal* or the *gastrointestinal tract,* is made up of several digestive organs. The organs connect to form a continuous passageway from the mouth to the anus (Figure 10-1). With the help of accessory organs the digestive tract prepares ingested food for use by the body cells and eliminates the solid waste products from the body.

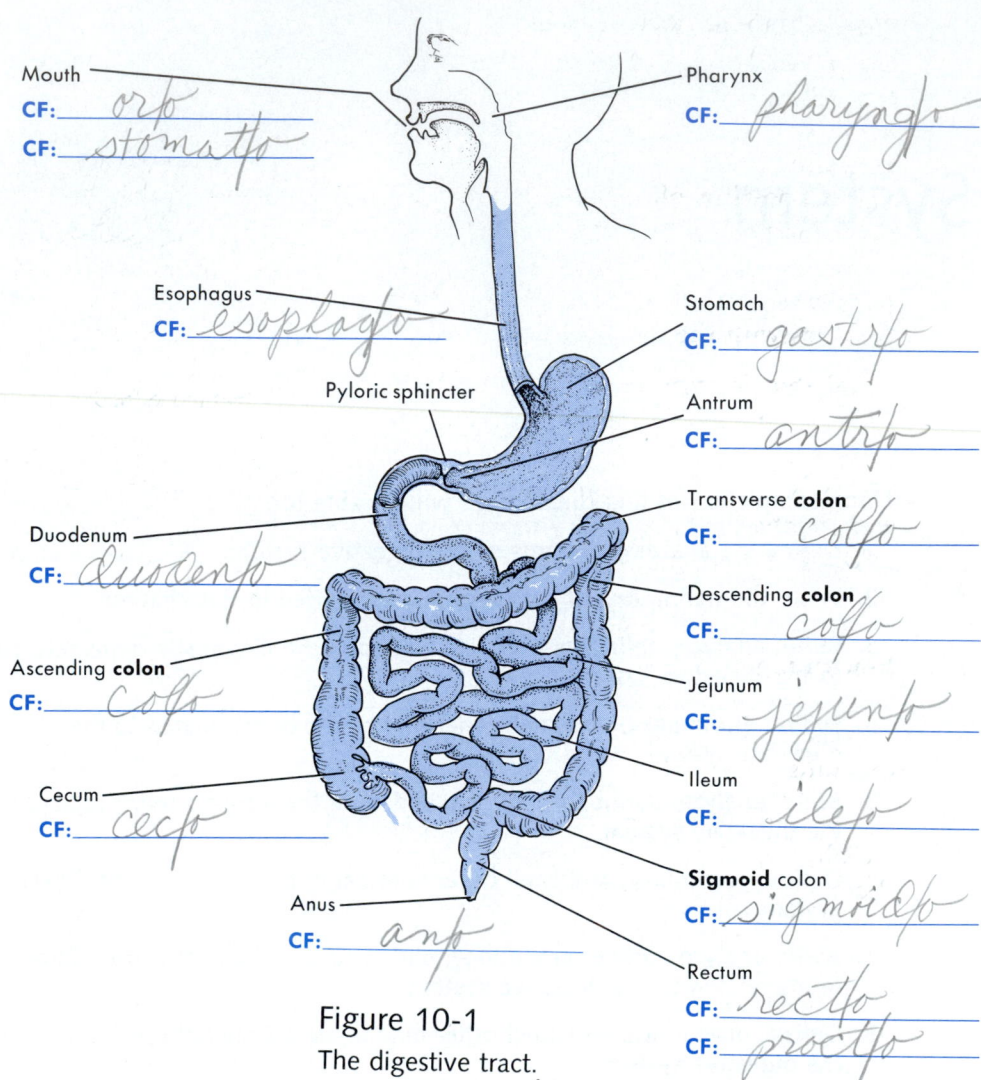

Mouth
CF: _orto_
CF: _stomato_

Pharynx
CF: _pharyngo_

Esophagus
CF: _esophago_

Pyloric sphincter

Stomach
CF: _gastro_

Antrum
CF: _antro_

Duodenum
CF: _duodeno_

Transverse **colon**
CF: _colo_

Descending **colon**
CF: _colo_

Ascending **colon**
CF: _colo_

Jejunum
CF: _jejuno_

Cecum
CF: _ceco_

Ileum
CF: _ileo_

Anus
CF: _ano_

**Sigmoid** colon
CF: _sigmoido_

Rectum
CF: _recto_
CF: _procto_

Figure 10-1
The digestive tract.

# ORGANS OF THE DIGESTIVE TRACT

1. mouth . . . . . . . . . . . . . . .  Opening through which food passes into the body
   a. palate . . . . . . . . . . . . .  Forms the roof of the mouth
   b. uvula . . . . . . . . . . . . .  Soft, V-shaped mass that hangs from the roof of the back of the mouth

2. pharynx or throat . . . . . .  Performs the swallowing action that passes food from the mouth to the esophagus

3. esophagus . . . . . . . . . . . .  Ten-inch (25 cm) tube that extends from the pharynx to the stomach

4. stomach . . . . . . . . . . . . .  Container for food
   a. antrum . . . . . . . . . . . .  Lower bulge of the stomach
   b. pyloric sphincter . . . .  Ring of muscles that guards the opening between the stomach and the duodenum

5. small intestine . . . . . . . . Twenty-foot (6 m) canal extending from the pyloric sphincter to the large intestine (Figure 10-1)

   a. duodenum . . . . . . . . First 10 to 12 inches (25 cm) of the small intestine

   b. jejunum . . . . . . . . . . Second portion of the small intestine, approximately 8 feet (2.4 m) long

   c. ileum . . . . . . . . . . . . Third portion of the small intestine, approximately 11 feet (3.3 m) long, which connects with the large intestine

6. large intestine . . . . . . . . Canal that is approximately 5 feet (1.5 m) long and which extends from the ileum to the anus

   a. cecum . . . . . . . . . . . First portion of the large intestine

   b. colon . . . . . . . . . . . . Next portion of the large intestine. The colon is divided into four parts: ascending colon, transverse colon, descending colon, and sigmoid colon (Figure 10-1)

   c. rectum . . . . . . . . . . . Remaining portion of the large intestine, approximately 8-10 inches (20 cm) long, extends from the sigmoid colon to the anus

7. anus . . . . . . . . . . . . . . . . Sphincter muscle (ringlike band of muscle fiber that keeps an opening tight) at the end of the digestive tract

**Duodenum** is derived from the Latin **duodeni,** meaning **twelve each,** a reference to its length. It was named in 240 BC by a Greek physician.

   **Jejunum** is derived from the Latin **jejunus,** meaning **empty;** it was so named because the early anatomists always found it empty.

   **Ileum** is derived from the Greek **eilein,** meaning **to roll,** a reference to the peristaltic waves that move food along the digestive tract. This term was first used in the early part of the seventeenth century.

## ACCESSORY ORGANS

1. salivary glands . . . . . . . . Produce saliva, which flows into the mouth (Figure 10-2)

2. liver . . . . . . . . . . . . . . . . Produces bile, which is necessary for the digestion of fats. The liver performs many other functions concerned with digestion

3. bile ducts . . . . . . . . . . . Passageways that carry bile: the hepatic duct is a passageway for bile from the liver, the cystic duct carries bile from the gallbladder. They join to form the common bile duct which conveys bile to the duodenum

4. gallbladder . . . . . . . . . . . Small saclike structure that stores bile

5. pancreas . . . . . . . . . . . . . Located behind the stomach. It produces pancreatic juice, which helps to digest all types of food

The pancreas has been described since 300 BC. It was so named because of its fleshy appearance. **Pancreas** derived from the Greek **pan,** meaning **all,** and **krea,** meaning **flesh.**

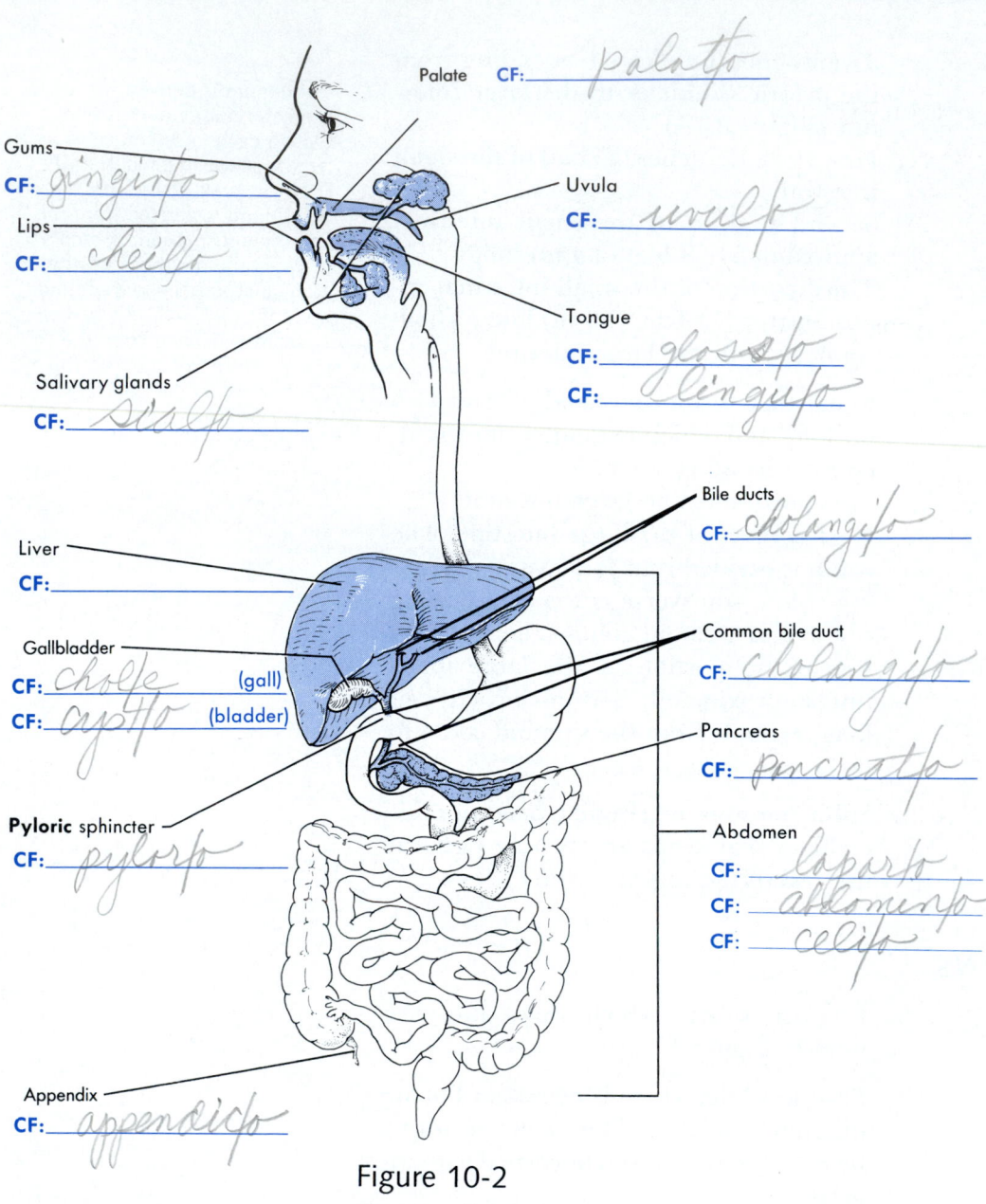

Palate    CF: _palato_

Gums
CF: _gingivo_

Lips
CF: _cheilo_

Uvula
CF: _uvulo_

Tongue
CF: _glosso_
CF: _linguo_

Salivary glands
CF: _sialo_

Bile ducts
CF: _cholangio_

Liver
CF:

Gallbladder
CF: _chole_    (gall)
CF: _cysto_    (bladder)

Common bile duct
CF: _cholangio_

Pancreas
CF: _pancreato_

**Pyloric** sphincter
CF: _pyloro_

Abdomen
CF: _laparo_
CF: _abdomino_
CF: _celio_

Appendix
CF: _appendico_

Figure 10-2
The digestive system.

## OTHER STRUCTURES

1.  peritoneum . . . . . . . . . . .    Lining of the abdominal and pelvic cavities

2.  appendix . . . . . . . . . . . .    Small pouch attached to the cecum, which has no known function

3.  abdomen . . . . . . . . . . . .    Portion of the body between the thorax and the pelvis

Learn the anatomical terms by completing the following exercises.

## EXERCISE 1

Fill in the blanks with the correct terms.

The digestive tract, also known as the (1) _alimentary_ _canal_ , and (2) _gastrointestinal tract_ , begins with the mouth, connects with the throat, or (3) _pharynx_ , and continues on to a 10-inch tube called the (4) _esophagus_ ; this connects with the (5) _stomach_ , the container for food.

The small intestine, the next portion of the digestive tract, is made up of three portions. They are called the (6) _duodenum_ , (7) _jejunum_ , and (8) _ileum_ . The small intestine connects with the first portion of the large intestine, the (9) _cecum_ , and then connects with the colon, which is divided into four parts called (10) _ascending colon_ , (11) _transverse colon_ , (12) _descending colon_ , and (13) _sigmoid colon_ . The (14) _rectum_ extends from the colon to the (15) _anus_ .

## EXERCISE 2

Match the definitions in the first column with the correct terms in the second column.

| | | |
|---|---|---|
| _l_ | 1. lower bulge of the stomach | a. salivary glands |
| _d_ | 2. hangs from the roof of the mouth | b. pancreas |
| _a_ | 3. produces saliva | c. peritoneum |
| _h_ | 4. produces bile | d. uvula |
| _f_ | 5. forms the roof of the mouth | e. gallbladder |
| _j_ | 6. guards the opening between the stomach and the duodenum | f. palate |
| | | g. abdomen |
| _b_ | 7. located behind the stomach | h. liver |
| _i_ | 8. small pouch, has no known function | i. appendix |
| _c_ | 9. lining of the abdominal and pelvic cavities | j. pyloric sphincter |
| | | k. cecum |
| | | l. antrum |

_____ 10. portion of the body
between the pelvis
and thorax

_____ 11. stores bile

Place a check mark (√) in the box to indicate that you have completed Objective 1.

☐ **DEFINE THE ANATOMICAL TERMS OF THE DIGESTIVE SYSTEM.**

# Objective 2   WRITE THE DEFINITIONS OF THE WORD PARTS INCLUDED IN THIS CHAPTER.

## Digestive Tract Word Parts

Study the word parts and their definitions listed as follows. Learning will
be made easier by completing the exercises that follow.

| COMBINING FORM | DEFINITION |
|---|---|
| 1. an/o | anus |
| 2. antr/o | antrum |
| 3. cec/o | cecum |
| 4. col/o | colon |
| 5. duoden/o | duodenum |
| 6. enter/o | intestines |
| 7. esophag/o (NOTE: *Esophag/o* was covered in Chapter 8.) | esophagus |
| 8. gastr/o | stomach |
| 9. ile/o | ileum |
| 10. jejun/o | jejunum |
| 11. proct/o rect/o | rectum |
| 12. sigmoid/o | sigmoid colon |
| 13. stomat/o or/o | mouth |

Learn the anatomical locations and definitions of the combining forms by
completing the following exercises.

### EXERCISE 3

Write the combining forms in the spaces marked **CF** on the diagram in
Figure 10-1, p. 364.

## EXERCISE 4

Write the definitions of the following combining forms.

1. proct/o _____ rectum _____
2. gastr/o _____ stomach _____
3. an/o _____ anus _____
4. cec/o _____ cecum _____
5. ile/o _____ ileum _____
6. stomat/o _____ mouth _____
7. duoden/o _____ duodenum _____
8. col/o _____ colon _____
9. or/o _____ mouth _____
10. enter/o _____ intestines _____
11. rect/o _____ rectum _____
12. antr/o _____ antrum _____
13. esophag/o _____ esophagus _____
14. jejun/o _____ jejunum _____
15. sigmoid/o _____ sigmoid colon _____

## EXERCISE 5

Write the combining form for each of the following.

1. cecum _____ cec/o _____
2. stomach _____ gastr/o _____
3. ileum _____ ile/o _____
4. jejunum _____ jejun/o _____
5. sigmoid colon _____ sigmoid/o _____
6. esophagus _____ esophag/o _____
7. rectum     a. _____ proct/o _____

     b. _____ rect/o _____

8. intestines       _enter/o_

9. duodenum       _duoden/o_

10. colon       _col/o_

11. mouth       a.       _stomat/o_

            b.       _or/o_

12. anus       _an/o_

13. antrum       _antr/o_

# Accessory Organs and Other Word Parts

| COMBINING FORM | DEFINITION |
|---|---|
| 1. appendic/o . . . . . . . . . . | appendix |
| 2. cheil/o. . . . . . . . . . . . . | lip |
| 3. chol/e . . . . . . . . . . . . . <br> (NOTE: The combining vowel is *e*.) | gall, bile |
| 4. cholangi/o. . . . . . . . . . . | bile duct |
| 5. choledoch/o . . . . . . . . . | common bile duct |
| 6. diverticul/o. . . . . . . . . . | diverticulum, or blind pouch extending from a hollow organ (*pl.* diverticula) (Figure 10-3) |
| 7. gingiv/o . . . . . . . . . . . . | gum |
| 8. gloss/o <br>    lingu/o . . . . . . . . . . . . . | tongue |
| 9. hepat/o . . . . . . . . . . . . | liver |

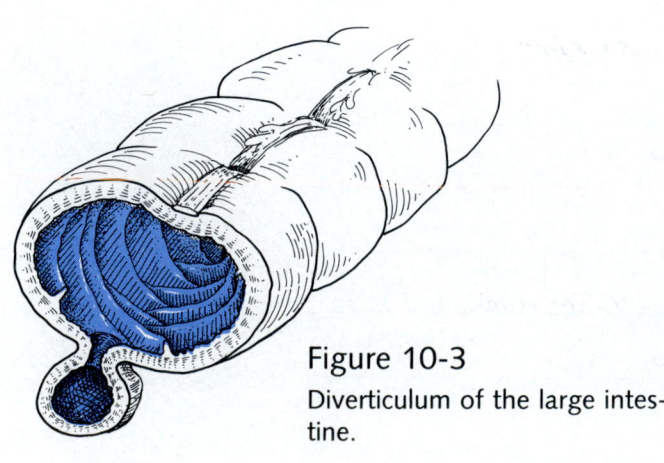

Figure 10-3
Diverticulum of the large intestine.

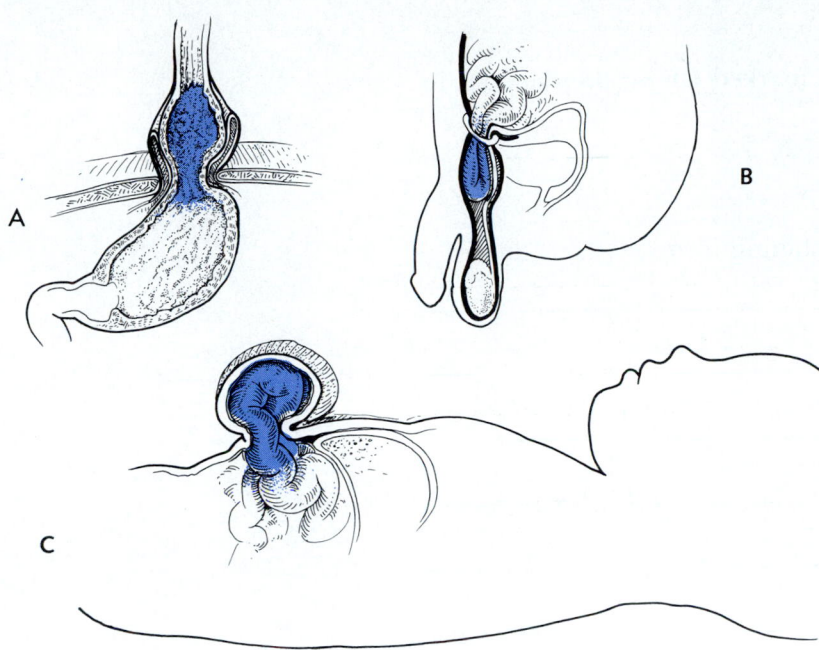

### Figure 10-4
Types of hernias. **A**, Hiatal. **B**, Inguinal. **C**, Umbilical.

| | | |
|---|---|---|
| 10. | herni/o . . . . . . . . . . . . . | hernia, or protrusion of an organ through a body wall. The layman's term for hernia is *rupture*. Types include abdominal hernia, hiatal or diaphragmatic hernia, inguinal hernia, and umbilical hernia (Figure 10-4). |
| 11. | lapar/o <br> abdomin/o <br> celi/o . . . . . . . . . . . . . . . | abdomen (abdominal cavity) |
| 12. | palat/o . . . . . . . . . . . . . | palate |
| 13. | pancreat/o . . . . . . . . . . . | pancreas |
| 14. | peritone/o . . . . . . . . . . . | peritoneum |
| 15. | pylor/o . . . . . . . . . . . . . <br> (NOTE: *Pylor/o* was covered in Chapter 8.) | pylorus, pyloric sphincter |
| 16. | polyp/o . . . . . . . . . . . . . | polyp, small growth |
| 17. | sial/o . . . . . . . . . . . . . . | saliva |
| 18. | uvul/o . . . . . . . . . . . . . | uvula |

Learn the anatomical locations and definitions of the combining forms by completing the following exercises.

## EXERCISE 6

Write the combining forms in the spaces marked **CF** on the diagram in Figure 10-2, p. 366.

## EXERCISE 7

Write the definitions of the following combining forms.

1. herni/o _____ *hernia*
2. abdomin/o _____ *abdomen*
3. sial/o _____ *saliva*
4. chol/e _____ *gall, bile*
5. diverticul/o _____ *diverticulum*
6. gingiv/o _____ *gum*
7. appendic/o _____ *appendix*
8. gloss/o _____ *tongue*
9. hepat/o _____ *liver*
10. cheil/o _____ *lip*
11. peritone/o _____ *peritoneum*
12. palat/o _____ *palate*
13. pancreat/o _____ *pancreas*
14. lapar/o _____ *abdomen*
15. lingu/o _____ *tongue*
16. choledoch/o _____ *common bile duct*
17. pylor/o _____ *pylorus*
18. uvul/o _____ *uvula*
19. cholangi/o _____ *bile duct*
20. polyp/o _____ *polyp, small growth*
21. celi/o _____ *abdomen*

## EXERCISE 8

Write the combining form for each of the following.

1. palate _____ *palato* _____

2. saliva _____ *sialo* _____

3. pancreas _____ *pancreato* _____

4. peritoneum _____ *peritoneo* _____

5. tongue    a. _____ *glosso* _____

 b. _____ *linguo* _____

6. gum _____ *gingivo* _____

7. pylorus _____ *pyloro* _____

8. liver _____ *hepato* _____

9. gall, bile _____ *chole* _____

10. abdomen    a. _____ *celio* _____

 b. _____ *abdomino* _____

 c. _____ *laparo* _____

11. hernia _____ *hernio* _____

12. diverticulum _____ *diverticulo* _____

13. lip _____ *cheilo* _____

14. appendix _____ *appendico* _____

15. uvula _____ *uvulo* _____

16. bile duct _____ *cholangio* _____

17. common bile duct _____ *choledocho* _____

18. small growth _____ *polypo* _____

# Suffix

**SUFFIX**                          **DEFINITION**

1.  -pepsia . . . . . . . . . . . . . .  digestion

Place a check mark (√) in the box to indicate that you have completed Objective 2.

☐ **WRITE THE DEFINITIONS OF THE WORD PARTS INCLUDED IN THIS CHAPTER.**

## Medical Terms

The terms you need to learn to complete this chapter are listed as follows. Now that you know the meaning of the word parts, the exercises found at the end of the list will assist you to learn the definition and the spelling of each word.

## Objective 3 | BUILD, ANALYZE, DEFINE, PRONOUNCE, AND SPELL THE DIAGNOSTIC TERMS RELATED TO THE DIGESTIVE SYSTEM.

## Diagnostic Terms

**TERM**
(built from word parts)

**DEFINITION**

1. **appendicitis** . . . . . . . . .
   (ap-*pen*-di-SĪ-tis)
   inflammation of the appendix (Figure 10-5)

2. **cholangioma** . . . . . . . . .
   (kō-lan-jē-Ō-ma)
   tumor of the bile duct

3. **cholecystitis** . . . . . . . . .
   (kō-lē-sis-TĪ-tis)
   inflammation of the gallbladder

4. **choledocholithiasis** . . . . .
   (kō-led-ō-kō-lith-Ī-a-sis)
   condition of stones in the common bile duct (Figure 10-6)

5. **cholelithiasis** . . . . . . . .
   (kō-lē-lith-Ī-a-sis)
   condition of gallstones (Figure 10-6)

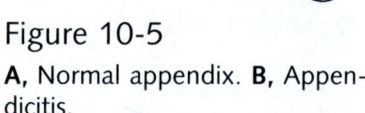

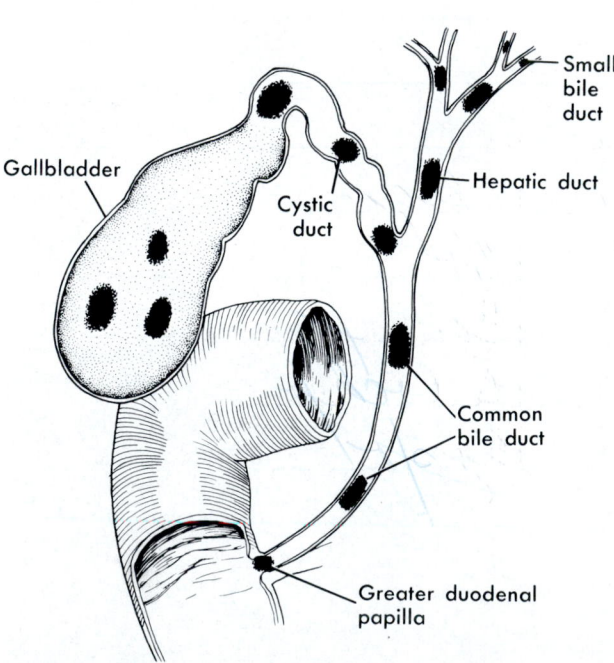

Gallbladder

Small bile duct

Hepatic duct

Cystic duct

Common bile duct

Greater duodenal papilla

**Figure 10-6**

Common sites of cholelithiasis and choledocholithiasis.

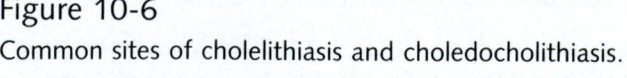
From Phipps WJ, Long BC, and Woods NF: *Shafer's medical-surgical nursing*, ed 7, St. Louis, 1980, Mosby.

A

B

**Figure 10-5**

**A,** Normal appendix. **B,** Appendicitis.

6.  diverticulitis . . . . . . . . .    inflammation of the diverticulum
    (dī-ver-tik-ū-LĪ-tis)

7.  diverticulosis . . . . . . . .    abnormal condition of having divertic-
    (dī-ver-tik-ū-LŌ-sis)    ula

8.  gastritis . . . . . . . . . . . .    inflammation of the stomach
    (gas-TRĪ-tis)

9.  gastroenteritis . . . . . . .    inflammation of the stomach and intes-
    (gas-trō-en-te-RĪ-tis)    tines

10. gastroenterocolitis . . . . .    inflammation of the stomach, intestines,
    (gas-trō-en-ter-ō-kō-LĪ-tis)    and colon

11. gingivitis . . . . . . . . . . .    inflammation of the gums
    (jin-ji-VĪ-tis)

12. hepatitis . . . . . . . . . . . .    inflammation of the liver
    (hep-a-TĪ-tis)

13. hepatoma . . . . . . . . . . .    tumor of the liver
    (hep-a-TŌ-ma)

14. palatitis . . . . . . . . . . . .    inflammation of the palate
    (pal-a-TĪ-tis)

15. pancreatitis . . . . . . . . . .    inflammation of the pancreas
    (pan-krē-a-TĪ-tis)

16. polyposis . . . . . . . . . . .    abnormal condition of (multiple) polyps
    (pol-ē-PŌ-sis)    (in the mucous membrane of the intes-
    tine, especially the colon, high potential
    for malignancy) (Figure 10-7)

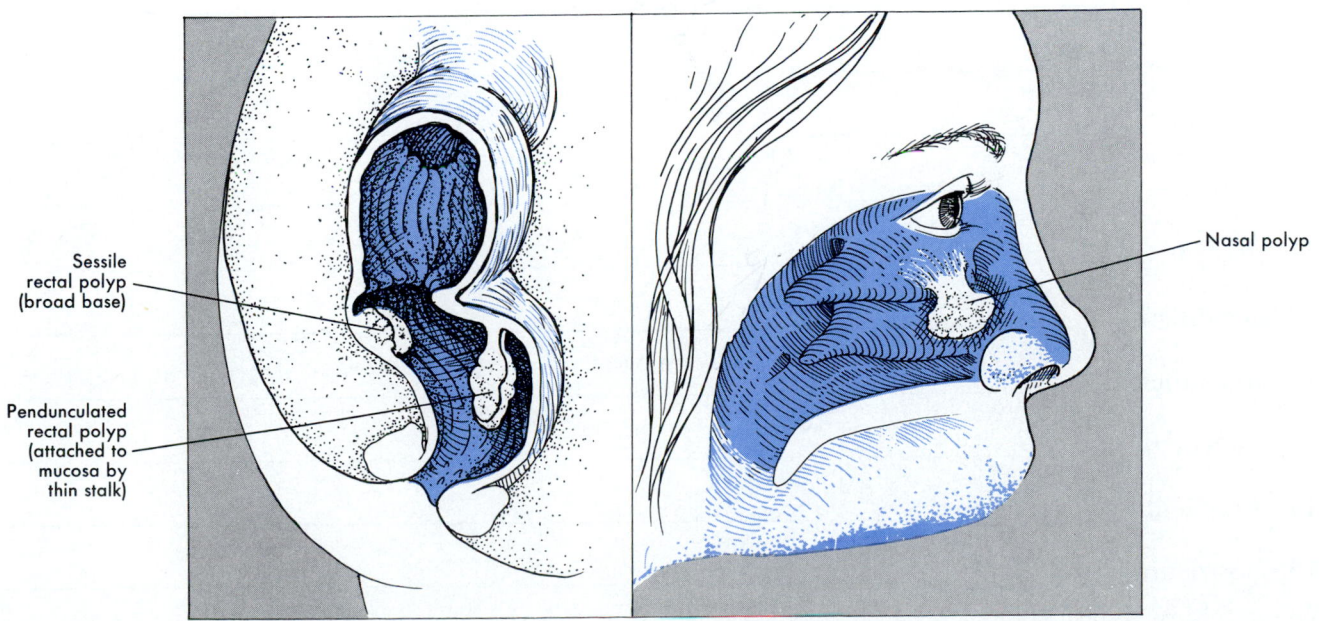

Sessile
rectal polyp
(broad base)

Pendunculated
rectal polyp
(attached to
mucosa by
thin stalk)

Nasal polyp

Figure 10-7
Polyp is a general term used to describe a protruding growth from a mucous membrane. Polyps are commonly found in the nose, uterus, intestines, and bladder.

17. proctoptosis . . . . . . . . .     prolapse of the rectum
    (*prok*-top-TŌ-sis)

18. rectocele. . . . . . . . . . . .     protrusion of the rectum (see Figure
    (REK-tō-sēl)                        7-11, *B*)

19. sialolith . . . . . . . . . . . .     salivary stone
    (sī-AL-ō-lith)

20. uvulitis . . . . . . . . . . . .     inflammation of the uvula
    (ū-vū-LĪ-tis)

Practice saying each of these terms aloud. To assist you in pronunciation,
obtain the audiotape designed for use in this text. Learn the definitions
and spellings of the diagnostic terms by completing the following exercises.

## EXERCISE 9

Analyze and define the following diagnostic terms.

1. cholelithiasis _____

2. diverticulosis _____

3. sialolith _____

4. hepatoma _____

5. uvulitis _____

6. pancreatitis _____

7. proctoptosis _____

8. gingivitis _____

9. gastritis _____

10. rectocele _____

11. palatitis _____

12. hepatitis _____

13. appendicitis _____

14. cholecystitis _____

15. diverticulitis _____

16. gastroenteritis _____

17. gastroenterocolitis _____

18. choledocholithiasis _____

19. cholangioma _____

20. polyposis _____

## EXERCISE 10

Build diagnostic terms for each of the following definitions by using the word parts you have learned.

1. tumor of the liver

   _____ *hepat* / *oma* _____
   WR      S

2. inflammation of the stomach

   _____ *gastr* *itis* _____
   WR      S

3. salivary stone

   _____ *sial* / *o* / *lith* _____
   WR    CV      WR

4. inflammation of the appendix

   _____ *appendic* / *itis* _____
   WR      S

5. inflammation of the diverticulum

   _____ *diverticul* *itis* _____
   WR      S

6. inflammation of the gallbladder

   _____ *chol* / *e* / *cyst* / *itis* _____
   WR    CV    WR      S

7. abnormal condition of having diverticula

   _____ *diverticul* *osis* _____
   WR      S

8. inflammation of the stomach and intestines

   _____ *gastr* / *o* / *enter* / *itis* _____
   WR    CV    WR      S

9. prolapse of the rectum

   _____ *proct* / *o* / *ptosis* _____
   WR    CV      S

10. protrusion of the rectum    _rect_ / _o_ / _cele_
    <br>WR   CV   S

11. inflammation of the uvula    _uvul_ / _itis_
    <br>WR   S

12. inflammation of the gums    _gingiv_ / _itis_
    <br>WR   S

13. inflammation of the liver    _hepat_ / _itis_
    <br>WR   S

14. inflammation of the palate    _palat_ / _itis_
    <br>WR   S

15. condition of gallstones    _chol_ / _e_ / _lith_ / _iasis_
    <br>WR   CV   WR   S

16. inflammation of the stomach, intestines, and colon    _gastr_ / _o_ / _enter_ / _o_ / _col_ / _itis_
    <br>WR   CV   WR   CV   WR   S

17. inflammation of the pancreas    _pancreat_ / _itis_
    <br>WR   S

18. tumor of the bile duct    _cholangi_ / _oma_
    <br>WR   S

19. condition of stones in the common bile duct    _choledoch_ / _o_ / _lith_ / _iasis_
    <br>WR   CV   WR   S

20. abnormal condition of (multiple) polyps    _polyp_ / _osis_
    <br>WR   S

## EXERCISE 11

Spell each of the diagnostic terms. Have someone dictate the terms on pp. 374 to 376 to you or say the words into a tape recorder; then spell the words from your recording as often as necessary. Think about the

word parts before attempting to write the word. Study any you have
spelled incorrectly.

1. _____     11. _____
2. _____     12. _____
3. _____     13. _____
4. _____     14. _____
5. _____     15. _____
6. _____     16. _____
7. _____     17. _____
8. _____     18. _____
9. _____     19. _____
10. _____     20. _____

Place a check mark (√) in the box to indicate that you have completed Objective 3.

☐ **BUILD, ANALYZE, DEFINE, PRONOUNCE, AND SPELL THE DIAGNOSTIC TERMS RELATED TO THE DIGESTIVE SYSTEM.**

# Objective 4    DEFINE, PRONOUNCE AND SPELL OTHER DIAGNOSTIC TERMS RELATED TO THE DIGESTIVE SYSTEM.

## Other Diagnostic Terms

| TERM | DEFINITION |
|---|---|
| 1. adhesion............<br>(ad-HĒ-zhun) | abnormal growing together of two surfaces that normally are separated (Figure 10-8). They may occur after abdominal surgery; surgical treatment is adhesiolysis or adhesiotomy. |

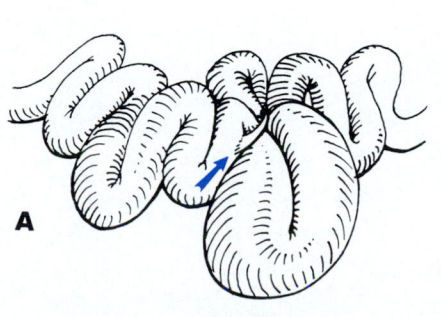
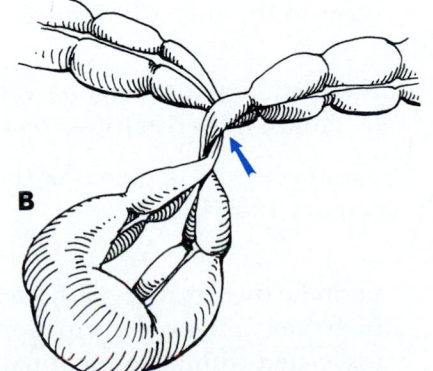
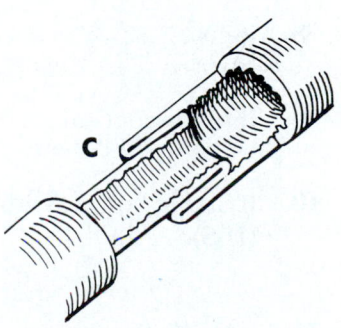

Figure 10-8

Some causes of intestinal obstruction. **A,** Constriction by adhesions. **B,** Volvulus. **C,** Intussusception.

Modified from Phipps WJ, Long BC, Woods NF and others: *Medical-surgical nursing*, ed 4, St. Louis, 1991, Mosby.

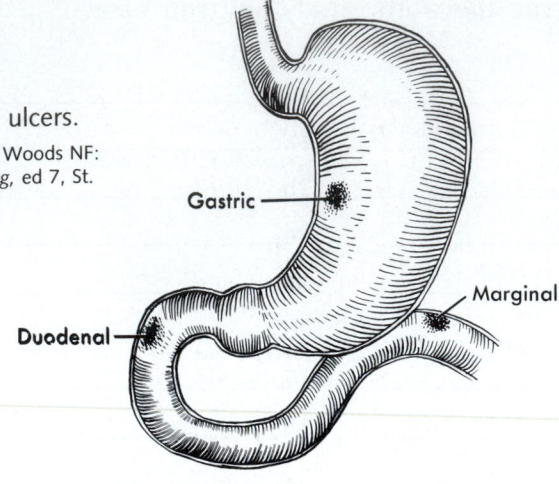

Figure 10-9

Common sites of peptic ulcers.

From Phipps WJ, Long BC, and Woods NF: *Shafer's medical-surgical nursing,* ed 7, St. Louis, 1980, Mosby.

2.  **anorexia nervosa** . . . . . .     psychoneurotic disorder characterized
    (*an*-ō-REK-sē-a) (ner-VŌ-sa)     by a prolonged refusal to eat, resulting
                                        in emaciation, amenorrhea, and abnor-
                                        mal fear of becoming obese. It occurs
                                        primarily in adolescents.

3.  **bulimia** . . . . . . . . . . . . .     gorging with food then inducing vomit-
    (bu-LIM-ē-a)                          ing

4.  **cirrhosis** . . . . . . . . . . . .     chronic disease of the liver with gradual
    (ser-RŌ-sis)                          destruction of cells, most commonly
                                        caused by alcoholism

5.  **Crohn's disease** . . . . . . .     chronic inflammation usually affecting
    (krōnz)                               the ileum and sometimes the colon,
                                        characterized by cobblestone ulcerations
                                        along the intestinal wall and the forma-
                                        tion of scar tissue. It may cause obstruc-
                                        tion. Also called regional ileitis or re-
                                        gional enteritis

6.  **duodenal ulcer** . . . . . . . .     ulcer in the duodenum (Figure 10-9)
    (*dū*-o-DĒ-nal)

7.  **gastric ulcer** . . . . . . . . . .     ulcer in the stomach (Figure 10-9)
    (GAS-trik)

8.  **ileus** . . . . . . . . . . . . . . .     obstruction of the intestine, often caused
    (IL-ē-us)                             by failure of peristalsis

9.  **intussusception** . . . . . . . .     telescoping of a segment of the intestine
    (*in*-tus-sus-SEP-shun)               (Figure 10-8)

10. **irritable bowel syndrome
    (IBS)** . . . . . . . . . . . . . .     periodic disturbances of bowel function
                                        (diarrhea and/or constipation) usually
                                        associated with abdominal pain

11. peptic ulcer . . . . . . . . . .    another name for gastric or duodenal ul-
    (PEP-tik)                            cer (Fig. 10-9)

12. polyp . . . . . . . . . . . . . .    tumor-like growth extending outward
    (POL-ip)                             from a mucous membrane. Usually be-
                                         nign, common sites are in the nose,
                                         throat, and intestines (Figure 10-7)

13. ulcerative colitis. . . . . . .      inflammation of the colon with the for-
    (UL-ser-a-tiv) (kol-LĪ-tis)          mation of ulcers. The main symptom is
                                         diarrhea: as many as 15 to 29 stools per
                                         day. An ileostomy may be performed in
                                         an attempt to cure the condition

14. volvulus . . . . . . . . . . . .     twisting or kinking of the intestine, caus-
    (VOL-vū-lus)                         ing intestinal obstruction (Figure 10-8)

Practice saying each of these terms aloud. To assist you in pronunciation, obtain the audiotape designed for use with this text. Learn the definitions and spellings of the other diagnostic terms by completing the following exercises.

## EXERCISE 12

Match the definitions in the first column with the correct terms in the second column.

_f_ 1. prolonged refusal to eat

_b_ 2. chronic disease of the liver

_e_ 3. chronic inflammation of the intestines

_c_ 4. abnormal growing together of two surfaces

_d_ 5. twisted intestine

_g_ 6. gastric or duodenal ulcer

_a_ 7. telescoping of a segment of the intestine

_k_ 8. tumor-like growth

_h_ 9. formation of ulcers in the colon

_j_ 10. gorging food, then inducing vomiting

_m_ 11. obstruction of the intestine

a. intussusception

b. cirrhosis

c. adhesion

d. volvulus

e. Crohn's disease

f. anorexia nervosa

g. peptic ulcer

h. ulcerative colitis

i. irritable bowel syndrome

j. bulimia

k. polyp

l. hernia

m. ileus

_____  12. periodic distur-
          bance of bowel
          function

## EXERCISE 13

Write the definitions of the following terms.

1. peptic ulcer _____

2. anorexia nervosa _____

3. Crohn's disease _____

4. volvulus _____

5. adhesion _____

6. cirrhosis _____

7. intussusception _____

8. gastric ulcer _____

9. duodenal ulcer _____

10. ulcerative colitis _____

11. bulimia _____

12. polyp _____

13. irritable bowel syndrome _____

14. ileus _____

## EXERCISE 14

Spell each of the other diagnostic terms. Have someone dictate the terms
on pp. 379 to 381 to you or say the words into a tape recorder; then spell
the words from your recording as often as necessary. Study any you have
spelled incorrectly.

1. _____        8. _____

2. _____        9. _____

3. _____        10. _____

4. _____        11. _____

5. _____        12. _____

6. _____        13. _____

7. _____        14. _____

Place a check mark (√) in the box to indicate that you have completed Objective 4.

☐ DEFINE, PRONOUNCE, AND SPELL OTHER DIAGNOSTIC TERMS RELATED TO THE DIGESTIVE SYSTEM.

# Objective 5    BUILD, ANALYZE, DEFINE, PRONOUNCE, AND SPELL THE SURGICAL TERMS RELATED TO THE DIGESTIVE SYSTEM.

# Surgical Terms

| TERM (built from word parts) | DEFINITION |
|---|---|
| 1. abdominoplasty ........ (ab-DOM-i-nō-plas-tē) | plastic repair of the abdomen |
| 2. anoplasty .......... (Ā-nō-*plas*-tē) | surgical repair of the anus |
| 3. antrectomy .......... (an-TREK-tō-mē) | excision of the antrum (Figure 10-10) |
| 4. appendectomy ....... (*ap*-en-DEK-tō-mē) | excision of the appendix |
| 5. celiotomy .......... (sē-lē-OT-ō-mē) | incision into the abdominal cavity |
| 6. cheilorrhaphy........ (kī-LOR-a-fē) | suture of the lips |
| 7. cholecystectomy ...... (kō-lē-sis-TEK-tō-mē) | excision of the gallbladder |

The first **cholecystectomy** was performed in 1882 by a German surgeon.
The first **laparoscopic cholecystectomy** was performed in 1987 in France.

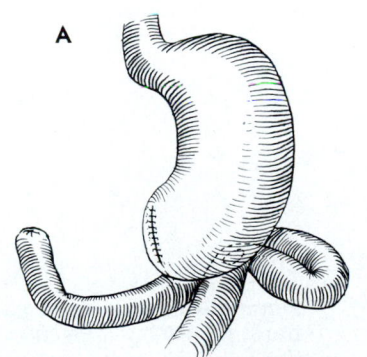 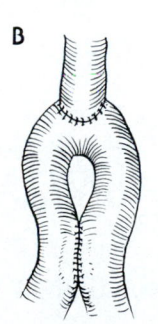 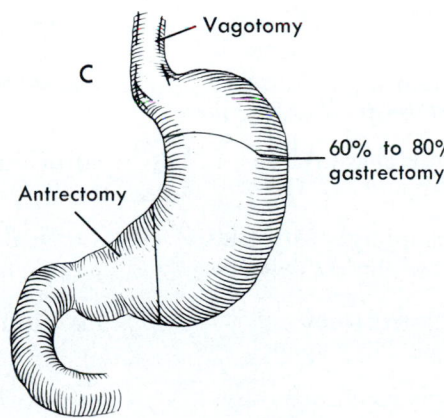

## Figure 10-10

**A,** Partial gastrectomy and gastrojejunostomy. **B,** Gastrectomy with anastomosis of esophagus to jejunum. **C,** Some surgical approaches used in treatment of peptic ulcers.

Modified from Phipps WJ, Long BC, and Woods NF: *Shafer's medical-surgical nursing,* ed 7, St. Louis, 1980, Mosby.

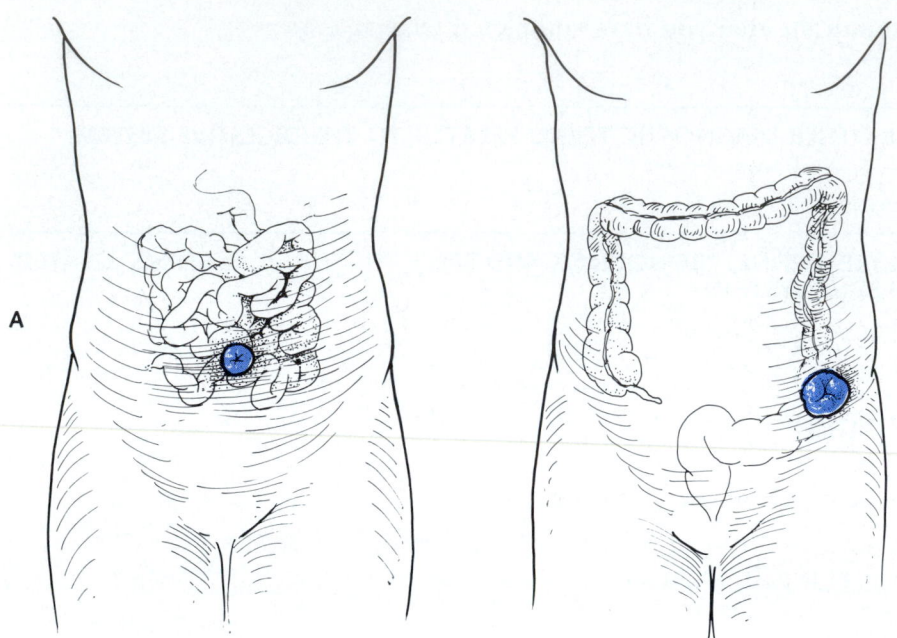

Figure 10-11
**A,** Ileostomy following total colectomy. **B,** Colostomy following abdominal perineal resection.

8. choledocholithotomy . . .  incision into the common bile duct to remove a stone
   (kō-led-ō-kō-li-THOT-ō-mē)

9. choledocholithotripsy. . .  surgical crushing of a stone in the common bile duct
   (kō-led-ō-kō-LITH-ō-trip-sē)

10. colectomy . . . . . . . . . . .  excision of the colon
    (kō-LEK-tō-mē)

11. colostomy . . . . . . . . . . .  artificial opening through the abdominal wall into the colon (used for the passage of stool. It is performed for cancer of the colon) (Figure 10-11)
    (kō-LOS-tō-mē)

12. diverticulectomy. . . . . . .  excision of a diverticulum
    (*dī*-ver-tik-ū-LEK-tō-mē)

13. enterorrhaphy . . . . . . . .  suture of the intestine
    (en-ter-ŌR-a-fē)

14. esophagogastroplasty . . .  surgical repair of the esophagus and the stomach
    (ē-*sof*-a-gō-GAS-trō-plas-tē)

15. gastrectomy . . . . . . . . .  excision of the stomach (Figure 10-10)
    (gas-TREK-tō-mē)

16. gastrojejunostomy . . . . .  creation of an artificial opening between the stomach and jejunum (Figure 10-10)
    (*gas*-trō-je-jū-NOS-tō-mē)

17. gastrostomy . . . . . . . . .  creation of an artificial opening through the abdominal wall into the stomach (a tube is inserted through the opening for administration of food when swallowing is impossible) (Figure 10-12)
    (gas-TROS-tō-mē)

**Percutaneous endoscopic gastrostomy (PEG)** (Figure 10-12) was first described in 1980. It is an alternative to traditional gastrostomy. An endoscope is used to place the tube in the stomach. Cost and discomfort to the patient is reduced when PEG is used rather than the traditional gastrostomy.

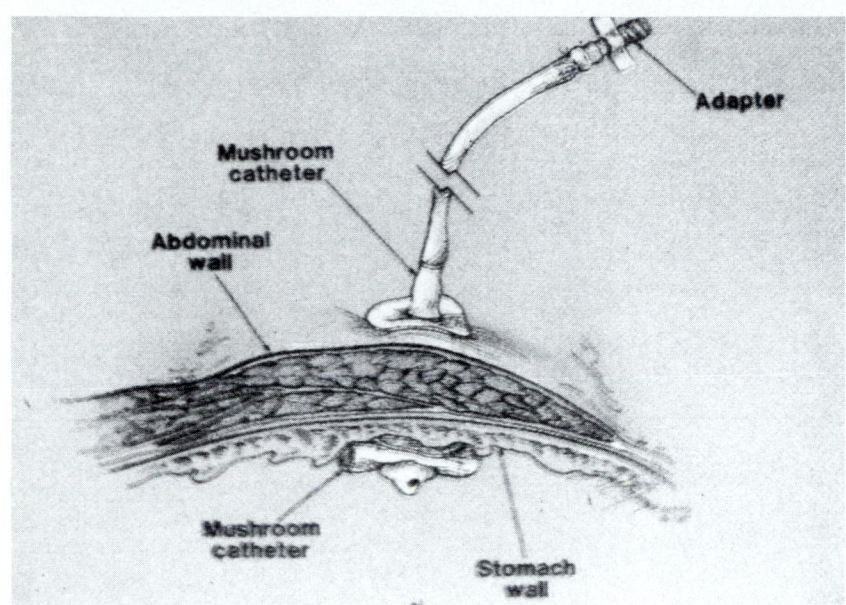

Figure 10-12
Tube placed by using percutaneous endoscopic gastrostomy (PEG) procedure.

18. **gingivectomy** . . . . . . . .    surgical removal of gum tissue
    (*jin*-ji-VEK-tō-mē)

19. **glossorrhaphy** . . . . . . . .    suture of the tongue
    (glo-SŌR-a-fē)

20. **herniorrhaphy** . . . . . . .    suturing (to repair) of a hernia
    (*her*-nē-ŌR-a-fē)

21. **ileostomy** . . . . . . . . . . .    creation of an artificial opening through
    (il-ē-OS-tō-mē)    the abdominal wall into the ileum (used
    for the passage of stool. It is performed
    for ulcerative colitis, Crohn's disease, or
    cancer) (Figure 10-11)

22. **laparotomy** . . . . . . . . . .    incision into the abdominal wall
    (*lap*-a-ROT-ō-mē)

23. **palatoplasty** . . . . . . . . . .    surgical repair of the palate
    (PAL-a-tō-*plas*-tē)

24. **polypectomy** . . . . . . . . . .    excision of a polyp
    (pol-ē-PEK-tō-mē)

25. **pyloromyotomy** . . . . . . .    incision into the pylorus muscle
    (pī-*lor*-ō-mī-OT-ō-mē)

26. **pyloroplasty** . . . . . . . . . .    surgical repair of the pylorus
    (pī-LOR-ō-plas-tē)

27. **uvulectomy** . . . . . . . . . .    excision of the uvula
    (ū-vū-LEK-tō-mē)

28. **uvulopalatopharyngo-
    plasty (UPPP)** . . . . . . . .    surgical repair of the uvula, palate, and
    (ū-vū-lō-*pal*-a-tō-*phar*-in-GŌ-    pharynx (performed to correct obstruc-
    plas-tē)    tive sleep apnea)

Practice saying each of these terms aloud. To assist you in pronunciation, obtain the audiotape designed for use with this text. Learn the definitions and spellings of the surgical terms by completing the following exercises.

## EXERCISE 15

Analyze and define the following surgical terms.

1. gastrectomy _____

2. esophagogastroplasty _____

3. diverticulectomy _____

4. antrectomy _____

5. palatoplasty _____

6. uvulectomy _____

7. gastrojejunostomy _____

8. cholecystectomy _____

9. colectomy _____

10. colostomy _____

11. pyloroplasty _____

12. anoplasty _____

13. appendectomy _____

14. cheilorrhaphy _____

15. gingivectomy _____

16. laparotomy _____

17. ileostomy _____

18. gastrostomy _____

19. herniorrhaphy _____

20. glossorrhaphy _____

21. choledocholithotomy _____

22. choledocholithotripsy _____

23. polypectomy _____

24. enterorrhaphy _____

25. abdominoplasty _____

26. pyloromyotomy _____

27. uvulopalatopharyngoplasty _____

28. celiotomy _____

## EXERCISE 16

Build surgical terms to match the following definitions.

1. excision of the appendix
   _____/_____
   WR        S

2. suture of the tongue
   _____/_____
   WR        S

3. surgical repair of the esophagus and stomach
   ____/____/____/____/____
   WR   CV   WR   CV   S

4. excision of a diverticulum
   _____/_____
   WR        S

5. artificial opening into the ileum
   _____/_____
   WR        S

6. surgical removal of the gum tissue
   _____/_____
   WR        S

7. incision into the abdominal wall
   _____/_____
   WR        S

8. surgical repair of the anus
   _____/____/_____
   WR   CV   S

9. excision of the antrum
   _____/_____
   WR        S

10. excision of the gallbladder

        _____ / _____ / _____ / _____
        WR   CV   WR   S

11. excision of the colon

        _____ / _____
        WR   S

12. creation of an artificial opening into the colon

        _____ / _____
        WR   S

13. excision of the stomach

        _____ / _____
        WR   S

14. creation of an artificial opening into the stomach

        _____ / _____
        WR   S

15. creation of an artificial opening between the stomach and jejunum

        _____ / _____ / _____ / _____
        WR   CV   WR   S

16. excision of the uvula

        _____ / _____
        WR   S

17. surgical repair of the palate

        _____ / _____ / _____
        WR   CV   S

18. surgical repair of the pylorus

        _____ / _____ / _____
        WR   CV   S

19. suture of a hernia

        _____ / _____
        WR   S

20. suture of the lip

        _____ / _____
        WR   S

21. surgical crushing of a
    stone in the common bile
    duct

    _____
      WR  /  CV  /  WR  /  CV  /   S

22. incision into the common
    bile duct to remove a
    stone

    _____
       WR  /  CV  /  WR  /   S

23. excision of a polyp

    _____
              WR  /   S

24. suture of the intestine

    _____
              WR  /   S

25. plastic repair of the ab-
    domen

    _____
            WR  /  CV  /   S

26. incision into the abdomi-
    nal cavity

    _____
              WR  /   S

27. incision into the pylorus
    muscle

    _____
           WR  /  CV  /  WR  /   S

28. surgical repair of the
    uvula, palate, and phar-
    ynx

    _____
      WR  /  CV  /  WR  /  CV  /  WR  /  CV  /   S

## EXERCISE 17

Spell each of the surgical terms. Have someone dictate the surgical terms
on pp. 383 to 385 to you or say the words into a tape recorder; then spell
the words from your recording as often as necessary. Think of the the
word parts before attempting to write the word. Study any you have
spelled incorrectly.

1. _____     5. _____

2. _____     6. _____

3. _____     7. _____

4. _____     8. _____

9. _____    19. _____
10. _____    20. _____
11. _____    21. _____
12. _____    22. _____
13. _____    23. _____
14. _____    24. _____
15. _____    25. _____
16. _____    26. _____
17. _____    27. _____
18. _____    28. _____

Place a check mark (√) in the box to indicate that you have completed Objective 5.

☐ **BUILD, ANALYZE, DEFINE, PRONOUNCE, AND SPELL THE SURGICAL TERMS RELATED TO THE DIGESTIVE SYSTEM.**

## Objective 6  DEFINE, PRONOUNCE, AND SPELL OTHER SURGICAL TERMS RELATED TO THE DIGESTIVE SYSTEM.

## Other Surgical Terms

| TERM | DEFINITION |
|------|------------|
| 1. abdominoperineal resection. . . . . . . . . . . . . . . . . (ab-*dom*-in-ō-pēr-i-NĒ-el) | removal of the colon and rectum |
| 2. anastomosis . . . . . . . . . . (a-*nas*-tō-MŌ-sis) | surgical connection between two normally distinct structures (Figure 10-10) |
| 3. vagotomy . . . . . . . . . . . (va-GOT-ō-mē) | cutting of certain branches of vagus nerve, performed with gastric surgery to reduce the amount of gastric acid produced and thus reduce the recurrence of ulcers (Figure 10-10) |

Practice saying these terms aloud. To assist you in pronunciation, obtain the audiotape designed for use with this text. Learn the definitions and spellings of the other surgical terms by completing the following exercises.

### EXERCISE 18

Write the term for each of the following definitions.

1. cutting certain branches of the vagus nerve _____*vagotomy*_____

2. surgical connection between two structures

*anastomosis*

3. removal of the colon and rectum

*abdominoperineal resection*

## EXERCISE 19

Spell each of the other surgical terms. Have someone dictate the terms on p. 390 to you or say the words into a tape recorder; then spell the words from your recording as often as necessary. Study any you have spelled incorrectly.

1. _____      3. _____

2. _____

Place a check mark (√) in the box to indicate that you have completed Objective 6.

☐ DEFINE, PRONOUNCE, AND SPELL OTHER SURGICAL TERMS RELATED TO THE DIGESTIVE SYSTEM.

## Objective 7  BUILD, ANALYZE, DEFINE, PRONOUNCE, AND SPELL THE DIAGNOSTIC PROCEDURAL TERMS RELATED TO THE DIGESTIVE SYSTEM.

## Diagnostic Procedural Terms

**TERM**
(built from word parts)

**DEFINITION**

1. cholangiogram (kō-LAN-je-ō-gram) — x-ray film of bile ducts. (An injection of radiopaque material is used to outline the ducts.)

2. cholecystogram (kō-lē-SIS-tō-gram) — x-ray film of the gallbladder (also known as a *G.B. Series*) (Figure 10-13)

3. colonoscope (kō-LON-ō-skōp) — instrument used for visual examination of the colon

4. colonoscopy (kō-lon-OS-kō-pē) — visual examination of the colon

5. endoscope (EN-dō-skōp) — instrument used for visual examination within hollow organ

6. endoscopy (en-DOS-kō-pē) — visual examination within a hollow organ

> Operative and postoperative **cholangiography** use the injection of contrast medium into the common bile duct. The dye is inserted through the drainage T-tube to discover any small remaining gallstones after surgery.

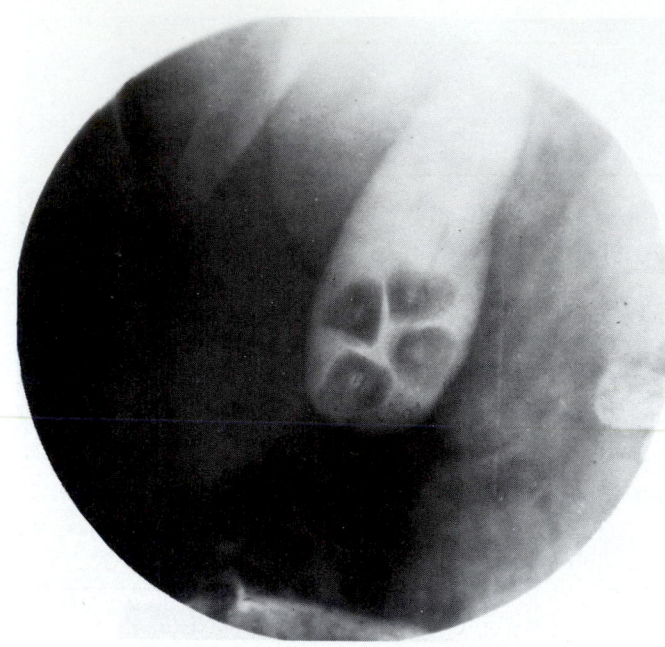

### Figure 10-13
Cholecystogram showing cholelithiasis.

From Ballinger PW: *Merrill's atlas of radiographic positions and radiologic procedures,* ed 7, St. Louis, 1991, Mosby.

7. **esophagogastro-
   duodenoscopy (EGD)** . . .    visual examination of the esophagus,
   (ē-*sof*-a-gō-*gas*-trō-dū-od-e-    stomach, and duodenum
   NOS-kō-pē)

8. **esophagoscope** . . . . . . .    instrument used for visual examination
   (ē-SOF-a-gō-skōp)    of the esophagus

9. **esophagoscopy** . . . . . . .    visual examination of the esophagus
   (ē-*sof*-a-GOS-kō-pē)

10. **gastroscope** . . . . . . . . . .    instrument used for visual examination
    (GAS-trō-skōp)    of the stomach (Figure 10-14)

11. **laparoscope** . . . . . . . . .    instrument for visual examination of the
    (LAP-a-rō-skōp)    abdominal cavity

12. **laparoscopy** . . . . . . . . .    visual examination of the abdominal
    (lap-a-ROS-kō-pē)    cavity

13. **gastroscopy** . . . . . . . . . .    visual examination of the stomach
    (gas-TROS-kō-pē)

14. **proctoscope** . . . . . . . . .    instrument used for visual examination
    (PROK-tō-skōp)    of the rectum

15. **proctoscopy** . . . . . . . . .    visual examination of the rectum
    (prok-TOS-kō-pē)

16. **sigmoidoscope** . . . . . . . .    instrument used for visual examination
    (sig-MOY-dō-skōp)    of the sigmoid colon

17. **sigmoidoscopy** . . . . . . . .    visual examination of the sigmoid colon
    (*sig*-moy-DOS-kō-pē)    (Figure 10-15)

The **laparoscope** is also the instrument used to perform laparoscopy surgery, a modern method that replaces open abdominal incisional surgery. Surgeries performed using a laparoscope include laparoscopic cholecystectomy, laparoscopic herniorrhaphy, and laparoscopic appendectomy.

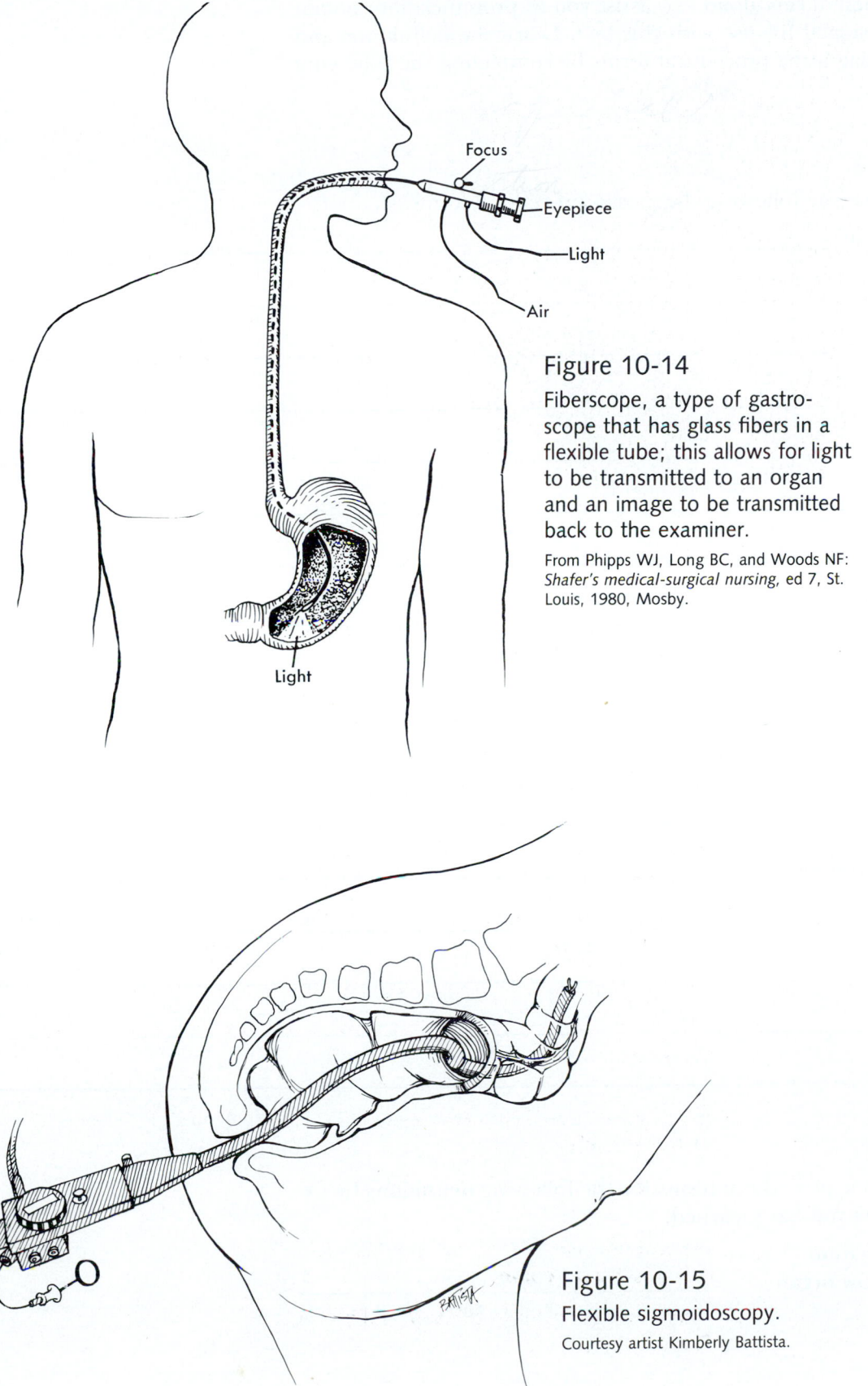

**Figure 10-14**

Fiberscope, a type of gastroscope that has glass fibers in a flexible tube; this allows for light to be transmitted to an organ and an image to be transmitted back to the examiner.

From Phipps WJ, Long BC, and Woods NF: *Shafer's medical-surgical nursing,* ed 7, St. Louis, 1980, Mosby.

**Figure 10-15**

Flexible sigmoidoscopy.

Courtesy artist Kimberly Battista.

Practice saying these terms aloud. To assist you in pronunciation, obtain the audiotape designed for use with this text. Learn the definitions and spellings of the diagnostic procedural terms by completing the following exercises.

## EXERCISE 20

Analyze and define the following diagnostic procedural terms.

1. esophagoscope _____

2. esophagoscopy _____

3. gastroscope _____

4. gastroscopy _____

5. proctoscope _____

6. proctoscopy _____

7. endoscope _____

8. endoscopy _____

9. sigmoidoscope _____

10. sigmoidoscopy _____

11. cholecystogram _____

12. cholangiogram _____

13. esophagogastroduodenoscopy _____

14. colonoscope _____

15. laparoscope _____

16. colonoscopy _____

17. laparoscopy _____

## EXERCISE 21

Build the diagnostic procedural terms for the following definitions by using the word parts you have learned.

1. visual examination
   within a hollow organ    ____endo_/_scopy____
                                P     S(WR)

2. instrument used for visual examination of the stomach

_gastr_ / _o_ / _scope_
WR / CV / S

3. instrument used for visual examination of the rectum

_proct_ / _o_ / _scope_
WR / CV / S

4. instrument used for visual examination of the sigmoid colon

_sigmoid_ / _o_ / _scope_
WR / CV / S

5. x-ray film of the gallbladder

_chol_ / _e_ / _cyst_ / _o_ / _gram_
WR / CV / WR / CV / S

6. instrument used for visual examination within a hollow organ

_endo_ / _scope_
P / S(WR)

7. instrument used for visual examination of the esophagus

_esophag_ / _o_ / _scope_
WR / CV / S

8. visual examination of the rectum

_proct_ / _o_ / _scope_
WR / CV / S

9. visual examination of the esophagus

_esophag_ / _o_ / _scopy_
WR / CV / S

10. visual examination of the sigmoid colon

_sigmoid_ / _o_ / _scopy_
WR / CV / S

11. x-ray of bile ducts

_cholangi_ / _o_ / _gram_
WR / CV / S

12. visual examination of the stomach

 gastr / o / scopy
 WR / CV / S

13. instrument used for visual examination of the abdominal cavity

 lapar / o / scope
 WR / CV / S

14. visual examination of the esophagus, stomach and duodenum

 esophag / o / gastr / o / duoden / o / scopy
 WR / CV / WR / CV / WR / CV / S

15. visual examination of the colon

 colon / o / scopy
 WR / CV / S

16. visual examination of the abdominal cavity

 lapar / o / scopy
 WR / CV / S

17. instrument used for visual examination of the colon

 colon / o / scope
 WR / CV / S

Test your spelling of the diagnostic procedural terms when you come to Exercise 23.

Place a check mark (√) in the box to indicate that you have completed Objective 7.

☐ **BUILD, ANALYZE, DEFINE, PRONOUNCE, AND SPELL THE DIAGNOSTIC PROCEDURAL TERMS RELATED TO THE DIGESTIVE SYSTEM.**

# Objective 8  DEFINE, PRONOUNCE, AND SPELL OTHER DIAGNOSTIC PROCEDURAL TERMS RELATED TO THE DIGESTIVE SYSTEM.

## Other Diagnostic Procedural Terms

| TERM | DEFINITION |
| --- | --- |
| 1. lower GI (gastrointestinal) series . . . . . . . . . . . . . . . | series of x-ray films taken of the large intestine after a barium enema has been administered (Figure 10-16) (also called *barium enema*) |

ERCP was first performed in 1968. ERCP is used to evaluate obstructions, pancreatic cancer, and unexplained pancreatitis. It is used to diagnose stone diseases, strictures, and pancreatic neoplasms.

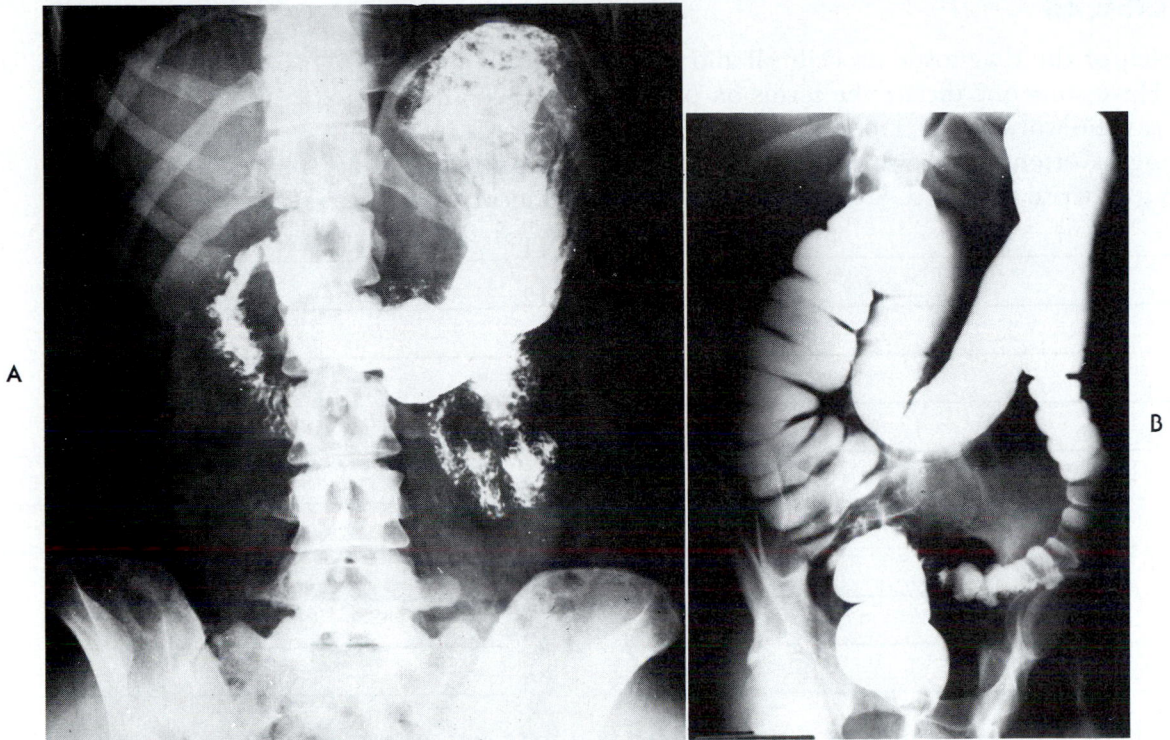

## Figure 10-16

X-ray films of **A,** upper GI, and **B,** lower GI (also called barium enema).

From Ballinger PW: *Merrill's atlas of radiographic positions and radiologic procedures,* ed 5, St. Louis, 1982, Mosby.

2. upper GI (gastrointestinal) series . . . . . . . . . . . . series of x-ray films taken of the stomach and duodenum after barium has been swallowed (Figure 10-16)

3. endoscopic retrograde cholangiopancreatography (ERCP) . . . . . . . . . (kō-lan-jē-ō-*pan*-krē-a-TOG-rah-fē) radiographic (x-ray) examination of the bile and pancreatic ducts using contrast medium, fluoroscopy, and endoscopy

## EXERCISE 22

Write definitions of the following terms.

1. upper GI series _X rays of stomach + duodenum after barium has been swallowed_

2. lower GI series _X rays of large intestine after barium enema_

3. endoscopic retrograde cholangiopancreatography _radiographic exam of bile + pancreatic ducts using contrast medium, fluoroscopy + endoscopy_

## EXERCISE 23

Spell each of the diagnostic procedural and other diagnostic procedural terms. Have someone dictate the terms on pp. 391, 392, 396 and 397 to you or say the words into a tape recorder; then spell the words from your recording as often as necessary. Think about the word parts before attempting to write the word. Study any you have spelled incorrectly.

1. _____
2. _____
3. _____
4. _____
5. _____
6. _____
7. _____
8. _____
9. _____
10. _____
11. _____
12. _____
13. _____
14. _____
15. _____
16. _____
17. _____
18. _____
19. _____
20. _____

Place a check mark (√) in the box to indicate that you have completed Objective 8.

☐ **DEFINE, PRONOUNCE, AND SPELL OTHER DIAGNOSTIC PROCEDURAL TERMS RELATED TO THE DIGESTIVE SYSTEM.**

# Objective 9  BUILD, ANALYZE, DEFINE, PRONOUNCE, AND SPELL THE ADDITIONAL TERMS RELATED TO THE DIGESTIVE SYSTEM.

## Additional Terms

| TERM (built from word parts) | DEFINITION |
|---|---|
| 1. abdominal (ab-DOM-i-nal) | pertaining to the abdomen |
| 2. abdominocentesis (ab-*dom*-i-nō-sen-TĒ-sis) | surgical puncture to remove fluid from the abdominal cavity (also called paracentesis) |
| 3. anal (Ā-nal) | pertaining to the anus |
| 4. apepsia (a-PĒP-sē-a) | without (lack of) digestion |
| 5. aphagia (a-FĀ-jē-a) | inability to swallow |
| 6. bradypepsia (*brād*-ē-PĒP-sē-a) | slow digestion |
| 7. dyspepsia (dis-PĒP-sē-a) | difficult digestion |

8. dysphagia . . . . . . . . . . . difficult swallowing
   (dis-FĀ-jē-a)

9. gastrodynia . . . . . . . . . . pain in the stomach
   (*gas*-trō-DĪN-ē-a)

10. gastromalacia . . . . . . . . softening of the stomach
    (*gas*-trō-ma-LĀ-shē-a)

11. glossopathy . . . . . . . . . . disease of the tongue
    (glo-SOP-a-thē)

12. ileocecal . . . . . . . . . . . . pertaining to the ileum and cecum
    (*il*-ē-ō-SĒ-kal)

13. nasogastric . . . . . . . . . . pertaining to the nose and stomach
    (*nā*-zō-GAS-trik)

14. oral . . . . . . . . . . . . . . . pertaining to the mouth
    (Ō-ral)

15. pancreatic . . . . . . . . . . . pertaining to the pancreas
    (*pan*-krē-AT-ik)

16. peritoneal . . . . . . . . . . . pertaining to the peritoneum
    (*pĕr*-i-tō-NĒ-al)

17. proctologist . . . . . . . . . physician who specializes in proctology
    (prok-TOL-ō-jist)

18. proctology . . . . . . . . . . branch of medicine concerned with dis-
    (prok-TOL-ō-jē)                orders of the rectum and anus

19. stomatogastric . . . . . . . pertaining to the mouth and stomach
    (*stō*-ma-tō-GAS-trik)

20. sublingual . . . . . . . . . . pertaining to under the tongue
    (sub-LING-gwal)

Practice saying each of these terms aloud. To assist you in pronunciation, obtain the audiotape designed for use with this text. Learn the definitions and spellings of the additional terms by completing the following exercises.

## EXERCISE 24

Analyze and define the following additional terms.

1. aphagia _____

2. dyspepsia _____

3. anal _____

4. dysphagia _____

5. glossopathy _____

6. ileocecal _____

7. oral _____

8. stomatogastric _____

9. bradypepsia _____

10. abdominocentesis _____

11. apepsia _____

12. gastromalacia _____

13. pancreatic _____

14. gastrodynia _____

15. peritoneal _____

16. sublingual _____

17. proctology _____

18. nasogastric _____

19. abdominal _____

20. proctologist _____

## EXERCISE 25

Build additional terms for the following definitions by using the word parts you have learned.

1. disease of the tongue

_____ gloss _/_ o _/_ pathy _____
　　　　　WR　　CV　　 S

2. inability to swallow

_____ a _/_ phagia _____
　　　　　P　　S(WR)

3. pertaining to under the tongue

_____ sub _/_ lingu _/_ al _____
　　　　　P　　WR　　S

4. pertaining to the nose and stomach

_____ nas _/_ o _/_ gastr _/_ ic _____
　　　WR　　CV　　WR　　S

5. pertaining to the mouth and stomach

_____ stomat _/_ o _/_ gastr _/_ ic _____
　　　WR　　CV　　WR　　S

6. pertaining to the anus

          an | al
          WR    S

7. surgical puncture to remove fluid from the abdominal cavity

          abdomin | o | centesis
          WR   CV   S

8. pertaining to the peritoneum

          peritone | al
          WR    S

9. pertaining to the abdomen

          abdomin | al
          WR    S

10. difficult swallowing

          dys | phagia
          P    S(WR)

11. pertaining to the ileum and cecum

          ile | o | cec | al
          WR  CV  WR  S

12. slow digestion

          brady | pepsia
          P    S(WR)

13. softening of the stomach

          gastr | o | malacia
          WR  CV  S

14. without (lack of) digestion

          a | pepsia
          P    S(WR)

15. pain in the stomach

          gastro | dynia
          WR    S

16. physician who specializes in proctology

          proctol | ogist
          WR    S

17. difficult digestion

          dys | pepsia
          P    S(WR)

18. pertaining to the pancreas

     *pancreat / ic*
        WR     S

19. branch of medicine concerned with disease of the rectum and anus

     *proct / ology*
        WR     S

20. pertaining to the mouth

     *or / al*
        WR     S

## EXERCISE 26

Spell each of the additional terms. Have someone dictate the terms on pp. 398 and 399 to you or say the words into a tape recorder; then spell the words from your recording as often as necessary. Think about the word parts before attempting to write the word. Study any you have spelled incorrectly.

1. _____
2. _____
3. _____
4. _____
5. _____
6. _____
7. _____
8. _____
9. _____
10. _____

11. _____
12. _____
13. _____
14. _____
15. _____
16. _____
17. _____
18. _____
19. _____
20. _____

Place a check mark (√) in the box to indicate that you have completed Objective 9.

☐ BUILD, ANALYZE, DEFINE, PRONOUNCE, AND SPELL ADDITIONAL TERMS RELATED TO THE DIGESTIVE SYSTEM.

# Objective 10    DEFINE, PRONOUNCE, AND SPELL THE OTHER ADDITIONAL TERMS RELATED TO THE DIGESTIVE SYSTEM.

## Other Additional Terms

**TERM**

1. ascites . . . . . . . . . . . . . . .
   (a-SĪ-tēz)

**DEFINITION**

abnormal collection of fluid in the peritoneal cavity

2. **diarrhea** . . . . . . . . . . . . .   frequent discharge of liquid stool
   (dī-a-RĒ-a)
   (NOTE: Diarrhea composed of *dia* meaning through and *orrhea* meaning flow. The "o" is dropped.)

3. **dysentery** . . . . . . . . . . . .   disorder that involves inflammation of
   (DIS-en-ter-ē)                          the intestine associated with diarrhea
                                           and abdominal pain

4. **feces** . . . . . . . . . . . . . . .   waste from the digestive tract expelled
   (FĒ-sēz)                                 through the rectum (also called a *bowel
                                            movement* or *stool*)

5. **flatus**. . . . . . . . . . . . . . .   gas in the digestive tract or expelled
   (FLĀ-tus)                                 through the anus

6. **gavage** . . . . . . . . . . . . . .   process of feeding a person through a
   (ga-VOZH)                                 nasogastric tube

7. **gastric lavage** . . . . . . . . . .   washing out of the stomach
   (la-VOZH)

8. **nausea** . . . . . . . . . . . . . .   urge to vomit
   (NAW-zē-a)

9. **vomit** . . . . . . . . . . . . . . .   matter expelled from the stomach
   (VOM-it)                                  through the mouth

Practice saying each of these terms aloud. To assist you in pronunciation, obtain the audiotape designed for use with this text. Learn the definitions and spellings of the terms by completing the following exercises.

## EXERCISE 27

Match the definitions in the first column with the correct terms in the second column.

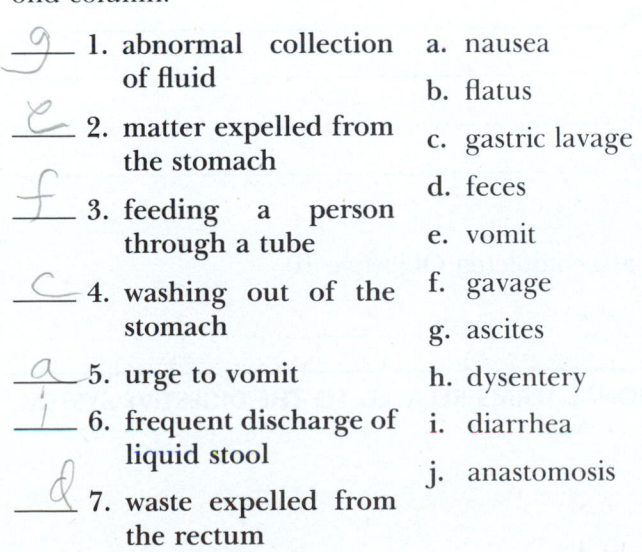

_g_ 1. abnormal collection of fluid

_e_ 2. matter expelled from the stomach

_f_ 3. feeding a person through a tube

_c_ 4. washing out of the stomach

_a_ 5. urge to vomit

_i_ 6. frequent discharge of liquid stool

_d_ 7. waste expelled from the rectum

a. nausea

b. flatus

c. gastric lavage

d. feces

e. vomit

f. gavage

g. ascites

h. dysentery

i. diarrhea

j. anastomosis

———— 8. inflammation of the
     intestine

———— 9. gas expelled through
     the anus

## EXERCISE 28

Write definitions for each of the following terms.

1. ascites _____

2. gavage _____

3. gastric lavage _____

4. feces _____

5. nausea _____

6. vomit _____

7. dysentery _____

8. diarrhea _____

9. flatus _____

## EXERCISE 29

Spell each of the other additional terms. Have someone dictate the terms
on pp. 402 and 403 to you or say the words into a tape recorder; then
spell the words from your recording as often as necessary. Study any you
have spelled incorrectly.

1. _____    6. _____
2. _____    7. _____
3. _____    8. _____
4. _____    9. _____
5. _____

Place a check mark (√) in the box to indicate that you have completed Objective 10.

☐ DEFINE, PRONOUNCE, AND SPELL THE OTHER ADDITIONAL TERMS RELATED TO THE DIGESTIVE SYSTEM.

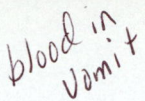
*blood in vomit*

**Case History:** This is a 40-year-old African-American female who was referred to endoscopy clinic for evaluation. Patient complains of persistent nausea and vomiting with upper abdominal pain. She has also had a problem with dyspepsia but denies any hematemesis. She has not used any alcohol or salicylates. She is currently on several medications but they do not appear to be ulcerogenic.

**Esophagogastroduodenoscopy:** the patient was prepared for the procedure by being given 2 mg of intravenous Versed along with Hurricaine spray. After the patient was placed in the left lateral decubitus position the Olympus gastroscope was passed into the esophagus without any difficulty. The esophagus in its entirety was essentially free of mucosal abnormalities. No evidence of reflux. The stomach was entered; some gastric juices were aspirated. The stomach, the body, the cardia, and antrum, proximally, were all free of mucosal abnormalities. In the distal antral area some mild erythematous changes were noted. The pylorus had normal peristaltic activity in opening. The first part of the duodenum, however, revealed evidence of ulcerations, both anterosuperiorly as well as posteroinferiorly, with surrounding tissue irritation noted. These ulcers were less than 1 mm in size. The second part of the duodenum, however, was free of mucosal abnormalities. Withdrawing the scope confirmed the findings upon entry. The patient, in fact, tolerated the procedure quite well. Vital signs will be taken every half hour for the next two hours.

**Postop Diagnosis:** Gastritis. Duodenal ulcerations.

## EXERCISE 30

To test your understanding of the terms introduced in this chapter, circle the words that correctly complete the sentences. The italicized words refer to the correct answer.

1. Mr. E. was admitted to the hospital with a diagnosis of *gallstones,* or (cholelithiasis, cholecystitis, sialolithiasis).
2. To confirm the diagnosis, his physician ordered an *x-ray film of his gallbladder,* or (GI series, cholecystography, cholecystogram).
3. The x-ray film confirmed the admitting diagnosis, and Mr. E. is now scheduled for an *excision of the gallbladder,* or (cholecystostomy, cholecystectomy, colectomy).
4. A *prolapse of the rectum* is (rectocele, intussusception, proctoptosis).
5. An *abnormal growing together of two surfaces* is (anastomosis, adhesion, amniocentesis).
6. Three surgical procedures are often performed on a patient with peptic ulcers: they are (a) *excision of the stomach,* or (gastrotomy, gastrostomy, gastrectomy); (b) *surgical repair of the pylorus,* or (pyloroplasty, cheilorrhaphy, gastrojejunostomy); and (c) *cutting of certain branches of the vagus nerve,* or (colostomy, vagotomy, gingivectomy).
7. *Difficult digestion* is (dyspepsia, bradypepsia, dysphagia).
8. *Feeding* a person *through a gastric tube* is called (lavage, gavage, gastrostomy).
9. The *surgical procedure to remove the colon and rectum and create an artificial opening into the colon* is (colectomy and colostomy; abdominal perineal resection and colostomy; abdominal perineal resection and ileostomy).

10. *Surgical crushing of a stone in the common bile duct* is (choledocholithot-
    ripsy, cholangiolithotripsy, cholecystolithotripsy).
11. To rule out cancer of the colon, the doctor performed a diagnostic
    procedure to *visually examine the colon* or (colonoscopy, colonoscope,
    colostomy).
12. The doctor diagnosed the patient as having *an obstruction of the intes-
    tine* or (polyp, irritable bowel syndrome, ileus).

## EXERCISE 31

Unscramble the following mixed-up terms. The words on the left indicate the *suffix* in each of the following.

1. suture

/ / /e/ / / / / / / / /h/ /
i r y r c l p a h h h e o

2. creation of an artificial
   opening

/ /l/ / / / / / / /
t i l m o y s o e

3. excision

/ / /n/ / /v/ / / / / / /
t g e v i n i g o y m c

4. softening

/ / /s/ / / /m/ / / / / / /
t s a g a i c l a r o m a

5. swallowing

/ / /s/ / / / / / /
d a p g y i s a h

6. digestion

/ /p/ / / / / /
p s p a a e i

7. surgical repair

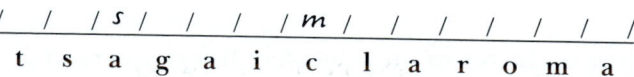

/ /v/ / / / / / / / /
y s n y h p p u v o l
/p/ / / / / / / / / / /
l a t o r a g p o l a a t

## EXERCISE 32

Test your knowledge on diagnostic procedural terms by circling the letter of each correct answer.

1. The physician did a visual examination of the vagina and cervix to note changes in the cells and capillary network. The procedure takes 10 minutes and is called a
   a. coloscopy
   b. colposcope
   c. sigmoidoscope
   d. colposcopy
   e. coloscope

2. The physician ordered x-ray films of the large intestine to rule out the presence of a tumor. He or she ordered a(n)
   a. upper GI series
   b. mammogram
   c. cholecystogram
   d. intravenous pyelogram
   e. barium enema

3. The patient was experiencing hematuria. To locate and control the source of the bleeding the doctor performed a
   a. bronchoscopy
   b. culdoscopy
   c. cystoscopy
   d. proctoscopy
   e. gastroscopy

4. The patient was scheduled for an x-ray film of a blood vessel, or
   a. arteriogram
   b. angiogram
   c. aortogram
   d. venogram
   e. nephrogram

5. A record of the electrical impulses of the heart is a(n)
   a. electrocardiogram
   b. echocardiogram
   c. electrocardiograph
   d. phonocardiograph
   e. electrocardiography

# COMBINING FORMS CROSSWORD PUZZLE

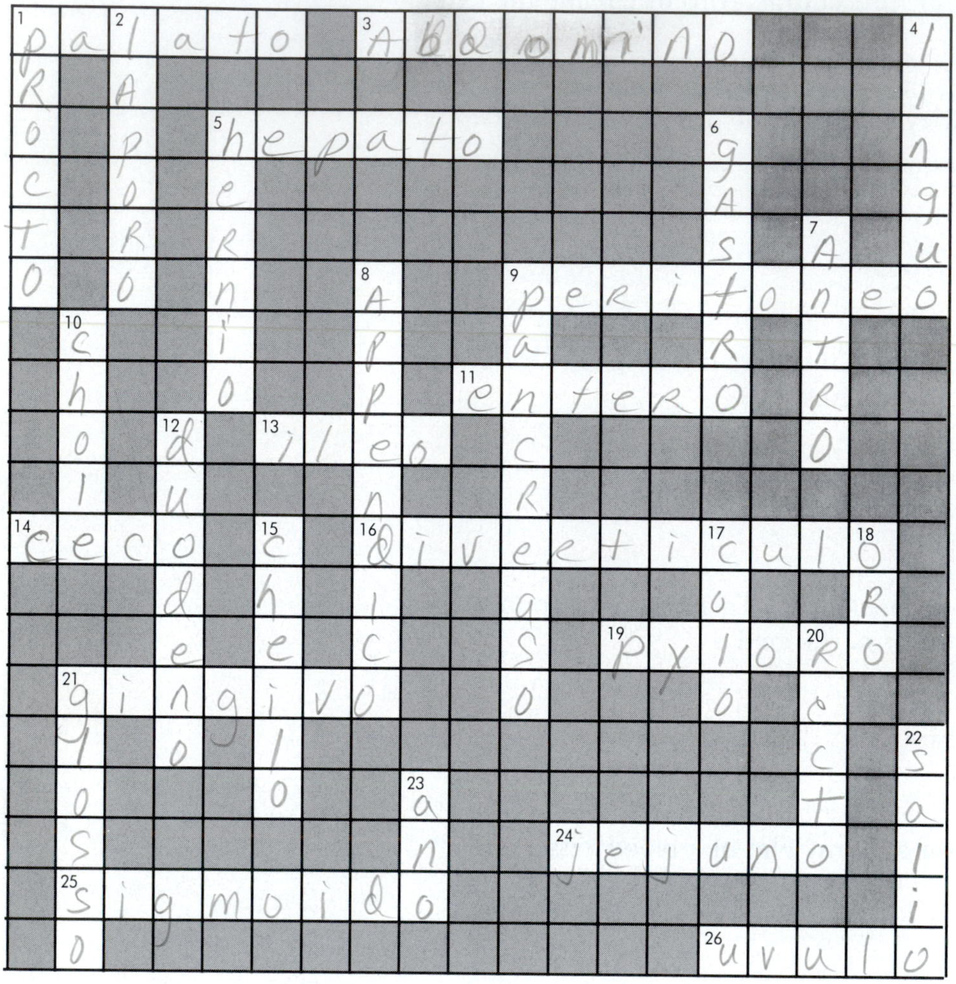

The crossword grid contains the following handwritten answers:

- Across 1: palato
- Across 3: ABDOMINO
- Across 5: hepato
- Across 9: peritoneo
- Across 11: entero
- Across 13: ileo
- Across 14: ceco
- Across 16: diveticulo
- Across 19: pyloro
- Across 21: gingivo
- Across 24: jejuno
- Across 25: sigmoido
- Across 26: uvulo
- Down 1: procto
- Down 2: palato
- Down 4: linguo
- Down 6: gastro
- Down 7: antro
- Down 9: pancreato
- Down 10: choli
- Down 12: duedeno
- Down 15: chilo
- Down 17: colo
- Down 18: R
- Down 20: recto
- Down 21: gloso
- Down 22: salai
- Down 23: ano

## Across Clues

1. palate
3. abdomen
5. liver
9. peritoneum
11. intestine
13. ileum
14. cecum
16. diverticulum
19. pylorus
21. gum
24. jejunum
25. sigmoid
26. uvula

## Down Clues

1. rectum
2. abdomen
4. tongue
5. hernia
6. stomach
7. antrum
8. appendix
9. pancreas
10. gall, bile
12. duodenum
15. lip
17. colon
18. mouth
20. rectum
21. tongue
22. saliva
23. anus

# Summary

Can you build, analyze, define, spell, and pronounce the following terms *built from word parts?*   yes ☐   no ☐

| DIAGNOSTIC | SURGICAL | PROCEDURAL | ADDITIONAL |
|---|---|---|---|
| appendicitis (ap-*pen*-di-SĪ-tis) | abdominoplasty (ab-DOM-i-nō-plas-tē) | cholangiogram (kō-LAN-je-ō-gram) | abdominal (ab-DOM-i-nal) |
| cholangioma (kō-lan-jē-Ō-ma) | anoplasty (Ā-nō-*plas*-tē) | cholecystogram (kō-lē-SĪS-tō-gram) | abdominocentesis (ab-*dom*-i-nō-sen-TĒ-sis) |
| cholecystitis (*kō*-lē-sis-TĪ-tis) | antrectomy (an-TREK-tō-mē) | colonoscope (kō-LON-ō-skōp) | anal (Ā-nal) |
| choledocholithiasis (kō-led-ō-kō-lith-Ī-a-sis) | appendectomy (*ap*-en-DEK-tō-mē) | colonoscopy (kō-lon-OS-kō-pē) | apepsia (a-PEP-sē-a) |
| cholelithiasis (*kō*-lē-lith-Ī-a-sis) | celiotomy (sē-lē-OT-ō-mē) | endoscope (EN-dō-skōp) | aphagia (a-FĀ-jē-a) |
| diverticulitis (*dī*-ver-tik-ū-LĪ-tis) | cheilorrhaphy (kī-LOR-a-fē) | endoscopy (en-DOS-kō-pē) | bradypepsia (*brād*-ē-PEP-sē-a) |
| diverticulosis (*dī*-ver-tik-ū-LŌ-sis) | cholecystectomy (*kō*-lē-sis-TEK-tō-mē) | esophagogastro-duodenoscopy (ē-*sof*-a-gō *gas*-trō-dū-od-e-NOS-kō-pē) | dyspepsia (dis-PEP-sē-a) |
| gastritis (gas-TRĪ-tis) | choledocholithotomy (kō-led-ō-kō-li-THOT-ō-mē) | esophagoscope (ē-SOF-a-gō-skōp) | dysphagia (dis-FĀ-jē-a) |
| gastroenteritis (*gas*-trō-en-te-RĪ-tis) | choledocholithotripsy (kō-led-ō-kō-LITH-ō-trip-sē) | esophagoscopy (ē-*sof*-a-GOS-kō-pē) | gastrodynia (*gas*-trō-DĬN-ē-a) |
| gastroenterocolitis (gas-trō-*en*-ter-ō-kō-LĪ-tis) | colectomy (kō-LEK-tō-mē) | gastroscope (GAS-trō-skōp) | gastromalacia (*gas*-trō-ma-LĀ-shē-a) |
| gingivitis (jin-ji̧-VĪ-tis) | colostomy (kō-LOS-tō-mē) | gastroscopy (gas-TROS-kō-pē) | glossopathy (glo-SOP-a-thē) |
| hepatitis (hep-a-TĪ-tis) | diverticulectomy (*dī*-ver-tik-ū-LEK-tō-mē) | laparoscope (LAP-a-rō-skōp) | ileocecal (*il*-ē-ō-SĒ-kal) |
| hepatoma (hep-a-TŌ-ma) | enterorrhaphy (en-ter-ŌR-a-fē) | laparoscopy (lap-a-ROS-kō-pē) | nasogastric (*nā*-zō-GAS-trik) |
| palatitis (pal-a-TĪ-tis) | esophagogastroplasty (ē-*sof*-a-gō-GAS-trō-plas-tē) | proctoscope (PROK-tō-skōp) | oral (Ō-ral) |
| pancreatitis (*pan*-krē-a-TĪ-tis) | gastrectomy (gas-TREK-tō-mē) | proctoscopy (prok-TOS-kō-pē) | pancreatic (*pan*-krē-AT-ik) |
| polyposis (pol-ē-PŌ-sis) | gastrojejunostomy (*gas*-trō-je-jū-NOS-tō-mē) | sigmoidoscope (sig-MOY-dō-skōp) | peritoneal (*pēr*-i-tō-NĒ-al) |
| proctoptosis (*prok*-top-TŌ-sis) | gastrostomy (gas-TROS-tō-mē) | sigmoidoscopy (*sig*-moy-DOS-kō-pē) | proctologist (prok-TOL-ō-jist) |
| rectocele (REK-tō-sēl) | gingivectomy (*jin*-ji-VEK-tō-mē) | | proctology (prok-TOL-ō-jē) |
| sialolith (sī-AL-ō-lith) | glossorrhaphy (glo-SŌR-a-fē) | | stomatogastric (*stō*-ma-tō-GAS-trik) |
| uvulitis (ū-vū-LĪ-tis) | | | sublingual (sub-LING-gwal) |

**SURGICAL   cont'd**

herniorrhaphy
(her-nē-ŌR-a-fē)

ileostomy
(il-ē-OS-tŏ-mē)

laparotomy
(lap-a-ROT-ŏ-mē)

palatoplasty
(PAL-a-tō-plas-tē)

polypectomy
(pol-ē-PEK-tō-mē)

pyloromyotomy
(pī-lor-ŏ-mī-OT-ŏ-mē)

pyloroplasty
(pī-LOR-ō-plas-tē)

uvulectomy
(ū-vū-LEK-tŏ-mē)

uvulopalatopharyngo-
plasty
(ū-vū-lŏ-pal-a-tō-phar-in-
GO-plast-tē)

# Summary

Can you define, pronounce, and spell the following terms *not built from word parts?*   yes ☐   no ☐

| DIAGNOSTIC | SURGICAL | PROCEDURAL | ADDITIONAL |
|---|---|---|---|
| adhesion<br>(ad-HĒ-zhun) | abdominoperineal<br>   resection<br>(ab-dom-in-ŏ-pēr-i-NĒ-el) | endoscopic retrograde<br>   cholangiopancreato-<br>   graphy<br>(kŏ-lan-jē-ŏ-pan-krē-a-TOG-<br>ra-fē) | ascites<br>(a-SĪ-tēz) |
| anorexia nervosa<br>(an-ŏ-REK-sē-a)<br>(ner-VŎ-sa) | anastomosis<br>(a-nas-tŏ-MŎ-sis) | | diarrhea<br>(dī-a-RĒ-a) |
| bulimia<br>(bu-LIM-ē-a) | vagotomy<br>(va-GOT-ŏ-mē) | lower GI<br>(gastrointestinal series)<br>upper GI<br>(gastrointestinal series) | dysentery<br>(DIS-en-ter-ē) |
| cirrhosis<br>(ser-RŎ-sis) | | | feces<br>(FĒ-sēz) |
| Crohn's disease<br>(krŏnz) | | | flatus<br>(FLĀ-tus) |
| duodenal ulcer<br>(dū-o-DĒ-nal) | | | gavage<br>(ga-VOZH) |
| gastric ulcer<br>(GAS-trik) | | | gastric lavage<br>(la-VOZH) |

## DIAGNOSTIC   cont'd

ileus
(IL-ē-us)

intussusception
(*in*-tus-sus-SEP-shun)

irritable bowel
syndrome
peptic ulcer
(PEP-tik)

polyp
(POL-ip)

ulcerative colitis
(UL-ser-a-tiv) (kol-LĪ-tis)

volvulus
(VOL-vū-lus)

## ADDITIONAL   cont'd

nausea
(NAW-zē-a)

vomit
(VOM-it)

# Answers

## Exercise 1

1. alimentary canal
2. gastrointestinal tract
3. pharynx
4. esophagus
5. stomach
6. duodenum
7. jejunum
8. ileum
9. cecum
10. ascending colon
11. transverse colon
12. descending colon
13. sigmoid colon
14. rectum
15. anus

## Exercise 2

| | | | |
|---|---|---|---|
| 1. l | 4. h | 7. b | 10. g |
| 2. d | 5. f | 8. i | 11. e |
| 3. a | 6. j | 9. c | |

## Exercise 3

### Figure 10-1

Mouth: stomat/o, or/o
Esophagus: esophag/o
Duodenum: duoden/o
Ascending colon: col/o
Cecum: cec/o
Anus: an/o
Pharynx: pharyng/o
Stomach: gastr/o

Antrum: antr/o
Transverse colon: col/o
Descending colon: col/o
Jejunum: jejun/o
Ileum: ile/o
Sigmoid colon: sigmoid/o
Rectum: proct/o, rect/o

## Exercise 4

1. rectum
2. stomach
3. anus
4. cecum
5. ileum
6. mouth
7. duodenum
8. colon
9. mouth
10. intestines
11. rectum
12. antrum
13. esophagus
14. jejunum
15. sigmoid colon

## Exercise 5

1. cec/o
2. gastr/o
3. ile/o
4. jejun/o
5. sigmoid/o
6. esophag/o
7. a. rect/o
   b. proct/o
8. enter/o
9. duoden/o
10. col/o
11. a. or/o
    b. stomat/o
12. an/o
13. antr/o

## Exercise 6

### Figure 10-2

Gums: gingiv/o
Lips: cheil/o
Salivary glands: sial/o
Liver: hepat/o
Gall bladder: chol/e (gall)
              cyst/o (blad-
              der)
Pyloric sphincter: pylor/o
Appendix: appendic/o

Palate: palat/o
Uvula: uvul/o
Tongue: gloss/o, lingu/o
Bile duct: cholangi/o
Common bile duct:
   choledoch/o
Pancreas: pancreat/o
Abdomen: lapar/o,
         abdomin/o
         cei/o

## Exercise 7

1. hernia
2. abdomen
3. saliva
4. gall, bile
5. diverticulum
6. gum
7. appendix
8. tongue
9. liver
10. lip
11. peritoneum
12. palate
13. pancreas
14. abdomen
15. tongue
16. common bile duct
17. pylorus
18. uvula
19. bile duct
20. polyp, small growth
21. abdomen

## Exercise 8

1. palat/o
2. sial/o
3. pancreat/o
4. peritone/o
5. a. lingu/o
   b. gloss/o
6. gingiv/o
7. pylor/o
8. hepat/o
9. chol/e
10. a. abdomin/o
    b. lapar/o
    c. celi/o
11. herni/o
12. diverticul/o
13. cheil/o
14. appendic/o
15. uvul/o
16. cholangi/o
17. choledoch/o
18. polyp/o

## Exercise 9

1. 
   WR CV WR S
   chol/ e /lith/iasis
        CF
   condition of gallstones

2. 
   WR      S
   diverticul/osis
   abnormal condition of
   having diverticula

3. 
   WR CV WR
   sial/ o /lith
        CF
   salivary stone

4. 
   WR   S
   hepat/oma
   tumor of the liver

5. 
   WR   S
   uvul/itis
   inflammation of the uvula

6. 
   WR      S
   pancreat/tis
   inflammation of the pancreas

7. 
   WR  CV   S
   proct/ o /ptosis
        CF
   prolapse of the rectum

8. 
   WR    S
   gingiv/itis
   inflammation of the gums

9. 
   WR   S
   gastr/itis
   inflammation of the stomach

10. 
    WR  CV   S
    rect/ o /cele
         CF
    protrusion of the rectum

11. 
    WR   S
    palat/itis
    inflammation of the pal-
    ate

12. 
    WR   S
    hepat/itis
    inflammation of the liver

13. 
    WR      S
    appendic/itis
    inflammation of the ap-
    pendix

14. 
    WR CV WR  S
    chol/ e /cyst/itis
         CF
    inflammation of the gall-
    bladder

15. 
    WR      S
    diverticul/itis
    inflammation of a diver-
    ticulum

16. 
    WR CV WR  S
    gastr/ o /enter/itis
         CF
    inflammation of the stom-
    ach and intestines

17. 
    WR  CV  WR  CV WR S
    gastr/ o /enter/ o /col/itis
         CF        CF
    inflammation of the stom-
    ach, intestines, and co-
    lon

18. 
    WR      CV WR  S
    choledoch/ o /lith/iasis
            CF
    condition of stones in the
    common bile duct

19. 
    WR     S
    cholangi/oma
    tumor of the bile duct

20. 
    WR   S
    polyp/osis
    abnormal condition of
    (multiple) polyps

## Exercise 10

1. hepat/oma
2. gastr/itis
3. sial/o/lith
4. appendic/itis
5. diverticul/itis
6. chol/e/cyst/itis
7. diverticul/osis
8. gastr/o/enter/itis
9. proct/o/ptosis
10. rect/o/cele
11. uvul/itis
12. gingiv/itis
13. hepat/itis
14. palat/itis
15. chol/e/lith/iasis
16. gastr/o/enter/o/col/itis
17. pancreat/itis
18. cholangi/oma
19. choledoch/o/lith/iasis
20. polyp/osis

## Exercise 11

Spelling exercise; *see* text, pp. 378, 379.

## Exercise 12

1. f   3. e   5. d   7. a   9. h   11. m
2. b   4. c   6. g   8. k   10. j  12. i

## Exercise 13

1. another name for gastric or duodenal ulcer
2. psychoneurotic disorder characterized by a prolonged refusal to eat
3. chronic inflammation of the small and/or large intestines
4. twisting or kinking of the intestine
5. abnormal growing together of two surfaces that normally are separated
6. chronic disease of the liver with gradual destruction of cells
7. telescoping of segment of the intestine
8. ulcer in the stomach
9. ulcer in the duodenum
10. inflammation of the colon with the formation of ulcers
11. gorging food then inducing vomiting
12. tumor-like growth extending out from a mucous membrane
13. disturbance of bowel function
14. obstruction of the intestine, often caused by failure of peristalsis

## Exercise 14

Spelling exercise; *see* text, p. 382.

## Exercise 15

WR　S
1. gastr/ectomy　　　　　excision of the stomach

WR　CV　WR　CV
2. esophag/ o /gastr/ o /　surgical repair of the
　　　CF　　　CF　　　　esophagus and the
　S　　　　　　　　　　stomach
plasty

WR　　S
3. diverticul/ectomy　　　excision of a diverticulum

WR　　S
4. antr/ectomy　　　　　excision of the antrum

WR　CV　S
5. palat/ o /plasty　　　　surgical repair of the pal-
　　CF　　　　　　　　ate

WR　　S
6. uvul/ectomy　　　　　excision of the uvula

WR　CV　WR　　S
7. gastr/ o /jejun/ostomy　creation of an artificial
　　CF　　　　　　　　opening between the
　　　　　　　　　　　stomach and the jeju-
　　　　　　　　　　　num

WR　CV　WR　　S
8. chol/ e /cyst/ectomy　　excision of the gallblad-
　　CF　　　　　　　　der

WR　　S
9. col/ectomy　　　　　excision of the colon

WR　　S
10. col/ostomy　　　　　creation of an artificial
　　　　　　　　　　　opening into the colon

WR　CV　S
11. pylor/ o /plasty　　　surgical repair of the py-
　　CF　　　　　　　　lorus

WR CV　S
12. an/ o /plasty　　　　surgical repair of the
　　CF　　　　　　　　anus

WR　　S
13. append/ectomy　　　excision of the appendix

WR　　S
14. cheil/orrhaphy　　　suture of the lips

WR　　S
15. gingiv/ectomy　　　surgical removal of gum
　　　　　　　　　　　tissue

WR　　S
16. lapar/otomy　　　　incision into the abdomi-
　　　　　　　　　　　nal wall

WR　　S
17. ile /ostomy　　　　　creation of an artificial
　　　　　　　　　　　opening into the ileum

WR　　S
18. gastr/ostomy　　　　creation of an artificial
　　　　　　　　　　　opening into the stom-
　　　　　　　　　　　ach

WR　　S
19. herni/orrhaphy　　　suturing of a hernia

WR　　S
20. gloss/orrhaphy　　　suture of the tongue

WR　CV WR
21. choledoch/ o /lith/　　incision into the common
　　　CF　　　　　　　bile duct to remove a
　S　　　　　　　　　stone
otomy

WR　CV WR CV
22. choledoch/ o /lith/ o /　surgical crushing of a
　　　CF　　　CF　　　stone in the common
　S　　　　　　　　　bile duct
tripsy

WR　　S
23. polyp/ectomy　　　excision of a polyp

WR　　S
24. enter/orrhaphy　　　suture of the intestine

WR　CV　S
25. abdomin/ o /plasty　　plastic repair of the ab-
　　　CF　　　　　　　domen

WR　CV WR　　S
26. pylor/ o /my/otomy　　incision into the
　　　CF　　　　　　　pylorus muscle

WR　CV　WR CV
27. uvul/ o /palat/ o /　　surgical repair
　　CF　　　CF　　　　of the uvula, palate,
WR　　CV　S　　　　and pharynx
pharyng/ o /plasty
　　　CF

WR　　S
28. celi/otomy　　　　incision into the
　　　　　　　　　　abdominal cavity

## Exercise 16

1. append/ectomy
2. gloss/orrhaphy
3. esophag/o/gastr/o/
　　plasty
4. diverticul/ectomy
5. ile/ostomy
6. gingiv/ectomy
7. lapar/otomy
8. an/o/plasty
9. antr/ectomy
10. chol/e/cyst/ectomy
11. col/ectomy
12. col/ostomy
13. gastr/ectomy
14. gastr/ostomy
15. gastr/o/jejun/ostomy

16. uvul/ectomy
17. palat/o/plasty
18. pylor/o/plasty
19. herni/orrhaphy
20. cheil/orrhaphy
21. choledoch/o/lith/o/
　　tripsy
22. choledoch/o/lith/
　　otomy
23. polyp/ectomy
24. enter/orrhaphy
25. abdomin/o/plasty
26. celi/otomy
27. pylor/o/my/o/tomy
28. uvul/o/palat/o/
　　pharyng/o/plasty

## Exercise 17

Spelling exercise; *see* text, p. 389.

## Exercise 18

1. vagotomy
2. anastomosis
3. abdominoperineal resection

## Exercise 19

Spelling exercise, *see* text, p. 390.

## Exercise 20

1. WR CV S
   esophag/ o /scope — instrument used for visual examination of the esophagus
   CF

2. WR CV S
   esophag/ o /scopy — visual examination of the esophagus
   CF

3. WR CV S
   gastr/ o /scope — instrument used for visual examination of the stomach
   CF

4. WR CV S
   gastr/ o /scopy — visual examination of the stomach
   CF

5. WR CV S
   proct/ o /scope — instrument used for visual examination of the rectum
   CF

6. WR CV S
   proct/ o /scopy — visual examination of the rectum
   CF

7. P S(WR)
   endo/scope — instrument used for visual examination within a hollow organ

8. P S(WR)
   endo/scopy — visual examination within a hollow organ

9. WR CV S
   sigmoid/ o /scope — instrument used for visual examination of the sigmoid colon
   CF

10. WR CV S
    sigmoid/ o /scopy — visual examination of the sigmoid colon
    CF

11. WR CV WR CV
    chol/ e /cyst/ o / — x-ray film of the gallbladder
    CF       CF
    S
    gram

12. WR CV S
    cholangi/ o /gram — x-ray film of bile ducts
    CF

13. WR CV WR
    esophag/ o /gastr/ — visual examination of the esophagus, stomach and duodenum
    CF       CF
    CV WR CV
    o /duoden/ o /
    CF
    S
    scopy

14. WR CV S
    colon/ o /scope — instrument used for visual examination of the colon
    CF

15. WR CV S
    lapar/ o /scope — instrument used for visual examination of the abdominal cavity
    CF

16. WR CV S
    colon/ o /scopy — visual examination of the colon
    CF

17. WR CV S
    lapar/ o /scopy — visual examination of the abdominal cavity
    CF

## Exercise 21

1. endo/scopy
2. gastr/o/scope
3. proct/o/scope
4. sigmoid/o/scope
5. chol/e/cyst/o/gram
6. endo/scope
7. esophag/o/scope
8. proct/o/scopy
9. esophag/o/scopy
10. sigmoid/o/scopy
11. cholangi/o/gram
12. gastr/o/scopy
13. lapar/o/scope
14. esophag/o/gastr/o/duoden/o/scopy
15. colon/o/scopy
16. lapar/o/scopy
17. colon/o/scope

## Exercise 22

1. series of x-ray films taken of the stomach and duodenum after barium has been swallowed
2. series of x-ray films taken of the large intestine after a barium enema has been administered
3. x-ray examination of the bile and pancreatic ducts

## Exercise 23

Spelling exercise; *see* text, p. 398.

## Exercise 24

```
     P   S(WR)
```
1. a/phagia                     inability to swallow
```
     P   S(WR)
```
2. dys/pepsia                   difficult digestion
```
     WR  S
```
3. an/al                        pertaining to the anus
```
     P   S(WR)
```
4. dys/phagia                   difficult swallowing
```
     WR  CV   S
```
5. gloss/ o /pathy              disease of the tongue
```
          CF
```
```
     WR  CV WR S
```
6. ile/ o /cec/al               pertaining to the ileum
```
          CF
```
                                and cecum
```
     WR  S
```
7. or /al                       pertaining to the mouth
```
     WR   CV  WR S
```
8. stomat/ o /gastr/ic          pertaining to the mouth
```
          CF
```
                                and stomach
```
     P   S(WR)
```
9. brady/pepsia                 slow digestion
```
     WR   CV    S
```
10. abdomin/ o /centesis         surgical puncture to re-
```
          CF
```
                                move fluid from the
                                abdominal cavity
```
     P   S(WR)
```
11. a/pepsia                     lack of digestion
```
     WR  CV    S
```
12. gastr/ o /malacia            softening of the stomach
```
          CF
```
```
     WR    S
```
13. pancreat/ic                  pertaining to the pan-
                                creas
```
     WR    S
```
14. gastr/odynia                 pain in the stomach
```
     WR    S
```
15. peritone/al                  pertaining to the perito-
                                neum
```
     P   WR  S
```
16. sub/lingu/al                 pertaining to under the
                                tongue

```
     WR   S
```
17. proct/ology                  branch of medicine con-
                                cerned with disorders
                                of the rectum and
                                anus
```
     WR CV  WR  S
```
18. nas/ o /gastr/ic             pertaining to the nose
```
          CF
```
                                and stomach
```
     WR     S
```
19. abdomin/al                   pertaining to the abdo-
                                men
```
     WR    S
```
20. proct/ologist                physician who special-
                                izes in proctology

## Exercise 25

1. gloss/o/pathy
2. a/phagia
3. sub/lingu/al
4. nas/o/gastr/ic
5. stomat/o/gastr/ic
6. an/al
7. abdomin/o/centesis
8. peritone/al
9. abdomin/al
10. dys/phagia
11. ile/o/cec/al
12. brady/pepsia
13. gastr/o/malacia
14. a/pepsia
15. gastr/odynia
16. proct/ologist
17. dys/pepsia
18. pancreat/ic
19. proct/ology
20. or/al

## Exercise 26

Spelling exercise; *see* text, p. 402.

## Exercise 27

1. g    3. f    5. a    7. d    9. b
2. e    4. c    6. i    8. h

## Exercise 28

1. abnormal collection of fluid in the peritoneal cavity
2. process of feeding a person through a nasogastric tube
3. washing out of the stomach
4. waste from the digestive tract expelled through the rectum
5. urge to vomit
6. matter expelled from the stomach through the mouth
7. disorder that involves inflammation of the intestine
8. frequent discharge of liquid stool
9. gas expelled through the anus

## Exercise 29

Spelling exercise; *see* text, p. 404.

## Exercise 30

1. cholelithiasis
2. cholecystogram
3. cholecystectomy
4. proctoptosis
5. adhesion
6. gastrectomy; pyloro-plasty; vagotomy
7. dyspepsia
8. gavage
9. abdominal perineal resection and colostomy
10. choledocholithotripsy
11. colonoscopy
12. ileus

## Exercise 31

1. cheilorrhaphy
2. ileostomy
3. gingivectomy
4. gastromalacia
5. dysphagia
6. apepsia
7. uvulopalatopharyngo-plasty

## Exercise 32

1. d  2. e  3. c  4. b  5. a

# Answers

```
P A L A T O   A B D O M I N O         L
R   A                                 I
O   P   H E P A T O         G         N
C   A   E                   A   A     G
T   R   R             S   A         U
O   O   N       A   P E R I T O N E O
  C     I       P       A     R   T
  H     O   P   E N T E R O     R
  O   D   I L E O   C         O
  L   U     N       R
C E C O   C   D I V E R T I C U L O
    D   H   I       A       A   R
    E   E   C       T   P Y L O R O
G I N G I V O       O       O   E
  L   O   L                     C   S
  O     O     A             T   I
  S       N       J E J U N O   A
S I G M O I D O                 L
O                       U V U L O
```

# 11

# Eye

## Objectives

Upon completion of this chapter you will be able to:

1. Define the anatomical terms of the eye.

2. Write the definitions of the word parts included in this chapter.

3. Build, analyze, define, pronounce, and spell the diagnostic terms related to the eye.

4. Define, pronounce, and spell other diagnostic terms related to the eye.

5. Build, analyze, define, pronounce, and spell the surgical terms related to the eye.

6. Define, pronounce, and spell other surgical terms related to the eye.

7. Build, analyze, define, pronounce, and spell the diagnostic procedural terms related to the eye.

8. Build, analyze, define, pronounce, and spell additional terms related to the eye.

9. Define, pronounce, and spell the other additional terms related to the eye.

## Objective 1   DEFINE THE ANATOMICAL TERMS RELATED TO THE EYE.

## Anatomical Terms

The eye is located in a bony protective cavity of the skull called the *orbit*.

### PARTS OF THE EYE (FIGURE 11-1)

| | | |
|---|---|---|
| 1. | sclera . . . . . . . . . . . . . . | Outer protective layer of the eye; anteriorly referred to as the white of the eye. |
| | a. cornea . . . . . . . . . . . | Transparent anterior part of the sclera, which lies over the iris. |
| 2. | choroid. . . . . . . . . . . . . | Middle layer of the eye, which is interlaced with many blood vessels. |
| | a. iris . . . . . . . . . . . . . | Muscular structure that gives the eye its color. |
| | b. pupil . . . . . . . . . | Opening in the center of the iris. |
| | c. lens . . . . . . . . . . . . | Lies directly behind the pupil. |

In Greek mythology, **Iris** was the special messenger of the Queen of Heaven. In this role she passed from heaven to earth over the rainbow while dressed in rainbow hues. Her name was applied to the circular eye muscle because of its varied colors.

**417**

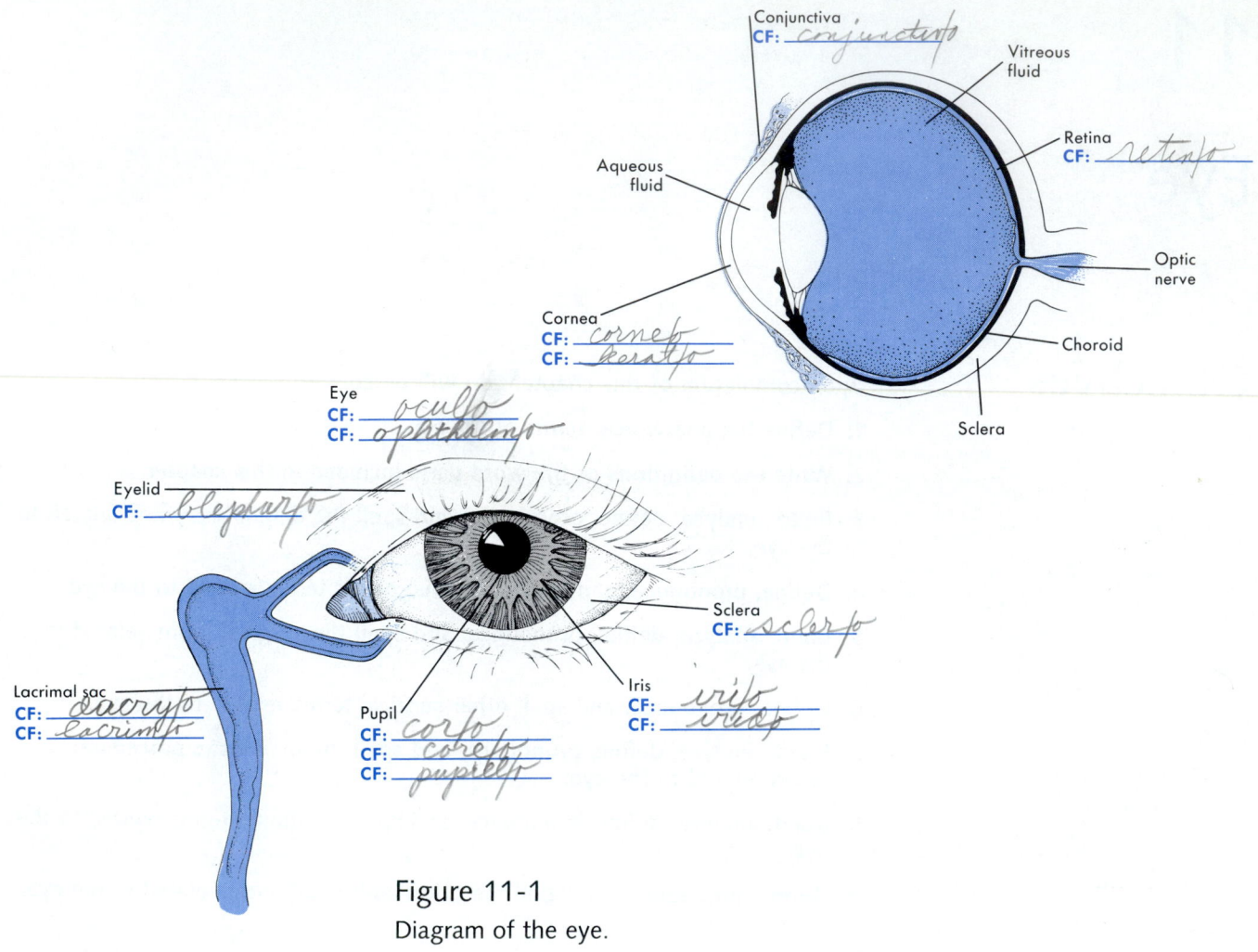

Conjunctiva
CF: _conjunctivo_

Vitreous fluid

Retina
CF: _retino_

Aqueous fluid

Optic nerve

Cornea
CF: _corneo_
CF: _kerato_

Choroid

Sclera

Eye
CF: _oculo_
CF: _ophthalmo_

Eyelid
CF: _blepharo_

Sclera
CF: _sclero_

Lacrimal sac
CF: _dacryo_
CF: _lacrimo_

Pupil
CF: _coro_
CF: _coreo_
CF: _pupillo_

Iris
CF: _irio_
CF: _irido_

**Figure 11-1**
Diagram of the eye.

3.  retina . . . . . . . . . . . . . .   Innermost layer of the eye, which contains the vision receptors.

4.  aqueous fluid . . . . . . . . .   Watery liquid found in the anterior cavity of the eye.

5.  vitreous fluid . . . . . . . . .   Jellylike liquid found behind the lens in the posterior cavity of the eye.

6.  meibomian glands . . . . . .   Oil glands found in the upper and lower edges of the eyelids that help lubricate the eye.

7.  lacrimal glands
    and ducts . . . . . . . . . . . .   Produce and drain tears.

8.  optic nerve . . . . . . . . . . .   Carries visual impulses from the retina to the brain.

9.  conjunctiva. . . . . . . . . . .    Mucous membrane lining the eyelids and covering the anterior portion of the sclera.

Learn the anatomical terms by completing the following exercises.

## EXERCISE 1A

Match the terms in the first column with the correct definitions in the second column.

_d_ 1. aqueous fluid
_c_ 2. choroid
_f_ 3. conjunctiva
_h_ 4. cornea
_b_ 5. iris
_e_ 6. lacrimal glands
_a_ 7. lens

a.  lies directly behind the pupil
b.  gives the eye its color
c.  middle layer of the eye
d.  watery liquid found in the anterior cavity of the eye
e.  produces tears
f.  mucous membrane lining the eyelids
g.  jellylike fluid behind the lens and in the posterior cavity
h.  transparent anterior part of the sclera

## EXERCISE 1B

Match the terms in the first column with the correct definitions in the second column.

_d_ 1. meibomian gland
_f_ 2. optic nerve
_h_ 3. orbit
_e_ 4. pupil
_b_ 5. retina
_a_ 6. sclera
_c_ 7. vitreous fluid

a.  outer protective layer of the eye
b.  innermost layer of the eye
c.  jellylike liquid found behind the lens and in the posterior cavity of the eye
d.  oil glands in eyelids that help lubricate the eye
e.  opening in the center of the iris
f.  carries visual impulses from retina to the brain
g.  middle layer of the eye
h.  bony protective cavity of the skull in which the eye lies

Place a check mark (√) in the box to indicate that you have completed Objective 1.

☐ DEFINE THE ANATOMICAL TERMS RELATED TO THE EYE.

# Objective 2    WRITE THE DEFINITIONS OF THE WORD PARTS INCLUDED IN THIS CHAPTER.

## Eye Word Parts

Study the word parts and their definitions as follows. Learning will be made easier by completing the exercises that follow.

| COMBINING FORM | DEFINITION |
|---|---|
| 1. blephar/o . . . . . . . . . . . | eyelid |
| 2. conjunctiv/o . . . . . . . . . | conjunctiva |
| 3. cor/o, core/o<br>   pupill/o. . . . . . . . . . . . | pupil |
| 4. corne/o<br>   kerat/o . . . . . . . . . . . . .<br>   (NOTE: *Kerat/io* also means *hard*<br>   or *horny tissue;* see Chapter 3.) | cornea |
| 5. dacry/o<br>   lacrim/o . . . . . . . . . . . . | tear, tear duct |
| 6. irid/o, iri/o . . . . . . . . . . | iris |
| 7. ocul/o<br>   ophthalm/o. . . . . . . . . . | eye |
| 8. opt/o. . . . . . . . . . . . . . . | vision |
| 9. retin/o. . . . . . . . . . . . . | retina |
| 10. scler/o. . . . . . . . . . . . . | sclera |

Learn the anatomical locations and definitions of the combining forms by completing the following exercises.

## EXERCISE 2

Write the combining forms in the spaces marked **CF** on the diagram in Figure 11-1, p. 418.

## EXERCISE 3

Write the definitions of the following combining forms.

1. ocul/o _____ *eye*
2. blephar/o _____ *eyelid*
3. corne/o _____ *cornea*
4. lacrim/o _____ *tear, tear duct*
5. retin/o _____ *retina*
6. pupill/o _____ *pupil*

7. scler/o _____ *sclera* _____

8. irid/o _____ *iris* _____

9. conjunctiv/o _____ *conjunctiva* _____

10. cor/o _____ *pupil* _____

11. ophthalm/o _____ *eye* _____

12. kerat/o _____ *cornea* _____

13. iri/o _____ *iris* _____

14. core/o _____ *pupil* _____

15. opt/o _____ *vision* _____

16. dacry/o _____ *tear, tear duct* _____

## EXERCISE 4

Write the combining form for each of the following.

1. eye            a. _____

                  b. _____

2. cornea         a. _____

                  b. _____

3. conjunctiva    _____

4. tear duct, tear   a. _____

                     b. _____

5. eyelid         _____

6. pupil          a. _____

                  b. _____

                  c. _____

7. sclera         _____

8. retina         _____

9. iris           a. _____

                  b. _____

10. vision        _____

# Related Word Parts

| COMBINING FORM | DEFINITION |
|---|---|
| 1. cry/o . . . . . . . . . . . . . . . | cold |
| 2. dipl/o . . . . . . . . . . . . . | two, double |
| 3. phot/o . . . . . . . . . . . . . | light |
| 4. ton/o . . . . . . . . . . . . . . | tension, pressure |

Learn the related combining forms by completing the following exercises.

## EXERCISE 5

Write the definitions of the following combining forms.

1. ton/o ___ *tension, pressure* ___
2. phot/o ___ *light* ___
3. cry/o ___ *cold* ___
4. dipl/o ___ *two, double* ___

## EXERCISE 6

Write the combining form for each of the following.

1. cold _____

2. tension, pressure _____

3. two, double _____

4. light _____

# Prefix and Suffixes

| PREFIX | DEFINITION |
|---|---|
| 1. bi-, bin- . . . . . . . . . . . . . | two |

| SUFFIX | DEFINITION |
|---|---|
| 1. -ician . . . . . . . . . . . . . . | one who |
| 2. -opia . . . . . . . . . . . . . . . | vision (condition) |
| 3. -phobia . . . . . . . . . . . . . | abnormal fear of or aversion to specific things |
| 4. -plegia . . . . . . . . . . . . . | paralysis |

## EXERCISE 7

Write the definitions of the following prefixes and suffixes.

1. -opia _____ *vision (condition)* _____

2. bi- _____ *two* _____

3. -plegia _____ *paralysis* _____

4. -ician _____ *one who* _____

5. -phobia _____ *abnormal fear of or aversion to specific things* _____

6. bin- _____ *two* _____

## EXERCISE 8

Write the prefix or suffixes for each of the following prefixes and suffixes.

1. one who                    _____

2. paralysis                  _____

3. two              a. _____

                    b. _____

4. abnormal fear of or
   aversion to specific
   things                     _____

5. vision (condition)         _____

Place a check mark (√) in the box to indicate that you have completed Objective 2.

☐ WRITE THE DEFINITIONS OF THE WORD PARTS INCLUDED IN THIS CHAPTER.

# Objective 3   BUILD, ANALYZE, DEFINE, PRONOUNCE, AND SPELL THE DIAGNOSTIC TERMS RELATED TO THE EYE.

## Medical Terms

The terms you need to learn to complete this chapter are listed as follows. Now that you know the meaning of the word parts, the exercises at the end of the list will assist you to learn the definition and the spelling of each word.

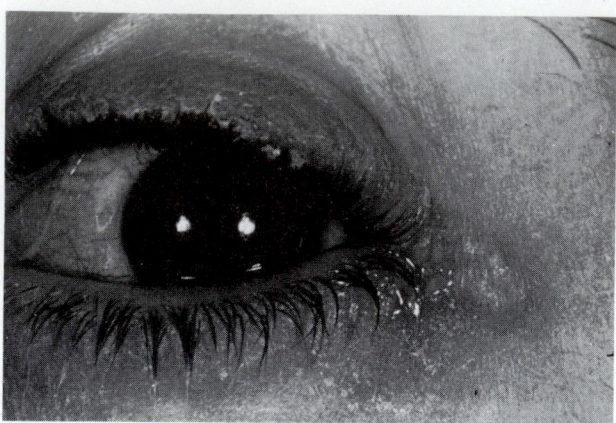

**Figure 11-2**
Blepharitis. Note crusting of left lid margin and lashes with redness at outer angle.

From Havener WH: *Synopsis of ophthalmology*, ed 6, St. Louis, 1984, Mosby.

# Diagnostic Terms

| **TERM** (built from word parts) | **DEFINITION** |
|---|---|
| 1. **blepharitis** . . . . . . . . . . (*blef*-a-RĪ-tis) | inflammation of the eyelids (Figure 11-2) |
| 2. **blepharoptosis** . . . . . . . (*blef*-ar-op-TŌ-sis) | drooping of the eyelid (Figure 11-3) |
| 3. **conjunctivitis** . . . . . . . . (kon-*junk*-ti-VĪ-tis) | inflammation of the conjunctiva |
| 4. **corneoiritis** . . . . . . . . . . (*kor*-nē-ō-ī-RĪ-tis) | inflammation of the cornea and the iris |
| 5. **dacryocystitis** . . . . . . . . (*dak*-rē-ō-sis-TĪ-tis) | inflammation of the tear (lacrimal) sac (Figure 11-4) |
| 6. **diplopia** . . . . . . . . . . . . (di-PLŌ-pē-a) | double vision |
| 7. **endophthalmitis** . . . . . . . (en-dof-thal-MĪ-tis) (NOTE: The "o" in endo is dropped.) | inflammation of (the contents of) the eye. |
| 8. **iridoplegia** . . . . . . . . . . (*ir*-i-dō-PLĒ-jē-a) | paralysis of the iris |
| 9. **iritis** . . . . . . . . . . . . . . (i-RĪ-tis) | inflammation of the iris |
| 10. **keratitis** . . . . . . . . . . . (ker-a-TĪ-tis) | inflammation of the cornea |
| 11. **leukocoria** . . . . . . . . . . (lū-kō-KŌ-rē-a) | condition of white pupil |

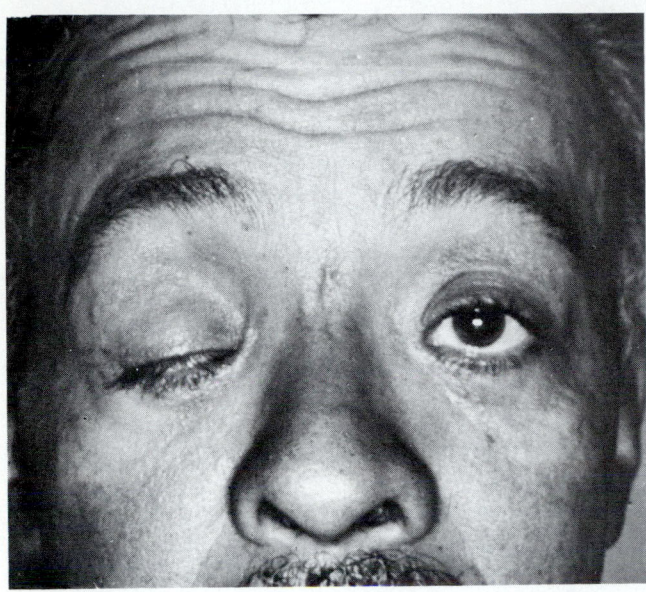

**Figure 11-3**

Blepharoptosis.

From Saunders WH and others: *Nursing care in eye, ear, nose, and throat disorders*, ed 4, St. Louis, 1979, Mosby.

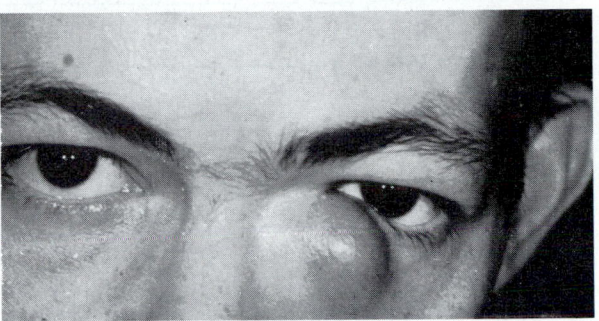

**Figure 11-4**

Dacryocystitis.

From Saunders WH and others: *Nursing care in eye, ear, nose, and throat disorders*, ed 4, St. Louis, 1979, Mosby.

12. oculomycosis . . . . . . . .    abnormal condition of the eye caused by
    (*ok*-ū-lō-mī-KŌ-sis)          a fungus

13. ophthalmalgia . . . . . . . .   pain in the eye
    (*of*-thal-MAL-jē-a)

14. ophthalmoplegia . . . . . .    paralysis of the eye (muscle)
    (of-thal-mō-PLĒ-jē-a)

15. ophthalmorrhagia . . . . .     hemorrhage from the eye
    (of-*thal*-mō-RĂ-jē-a)

16. photophobia . . . . . . . . .    abnormal fear of (sensitivity to) light
    (*fō*-tō-FŌ-bē-a)

17. photoretinitis . . . . . . . .   inflammation of retina caused by (ex-
    (*fō*-tō-*ret*-i-NĪ-tis)         treme) light

18. retinoblastoma . . . . . . . .   tumor arising from the developing reti-
    (ret-i-nō-blas-TŌ-ma)            nal cell

19. sclerokeratitis . . . . . . . .  inflammation of the sclera and cornea
    (*skle*-rō-kār-a-TĪ-tis)

20. scleromalacia . . . . . . . .   softening of the sclera
    (*skle*-rō-ma-LĂ-shē-a)

Practice saying each of these terms aloud. To assist you in pronunciation, obtain the audiotape designed for use with this text. Learn the definitions and the spellings of the diagnostic terms by completing the following exercises.

## EXERCISE 9

Analyze and define the following diagnostic terms.

1. sclerokeratitis _____

2. ophthalmalgia _____

3. corneoiritis _____

4. blepharoptosis _____

5. diplopia _____

6. ophthalmorrhagia _____

7. conjunctivitis _____

8. leukocoria _____

9. iridoplegia _____

10. scleromalacia _____

11. photophobia _____

12. blepharitis _____

13. oculomycosis _____

14. photoretinitis _____

15. dacryocystitis _____

16. endophthalmitis _____

17. iritis _____

18. retinoblastoma _____

19. keratitis _____

20. ophthalmoplegia _____

## EXERCISE 10

Build medical terms for each of the following definitions by using the word
parts you have learned.

1. inflammation of the conjunctiva        ____conjunctivitis____
                      WR    S

2. abnormal eye condition caused by a fungus

ocul | o | myc | osis
WR | CV | WR | S

3. pain in the eye

ophthalm | algia
WR | S

4. inflammation of the retina caused by light

phot | o | retin | itis
WR | CV | WR | S

5. double vision

dipl | opia
WR | S

6. inflammation of the eyelids

blephar | itis
WR | S

7. condition of white pupil

leuk | o | cor | ia
WR | CV | WR | S

8. paralysis of the iris

irid | o | plegia
WR | CV | S

9. inflammation of the cornea and the iris

corne | o | iri | itis
WR | CV | WR | S

10. drooping of the eyelids

blephar | o | ptosis
WR | CV | S

11. inflammation of the iris

iri | itis
WR | S

12. tumor arising from developing retinal cell

retin | o | blast | oma
WR | CV | WR | S

13. softening of the sclera

scler | o | malacia
WR | CV | S

14. inflammation of a tear (lacrimal) sac

_dacry o cyst itis_
WR / CV / WR / S

15. hemorrhage from the eye

_opthalm orrhagia_
WR / S

16. inflammation of the sclera and cornea

_scler o kerat itis_
WR / CV / WR / S

17. abnormal fear of (sensitivity to) light

_phot o phobia_
WR / CV / S

18. inflammation of the cornea

_kerat itis_
WR / S

19. inflammation of (the contents of) the eye

_end opthalm itis_
P / WR / S

20. paralysis of the eye (muscle)

_opthalm o plegia_
WR / CV / S

## EXERCISE 11

Spell each of the diagnostic terms. Have someone dictate the terms on pp. 424, 425 to you or say the words into a tape recorder; then spell the words from your recording as often as necessary. Think about the word parts before attempting to write the word. Study those you have spelled incorrectly.

1. _____     9. _____

2. _____     10. _____

3. _____     11. _____

4. _____     12. _____

5. _____     13. _____

6. _____     14. _____

7. _____     15. _____

8. _____     16. _____

17. _____    19. _____

18. _____    20. _____

Place a check mark (√) in the box to indicate that you have completed Objective 3.

☐ BUILD, ANALYZE, DEFINE, PRONOUNCE, AND SPELL THE DIAGNOSTIC TERMS RELATED TO THE EYE.

# Objective 4   DEFINE, PRONOUNCE, AND SPELL OTHER DIAGNOSTIC TERMS RELATED TO THE EYE.

## Other Diagnostic Terms

| TERM | DEFINITION |
|---|---|
| 1. astigmatism <br>(a-STIG-ma-tizm) | defective curvature of the refractive surface of the eye |
| 2. cataract <br>(KAT-a-rakt) | clouding of the lens of the eye (Figure 11-5) |
| 3. chalazion (meibomian cyst) <br>(ka-LĀ-zē-on) | obstruction of the oil gland of the eyelid (Figure 11-6) |
| 4. detached retina | separation of the retina from choroid in back of the eye (Figure 11-7) |
| 5. emmetropia <br>(em-e-TRŌ-pē-a) | normal condition of the eye |

**Cataract** is derived from the Greek **kato**, meaning **down**, and **raktos**, meaning **precipice**. Together, the words were interpreted as **waterfall**. The cataract sufferer sees things as through a watery veil of mist, or waterfall.

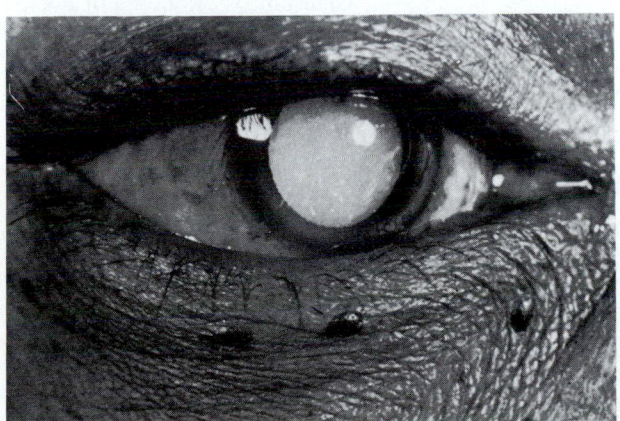

### Figure 11-5
Cataract, visible as the large white area behind the pupil.

From Havener WH: *Synopsis of ophthalmology*, ed 6, St. Louis, 1984, Mosby.

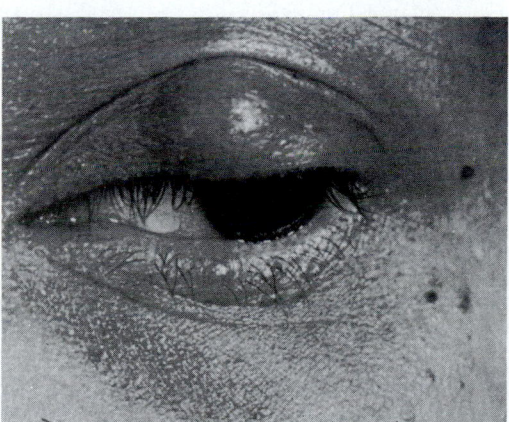

### Figure 11-6
Chalazion, appearing on the upper lid; a hordeolum, or sty, appears on the lower lid.

From Havener WH: *Synopsis of ophthalmology*, ed 6, St. Louis, 1984, Mosby.

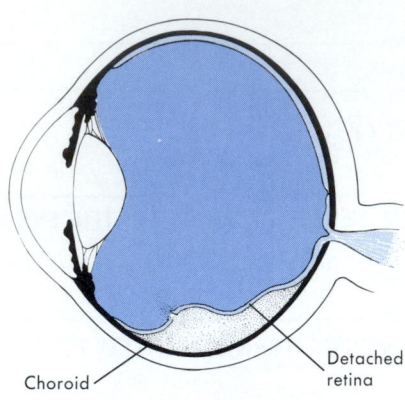

### Figure 11-7
Detached retina. Vitreous fluid has seeped through a break in retina, causing choroid coat and retina to separate.

Choroid

Detached retina

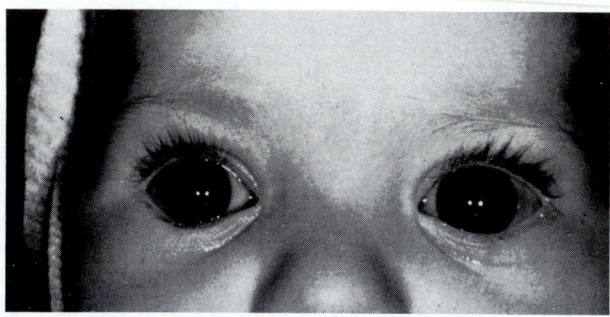

### Figure 11-8
Glaucoma. Congenital glaucoma increases the size of infant's eyes.

From Havener WH: *Synopsis of ophthalmology*, ed 6, St. Louis, 1984, Mosby.

| | | |
|---|---|---|
| 6. | glaucoma . . . . . . . . . . . (glaw-KŌ-ma) | abnormally increased intraocular tension (Figure 11-8) |
| 7. | hyperopia . . . . . . . . . . . (hī-per-Ō-pē-a) | farsightedness |
| 8. | myopia . . . . . . . . . . . . . (mī-Ō-pē-a) | nearsightedness |
| 9. | nyctalopia . . . . . . . . . . . (nik-ta-LŌ-pē-a) | poor vision at night or in faint light |
| 10. | nystagmus . . . . . . . . . . (nis-TAG-mus) | involuntary, rhythmic movements of the eyes |
| 11. | presbyopia . . . . . . . . . . (*pres*-bē-Ō-pē-a) | impaired vision as a result of aging |
| 12. | pterygium . . . . . . . . . . . (te-RIJ-ē-um) | abnormal fold of membrane extending from conjunctiva to cornea |
| 13. | retinitis pigmentosa . . . . (ret-i-NĪ-tis) (pig-men-TŌ-sa) | hereditary progressive disease marked by night blindness with atrophy and retinal pigment changes |

**Glaucoma** is composed of the Greek **glaukos,** meaning **blue-gray** or **sea green,** and **oma,** meaning a morbid condition. The term was given to any condition in which gray or green replaced the black in the pupil.

14. **strabismus** . . . . . . . . . . abnormal condition of squint or crossed-
    (stra-BIZ-mus)             eyes caused by the visual axes not meet-
                               ing at the same point
15. **sty (hordeolum)** . . . . . . . infection of the oil gland of the eyelid
    (stī) (hōr-DĒ-ō-lum)       (Figure 11-6)

Practice saying each of these terms aloud. To assist you in pronunciation,
obtain the audiotape designed for use with this text. Learn the definitions
and spellings of the other diagnostic terms by completing the following
exercises.

## EXERCISE 12

Fill in the blanks with the correct terms.

1. Another name for nearsightedness is ___myopia___.
2. Impaired vision as a result of aging is ___presbyopia___.
3. The abnormal condition of squint or crossed-eyes caused by visual axes not meeting at the same point
   is called ___strabismus___.
4. An obstruction of the oil gland of the eyelid is called a(n) ___chalazion___.
5. A defective curvature of the refractive surface of the eye causes a condition known as
   ___astigmatism___.
6. ___nystagmus___ is the name given to involuntary, rhythmic movements of the eye.
7. A clouding of the lens of the eye is called a(n) ___cataract___.
8. ___sty___ is the name given to an infection of the oil gland of the eyelids.
9. A condition of abnormally increased intraocular tension is ___glaucoma___.
10. A(n) ___detached___ ___retina___ is a separation of the retina from the cho-
    roid in the back of the eye.
11. Another name for farsightedness is ___hyperopia___.
12. Normal condition of the eye is called ___emmetropia___.
13. ___Retinitis___ ___pigmentosa___ is a hereditary progressive disease causing night
    blindness with retinal pigment changes and atrophy.
14. Poor vision at night or in faint light is called ___nyctalopia___.
15. A ___pterygium___ is an abnormal fold of membrane extending from conjunctiva to cornea.

## EXERCISE 13

Match the terms in the first column with the correct definitions in the second column.

___f___ 1. astigmatism      a. infection of the oil gland of the eye-
___h___ 2. cataract             lid
___k___ 3. chalazion         b. farsightedness

_n_ 4. detached retina

_m_ 5. glaucoma

_j_ 6. myopia

_d_ 7. nystagmus

_b_ 8. hyperopia

_e_ 9. presbyopia

_c_ 10. strabismus

_a_ 11. sty

_l_ 12. pterygium

_i_ 13. retinitis pigmentosa

_o_ 14. nyctalopia

_g_ 15. emmetropia

c. crossed-eyes or squint caused by visual axes not meeting at the same point

d. involuntary, rhythmic movements of the eye

e. impaired vision caused by aging

f. defective curvature of the refractive surface of the eye

g. normal condition of the eye

h. clouding of a lens of the eye

i. hereditary progressive disease marked by night blindness

j. nearsightedness

k. obstruction of the oil gland of the eye

l. abnormal fold of membrane extending from conjunctiva to cornea

m. increased intraocular tension

n. separation of retina from choroid in the back of the eye

o. poor vision at night or in faint light

## EXERCISE 14

Have someone dictate the other diagnostic terms on pp. 429 and 431 to you or say the words into a tape recorder; then spell the words from your recording as often as necessary. Study any you have spelled incorrectly.

1. _____    9. _____

2. _____    10. _____

3. _____    11. _____

4. _____    12. _____

5. _____    13. _____

6. _____    14. _____

7. _____    15. _____

8. _____

Place a check mark (✓) in the box to indicate that you have completed Objective 4.

☐ DEFINE, PRONOUNCE, AND SPELL OTHER DIAGNOSTIC TERMS RELATED TO THE EYE.

# Objective 5

**BUILD, ANALYZE, DEFINE, PRONOUNCE, AND SPELL THE SURGICAL TERMS RELATED TO THE EYE.**

## Surgical Terms

| TERM (built from word parts) | DEFINITION |
|---|---|
| 1. blepharoplasty (BLEF-a-rō-plast-tē) | surgical repair of the eyelid |
| 2. cryoretinopexy (*krī-ō-re*-tin-ō-PEK-sē) | fixation of the retina to the choroid by extreme cold (liquid nitrogen) |
| 3. dacryocystorhinostomy (*dak*-rē-ō-*sis*-tō-rī-NOS-tō-mē) | creation of an artificial opening between the tear (lacrimal) sac and the nose to restore drainage into the nose when the nasolacrimal duct is obstructed or obliterated |
| 4. dacryocystotomy (*dak*-rē-ō-sis-TOT-ō-mē) | incision into the tear sac |
| 5. iridectomy (ir-i-DEK-tō-mē) | excision (of part) of the iris |
| 6. iridosclerotomy (ir-ī-dō-skle-ROT-tō-mē) | incision into the edge of the iris and into the sclera |
| 7. keratoplasty (KĀR-a-tō-plas-tē) | surgical repair of the cornea (corneal transplant) |
| 8. sclerotomy (skle-ROT-ō-mē) | incision into the sclera |

Practice saying each of these terms aloud. To assist you in pronunciation, obtain the audiotape designed for use with this text. Learn the definitions and spellings of the surgical terms by completing the following exercises.

## EXERCISE 15

Analyze and define the following surgical terms.

1. keratoplasty _____

2. sclerotomy _____

3. dacryocystotomy _____

4. cryoretinopexy _____

5. iridosclerotomy _____

6. blepharoplasty _____

7. iridectomy _____

8. dacryocystorhinostomy _____

## EXERCISE 16

Build surgical terms for the following definitions by using the word parts you have learned.

1. artificial opening between the tear (lacrimal) sac and the nose to restore drainage when the nasolacrimal duct is obstructed

   dacry / o / cyst / o / rhin / ostomy
   WR / CV / WR / CV / WR / S

2. excision of the iris

   irid / ectomy
   WR / S

3. surgical repair of the cornea

   kerat / o / plasty
   WR / CV / S

4. incision into the sclera

   scler / otomy
   WR / S

5. surgical repair of the eyelid

   blephar / o / plasty
   WR / CV / S

6. fixation of the retina by a method utilizing extreme cold

   cry / o / retin / o / pexy
   WR / CV / WR / CV / S

7. incision into the tear sac

   dacry / o / cyst / otomy
   WR / CV / WR / S

8. incision into the edge of the iris and into the sclera

   irid / o / scler / otomy
   WR / CV / WR / S

## EXERCISE 17

Spell each of the surgical terms. Have someone dictate the terms on p. 433 to you or say the words into a tape recorder; then spell the words from your recording as often as necessary. Think about the word parts before attempting to write the word. Study any you have spelled incorrectly.

1. _____    5. _____

2. _____    6. _____

3. _____    7. _____

4. _____    8. _____

Place a check mark (√) in the box to indicate that you have completed Objective 5.

☐ BUILD, ANALYZE, DEFINE, PRONOUNCE, AND SPELL THE SURGICAL TERMS RELATED TO THE EYE.

## Objective 6    DEFINE, PRONOUNCE, AND SPELL OTHER SURGICAL TERMS RELATED TO THE EYE.

## Other Surgical Terms

| TERM | DEFINITION |
|---|---|
| 1. cryoextraction of the lens. (krī-ō-eks-TRAK-shun) | procedure in which a cataract is lifted from the eye with an extremely cold probe (cryoprobe) (Figure 11-9) |
| 2. enucleation. . . . . . . . . . (e-nū-klē-Ā-shun) | surgical removal of the eye (also, the removal of any organ that comes out clean and whole) |

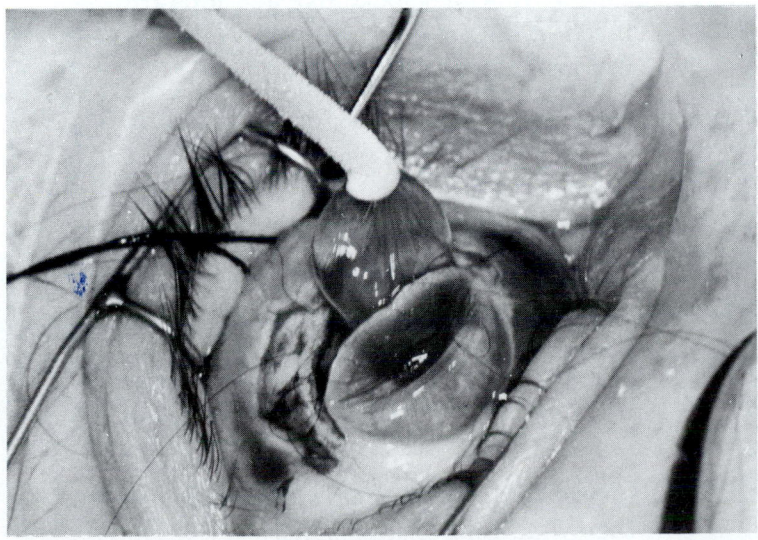

## Figure 11-9

Cryoextraction of lens. Cryoprobe freezes to surface of cataract and makes it easy to remove.

From Saunders WH and others: *Nursing care in eye, ear, nose, and throat disorders,* ed 4, St. Louis, 1979, Mosby.

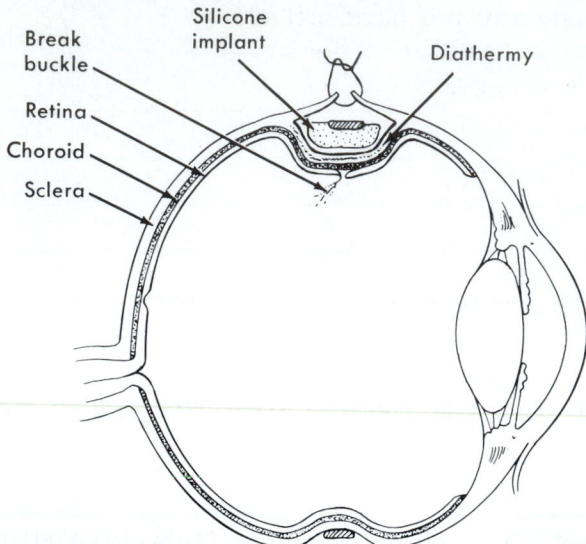

**Figure 11-10**

Scleral buckling. Diagram shows one of the methods used in this type of surgery.

From Phipps WJ, Long BC, and Woods NF: *Shafer's medical-surgical nursing*, ed 7, St. Louis, 1980, Mosby.

3. **phacoemulsification** . . . . .
   (fā-kō-ē-*mul*-si-fi-KĀ-shun)

   method to remove cataracts in which an ultrasonic needle probe breaks up the lens, which is then aspirated

4. **radial keratotomy** . . . . . .
   (ker-a-TOT-ō-mē)

   surgery in which spoke-like incisions are made to flatten the cornea thus correcting nearsightedness

5. **retinal photocoagulation** .
   (RET-in-al)   (fō-tō-kō-*ag*-ū-LĀ-shun)

   procedure to repair tears in the retina by use of an intense, precisely focused light beam, which causes coagulation of the tissue protein; used to repair retinal detachment

6. **scleral buckling** . . . . . . . .
   (SKLE-ral) (BUK-ling)

   repair of a detached retina. A strip of sclera is resected, or a fold is made in the sclera. An implant is inserted with sutures to hold and buckle the sclera (Figure 11-10)

7. **strabotomy** . . . . . . . . . . .
   (stra-BOT-ō-mē)

   incision into the tendon of a muscle of the eye to relieve strabismus

8. **trabeculectomy** . . . . . . . .
   (tra-bek-ū-LEK-tō-mē)

   surgical creation of a drain to reduce intraocular pressure

9. **vitrectomy** . . . . . . . . . . .
   (vi-TREK-tō-mē)

   surgical removal of all or part of the vitreous fluid

Practice saying each of these terms aloud. To assist you in pronunciation, obtain the audiotape designed for use with this text. Learn the definitions and spellings of the other surgical terms by completing the following exercises.

## EXERCISE 18

Fill in the blanks with the correct terms.

1. The procedure performed to repair tears in the retina is called _____

   _____ .

2. _____ is the name given to the procedure in which the cataract is lifted from the eye by an extremely cold probe.

3. Surgical removal of an eye is called a(n) _____ .

4. _____ is the name given to the procedure that breaks up the lens with ultrasound and then aspirates it.

5. An incision into the tendon of a muscle to relieve a crossed-eyed condition is a(n)

   _____ .

6. _____ is the surgical creation of a drain to reduce intraocular pressure.

7. An operation to repair a detached retina in which the sclera is folded or resected, an implant inserted, and sutures made to hold the sclera is called _____ _____ .

8. Surgery in which spoke-like incisions are made to flatten the cornea thus correcting nearsightedness is called a _____ _____ .

9. Surgery to remove vitreous fluid from the eye is called _____ .

## EXERCISE 19

Match the terms in the first column with the correct definitions in the second column.

_____ 1. strabotomy

_____ 2. enucleation

_____ 3. trabeculectomy

_____ 4. retinal photocoagulation

_____ 5. cryoextraction of lens

_____ 6. phacoemulsification

_____ 7. scleral buckling surgery

_____ 8. radial keratotomy

_____ 9. vitrectomy

a. a surgery to flatten the cornea thus correcting nearsightedness

b. surgical creation of a permanent drain to reduce intraocular pressure

c. procedure to repair tears in the retina

d. procedure in which the lens is broken up by ultrasound and aspirated

e. incision into muscle tendon to relieve crossed eyes

f. surgical removal of an eye

g. surgical removal of vitreous fluid

h. operation in which a cataract is lifted from the eye with an extremely cold probe

    i.  detached retina surgery in which the sclera is folded, an implant inserted, and sutures made to hold the sclera

    j.  surgical incision into the sclera

## EXERCISE 20

Spell each of the other surgical terms. Have someone dictate the terms on pp. 435, 436 to you. Study any you have spelled incorrectly.

1. _____     6. _____

2. _____     7. _____

3. _____     8. _____

4. _____     9. _____

5. _____

Place a check mark (√) in the box to indicate that you have completed Objective 6.

☐ **DEFINE, PRONOUNCE, AND SPELL OTHER SURGICAL TERMS RELATED TO THE EYE.**

# Objective 7    BUILD, ANALYZE, DEFINE, PRONOUNCE, AND SPELL THE DIAGNOSTIC PROCEDURAL TERMS RELATED TO THE EYE.

## Diagnostic Procedural Terms

| **TERM** (built from word parts) | **DEFINITION** |
|---|---|
| 1. fluorescein angiography. (flō-RES-ē-in)(an-jē-OG-ra-fē) | process of x-ray filming the blood vessels of the eye using fluoresing dye |
| 2. keratometer . . . . . . . . . (kār-a-TOM-e-ter) | instrument that measures (the curvature of) the cornea (used for fitting contact lenses) |
| 3. ophthalmoscope . . . . . . . (of-THAL-mō-skōp) | instrument that examines the interior of the eye (Figure 11-11) |
| 4. ophthalmoscopy . . . . . . . (of-thal-MOS-kō-pē) | visual examination of the eye |
| 5. optometer . . . . . . . . . . . (op-TOM-e-ter) | instrument that measures (power and range of) vision |
| 6. optometry . . . . . . . . . . . (op-TOM-e-trē) | measurement of visual acuity and the prescribing of corrective lenses |
| 7. optomyometer . . . . . . . . (op-tom-ī-OM-e-ter) | instrument that measures the power of the muscles of vision |

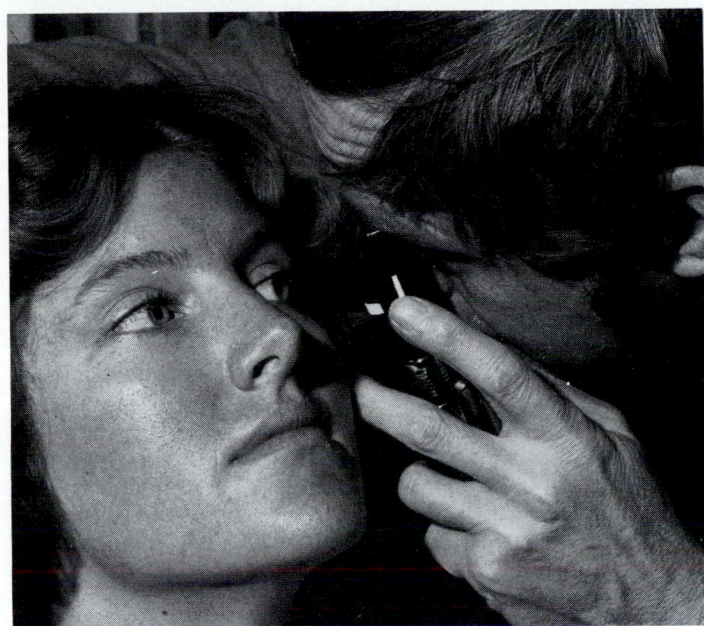

**Figure 11-11**
Ophthalmoscope, used to view the retina.

From Havener WH: *Synopsis of ophthalmology*, ed 6, St. Louis, 1984, Mosby.

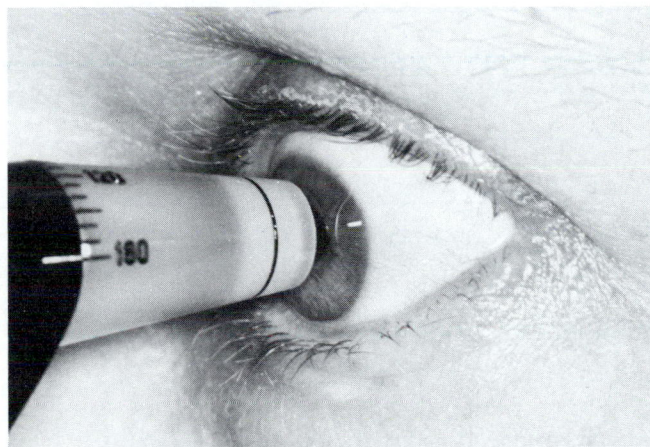

**Figure 11-12**
Tonometer, used to measure intraocular pressure.

From Saunders WH and others: *Nursing care in eye, ear, nose, and throat disorders*, ed 4, St. Louis, 1979, Mosby.

| | | |
|---|---|---|
| 8. | pupillometer . . . . . . . . <br> (pū-pil-OM-e-ter) | instrument that measures the width and diameter of the pupil |
| 9. | pupilloscope . . . . . . . . . <br> (pū-PIL-ō-skōp) | instrument that examines (the reactions of) the pupil |
| 10. | tonometer . . . . . . . . . . . <br> (ton-OM-e-ter) | instrument that measures the pressure within the eye (used to diagnose glaucoma) (Figure 11-12) |
| 11. | tonometry . . . . . . . . . . . <br> (ton-OM-e-trē) | measurement of pressure within the eye |

Practice saying each of these terms aloud. To assist you in pronunciation, obtain the audiotape designed for use with this text. Learn the definitions and spellings of the diagnostic procedural terms by completing the following exercises.

## EXERCISE 21

Analyze and define the following diagnostic procedural terms.

1. optometer _instrument that measures vision_

2. pupilloscope _instrument that examines the pupil_

3. optometry _measurement of visual acuity & prescribing of corrective lenses_

4. ophthalmoscope _instrument that examines the interior of the eye_

5. tonometry _measurement of pressure within the eye_

6. pupillometer _instrument that measures the width & diameter of the pupil_

7. optomyometer _instrument that measures the power of the muscles of vision_

8. tonometer _instrument that measures the pressure in the eye_

9. keratometer _instrument that measures the curvature of the cornea_

10. ophthalmoscopy _visual examination of the eye_

11. fluorescein angiography _process of x-ray filming the blood vessels of the eye using fluoresing dye_

## EXERCISE 22

Build diagnostic terms for the following definitions by using the word parts you have learned.

1. instrument that measures the power and range of vision

   _____/___/___
   WR   CV   S

2. measurement of pressure within the eye

   _____/___/___
   WR   CV   S

3. instrument that measures (the width and diameter of) the pupil

   _____/___/___
   WR   CV   S

4. instrument that measures
(the curvature of) the cornea

_____
WR / CV / S

5. measurement of visual acuity and the prescribing of corrective lenses

_____
WR / CV / S

6. instrument that measures the power of the muscles of vision

_____
WR / CV / WR / CV / S

7. instrument that examines the interior of the eye

_____
WR / CV / S

8. instrument that measures pressure within the eye

_____
WR / CV / S

9. instrument that examines the reaction of the pupil

_____
WR / CV / S

10. visual examination of the eye

_____
WR / CV / S

11. process of x-ray filming of the blood vessels of the eye using fluorescing dye

_____

_____
WR / CV / S

## EXERCISE 23

Spell each of the diagnostic procedural terms. Have someone dictate the terms on pp. 438, 439 to you. Think about the word parts before attempting to write the word. Study any you have spelled incorrectly.

1. _____   3. _____

2. _____   4. _____

5. _____   9. _____

6. _____   10. _____

7. _____   11. _____

8. _____

Place a check mark (√) in the box to indicate that you have completed Objective 7.

☐ **BUILD, ANALYZE, DEFINE, PRONOUNCE, AND SPELL DIAGNOSTIC PROCEDURAL TERMS RELATED TO THE EYE.**

# Objective 8   BUILD, ANALYZE, DEFINE, PRONOUNCE, AND SPELL ADDITIONAL TERMS RELATED TO THE EYE.

## Additional Terms

| TERM | DEFINITION |
|---|---|
| **(built from word parts)** | |
| 1. **binocular** . . . . . . . . . . . <br>(bin-OK-ū-lar) | pertaining to two or both eyes |
| 2. **corneal** . . . . . . . . . . . . <br>(KŌR-nē-al) | pertaining to the cornea |
| 3. **intraocular** . . . . . . . . . <br>(*in*-tra-OK-ū-lar) | pertaining to within the eye |
| 4. **lacrimal** . . . . . . . . . . . <br>(LAK-ri-mal) | pertaining to tears or tear ducts |
| 5. **nasolacrimal** . . . . . . . . <br>(nā-zō-LAK-ri-mal) | pertaining to the nose and tear ducts |
| 6. **ophthalmic** . . . . . . . . . . <br>(of-THAL-mik) | pertaining to the eye |
| 7. **ophthalmologist** . . . . . . . <br>(*of*-thal-MOL-ō-jist) | physician who specializes in ophthalmology |
| 8. **ophthalmology** . . . . . . . <br>(*of*-thal-MOL-ō-jē) | study of diseases and treatment of the eye |
| 9. **ophthalmopathy** . . . . . . . <br>(*of*-thal-MOP-a-thē) | any disease of the eye |
| 10. **optic** . . . . . . . . . . . . . . <br>(ŌP-tik) | pertaining to vision |
| 11. **optician** . . . . . . . . . . . . <br>(op-TISH-in) | one who is skilled in filling prescriptions for lenses |
| 12. **pupillary** . . . . . . . . . . . <br>(PŪ-pi-lār-ē) | pertaining to the pupil of the eye |
| 13. **retinal** . . . . . . . . . . . . . <br>(RET-i-nal) | pertaining to the retina |

14. retinopathy . . . . . . . . . . (any noninflammatory) disease of the
    (*ret*-i-NOP-a-thē)     retina (such as diabetic retinopathy)

Practice saying each of these terms aloud. To assist you in pronunciation, obtain the audiotape designed for use with this text. Learn the definitions and spellings of the additional terms by completing the following exercises.

## EXERCISE 24

Analyze and define the following additional terms.

1. ophthalmology _____

2. binocular _____

3. optician _____

4. lacrimal _____

5. pupillary _____

6. retinopathy _____

7. ophthalmologist _____

8. corneal _____

9. ophthalmic _____

10. nasolacrimal _____

11. optic _____

12. intraocular _____

13. retinal _____

14. ophthalmopathy _____

## EXERCISE 25

Build additional terms for the following definitions by using the word parts you have learned.

1. study of diseases and
    treatment of the eye

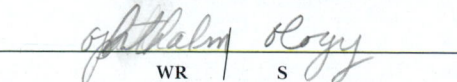
WR      S

2. pertaining to two or both
    eyes

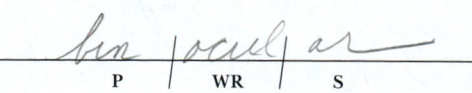
P      WR      S

3. pertaining to the retina

            retin / al
                WR    S

4. pertaining to within the eye

            intra / ocul / ar
                P    WR    S

5. physician who specializes in ophthalmology

            ophtham / ologist
                WR    S

6. pertaining to tears or tear ducts

            lacrim / al
                WR    S

7. pertaining to vision

            opt / ic
                WR    S

8. one who is skilled in filling prescriptions for lenses

            opt / ician
                WR    S

9. (any noninflammatory) disease of the retina

            retin / o / pathy
                WR    CV    S

10. pertaining to the cornea

            corne / al
                WR    S

11. pertaining to the nose and tear ducts

            nas / o / lacrim / al
                WR    CV    WR    S

12. any disease of the eye

            ophthalm / o / pathy
                WR    CV    S

13. pertaining to the pupil of the eye

            pupill / ary
                WR    S

## EXERCISE 26

Spell each of the additional terms. Have someone dictate the terms on pp. 442, 443 to you or say the words into a tape recorder; then spell the words from your recording as often as necessary. Think about the word parts before attempting to write the word. Study any you have spelled incorrectly.

1. _____     8. _____

2. _____     9. _____

3. _____     10. _____

4. _____     11. _____

5. _____     12. _____

6. _____     13. _____

7. _____     14. _____

Place a check mark (√) in the box to indicate that you have completed Objective 8.

☐ BUILD, ANALYZE, DEFINE, PRONOUNCE, AND SPELL ADDITIONAL TERMS RELATED TO THE EYE.

## Objective 9 DEFINE, PRONOUNCE, AND SPELL THE OTHER ADDITIONAL TERMS RELATED TO THE EYE.

## Other Additional Terms

| TERM | DEFINITION |
|---|---|
| 1. miotic................<br>(mī-OT-ik) | agent that constricts the pupil |
| 2. mydriatic ............<br>(mid-rē-AT-ik) | agent that dilates the pupil |
| 3. oculus dexter (OD) .....<br>(OK-ū-lus) (DEX-ter) | medical term for right eye |
| 4. oculus sinister (OS) .....<br>(OK-ū-lus) (sin-IS-ter) | medical term for left eye |
| 5. oculus uterque (OU) ....<br>(OK-ū-lus) (ū-TERK) | medical term for each eye |
| 6. optometrist...........<br>(op-TOM-e-trist) | a health professional who prescribes corrective lenses and/or eye exercises |
| 7. visual acuity ..........<br>(VIZH-ū-al) (a-KŪ-i-tē) | testing sharpness of central vision for either distance or nearness |

> **Optometrist** is derived from the Greek **optikos,** meaning **sight,** and **metron,** meaning **measure.** Literally, an optometrist is a person who measures sight.

Practice saying each of these terms aloud. To assist you in pronunciation, obtain the audiotape designed for use with this text. Learn the definitions and spellings of the other additional terms by completing the following exercises.

## EXERCISE 27

Write the definitions of the following terms.

1. oculus sinister _____

2. optometrist _____

3. mydriatic _____

4. oculus uterque _____

5. visual acuity _____

6. miotic _____

7. oculus dexter _____

## EXERCISE 28

Fill in the blanks with the correct terms.

1. The medical term for the left eye is _oculus_ _sinister_ .
2. An agent that dilates a pupil is a(n) _mydriatic_ .
3. _oculus_ _uterque_ means each eye.
4. An agent that constricts a pupil is a(n) _miotic_ .
5. The medical term for the right eye is _oculus dexter_
6. A health professional who prescribes corrective lenses and/or eye exercises is
   a(n) _optometrist_ .
7. Another term for sharpness of vision is _visual_ _acuity_ .

## EXERCISE 29

Spell each of the other additional terms. Have someone dictate the terms on p. 445 to you or say the words into a tape recorder; then spell the words from your recording as often as necessary. Study any you have spelled incorrectly.

1. _____     5. _____

2. _____     6. _____

3. _____     7. _____

4. _____

Place a check mark (√) in the box to indicate that you have completed Objective 9.

☐ **DEFINE, PRONOUNCE, AND SPELL THE OTHER ADDITIONAL TERMS RELATED TO THE EYE.**

---

**Case History:** This is a 66-year-old Mexican-American male, hypertensive and diabetic, on oral medication, Micronase and Lopressor. Previous history of a pterygium, excised without complication.
Family history of glaucoma (brother).

---

**EXAMINATION**
**Visual Acuities:** Aided: OD 20/25-2   OS 20/30-1   OU 20/25
             Unaided: OD 20/100   OS 20/80-1   OU 20/80
**Externals:** 2 mm blepharoptosis OD PERRLA (pupils equal, round, responsive to
       light and accommodation)
       Ocular motility normal
**Ophthalmoscopic:** Lens: OS showed early cortical spokes
             Disk: margins normal
             Cup to disk ratio: .2 OU
             Fundus:   copper wire appearance to arteries along with
                   marked arteriovenous compression. Pronounced nar-
                   rowing of the arterioles. A-V ratio 1 to 2. Several
                   punctate hemorrhages and hard yellow exudates
                   noted in macular area of both eyes.
             **Refraction:**  OD −1.00 −0.50 × 90 20/20
                       OS −0.75 −0.50 × 85 20/25
             **Tonometry:** 14 mm/Hg OD   13 mm/Hg OS
**Visual Field:** Negative OU
**Diagnosis:** Patient is a compound myopic astigmat and presbyope with stage 1
       diabetic retinopathy and grade II hypertension and arteriolar sclerosis.
       He also shows an early cataract in left eye.
**Treatment:** Provide prescription for corrective lenses. See patient for follow-up
       visit in 6 months to reevaluate diabetic retinopathy and cataract.
       Counsel patient to report any sudden changes in vision.

---

# EXERCISE 30

To test your understanding of the terms introduced in this chapter, circle the words that correctly complete the sentences. The italicized words refer to the correct answer.

1. The patient's *pupils* needed to be *dilated,* therefore the doctor requested that a (miotic, mydriatic, miopic) medication be placed in each eye.
2. A person with a *defective curvature of the refractive surface* of the eye has a(n) (astigmatism, glaucoma, strabismus).
3. The doctor diagnosed the patient with the *clouded lens* of the eye as having a(n) (nystagmus, astigmatism, cataract).
4. To *measure the pressure within the patient's eye,* the physician used a(n) (optomyometer, pupillometer, tonometer).
5. A person who is *farsighted* has (hyperopia, myopia, diplopia).
6. An *obstruction of the oil gland of the eyelid* is called a(n) (sty, chalazion, conjunctivitis).
7. A patient with an *involuntary rhythmic movement of the eyes* has a condition known as (astigmatism, strabismus, nystagmus).

8. The name of the *surgery performed to create a permanent drain to reduce intraocular pressure* is (trabeculectomy, strabotomy, phacoemulsification).

9. The doctor ordered an *x-ray filming of the blood vessels of the eye* or a/an (ophthalmoscopy, fluorescein angiography, optometer).

## EXERCISE 31

Unscramble the following mixed-up terms. The word on the left gives a hint to the word root in each of the opposite scrambled words.

1. eye

/ / / / / / / m / / / / / a /
g a l l t o h a p a m h i

2. iris

/ / / / / / / / / /
m o d r e c y i i t

3. eyelid

/ / / / / / / / / / /
r a l e i b h i s p t

4. eye

/ / / / / a / / / / c / / / /
s o o l m o t h c a p p e h

5. retina

/ / / / / / p / / / /
n o t e r p h y i a t

## EXERCISE 32

The following words did not appear in this chapter but are composed of word parts studied in this or the previous chapters. Find their definitions by translating the word parts literally.

1. **endonasal**
   (*en*-do-NĀ-zal) _____
2. **erythropoiesis**
   (e-*rith*-rō-poy-Ē-sis) _____
3. **esophagocele**
   (e-SOF-a-gō-sēl) _____
4. **fibrogenic**
   (*fi*-brō-JEN-ik) _____
5. **glomerulosclerosis**
   (glo-*mer*-u-lō-skle-RO-sis) _____
6. **hematorrhea**
   (*hem*-a-tō-RĒ-a) _____
7. **hepatolith**
   (HEP-a-tō-lith) _____
8. **histolysis**
   (his-TOL-i-sis) _____
9. **hydropyonephrosis**
   (hī-drō-*pī*-ō-ne-FRŌ-sis) _____
10. **hypermyotrophy**
    (hī-per-mī-OT-rō-fē) _____

# Summary

Can you build, analyze, define, spell, and pronounce the following terms *built from word parts?*   yes ☐   no ☐

## DIAGNOSTIC

blepharitis
(*blef*-a-RĪ-tis)

blepharoptosis
(*blef*-ar-op-TŌ-sis)

conjunctivitis
(kon-*junk*-ti-VĪ-tis)

corneoiritis
(*kor*-nē-ō-i-RĪ-tis)

dacryocystitis
(*dak*-rē-ō-sis-TĪ-tis)

diplopia
(di-PLŌ-pē-a)

endophthalmitis
(en-dof-thal-MĪ-tis)

iridoplegia
(*ir*-i-dō-PLĒ-jē-a)

iritis
(i-RĪ-tis)

keratitis
(ker-a-TĪ-tis)

leukocoria
(lū-kō-KŌ-rē-a)

oculomycosis
(*ok*-ū-lō-mī-KŌ-sis)

ophthalmalgia
(*of*-thal-MAL-jē-a)

ophthalmoplegia
(of-thal-mō-PLĒ-jē-a)

ophthalmorrhagia
(of-*thal*-mō-RA-jē-a)

photophobia
(*fō*-tō-FŌ-bē-a)

photoretinitis
(*fō*-tō-*ret*-i-NĪ-tis)

retinoblastoma
(ret-i-no-blas-TŌ-ma)

sclerokeratitis
(skle-rō-kār-a-TĪ-tis)

scleromalacia
(skle-rō-ma-LĀ-shē-a)

## SURGICAL

blepharoplasty
(BLEF-a-rō-plas-tē)

cryoretinopexy
(krī-ō-*re*-tin-ō-PEK-sē)

dacryocystorhinostomy
(dak-rē-ō-*sis*-tō-rī-NOS-tō-mē)

dacryocystotomy
(dak-rē-ō-sis-TOT-ō-mē)

iridectomy
(ir-i-DEK-tō-mē)

iridosclerotomy
(ir-i-dō-skle-ROT-tō-mē)

keratoplasty
(KĀR-a-tō-plas-tē)

sclerotomy
(skle-ROT-ō-mē)

## PROCEDURAL

fluorescein
(flo-RES-ē-in)
angiography
(an-jē-OG-ra-fē)

keratometer
(kār-a-TOM-e-ter)

ophthalmoscope
(of-THAL-mō-skōp)

ophthalmoscopy
(of-thal-MOS-kō-pē)

optometer
(op-TOM-e-ter)

optometry
(op-TOM-e-trē)

optomyometer
(*op*-tom-ī-OM-e-ter)

pupillometer
(pū-pil-OM-e-ter)

pupilloscope
(pū-PIL-ō-skōp)

tonometer
(ton-OM-e-ter)

tonometry
(ton-OM-e-trē)

## ADDITIONAL

binocular
(bin-OK-ū-lar)

corneal
(KŌR-nē-al)

intraocular
(*in*-tra-OK-ū-lar)

lacrimal
(LAK-ri-mal)

nasolacrimal
(nā-zō-LAK-ri-mal)

ophthalmic
(of-THAL-mik)

ophthalmologist
(*of*-thal-MOL-ō-jist)

ophthalmology
(*of*-thal-MOL-ō-jē)

ophthalmopathy
(*of*-thal-MOP-a-thē)

optic
(OP-tik)

optician
(op-TISH-in)

pupillary
(PŪ-pi-lār-ē)

retinal
(RET-i-nal)

retinopathy
(*ret*-i-NOP-a-thē)

# Summary

Can you define, pronounce, and spell the following terms *not built from word parts?*  yes ☐  no ☐

### DIAGNOSTIC

astigmatism
(a-STIG-ma-tizm)

cataract
(KAT-a-rakt)

chalazion
(ka-LĀ-zē-on)

detached retina

emmetropia
(em-e-TRŌ-pē-a)

glaucoma
(glaw-KŌ-ma)

hyperopia
(*hī*-per-Ō-pē-a)

myopia
(mī-Ō-pē-a)

nyctalopia
(nik-ta-LŌ-pē-a)

nystagmus
(nis-TAG-mus)

presbyopia
(*pres*-bē-Ō-pē-a)

pterygium
(te-RIJ-ē-um)

retinitis pigmentosa
(ret-i-NĪ-tis)
(pig-MEN-tō-sa)

strabismus
(stra-BIZ-mus)

sty (hordeolum)
(stī) (hōr-DĒ-ō-lum)

### SURGICAL

cryoextraction of the
  lens
(*krī*-ō-eks-TRAK-shun)

enucleation
(e-*nū*-klē-Ā-shun)

phacoemulsification
(*fa*-kō-ē-*mul*-si-fi-KĀ-shun)

radial keratotomy
(ker-a-TOT-ō-mē)

retinal photocoagulation
(RET-in-al) (*fō*-tō-kō-*ag*-ū-LĀ-shun)

scleral buckling
(SKLE-ral) (BUK-ling)

strabotomy
(stra-BOT-ō-mē)

trabeculectomy
(tra-bek-ū-LEK-tō-mē)

vitrectomy
(vi-TREK-tō-mē)

### ADDITIONAL

miotic
(mī-OT-ik)

mydriatic
(*mid*-rē-AT-ik)

oculus dexter (OD)
(OK-ū-lus) (DEX-ter)

oculus sinister (OS)
(OK-ū-lus) (sin-IS-ter)

oculus uterque (OU)
(OK-ū-lus) (ū-TERK)

optometrist
(op-TOM-e-trist)

visual acuity
(VIZH-ū-al) (a-KŪ-i-tē)

# Answers

## Exercise 1A

1. d   3. f   5. b   7. a
2. c   4. h   6. e

## Exercise 1B

1. d   3. h   5. b   7. c
2. f   4. e   6. a

## Exercise 2

**Figure 11-1**

Eye: ocul/o, ophthalm/o
Eyelid: blephar/o
Lacrimal sac: dacry/o,
   lacrim/o
Conjunctiva: conjunctiv/o
Cornea: corne/o, kerat/o

Pupil: cor/o, core/o,
   pupill/o
Retina: retin/o
Sclera: scler/o
Iris: irid/o, iri/o

## Exercise 3

1. eye
2. eyelid
3. cornea
4. tear, tear duct
5. retina
6. pupil
7. sclera
8. iris
9. conjunctiva
10. pupil
11. eye
12. cornea
13. iris
14. pupil
15. vision
16. tear, tear duct

## Exercise 4

1. a. ocul/o
   b. ophthalm/o
2. a. corne/o
   b. kerat/o
3. conjunctiv/o
4. a. lacrim/o
   b. dacry/o
5. blephar/o
6. a. cor/o
   b. core/o
   c. pupill/o
7. scler/o
8. retin/o
9. a. iri/o
   b. irid/o
10. opt/o

## Exercise 5

1. tension, pressure
2. light
3. cold
4. two, double

## Exercise 6

1. cry/o   3. dipl/o
2. ton/o   4. phot/o

## Exercise 7

1. vision (condition)
2. two
3. paralysis
4. one who
5. abnormal fear of or
   aversion to specific
   things
6. two

## Exercise 8

1. -ician     3. a. bi-     4. -phobia
2. -plegia       b. bin-    5. -opia

## Exercise 9

1. scler/o /kerat/itis (WR CV WR S, CF) — inflammation of the sclera and the cornea
2. ophthalm/algia (WR S) — pain in the eye
3. corne/o / ir /itis (WR CV WR S, CF) — inflammation of the cornea and the iris
4. blephar/o /ptosis (WR CV S, CF) — drooping of the eyelid
5. dipl/opia (WR S) — double vision
6. ophthalm/orrhagia (WR S) — hemorrhage from the eye
7. conjunctiv/itis (WR S) — inflammation of the conjunctiva
8. leuk/o /cor/ia (WR CV WR S, CF) — condition of white pupil
9. irid/o /plegia (WR CV S, CF) — paralysis of the iris
10. scler/o /malacia (WR CV S, CF) — softening of the sclera
11. phot/o /phobia (WR CV S, CF) — abnormal fear of (sensitivity to) light
12. blephar/itis (WR S) — inflammation of the eyelid
13. ocul/o / myc/ osis (WR CV WR S, CF) — abnormal condition of the eye caused by a fungus
14. phot/o /retin/itis (WR CV WR S, CF) — inflammation of the retina caused by light
15. dacry/o /cyst/itis (WR CV WR S, CF) — inflammation of the tear (lacrimal) sac
16. end/ophthalm/itis (P WR S) — inflammation of (the contents of) the eye
17. ir /itis (WR S) — inflammation of the iris
18. retin/o /blast/oma (WR CV WR S, CF) — tumor arising from developing retinal cell

     WR   S
19. kerat/itis             inflammation of the cornea

      WR    CV  S
20. ophthalm/ o /plegia     paralysis of the eye (muscles)
          CF

## Exercise 10

| | |
|---|---|
| 1. conjunctiv/itis | 11. ir/itis |
| 2. ocul/o/myc/osis | 12. retin/o/blast/oma |
| 3. ophthmal/algia | 13. scler/o/malacia |
| 4. phot/o/retin/itis | 14. dacry/o/cyst/itis |
| 5. dipl/opia | 15. ophthalm/orrhagia |
| 6. blephar/itis | 16. scler/o/kerat/itis |
| 7. leuk/o/cor/ia | 17. phot/o/phobia |
| 8. irid/o/plegia | 18. kerat/itis |
| 9. corne/o/ir/itis | 19. end/ophthalm/itis |
| 10. blephar/o/ptosis | 20. ophthalm/o/plegia |

## Exercise 11

Spelling exercise, *see* text, pp. 428, 429.

## Exercise 12

| | |
|---|---|
| 1. myopia | 9. glaucoma |
| 2. presbyopia | 10. detached retina |
| 3. strabismus | 11. hyperopia |
| 4. chalazion | 12. emmetropia |
| 5. astigmatism | 13. retinitis pigmentosa |
| 6. nystagmus | 14. nyctalopia |
| 7. cataract | 15. pterygium |
| 8. sty (hordeolum) | |

## Exercise 13

| | | | | |
|---|---|---|---|---|
| 1. f | 4. n | 7. d | 10. c | 13. i |
| 2. h | 5. m | 8. b | 11. a | 14. o |
| 3. k | 6. j | 9. e | 12. l | 15. g |

## Exercise 14

Spelling exercise; *see* text, p. 432.

## Exercise 15

    WR  CV  S
1. kerat/ o /plasty      surgical repair of the
      CF                  cornea

    WR   S
2. scler/otomy         incision into the sclera

    WR  CV WR  S
3. dacry/ o /cyst/otomy    incision into the tear
      CF               sac

    WR CV  WR CV  S
4. cry/ o /retin/ o /pexy     fixation of the retina
      CF      CF          by extreme cold

    WR CV WR   S
5. irid/ o /scler/otomy     incision into the edge
      CF                of the iris and into
                        the sclera

    WR   CV  S
6. blephar/ o /plasty     surgical repair of the
      CF               eyelids

    WR   S
7. irid/ectomy         excision of part of the
                       iris

    WR  CV WR CV WR    S
8. dacry/ o /cyst/ o /rhin/ostomy   creation of an artifi-
      CF     CF          cial opening be-
                        tween the tear (lac-
                        rimal) sac and the
                        nose

## Exercise 16

1. dacry/o/cyst/o/rhin/ostomy
2. irid/ectomy
3. kerat/o/plasty
4. scler/otomy
5. blephar/o/plasty
6. cry/o/retin/o/pexy
7. dacry/o/cyst/otomy
8. irid/o/scler/otomy

## Exercise 17

Spelling exercise; *see* text, pp. 434, 435.

## Exercise 18

| | |
|---|---|
| 1. retinal photocoagulation | 5. strabotomy |
| 2. cryoextraction of the lens | 6. trabeculectomy |
| 3. enucleation | 7. scleral buckling |
| 4. phacoemulsification | 8. radial keratotomy |
| | 9. vitrectomy |

## Exercise 19

| | | | | |
|---|---|---|---|---|
| 1. e | 3. b | 5. h | 7. i | 9. g |
| 2. f | 4. c | 6. d | 8. a | |

## Exercise 20

Spelling exercise; *see* text, p. 438.

## Exercise 21

WR CV S
1. opt/ o /meter — instrument that measures power and range of vision
CF

WR CV S
2. pupill/ o /scope — instrument that measures the reaction of the pupil
CF

WR CV S
3. opt/ o /metry — measurement of visual acuity and the prescribing of corrective lenses
CF

WR CV S
4. ophthalm/ o /scope — instrument that examines the interior of the eye
CF

WR CV S
5. ton/ o /metry — measurement of pressure within the eye
CF

WR CV S
6. pupill/ o /meter — instrument that measures the width and diameter of the pupil
CF

WR CV WR CV S
7. opt/ o /my/ o /meter — instrument that measures the power of the muscles of vision
CF  CF

WR CV S
8. ton/ o /meter — instrument that measures pressure within the eye
CF

WR CV S
9. kerat/ o /meter — instrument that measures (the curvature of) the cornea
CF

WR CV S
10. ophthalm/ o /scopy — visual examination of the eye
CF

WR CV S
11. angi/ o /graphy — process of x-ray filming the blood vessels of the eye using fluorescing dye
CF

## Exercise 22

1. opt/o/meter
2. ton/o/metry
3. pupill/o/meter
4. kerat/o/meter
5. opt/o/metry
6. opt/o/my/o/meter
7. ophthalm/o/scope
8. ton/o/meter
9. pupill/o/scope
10. ophthalm/o/scopy
11. fluorescein angi/o/graphy

## Exercise 23

Spelling exercises; *see* text, p. 446.

## Exercise 24

WR S
1. ophthalm/ology — study of diseases and treatment of the eye

P WR S
2. bin/ocul/ar — pertaining to two or both eyes

WR S
3. opt/ician — one who is skilled in filling prescriptions for lenses

WR S
4. lacrim/al — pertaining to tears or tear ducts

WR S
5. pupill/ary — pertaining to the pupil of the eye

WR CV S
6. retin/ o /pathy — (any noninflammatory) disease of the retina
CF

WR S
7. ophthalm/ologist — physician who specializes in ophthalmology

WR S
8. corne/al — pertaining to the cornea

WR S
9. ophthalm/ic — pertaining to the eye

WR CV WR S
10. nas/ o /lacrim/al — pertaining to the nose and tear ducts
CF

WR S
11. opt/ic — pertaining to vision

P WR S
12. intra/ocul/ar — pertaining to within the eye

WR S
13. retin/al — pertaining to the retina

WR CV S
14. ophthalm/ o /pathy — any disease of the eye
CF

## Exercise 25

1. opthalm/ology
2. bin/ocul/ar
3. retin/al
4. intra/ocul/ar
5. ophthalm/ologist
6. lacrim/al
7. opt/ic
8. opt/ician
9. retin/o/pathy
10. corne/al
11. nas/o/lacrim/al
12. ophthalm/o/pathy
13. pupill/ary

## Exercise 26

Spelling exercise; *see* text, pp. 442 and 443.

## Exercise 27

1. left eye
2. a health professional who prescribes corrective lenses and/or eye exercises
3. agent that dilates the pupil
4. each eye
5. sharpness of vision
6. agent that constricts the pupil
7. right eye

## Exercise 28

| | | |
|---|---|---|
| 1. oculus sinister | 4. miotic | 7. visual acuity |
| 2. mydriatic | 5. oculus dexter | |
| 3. oculus uterque | 6. optometrist | |

## Exercise 29

Spelling exercise; *see* text, p. 445.

## Exercise 30

| | | |
|---|---|---|
| 1. mydriatic | 4. tonometer | 7. nystagmus |
| 2. astigmatism | 5. hyperopia | 8. trabeculectomy |
| 3. cataract | 6. chalazion | 9. fluorescein angiography |

## Exercise 31

| | | |
|---|---|---|
| 1. ophthalmalgia | 3. blepharitis | 5. retinopathy |
| 2. iridectomy | 4. ophthalmoscope | |

## Exercise 32

1. pertaining to within the nose
2. formation of red blood cells
3. hernia of the esophagus
4. producing fibers
5. hardening (caused by scarring) of the glomeruli
6. excessive flow of blood
7. stone in the liver
8. dissolution or breaking down of tissue
9. abnormal condition of water and pus in the kidney
10. excessive development of muscle tissue

# 12

# Ear

## Objectives

**Upon completion of this chapter you will be able to:**

1. Define the anatomical terms of the ear.

2. Write the definitions of the word parts included in this chapter.

3. Build, analyze, define, pronounce, and spell the diagnostic terms related to the ear.

4. Define, pronounce, and spell other diagnostic terms related to the ear.

5. Build, analyze, define, pronounce, and spell the surgical terms related to the ear.

6. Build, analyze, define, pronounce, and spell the diagnostic procedural terms related to the ear.

7. Build, analyze, define, pronounce, and spell additional terms related to the ear.

## Objective 1 — DEFINE THE ANATOMICAL TERMS OF THE EAR.

## Anatomical Terms

The two functions of the ear are to hear and to provide the sense of balance. The ear is made up of three parts: the *external ear*, the *middle ear*, and the *inner ear*. We hear because sound waves vibrate through the ear, where they are transformed into nerve impulses that are then carried to the brain.

### EAR PARTS

1. External ear
   a. auricle, or pinna . . . . Located on either side of the head. The auricle directs sound waves into the external auditory meatus.

   b. external auditory meatus . . . . . . . . . . . . . Short tube that ends at the tympanic membrane. The inner part lies within the temporal bone of the skull and contains the glands that secrete earwax (cerumen).

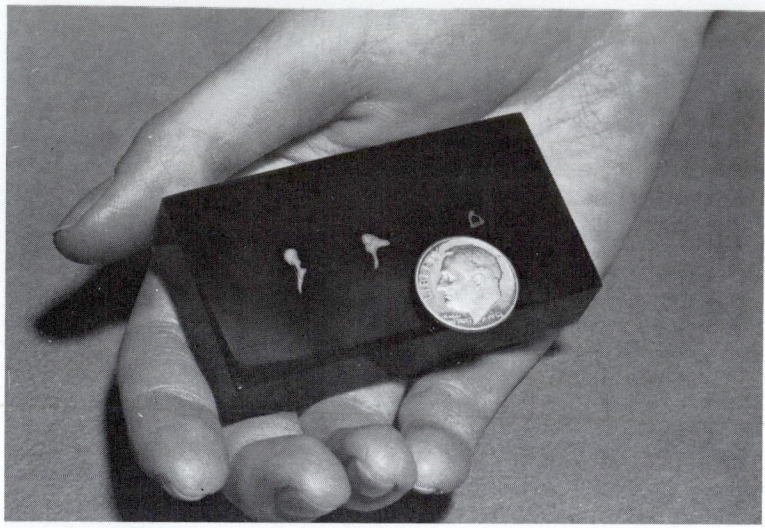

Figure 12-1

Human malleus, incus, and stapes, mounted in plastic and comparable in size to a dime.

From Saunders WH and others: *Nursing care in eye, ear, nose, and throat disorders,* ed 4, St. Louis, 1979, Mosby

2.  Middle ear
    a.  tympanic membrane, or eardrum . . . . . . .   Semitransparent membrane that separates the external auditory meatus and the middle ear cavity.
    b.  eustachian tube . . . . .   Connects the middle ear and the pharynx. It equalizes air pressure on either side of the eardrum.
    c.  ossicles. . . . . . . . . . .   Bones of the middle ear that carry sound vibrations. The ossicles comprise the malleus (hammer), incus (anvil), and stapes (stirrup). The stapes connects to the *oval window,* which carries the sound vibrations to the inner ear (Figure 12-1).

3.  Inner ear, or labyrinth. . .   Bony spaces within the temporal bone of the skull. It contains the following:
    a.  cochlea. . . . . . . . . . .   Is snail shaped and contains the organ of hearing. The cochlea connects to the oval window in the middle ear.
    b.  semicircular canals . .   Contain receptors and endolymph that help the body to maintain its sense of balance (equilibrium).

4.  mastoid bone and cells . .   Located in the skull bone behind the external auditory meatus.

The **tympanic membrane**'s name is derived from the Greek **tympanon,** meaning **drum,** because of its resemblance to a drum or tambourine.

**Stapes** is Latin for **stirrup.** The anatomical stapes was so named for its stirruplike shape.

Learn the anatomical terms by completing the following exercises.

## EXERCISE 1

Match the terms in the first column with the correct definitions in the second column.

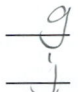

| | |
|---|---|
| _g_ | 1. auricle |
| _j_ | 2. cochlea |
| _b_ | 3. eustachian tube |
| _f_ | 4. external auditory meatus |
| _h_ | 5. labyrinth |
| _k_ | 6. mastoid bone |
| _d_ | 7. ossicles |
| _e_ | 8. oval window |
| _a_ | 9. semicircular canals |
| _c_ | 10. tympanic membrane |

a. contains receptors and endolymph, which help to maintain equilibrium

b. equalizes air pressure on both sides of eardrum

c. separates external auditory meatus and middle ear cavity

d. malleus, incus, and stapes

e. carries sound vibration to the inner ear

f. contains glands that secrete earwax

g. one located on either side of head

h. bony spaces in the inner ear

i. relays messages to the brain

j. contains the organ of hearing

k. located in skull behind external auditory meatus

Place a check mark (√) in the box to indicate that you have completed Objective 1.

☐ **DEFINE THE ANATOMICAL TERMS OF THE EAR.**

# Objective 2   WRITE THE DEFINITIONS FOR THE WORD PARTS INCLUDED IN THIS CHAPTER.

# Ear Word Parts

Study the word parts and their definitions listed as follows. Learning will be made easier by completing the exercises that follow.

| COMBINING FORM | DEFINITION |
|---|---|
| 1. acou/o<br>   audi/o | hearing |
| 2. aur/i, aur/o | ear |
| 3. labyrinth/o | labyrinth |
| 4. mastoid/o | mastoid |
| 5. myring/o | tympanic membrane (eardrum) |
| 6. ot/o | ear |
| 7. staped/o | stapes (middle ear bone) |
| 8. tympan/o | eardrum, middle ear |

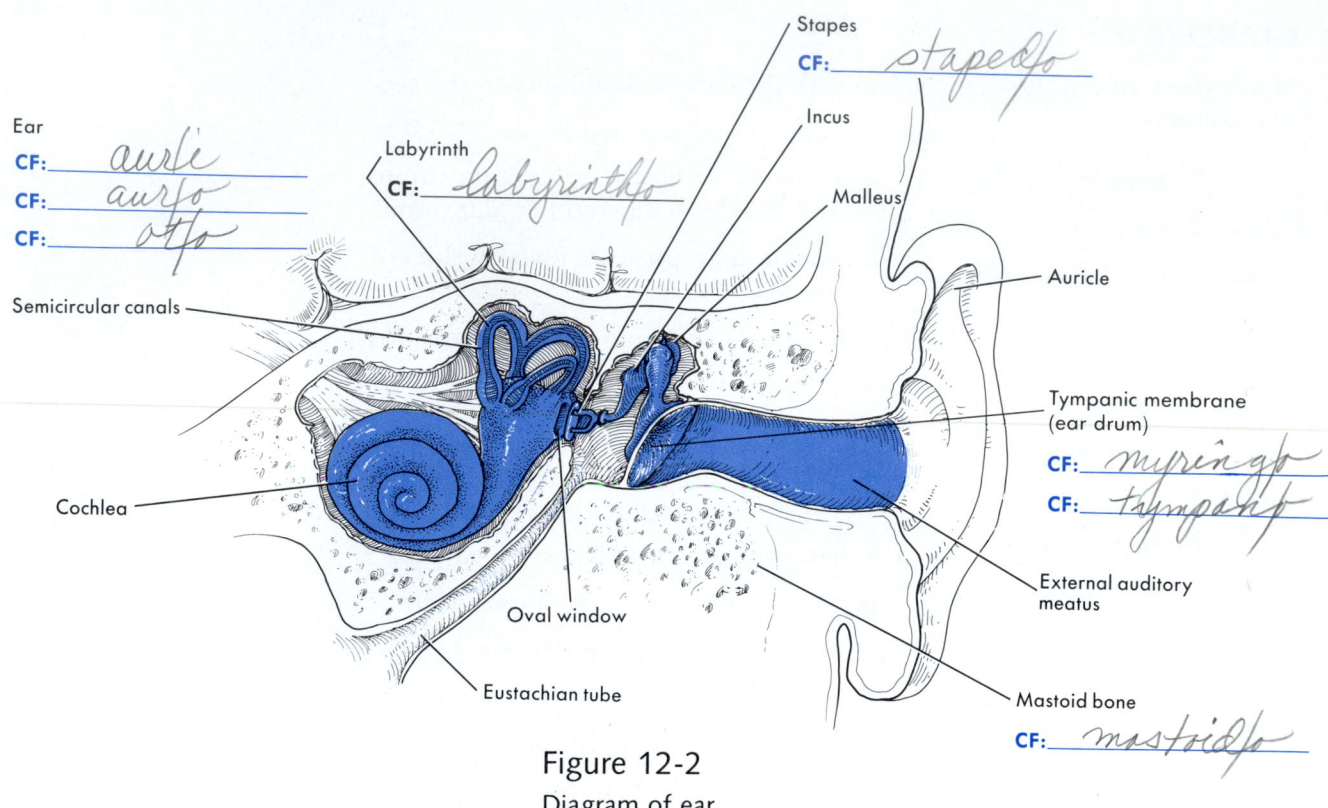

Ear
CF: _auri_
CF: _aur/o_
CF: _ot/o_

Labyrinth
CF: _labyrinth/o_

Stapes
CF: _staped/o_

Incus

Malleus

Semicircular canals

Auricle

Cochlea

Tympanic membrane (ear drum)
CF: _myring/o_
CF: _tympan/o_

External auditory meatus

Oval window

Eustachian tube

Mastoid bone
CF: _mastoid/o_

Figure 12-2
Diagram of ear

## EXERCISE 2

Write the combining forms in the spaces marked **CF** on the diagram in Figure 12-2 above.

## EXERCISE 3

Write the definitions of the following combining forms.

1. staped/o _____ stapes _____

2. mastoid/o _____ mastoid bone _____

3. audi/o _____ hearing _____

4. ot/o _____ ear _____

5. tympan/o _____ ear drum _____

6. aur/o, aur/i _____ ear _____

7. acou/o _____ hearing _____

8. labyrinth/o _____ labyrinth _____

9. myring/o _____ ear drum _____

## EXERCISE 4

Write the combining form for each of the following.

1. ear
   a. _____
   b. _____
   c. _____

2. mastoid _____

3. stapes _____

4. eardrum, middle ear _____

5. labyrinth _____

6. hearing
   a. _____
   b. _____

7. tympanic membrane (eardrum) _____

Place a check mark (√) in the box to indicate that you have completed Objective 2.

☐ WRITE THE DEFINITIONS OF THE WORD PARTS INCLUDED IN THIS CHAPTER.

## Medical Terms

The terms you need to learn to complete this chapter are listed as follows. Now that you know the meaning of the word parts, the exercises found at the end of this list will assist you to learn the definition and the spelling of each word.

## Objective 3 — BUILD, ANALYZE, DEFINE, PRONOUNCE, AND SPELL THE DIAGNOSTIC TERMS RELATED TO THE EAR.

## Diagnostic Terms

| TERM (built from word parts) | DEFINITION |
|---|---|
| 1. labyrinthitis (lab-i-rin-THĪ-tis) | inflammation of the labyrinth (in the inner ear, also called *otitis interna*) |
| 2. mastoiditis (mas-toyd-Ī-tis) | inflammation of the mastoid bone (and cells) |

3. myringitis . . . . . . . . . . . .     inflammation of the tympanic mem-
    (mīr-in-JĪ-tis)            brane (eardrum)

4. otalgia . . . . . . . . . . . . . .     pain in the ear
    (ō-TĂL-jē-a)

5. otomastoiditis . . . . . . . .     inflammation of the ear and the mastoid
    (ō-tō-*mas*-toyd-Ī-tis)     bone

6. otomycosis . . . . . . . . . .     condition of a fungal infection of the ear
    (ō-tō-mī-KŌ-sis)        (it usually affects the external auditory
                                meatus)

7. otopyorrhea . . . . . . . . . .     discharge of pus from the ear
    (ō-tō-pī-ō-RĒ-a)

8. otosclerosis . . . . . . . . . . .     hardening of the ear (stapes) (caused by
    (ō-tō-skle-RŌ-sis)       irregular bone development and result-
                                ing in hearing loss)

9. tympanitis . . . . . . . . . . .     inflammation of the middle ear (also
    (tim-pan-Ī-tis)         called *otitis media*)

Practice saying each of these terms aloud. To assist you in pronunciation, obtain the audiotape designed for use with this text. Learn the definitions and spellings of the diagnostic terms by completing the following exercises.

## EXERCISE 5

Analyze and define the following medical terms.

1. otomycosis _____

2. tympanitis _____

3. otomastoiditis _____

4. otalgia _____

5. labyrinthitis _____

6. myringitis _____

7. otosclerosis _____

8. mastoiditis _____

9. otopyorrhea _____

## EXERCISE 6

Build medical terms for the following definitions by using the word parts you have learned.

1. inflammation of the tym-
   panic membrane        _____ *myring* / *itis* _____
                                           WR     S

2. discharge of pus from the ear

    _ot_ / _o_ / _py_ / _orrhea_
    WR   CV   WR   S

3. inflammation of the mastoid bone

    _mastoid_ / _itis_
    WR   S

4. pain in the ear

    _ot_ / _algia_
    WR   S

5. hardening of the (ear) stapes

    _ot_ / _o_ / _sclerosis_
    WR   CV   S

6. condition of fungal infection of the ear

    _ot_ / _o_ / _myc_ / _osis_
    WR   CV   WR   S

7. inflammation of the ear and the mastoid bone

    _ot_ / _o_ / _mastoid_ / _itis_
    WR   CV   WR   S

8. inflammation of the labyrinth

    _labyrinth_ / _itis_
    WR   S

9. inflammation of the middle ear

    _tympan_ / _itis_
    WR   S

## EXERCISE 7

Spell each of the diagnostic terms. Have someone dictate the terms on pp. 459 and 460 to you or say the words into a tape recorder; then spell the words from your recording as often as necessary. Think about the word parts before attempting to write the word. Study any you have spelled incorrectly.

1. _____     6. _____

2. _____     7. _____

3. _____     8. _____

4. _____     9. _____

5. _____

Place a check mark (√) in the box to indicate that you have completed Objective 3.

☐ **BUILD, ANALYZE, DEFINE, PRONOUNCE, AND SPELL THE DIAGNOSTIC TERMS RELATED TO THE EAR.**

## Objective 4   **DEFINE, PRONOUNCE, AND SPELL OTHER DIAGNOSTIC TERMS RELATED TO THE EAR.**

## Other Diagnostic Terms

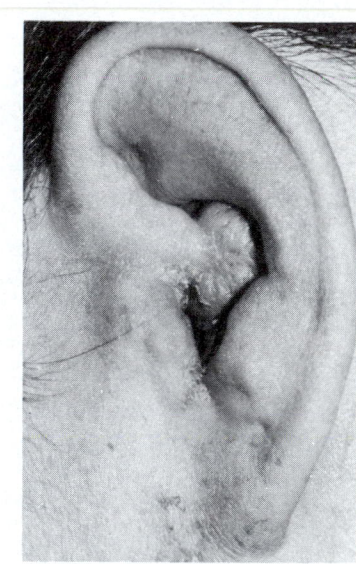

**Figure 12-3**

Chronic severe otitis externa.

From Saunders WH and others: *Nursing care in eye, ear, nose, and throat disorders,* ed 4, St. Louis, 1979, Mosby.

| TERM | DEFINITION |
|---|---|
| 1. acoustic neuroma.......<br>(a-KOOS-tik) (nū-RŌ-ma) | benign tumor within auditory canal growing from the acoustic nerve. May cause hearing loss |
| 2. ceruminoma..........<br>(se-roo-mi-NŌ-ma)<br>(NOTE: Although *cerumen* is spelled with an *e*, the word root is *cerumin/o.*) | tumor of the glands that secrete earwax (cerumen) |
| 3. Ménière's disease.......<br>(MEN-ē-ārz) | chronic disease of the inner ear characterized by dizziness and ringing in the ear |
| 4. otitis externa .........<br>(ō-TĪ-tis) (ex-TER-na) | inflammation of the outer ear (Figure 12-3) |
| 5. otitis media ..........<br>(ō-TĪ-tis) (MĒ-dia) | inflammation of the middle ear (Figure 12-4) |

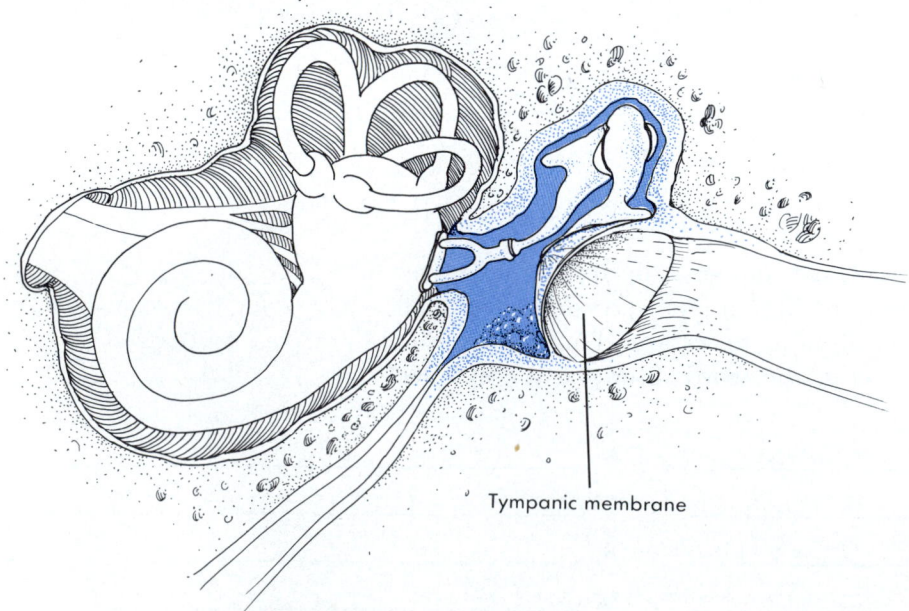

Tympanic membrane

**Figure 12-4**

Otitis media. Bulging, perforated, reddened, or retracted tympanic membrane.

6. **presbycusis** . . . . . . . . . . . hearing impairment in old age
(prez-bi-KŪ-sis)

7. **tinnitus** . . . . . . . . . . . . . . ringing in the ears
(tin-NĪ-tus)

8. **vertigo** . . . . . . . . . . . . . . dizziness
(VER-tig-ō)

Practice saying each of these terms aloud. To assist you in pronunciation, obtain the audiotape designed for use with this text. Learn the definitions and spellings of the other diagnostic terms by completing the following exercises.

## EXERCISE 8

Fill in the blanks with the correct terms.

1. The patient complained of dizziness, or _____*vertigo*_____ , and ringing in the ears, or _____*tinnitus*_____ .

2. A chronic ear disease characterized by dizziness and ringing in the ears is called _____*Ménière's*_____ disease.

3. Inflammation of the middle ear is called _____*otitis media*_____ .

4. _____*Ceruminoma*_____ is the name given to a tumor of the glands that secrete earwax.

5. _____*Otitis externa*_____ means inflammation of the outer ear.

6. A benign tumor arising from the acoustic nerve is called a(n) _____*acoustic neuroma*_____ .

7. _____*presbycusis*_____ is hearing impairment in old age.

## EXERCISE 9

Match the term in the first column with its correct definition in the second column.

_e_ 1. vertigo

_b_ 2. ceruminoma

_g_ 3. tinnitus

_c_ 4. Ménière's disease

_h_ 5. otitis externa

_d_ 6. acoustic neuroma

_a_ 7. otitis media

_i_ 8. presbycusis

a. inflammation of the middle ear

b. tumor of the glands that secrete earwax

c. chronic ear problem characterized by vertigo and tinnitus

d. benign tumor arising from acoustic nerve

e. dizziness

f. hardening of the oval window

g. ringing in the ears

h. inflammation of the outer ear

i. hearing impairment in old age

## EXERCISE 10

Spell each of the other diagnostic terms. Have someone dictate the terms on pp. 462 and 463 to you. Study any you have spelled incorrectly.

1. _____    5. _____

2. _____    6. _____

3. _____    7. _____

4. _____    8. _____

Place a check mark (√) in the box to indicate that you have completed Objective 4.

☐ DEFINE, PRONOUNCE, AND SPELL OTHER DIAGNOSTIC TERMS RELATED TO THE EAR.

# Objective 5    BUILD, ANALYZE, DEFINE, PRONOUNCE, AND SPELL THE SURGICAL TERMS RELATED TO THE EAR.

## Surgical Terms

**TERM**
(built from word parts)

**DEFINITION**

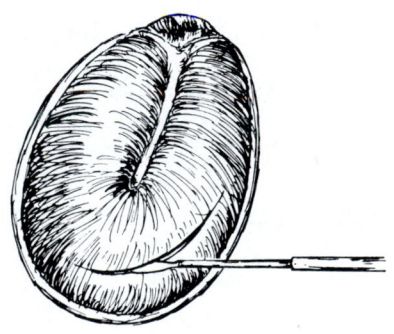

1. labyrinthectomy . . . . . . . .
   (*lab*-i-rin-THEK-tŏ-mē)
   excision of the labyrinth

2. mastoidectomy . . . . . . . . .
   (*mas*-toy-DEK-tŏ-mē)
   excision of the mastoid

3. mastoidotomy . . . . . . . . . .
   (*mas*-toy-DOT-ŏ-mē)
   incision into the mastoid

4. myringoplasty . . . . . . . .
   (mi-RING-gō-*plas*-tē)
   surgical repair of the tympanic membrane

5. myringotomy . . . . . . . . . .
   (mir-in-GOT-ŏ-mē)
   incision into tympanic membrane (performed to release pus and relieve pressure in the middle ear) (Figure 12-5)

**Figure 12-5**

Myringotomy: incision to release pus from tympanic membrane in acute otitis media.

From Saunders WH and others: *Nursing care in eye, ear, nose, and throat disorders*, ed 4, St. Louis, 1979, Mosby.

6. tympanoplasty . . . . . . . .
   (tim-pan-ō-PLAS-tē)
   surgical repair of the middle ear

Practice saying each of these terms aloud. To assist you in pronunciation, obtain the audiotape designed for use with this text. Learn the definitions and spellings of the surgical terms by completing the following exercises.

## EXERCISE 11

Analyze and define the following surgical terms.

1. mastoidectomy _____

2. myringotomy _____

3. labyrinthectomy _____

4. mastoidotomy _____

5. tympanoplasty _____

6. myringoplasty _____

## EXERCISE 12

Build surgical terms for the following definitions.

1. incision into the mastoid

   _mastoid / otomy_
   WR    S

2. excision of the labyrinth

   _labyrinth / ectomy_
   WR    S

3. surgical repair of the middle ear

   _tympan / o / plasty_
   WR   CV   S

4. excision of the mastoid

   _mastoid / ectomy_
   WR    S

5. incision into the tympanic membrane

   _myring / otomy_
   WR    S

6. surgical repair of the middle ear

   _tympan / o / plasty_
   WR   CV   S

## EXERCISE 13

Spell each of the surgical terms. Have someone dictate the terms on p. 464 to you or say the words into a tape recorder; then spell the words from your recording as often as necessary. Think about the word parts before attempting to spell the word. Study any you have spelled incorrectly.

1. _____    4. _____

2. _____    5. _____

3. _____    6. _____

Place a check mark (√) in the box to indicate that you have completed Objective 5.

☐ BUILD, ANALYZE, DEFINE, PRONOUNCE, AND SPELL THE SURGICAL TERMS RELATED TO THE EAR.

# Objective 6   BUILD, ANALYZE, DEFINE, PRONOUNCE, AND SPELL DIAGNOSTIC PROCEDURAL TERMS RELATED TO THE EAR.

# Diagnostic Procedural Terms

| TERM<br>(built from word parts) | DEFINITION |
|---|---|
| 1. acoumeter<br>(a-KOO-mē-ter) | instrument used to measure acuteness of hearing |
| 2. audiogram<br>(AW-dē-ō-gram) | graphic record of a hearing test |
| 3. audiometer<br>(*aw*-dē-OM-e-ter) | instrument used to measure hearing |
| 4. audiometry<br>(*aw*-dē-OM-e-trē) | measurement of hearing (Figure 12-6) |
| 5. otoscope<br>(Ō-tō-skōp) | instrument used for visual examination of the ear |
| 6. otoscopy<br>(ō-TOS-kō-pē) | visual examination of the ear |
| 7. tympanometer<br>(tim-pa-NOM-e-ter) | instrument to measure middle ear function |

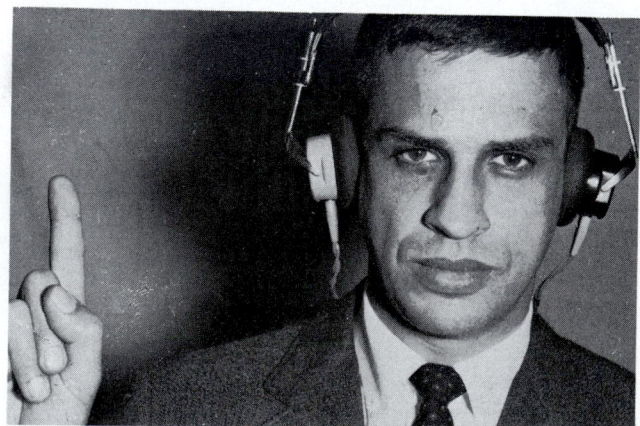

Figure 12-6

Audiometry. One earphone emits test sound while other earphone emits masking noise. Patient is told to signal (raise hand) when test sound occurs.

From Saunders WH and others: *Nursing care in eye, ear, nose, and throat disorders*, ed 4, St. Louis, 1979, Mosby.

8.　tympanometry . . . . . . . .　measurement (of the movement) of the
　　(tim-pa-NOM-e-trē)　　　　tympanic membrane

Practice saying each of these terms aloud. To assist you in pronunciation, obtain the audiotape designed for use with this text. Learn the definitions and spellings of the diagnostic procedural terms by completing the following exercises.

## EXERCISE 14

Analyze and define the following diagnostic procedural terms.

1. otoscope _____

2. audiometry _____

3. audiogram _____

4. otoscopy _____

5. audiometer _____

6. tympanometry _____

7. acoumeter _____

8. tympanometer _____

## EXERCISE 15

Build diagnostic procedural terms for the following definitions.

1. measurement (of move-
   ment) of the tympanic
   membrane

   _tympan_ / _o_ / _metry_
   　　WR 　 CV 　 S

2. instrument used to measure hearing

   _audio_ / _o_ / _meter_
   　　WR 　 CV 　 S

3. examination of the ear

   _ot_ / _o_ / _scopy_
   　WR 　 CV 　 S

4. graphic record of a hearing test

   _audi_ / _o_ / _gram_
   　WR 　 CV 　 S

5. instrument used for visual examination of the ear

_ot_ / _o_ / _scope_
WR / CV / S

6. measurement of hearing

_audi_ / _o_ / _metry_
WR / CV / S

7. instrument used to measure (acuteness of) hearing

_acou_ / _meter_
WR / S

8. instrument to measure middle ear function

_tympan_ / _o_ / _meter_
WR / CV / S

## EXERCISE 16

Spell each of the diagnostic procedural terms. Have someone dictate the terms on pp. 466 and 467 to you or say the words into a tape recorder; then spell the words from your recording as often as necessary. Think about the word parts before attempting to write the word. Study any you have spelled incorrectly.

1. _____   5. _____
2. _____   6. _____
3. _____   7. _____
4. _____   8. _____

Place a check mark (✓) in the box to indicate that you have completed Objective 6.

☐ **BUILD, ANALYZE, DEFINE, PRONOUNCE, AND SPELL THE DIAGNOSTIC PROCEDURAL TERMS RELATED TO THE EAR.**

# Objective 7   BUILD, ANALYZE, DEFINE, PRONOUNCE, AND SPELL ADDITIONAL TERMS RELATED TO THE EAR.

## Additional Terms

| TERM (built from word parts) | DEFINITION |
| --- | --- |
| 1. audiologist . . . . . . . . . . . (aw-dē-OL-ō-jist) | one who is skilled in and specializes in audiology |
| 2. audiology . . . . . . . . . . . . (aw-dē-OL-ō-jē) | study of hearing |

3. aural................ pertaining to the ear
   (AW-rul)

4. otologist ............. physician who studies and treats diseases
   (ō-TOL-ō-jist)           of the ear

5. otology .............. study of the ear
   (ō-TOL-ō-jē)

6. otorhinolaryngologist. . . . physician who studies and treats diseases
   (ō-tō-rī-nō-*lār*-in-GOL-ō-jist)   and disorders of the ear, nose, and
                             throat, also called otolaryngologist

Practice saying each of these terms aloud. To assist you in pronunciation, obtain the audiotape designed for use with this text. Learn the definitions and spellings of the additional terms by completing the following exercises.

## EXERCISE 17

Analyze and define the following terms.

1. otology _____

2. audiologist _____

3. otorhinolaryngologist _____

4. audiology _____

5. otologist _____

6. aural _____

## EXERCISE 18

Build terms for the following definitions.

1. study of hearing        _____ *audi* / *ology* _____
                                  WR      S

2. physician who studies and treats diseases and disorders of the ear, nose, and throat
   *ot* / *o* / *rhin* / *o* / *laryng* / *ologist*
   WR   CV   WR   CV    WR      S

3. study of the ear        _____ *ot* / *ology* _____
                                  WR      S

4. one who is skilled in audiology     *audi* / *ologist*
                                        WR      S

5. physician who studies and treats diseases of the ear

_ot_ | _ologist_
WR | S

6. pertaining to the ear

_aur_ | _al_
WR | S

Practice saying each of these terms aloud. To assist you in pronunciation, obtain the audiotape designed for use with this text. Learn the definitions and spellings of the additional terms by completing the following exercises.

## EXERCISE 19

Spell each of the additional terms. Have someone dictate the terms on pp. 469 and 470 to you. Think about the word parts before attempting to write the word. Study any you have spelled incorrectly.

1. _____        4. _____

2. _____        5. _____

3. _____        6. _____

Place a check mark (√) in the box to indicate that you have completed Objective 7.

☐ **BUILD, ANALYZE, DEFINE, PRONOUNCE, AND SPELL ADDITIONAL TERMS RELATED TO THE EAR.**

---

**Case History:** This 62-year-old American Indian male, appearing younger than age, was brought into the ENT clinic by his daughter who states that he is unable to hear what is being said to him by family members. She states that this problem has been existing for at least 30 years, but that it appears to be getting markedly worse. Patient states that he had several episodes of ear infection as a child and young adult. He denies any change in hearing. Otoscopy reveals there is scarring of tympanic membranes bilaterally. Both auditory canals are normal. He will be referred for audiometry.

---

**Results of Audiometry:** Auditory acuity at 500 Hz, 1000 Hz, 2000 Hz and 4000 Hz cycles per second in both right and left ear is markedly diminished. The patient is only hearing at 40 and 60 db at both 1000 and 500 cycles per second. He did not hear anything at 4000 or 2000 cycles per second.

**Impression:** Severe loss of hearing bilaterally, probably secondary to otitis media as a child. Some loss may be attributed to presbycusis.

## EXERCISE 20

To test your understanding of the terms introduced in this chapter, circle the words that correctly complete the sentences. The italicized phrase is the definition of the term.

1. *Inflammation of the eardrum* is (labyrinthitis, mastoiditis, myringitis).
2. The patient complained of *ringing in the ears,* or (tinnitus, vertigo, tympanitis).
3. The patient seeking a *specialist for his labyrinthitis* consulted an (optometrist, audiologist, otologist).
4. The physician planned to release the pus from the middle ear by making an *incision into the tympanic membrane*, or performing a (mastoidotomy, myringotomy, labyrinthectomy).

## EXERCISE 21

Unscramble the following mixed-up terms. The word on the left indicates a word part in each of the following.

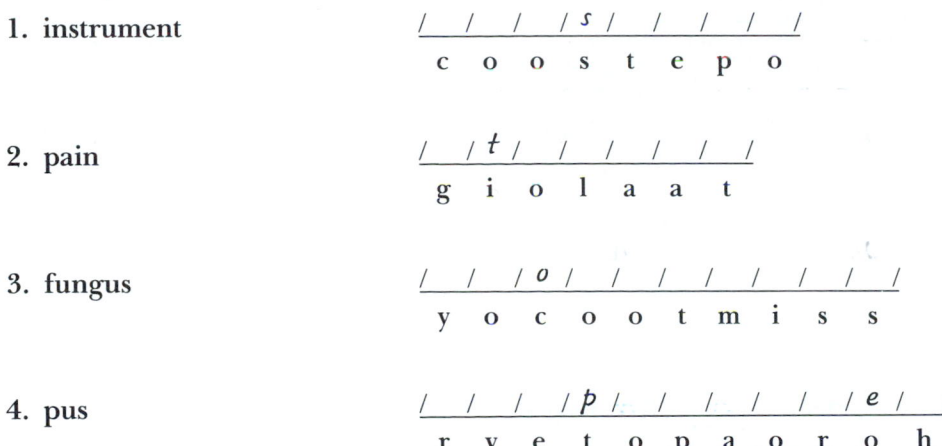

1. instrument

/ / / / s / / / / /
c  o  o  s  t  e  p  o

2. pain

/ / t / / / / / /
g  i  o  l  a  a  t

3. fungus

/ / / o / / / / / / /
y  o  c  o  o  t  m  i  s  s

4. pus

/ / / / p / / / / / / e / /
r  y  e  t  o  p  a  o  r  o  h

## EXERCISE 22

The following words did not appear in this chapter but are composed of word parts studied in this or the previous chapters. Find their definitions by translating the word parts literally.

1. **aglycemia**
   (*a*-glī-SĒ-mē-a) _____
2. **cardionephric**
   (*kar*-dē-ō-NEF-rik) _____
3. **cholecystogastric**
   (*kōlē*-*sis*-tō-GAS-trik) _____
4. **chromatometer**
   (*krō*-ma-TOM-e-ter) _____
5. **cystoplegia**
   (*sis*-tō-PLE-jē-a) _____
6. **dacryosinusitis**
   (*dak*-rē-ō-sī-nus-Ī-tis) _____
7. **gastroenterocolitis**
   (*gas*-trō-*en*-ter-ō-kō-LĪ-tis) _____

8. **hemocytolysis**
   (hē-mō-sī-TOL-i-sis) _____

9. **hysteroptosis**
   (*his*-ter-op-TŌ-sis) _____

10. **osteofibroma**
    (*os*-tē-ō-fī-BRO-ma) _____

11. **parasalpingeal**
    (*pār*-a-sal-PIN-jē-al) _____

12. **pericephalic**
    (*pār*-i-se-FAL-ik) _____

## COMBINING FORMS CROSSWORD PUZZLE

### Across Clues

1. hearing
4. cornea
6. light
9. abbreviation for Medical Corps
12. labyrinth
14. by mouth (medical abbreviation)
15. abbreviation for aortic regurgitation
17. abbreviation for number
18. conjunctiva
20. mastoid
22. tear duct
24. cornea
25. retina
27. double
28. vision

### Down Clues

2. ear
3. cold
5. eardrum, middle ear
7. tension
8. eyelid
10. pupil
11. eardrum
13. eye
16. sclera
19. stapes
21. tear
23. hearing
25. respiratory therapist (abbreviation)
26. abbreviation for ethylene oxide

# Summary

Can you build, analyze, define, spell, and pronounce the following terms *built from word parts?*   yes ☐   no ☐

| DIAGNOSTIC | SURGICAL | PROCEDURAL | ADDITIONAL |
|---|---|---|---|
| labyrinthitis<br>(*lab*-i-rin-THĪ-tis) | labyrinthectomy<br>(*lab*-i-rin-THEK-tŏ-mē) | acoumeter<br>(a-KOO-mē-ter) | audiologist<br>(aw-dē-OL-ō-jist) |
| mastoiditis<br>(*mas*-toyd-Ī-tis) | mastoidectomy<br>(*mas*-toy-DEK-tŏ-mē) | audiogram<br>(AW-dē-ō-gram) | audiology<br>(aw-dē-OL-ō-jē) |
| myringitis<br>(mĭr-in-JĪ-tis) | mastoidotomy<br>(*mas*-toy-DOT-ŏ-mē) | audiometer<br>(*aw*-dē-OM-e-ter) | aural<br>(AW-rul) |
| otalgia<br>(ō-TAL-jē-a) | myringoplasty<br>(mī-RING-gō-*plas*-tē) | audiometry<br>(*aw*-dē-OM-e-trē) | otologist<br>(ō-TOL-ō-jist) |
| otomastoiditis<br>(ō-tō-*mas*-toyd-Ī-tis) | myringotomy<br>(mir-in-GOT-ŏ-mē) | otoscope<br>(Ō-tō-skōp) | otology<br>(ō-TOL-ō-jē) |
| otomycosis<br>(ō-tō-mī-KŌ-sis) | tympanoplasty<br>(tim-pan-ō-PLAS-tē) | otoscopy<br>(ō-TOS-kō-pē) | otorhinolaryngologist<br>(ō-tō-*rī*-nō-*lăr*-in-GOL-ĕ-jist) |
| otopyorrhea<br>(ō-tō-pī-ō-RĒ-a) | | tympanometer<br>(tim-pa-NOM-e-ter) | |
| otosclerosis<br>(ō-tō-skle-RŌ-sis) | | tympanometry<br>(tim-pa-NOM-e-trē) | |
| tympanitis<br>(tim-pan-Ī-tis) | | | |

# Summary

Can you define, pronounce, and spell the following terms *not built from word parts?*   yes ☐   no ☐

## DIAGNOSTIC

acoustic neuroma
(a-KOOS-tik) (nū-RO-mah)

ceruminoma
(*se*-roo-mi-NŌ-ma)

Ménière's disease
(MEN-ē-ārz)

otitis externa
(ō-TĪ-tis) (ex-TER-na)

otitis media
(ō-TĪ-tis (MĒ-dia)

presbycusis
(prez-bi-KŪ-sis)

tinnitus
(tin-NĪ-tus)

vertigo
(VER-tig-ō)

# Answers

## Exercise 1
1. g  3. b  5. h  7. d  9. a
2. j  4. f  6. k  8. e  10. c

## Exercise 2
**Figure 12-2**
Ear: aur/i, aur/o, ot/o   Stapes: staped/o
Labyrinth: labyrinth/o   Tympanic membrane:
                             tympan/o, myring/o
                             Mastoid bone: mastoid/o

## Exercise 3
1. stapes  4. ear  7. hearing
2. mastoid  5. eardrum, middle ear  8. labyrinth
3. hearing  6. ear  9. tympanic membrane

## Exercise 4
1. a. aur/o  3. staped/o  6. a. acou/o
   b. aur/i  4. tympan/o     b. audi/o
   c. ot/o  5. labyrinth/o  7. myring/o
2. mastoid/o

## Exercise 5
1. ot/o/myc/osis (WRCV WR S, CF) — abnormal condition of a fungus infection of the ear
2. tympan/itis (WR S) — inflammation of the middle ear
3. ot/o/mastoid/itis (WR CV WR S, CF) — inflammation of the ear and the mastoid bone
4. ot/algia (WR S) — pain in the ear
5. labyrinth/itis (WR S) — inflammation of the labyrinth
6. myring/itis (WR S) — inflammation of the tympanic membrane
7. ot/o/sclerosis (WR CV S, CF) — hardening of the ear (stapes) (caused by irregular bone development)
8. mastoid/itis (WR S) — inflammation of the mastoid
9. ot/o/py/orrhea (WR CV WR S, CF) — discharge of pus from the ear

## Exercise 6
1. myring/itis  4. ot/algia  7. ot/o/mastoid/itis
2. ot/o/py/orrhea  5. ot/o/sclerosis  8. labyrinth/itis
3. mastoid/itis  6. ot/o/myc/osis  9. tympan/itis

## Exercise 7
Spelling exercise; *see* text, p. 461.

## Exercise 8
1. vertigo, tinnitus  5. otitis externa
2. Ménière's  6. acoustic neuroma
3. otitis media  7. presbycusis
4. ceruminoma

## Exercise 9
1. e  2. b  3. g  4. c  5. h  6. d  7. a  8. i

## Exercise 10
Spelling exercise; *see* text, pp. 462 and 463.

## Exercise 11
1. mastoid/ectomy (WR S) — excision of the mastoid
2. myring/otomy (WR S) — incision into the tympanic membrane
3. labyrinth/ectomy (WR S) — excision of the labyrinth
4. mastoid/otomy (WR S) — incision into the mastoid
5. tympan/o/plasty (WR CV S, CF) — surgical repair of the middle ear
6. myring/o/plasty (WR CV S, CF) — surgical repair of the tympanic membrane

## Exercise 12
1. mastoid/otomy  4. mastoid/ectomy
2. labyrinth/ectomy  5. myring/otomy
3. tympan/o/plasty  6. myring/o/plasty

## Exercise 13
Spelling exercise; *see* text, p. 465.

## Exercise 14
1. ot/o/scope (WR CV S, CF) — instrument used for the visual examination of the ear

     WR  CV   S
2. audi/ o /metry       measurement of hearing
        CF

     WR  CV   S
3. audi/ o /gram       graphic record of a hear-
        CF                ing test

     WR CV   S
4. ot / o /scopy       examination of the ear
        CF

     WR  CV   S
5. audi/ o /meter       instrument used to mea-
        CF                sure hearing

      WR   CV   S
6. tympan/ o /metry       measurement of move-
         CF                ment of the tympanic
                                membrane

     WR     S
7. acou/meter       instrument used to mea-
                           sure acuteness of hear-
                           ing

      WR   CV   S
8. tympan/ o /meter       instrument to measure
         CF                middle ear function

## Exercise 15

1. tympan/o/metry     4. audi/o/gram     7. acou/meter
2. audi/o/meter        5. ot/o/scope      8. tympan/o/meter
3. ot/o/scopy           6. audi/o/metry

## Exercise 16

Spelling exercise; *see* text, p. 468.

## Exercise 17

   WR   S
1. ot /ology                  study of the ear

   WR     S
2. audi/ologist              one who is skilled in
                             and specializes in au-
                             diology

   WR CV WR CV  WR    S
3. ot / o /rhin/ o /laryng/ologist      physician who studies
     CF      CF                 and treats diseases of
                               the ear, nose, and
                               throat

    WR    S
4. audi/ology                study of hearing

    WR    S
5. ot /ologist                physician who studies
                             and treats diseases of
                             the ear

    WR S
6. aur/al                  pertaining to the ear

## Exercise 18

1. audi/ology           4. audi/ologist
2. ot/o/rhin/o/laryng/    5. ot/ologist
   ologist                6. aur/al
3. ot/ology

## Exercise 19

Spelling exercise; *see* text, p. 470.

## Exercise 20

1. myringitis     3. otologist
2. tinnitus        4. myringotomy

## Exercise 21

1. otoscope     3. otomycosis
2. otalgia       4. otopyorrhea

## Exercise 22

1. absence of sugar in the blood
2. pertaining to the heart and the kidney
3. pertaining to the gallbladder and the stomach
4. instrument to measure color
5. paralysis of the bladder
6. inflammation of the tear sac and the sinuses
7. inflammation of the stomach, small intestine, and colon
8. separating of blood cells
9. prolapse of the uterus
10. tumor of the bone and fibrous tissue
11. pertaining to around (or in the wall of) the fallopian tube
12. pertaining to surrounding the head

# 13

# Musculoskeletal System

## Objectives

Upon completion of this chapter you will be able to:

1. Define the anatomical terms of the musculoskeletal system.

2. Write the definitions of the word parts included in this chapter.

3. Build, analyze, define, pronounce, and spell the diagnostic terms related to the musculoskeletal system.

4. Define, pronounce, and spell other diagnostic terms related to the musculoskeletal system.

5. Build, analyze, define, pronounce, and spell the surgical terms related to the musculoskeletal system.

6. Build, analyze define, pronounce, and spell the diagnostic procedural terms related to the musculoskeletal system.

7. Build, analyze, define, pronounce, and spell additional terms related to the musculoskeletal system.

8. Define, pronounce, and spell other additional terms related to the musculoskeletal system.

## Objective 1   DEFINE THE ANATOMICAL TERMS OF THE MUSCULOSKELETAL SYSTEM.

## Anatomical Terms

The musculoskeletal system is made up of bones, muscles, and joints. The body contains 206 bones, which are the framework of the body, and more than 500 muscles, which are responsible for movement. Joints are any place in the body at which two or more bones meet.

### BONE STRUCTURE

1. periosteum . . . . . . . . . . .   Outermost layer of the bone, made up of fibrous tissue (Figure 13-1).

2. compact bone . . . . . . . . .   Dense, hard layers of bone tissue that lie underneath the periosteum.

> **Periosteum** is composed of the prefix **peri**, meaning **surrounding**, and the word root **oste**, meaning **bone**.

476

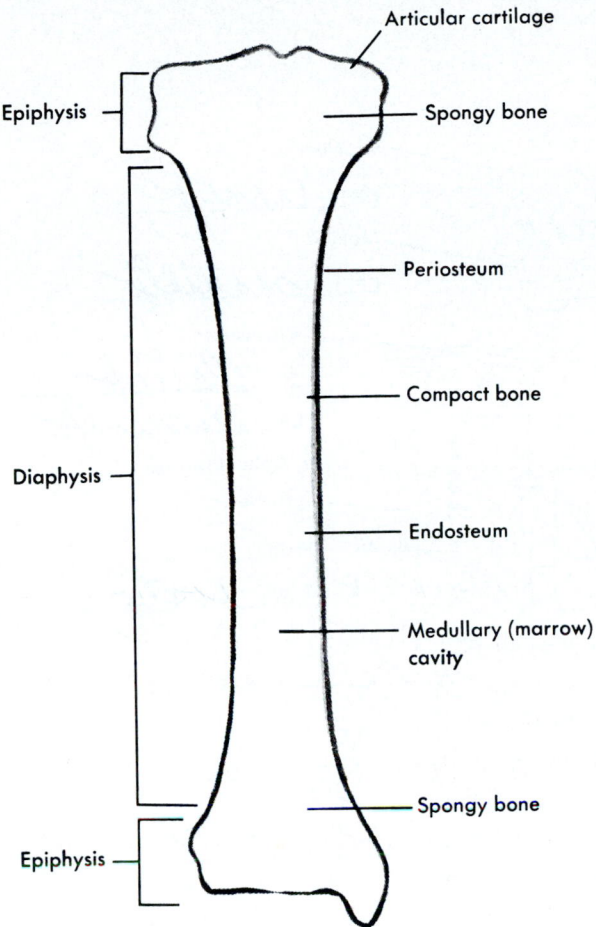

### Figure 13-1
Bone structure.

From Anthony CP and Thibodeau GA:
*Structure and function of the body,* ed 7,
St. Louis, 1984, Mosby.

3. cancellous (spongy) bone . Contains little spaces as in a sponge and is encased in the layers of compact bone.

4. endosteum . . . . . . . . . . . Membranous lining of the hollow cavity of the bone.

5. diaphysis . . . . . . . . . . . . Shaft of the long bones.

6. epiphysis . . . . . . . . . . . . Ends of the long bones.

7. bone marrow . . . . . . . . . Soft, spongelike material found in the cavities of bones.

## SKELETAL BONES

1. maxilla . . . . . . . . . . . . . . Upper jawbones (Figure 13-2).

2. mandible . . . . . . . . . . . Lower jawbone.

**Endosteum** is composed of the prefix **endo,** meaning **within,** and the word root **osteo,** meaning **bone.**

**Diaphysis** comes from the Greek **diaphusis,** meaning **state of growing between.**

**Epiphysis** has been used in the English language since the 1600s and still retains the meaning given to it by a Greco-Roman physician. It means a portion of bone attached for a time to another bone by a cartilage but which later combines with the principal bone. During the period of growth the epiphysis is separated from the main portion of the bone by cartilage.

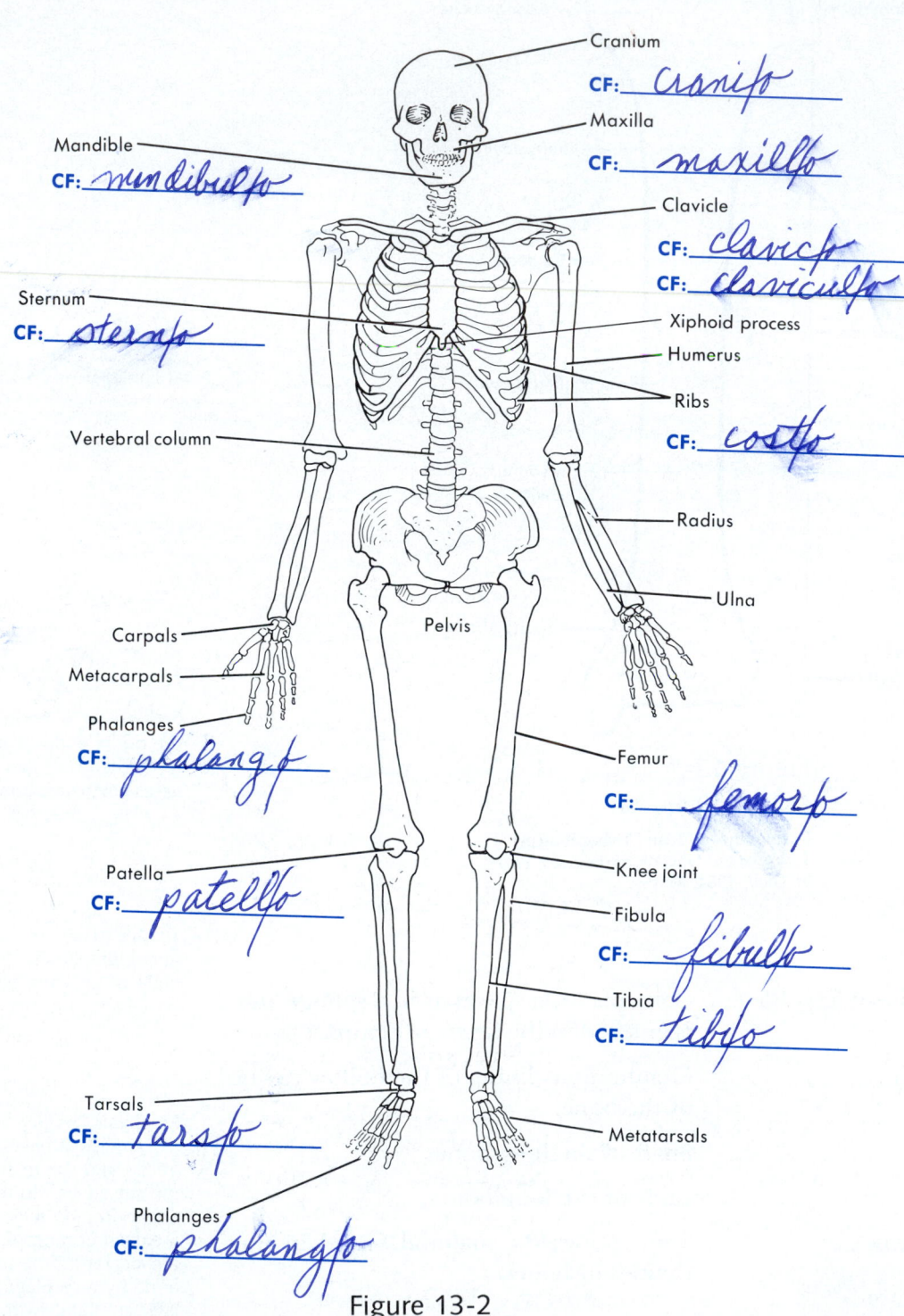

Cranium
CF: _cranio_

Maxilla
CF: _maxillo_

Mandible
CF: _mandibulo_

Clavicle
CF: _clavico_
CF: _claviculo_

Sternum
CF: _sterno_

Xiphoid process

Humerus

Ribs
CF: _costo_

Vertebral column

Radius

Ulna

Carpals

Pelvis

Metacarpals

Phalanges
CF: _phalango_

Femur
CF: _femoro_

Patella
CF: _patello_

Knee joint

Fibula
CF: _fibulo_

Tibia
CF: _tibio_

Tarsals
CF: _tarso_

Metatarsals

Phalanges
CF: _phalango_

Figure 13-2
Skeleton, anterior view.

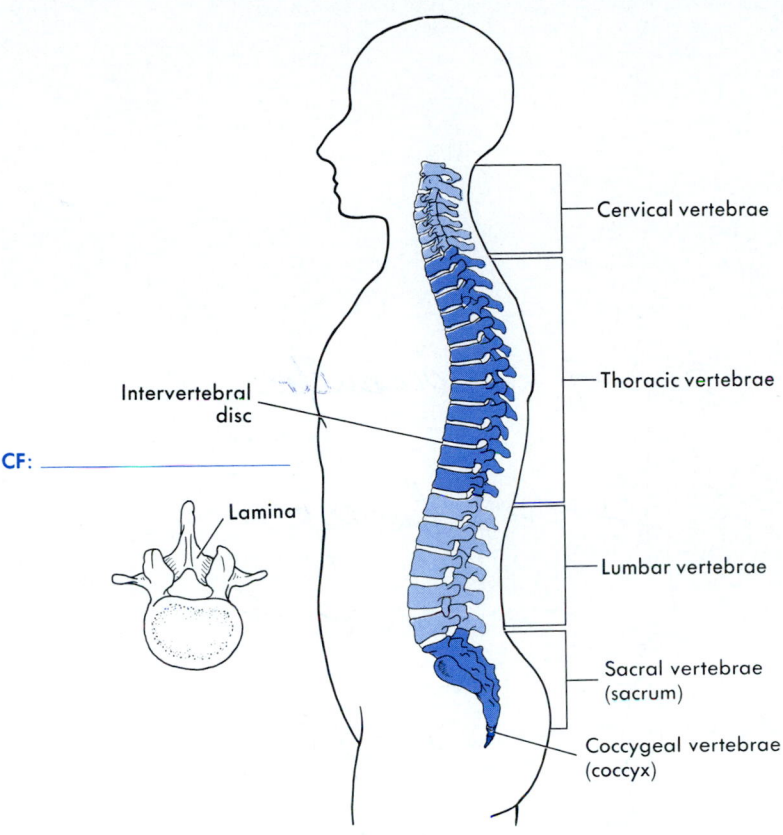

Cervical vertebrae

Thoracic vertebrae

Lumbar vertebrae

Sacral vertebrae (sacrum)

Coccygeal vertebrae (coccyx)

Intervertebral disc

CF: _____

Lamina

**Figure 13-3**
Vertebral column.

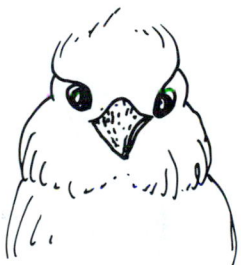

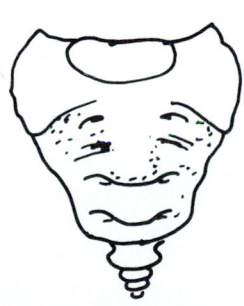

**Figure 13-4**
**Coccyx** is derived from the Greek word for **cuckoo** because of its resemblance to a cuckoo's beak.

3. vertebral column . . . . . . — Made up of bones called *vertebrae (pl.)* or *vertebra (sing.)* (Figure 13-3).

   a. cervical vertebrae . . — First set of seven bones, forming the neck.

   b. thoracic vertebrae . . — Second set of twelve vertebrae; they articulate with the twelve pairs of ribs to form the outward curve of the spine.

   c. lumbar vertebrae . . . — Third set of five larger vertebrae, which forms the inward curve of the spine.

   d. sacrum . . . . . . . . . . — Next four vertebrae, which fuse together in the young child.

   e. coccyx . . . . . . . . . . — Five vertebrae fused together to form the tailbone (Figure 13-4).

   f. lamina (*pl.* laminae). — Part of the vertebral arch (Figure 13-3).

4. clavicle . . . . . . . . . . . . . — Collarbone (Figure 13-2).

5. scapula . . . . . . . . . . . . . — Shoulder blade.

   a. acromion . . . . . . . . — Extension of the scapula, which forms the high point of the shoulder.

6. sternum . . . . . . . . . . . . — Breastbone.

   a. xiphoid process . . . . — Lower portion of the sternum.

7. humerus . . . . . . . . . . . . — Upper arm bone.

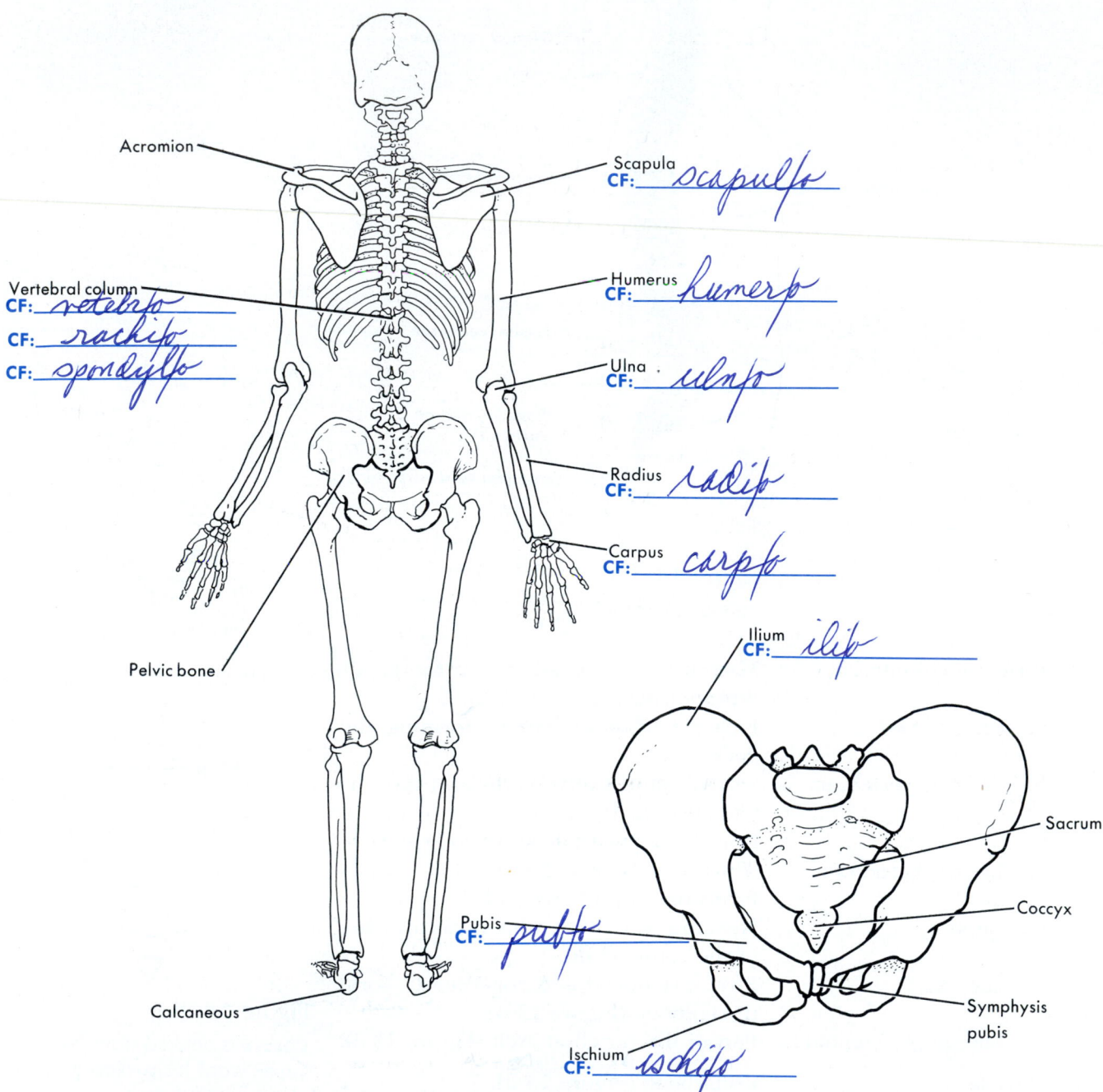

Acromion

Scapula
CF: _scapulo_

Vertebral column
CF: _vertebro_
CF: _rachio_
CF: _spondylo_

Humerus
CF: _humero_

Ulna
CF: _ulno_

Radius
CF: _radio_

Carpus
CF: _carpo_

Pelvic bone

Ilium
CF: _ilio_

Sacrum

Coccyx

Symphysis
pubis

Pubis
CF: _pubo_

Ischium
CF: _ischio_

Calcaneous

Figure 13-5
Skeleton, posterior view.

8. ulna and radius . . . . . . .   Lower arm bones (Figure 13-2).

9. carpal bones. . . . . . . . . .   Wrist bones.

10. metacarpal bones . . . . . .   Hand bones.

11. phalanges (*sing.* pha-
    lanx). . . . . . . . . . . . . . .   Finger and toe bones.

12. pelvic bone, or hip bone.   Made up of three bones fused together
    (Figure 13-5).
    a. ischium . . . . . . . . . .   Lower, rear portion on which one sits.
    b. ilium . . . . . . . . . . . .   Upper, wing-shaped part on each side.
    c. pubis . . . . . . . . . . .   Anterior portion of the pelvic bone.

13. acetabulum. . . . . . . . . .   Large socket in the pelvic bone for the
    head of the femur.

14. femur . . . . . . . . . . . . . .   Upper leg bone.

15. tibia and fibula. . . . . . .   Lower leg bones.

16. patella . . . . . . . . . . . . .   Kneecap.

17. tarsal bones . . . . . . . . .   Ankle bones (Figure 13-2).
    a. calcaneus . . . . . . . .   Heel bone.

18. metatarsal bones . . . . . .   Foot bones.

> **Metacarpus** literally means **beyond the wrist.** It is composed of the prefix **meta-**, meaning **beyond**, and **carpus**, meaning **wrist**.

## JOINTS

Joints, also called *articulations*, hold our bones together and make movement possible (Figure 13-6).

1. articular cartilage. . . . . .   Smooth layer of gristle covering the contacting surface of joints.
   a. meniscus . . . . . . . . .   Crescent-shaped cartilage found in the knee.
   b. intervertebral disc . . .   Cartilaginous disc found between each vertebra in the spine.
   c. symphysis pubis. . . . .   Cartilaginous joint at which two pubic bones fuse together.

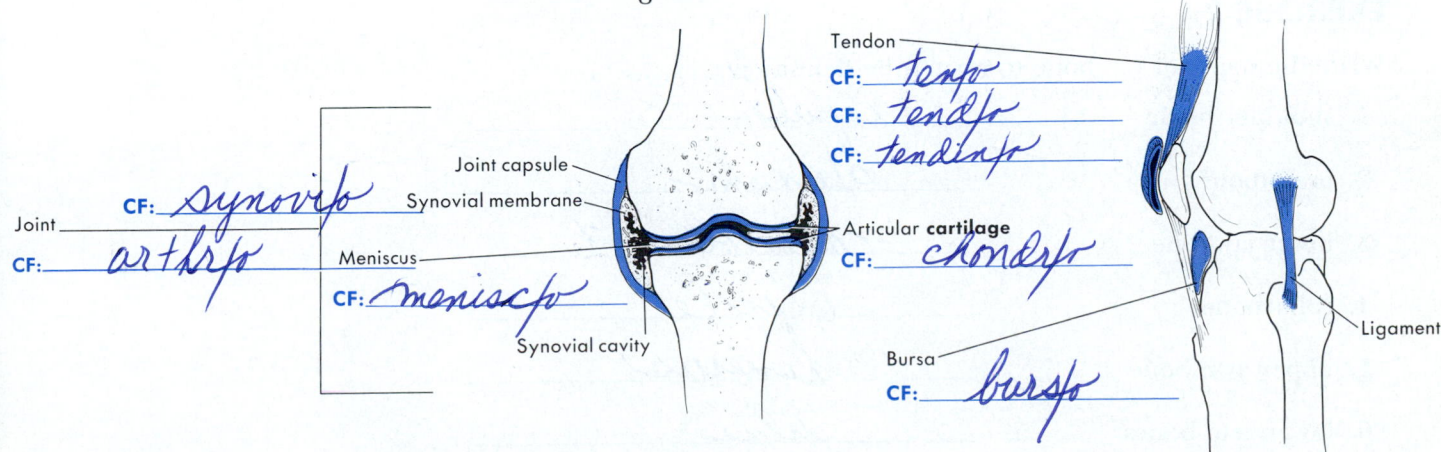

Figure 13-6
Joint.

2. synovia . . . . . . . . . . . . .    Fluid secreted by the synovial membrane and found in joint cavities.

3. bursa . . . . . . . . . . . .    Small, fluid-filled sac that allows for easy movement of one part of a joint over another.

4. ligament . . . . . . . . . . . .    Flexible, tough band of fibrous tissue that connects various bones and cartilages (see Figure 13-6).

5. tendon . . . . . . . . . . . . .    Band of tissue that attaches muscle to bone (see Figure 13-6).

6. aponeurosis . . . . . . . . . .    Strong sheet of tissue that acts as a tendon to attach muscles to bone.

Learn the anatomical terms by completing the following exercises.

## EXERCISE 1

Match the definitions in the first column with the correct terms in the second column.

_d_ 1. shaft of a bone     a. bone marrow

_c_ 2. hard layer of bone tissue     b. cancellous bone

    c. compact bone

_h_ 3. outermost layer of bone     d. diaphysis

_a_ 4. found in bone cavities     e. endometrium

    f. endosteum

_f_ 5. lining of the bone cavity     g. epiphysis

    h. periosteum

_g_ 6. ends of bones

_b_ 7. contains little spaces

## EXERCISE 2

Write the name of the bone to match the definition.

1. shoulder blade     _scapula_

2. breastbone     _sternum_

3. lower jawbone     _mandible_

4. collarbone     _clavicle_

5. upper arm bone     _humerus_

6. lower arm bones     a. _ulna_

    b. _radius_

7. ankle bones  _____ *tarsal bones*

8. finger, toe bones  _____ *phalanges*

9. foot bones  _____ *metatarsal*

10. hand bones  _____ *metacarpal*

11. upper leg bone  _____ *femur*

12. lower leg bones  a.  _____ *tibia*

                    b.  _____ *fibula*

13. kneecap  _____ *patella*

14. neck  _____ *cervical vertebrae*

15. third set of vertebrae  _____ *lumbar vertebrae*

16. anterior portion of the pelvic bone  _____ *pubis*

17. four vertebrae fused together  _____ *sacrum*

18. lower rear portion of the pelvic bone  _____ *ischium*

19. tailbone  _____ *coccyx*

20. upper, wing-shaped part of the pelvic bone  _____ *ilium*

21. wrist bones  _____ *carpal*

## EXERCISE 3

Match the definitions in the first column with the correct terms in the second column.

_m b_ 1. attaches muscle to bone

_C_ 2. fluid-filled sac

_e_ 3. smooth layer of gristle

_a_ 4. socket in the pelvic bone

_l_ 5. fluid

_d_ 6. heel bone

a. acetabulum

b. aponeurosis

c. bursa

d. calcaneus

e. cartilage

f. intervertebral disc

g. lamina

h. ligament

_h_ 7. connects bones to bone

_l_ 8. cartilage found in the knee

_k_ 9. pubic bone joint

_b_ 10. acts as a tendon

_f_ 11. found between each vertebra

_g_ 12. part of the arch of the vertebra

i. meniscus

j. periosteum

k. symphysis pubis

l. synovia

m. tendon

Place a check mark (√) in the box to indicate that you have completed Objective 1.

☐ **DEFINE THE ANATOMICAL TERMS OF THE MUSCULOSKELETAL SYSTEM.**

## Objective 2  WRITE THE DEFINITIONS OF THE WORD PARTS INCLUDED IN THIS CHAPTER.

# Musculoskeletal System Word Parts

At first glance the number of word parts introduced in this chapter may seem overwhelming to you; but notice that many of them are names for bones already learned in the anatomical section. The definitions of the word parts include both anatomical terms and commonly used words. For example, both *carpal* and *wrist bone* are given as the definition of the word root *carp/o.*

**COMBINING FORMING**                    **DEFINITION**

**LIST A**

1. carp/o . . . . . . . . . . . . . . . carpals (wrist bones)

2. clavic/o, clavicul/o . . . . . clavicle (collarbone)

3. cost/o . . . . . . . . . . . . . . . rib

4. crani/o . . . . . . . . . . . . . . cranium (skull)

5. femor/o. . . . . . . . . . . . . . femur (upper leg bone)

6. fibul/o. . . . . . . . . . . . . . . fibula (lower leg bone)

7. humer/o . . . . . . . . . . . . . humerus (upper arm bone)

8. ili/o. . . . . . . . . . . . . . . . . ilium

9. ischi/o. . . . . . . . . . . . . . . ischium

10. mandibul/o. . . . . . . . . . . mandible (lower jawbone)

**LIST B**

1. maxill/o . . . . . . . . . . . . . maxilla (upper jawbone)
2. patell/o . . . . . . . . . . . . . patella (kneecap)
3. phalang/o . . . . . . . . . . . phalanges (finger or toe bones)
4. pub/o . . . . . . . . . . . . . . pubis
5. radi/o . . . . . . . . . . . . . . radius (lower arm bone)
6. scapul/o . . . . . . . . . . . . scapula (shoulder blade)
7. stern/o . . . . . . . . . . . . . sternum (breastbone)
8. tars/o . . . . . . . . . . . . . . tarsals (ankle bones)
9. tibi/o . . . . . . . . . . . . . . tibia (lower leg bone)
10. uln/o . . . . . . . . . . . . . . ulna (lower arm bone)
11. vertebr/o
    rachi/o
    spondyl/o . . . . . . . . . . . vertebra, spinal, or vertebral column

Learn the anatomical locations and definitions of the combining forms by completing the following exercises.

## EXERCISE 4

Write the combining forms *from List A* in the spaces marked **CF** on the diagrams in Figures 13-2 and 13-5, pp. 478 and 480.

## EXERCISE 5

Write the definitions of the following combining forms.

1. clavic/o ___clavicle (collarbone)___
2. cost/o ___rib___
3. crani/o ___cranium___
4. femor/o ___femor (upper leg bone)___
5. clavicul/o ___clavicle (collarbone)___
6. humer/o ___humerus (upper arm bone)___
7. ili/o ___ilium___
8. ischi/o ___ischium___
9. carp/o ___carpals (wrist bones)___
10. fibul/o ___fibula (lower leg bone)___
11. mandibul/o ___mandible (lower jawbone)___

## EXERCISE 6

Write the combining form for each of the following.

1. clavicle      a. _____ clavic/o _____

           b. _____ clavicul/o _____

2. rib _____ cost/o _____

3. cranium _____ crani/o _____

4. femur _____ femor/o _____

5. humerus _____ humer/o _____

6. carpals _____ carp/o _____

7. ischium _____ ischi/o _____

8. fibula _____ fibul/o _____

9. ilium _____ ili/o _____

10. mandible _____ mandibul/o _____

## EXERCISE 7

Write the combining forms *from list B* in the spaces marked **CF** on the diagrams in Figures 13-2 and 13-5, pp. 478 and 480.

## EXERCISE 8

Write the definitions of the following combining forms.

1. rachi/o _____ vertebra, spinal or vetebral column _____

2. patell/o _____ patella, knee cap _____

3. spondyl/o _____ vertebra, spinal or vetebral column _____

4. maxill/o _____ maxilla, upper jawbone _____

5. phalang/o _____ phalanges, finger or toe bones _____

6. uln/o _____ ulna (lower arm bone) _____

7. radi/o _____ radius (lower arm bone) _____

8. tibi/o _____ tibia (lower leg bone) _____

9. pub/o _____ pubis _____

10. tars/o _____ tarsals (ankle bones) _____

11. scapul/o ___ *scapula shoulder blade*
12. stern/o ___ *sternum breastbone*
13. vertebr/o ___ *vertebra spinal or vertebral column*

## EXERCISE 9

Write the combining form for each of the following.

1. maxilla ___ *maxill/o*
2. ulna ___ *uln/o*
3. radius ___ *radi/o*
4. tibia ___ *tibi/o*
5. pubis ___ *pub/o*
6. tarsals ___ *tars/o*
7. vertebra
   a. ___ *vertebr/o*
   b. ___ *rachi/o*
   c. ___ *spondyl/o*
8. sternum ___ *stern/o*
9. scapula ___ *scapul/o*
10. patella ___ *patell/o*
11. phalanges ___ *phalang/o*

# Joints

| COMBINING FORM | DEFINITION |
| --- | --- |
| 1. aponeur/o . . . . . . . . . . . . . | aponeurosis |
| 2. arthr/o . . . . . . . . . . . . . . | joint |
| 3. burs/o . . . . . . . . . . . . . . | bursa (cavity) |
| 4. chondr/o . . . . . . . . . . . . . | cartilage |
| 5. disk/o . . . . . . . . . . . . . | intervertebral disk |
| 6. menisc/o . . . . . . . . . . . . . | meniscus (crescent) |
| 7. synovi/o . . . . . . . . . . . . . | synovia, synovial membrane |
| 8. ten/o, tend/o, tendin/o . . . | tendon |

Learn the anatomical locations and definitions of the combining forms by completing the following exercises.

## EXERCISE 10

Write the combining forms in the spaces marked **CF** on the diagram in Figures 13-3 and 13-6, pp. 479 and 481.

## EXERCISE 11

Write the definitions of the following combining forms.

1. arthr/o _____ *joint* _____

2. aponeur/o _____ *aponeurosis* _____

3. menisc/o _____ *meniscus (crescent)* _____

4. tendin/o _____ *tendon* _____

5. chondr/o _____ *cartilage* _____

6. ten/o _____ *tendon* _____

7. burs/o _____ *bursa (cavity)* _____

8. tend/o _____ *tendon* _____

9. synovi/o _____ *synovia   synovial membrane* _____

10. disk/o _____ *intervetebral disc* _____

## EXERCISE 12

Write the combining form for each of the following.

1. meniscus _____ *menisc/o* _____

2. aponeurosis _____ *aponeur/o* _____

3. joint _____ *arthr/o* _____

4. cartilage _____ *chondr/o* _____

5. tendon    a. _____ *ten/o* _____

   b. _____ *tend/o* _____

   c. _____ *tendin/o* _____

6. bursa _____ *burs/o* _____

7. synovia, synovial
   membrane _____ *synovi/o* _____

8. intervertebral disk _____ *disk/o* _____

# Other Word Parts

| COMBINING FORM | DEFINITION |
|---|---|
| 1. ankyl/o . . . . . . . . . . . . . | crooked, stiff, bent |
| 2. kinesi/o. . . . . . . . . . . . | movement, motion |
| 3. kyph/o . . . . . . . . . . . . | hump |
| 4. lamin/o. . . . . . . . . . . . | lamina (thin, flat plate or layer) |
| 5. lord/o . . . . . . . . . . . . . | bent forward |
| 6. myel/o, myelon/o . . . . . . | bone marrow |
| 7. my/o, myos/o . . . . . . . . | muscle |

(NOTE: *My/o* was introduced in Chapter 2.)

| | |
|---|---|
| 8. oste/o . . . . . . . . . . . . . | bone |
| 9. petr/o . . . . . . . . . . . . . | stone |

(NOTE: *Lith/o,* also a combining form for *stone,* was introduced in Chapter 5.)

| | |
|---|---|
| 10. scoli/o. . . . . . . . . . . . . | crooked, curved |

Learn the anatomical locations and definitions of the other combining forms by completing the following exercises.

## EXERCISE 13

Write the definitions of the following combining forms.

1. my/o _____ muscle _____
2. petr/o _____ stone _____
3. kinesi/o _____ movement, motion _____
4. oste/o _____ bone _____
5. lamin/o _____ lamina _____
6. myel/o _____ bone marrow _____
7. kyph/o _____ hump _____
8. ankyl/o _____ crooked stiff, bent _____
9. scoli/o _____ curved, crooked _____
10. myelon/o _____ bone marrow _____
11. myos/o _____ muscle _____
12. lord/o _____ bent forward _____

## EXERCISE 14

Write the combining form for each of the following.

1. muscle     a. _____ *myo* _____
            b. _____ *myos/o* _____

2. stone _____ *petr/o* _____

3. movement, motion _____ *kinesi/o* _____

4. bone _____ *oste/o* _____

5. lamina _____ *lamin/o* _____

6. bone marrow     a. _____ *myel/o* _____
            b. _____ *myelon/o* _____

7. hump _____ *kyph/o* _____

8. crooked, stiff, bent _____ *ankyl/o* _____

9. crooked, curved _____ *scoli/o* _____

10. bent forward _____ *lord/o* _____

# Prefixes

| PREFIX | DEFINITION |
|---|---|
| 1. inter- . . . . . . . . . . . . . . . | between |
| 2. supra- . . . . . . . . . . . . . . . | above |
| 3. syn-, sym- . . . . . . . . . . . . | together, joined |

Learn the prefixes by completing the following exercises.

## EXERCISE 15

Write the definitions of the following.

1. supra- _____ *above* _____

2. syn-, sym- _____ *together, joined* _____

3. inter- _____ *between* _____

## EXERCISE 16

Write the prefix for each of the following.

1. together, joined _____ *syn- syn-* _____

2. between _____ *inter-* _____

3. above _____ *supra-* _____

# Suffixes

| SUFFIX | DEFINITION |
|---|---|
| 1. -asthenia............ | weakness |
| 2. -clasis, -clast, -clasia..... | break |
| 3. -desis ............... | surgical fixation, fusion |
| 4. -physis .............. | growth |
| 5. -schisis .............. | split, fissure |

Learn the suffixes by completing the following exercises.

## EXERCISE 17

Write the definitions for the following.

1. -physis _____ *growth* _____

2. -clasis _____ *break* _____

3. -desis _____ *surgical fixation, fusion* _____

4. -clast _____ *break* _____

5. -schisis _____ *split, fissure* _____

6. -clasia _____ *break* _____

7. -asthenia _____ *weakness* _____

## EXERCISE 18

Write the suffix for each of the following.

1. growth _____ *physis* _____

2. weakness _____ *asthenia* _____

3. break
   a. _____ *clasis* _____
   b. _____ *clast* _____
   c. _____ *clasia* _____

4. surgical fixation, fu-
sion                                   *desis*

5. split, fissure                      *schisis*

Place a check mark (√) in the box to indicate that you have completed Objective 2.

---

☐ **WRITE THE DEFINITIONS OF THE WORD PARTS INCLUDED IN THIS CHAPTER.**

## Medical Terms

The terms you need to learn to complete this chapter are listed as follows. Now that you know the meaning of the word parts, the exercises
found at the end of the list will assist you to learn the definition and the
spelling of each word.

## Objective 3  BUILD, ANALYZE, DEFINE, PRONOUNCE, AND SPELL THE DIAGNOSTIC TERMS RELATED TO THE MUSCULOSKELETAL SYSTEM

## Diagnostic Terms

| TERM (built from word parts) | DEFINITION |
|---|---|
| 1. ankylosis (an-kil-Ō-sis) | abnormal condition of stiffness, (often referring to a joint, such as the result of chronic rheumatoid arthritis) |
| 2. arthritis (ar-THRĪ-tis) | inflammation of a joint, the two most common forms of arthritis being rheumatoid arthritis and osteoarthritis (Figure 13-7) |
| 3. arthrochondritis (ar-thrō-kon-DRĪ-tis) | inflammation of joint cartilages |
| 4. bursitis (bur-SĪ-tis) | inflammation of a bursa |
| 5. bursolith (BER-sō-lith) | stone in a bursa |
| 6. carpoptosis (kar-pōp-TŌ-sis) | drooping wrist (wristdrop) |
| 7. chondromalacia (kon-drō-ma-LĀ-shē-a) | softening of cartilage |
| 8. cranioschisis (krā-nē-OS-ki-sis) | (congenital) fissure of the skull |
| 9. diskitis (dis-KĪ-tis) | inflammation of an intervertebral disk |

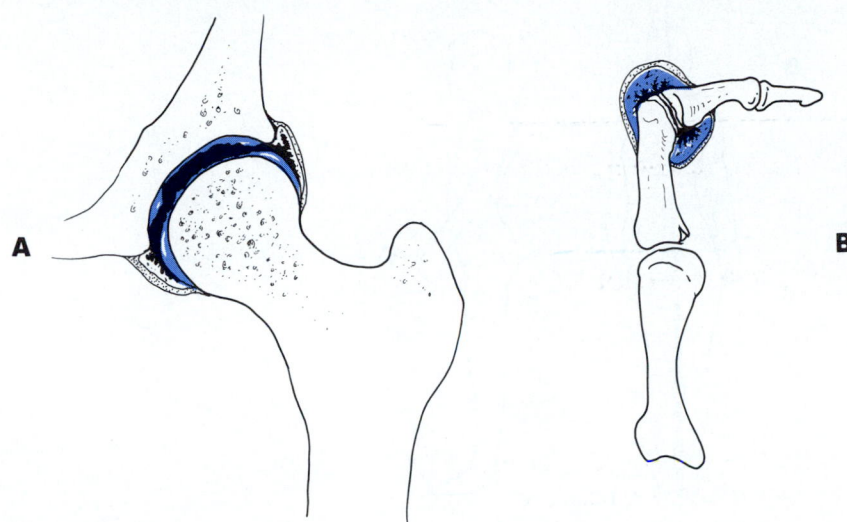

A                                    B

## Figure 13-7

**A,** Example of osteoarthritis, a degenerative disease of joints with deterioration of articular cartilage. Generally a disease of later life, osteoarthritis affects the spine and weight-bearing joints, especially the hips. **B,** Example of rheumatoid arthritis, a chronic systemic disease, which may lead to ankylosis and deformity. Small joints of the hands and feet are commonly affected. Most often it affects people between 36 and 50 years of age, more commonly women.

10. **kyphosis** . . . . . . . . . . . .  abnormal hump (of the thoracic spine);
    (kī-FŌ-sis)                        also called *hunchback* (Figure 13-8, *A*)

11. **lordosis** . . . . . . . . . . . .  abnormal condition of bending forward
    (lōr-DŌ-sis)                       (forward curvature of the lumbar spine)

12. **maxillitis** . . . . . . . . . . .  inflammation of the maxilla
    (*mak*-si-LĪ-tis)

13. **meniscitis** . . . . . . . . . . .  inflammation of the meniscus
    (*men*-i-SĪ-tis)

14. **myasthenia** . . . . . . . . . .  muscle weakness
    (mī-as-THĒ-nē-a)

15. **myeloma** . . . . . . . . . . . .  (malignant) tumor in the bone marrow
    (mī-e-LŌ-ma)

16. **osteitis** . . . . . . . . . . . . .  inflammation of the bone
    (*os*-tē-Ī-tis)

17. **osteocarcinoma** . . . . . . .  cancerous tumor of the bone
    (*os*-tē-ō-*kar*-si-NŌ-ma)

18. **osteochondritis** . . . . . . .  inflammation of the bone and cartilage
    (*os*-tē-ō-kon-DRĪ-tis)

19. **osteofibroma** . . . . . . . . .  tumor of the bone and fibrous tissue
    (*os*-tē-ō-fī-BRŌ-ma)

20. **osteomalacia** . . . . . . . . .  softening of bones
    (*os*-tē-ō-ma-LĀ-shē-a)

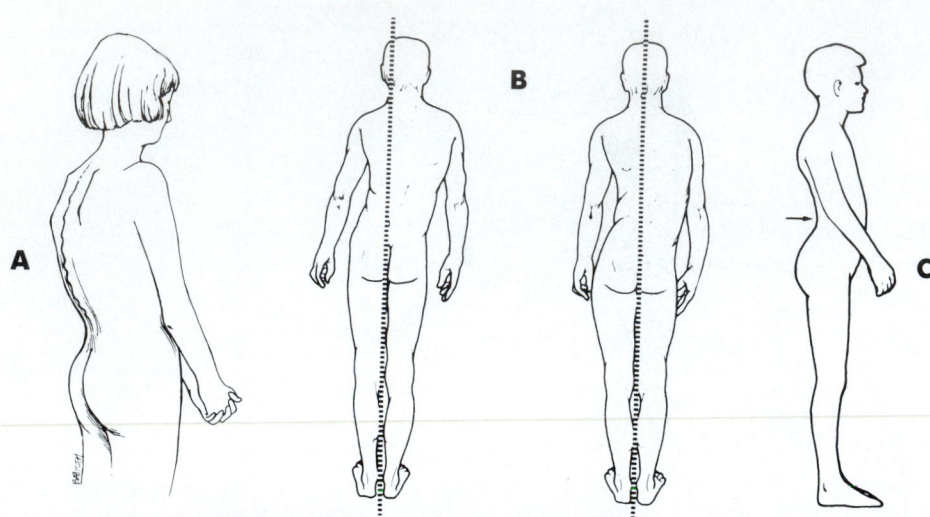

## Figure 13-8

**A,** Kyphosis. **B,** Scoliosis. **C,** Lordosis.

**A,** Courtesy artist Kimberly Battista. **B,** From the American Orthopaedic Association: *Manual of orthopaedic surgery,* ed 5, Chicago, 1979, The Association. **C,** From *Mosby's medical, nursing & allied health dictionary,* ed 3, St. Louis, 1990, Mosby.

21. osteomyelitis. . . . . . . . .      inflammation of the bone and bone marrow
    (*os*-tē-ō-*mī*-e-LĪ-tis)

22. osteopetrosis. . . . . . . . .      abnormal condition of stone (marblelike
    (*os*-tē-ō̱-pe-TRŌ-sis)              bones caused by increased formation of
                                         bone)

23. osteosarcoma . . . . . . . .        malignant tumor of the bone
    (os-tē-ō-sar-KŌ-ma)

24. polymyositis . . . . . . . . .      inflammation of many muscles
    (*pol*-ē-mī-ō-SĪ-tis)

25. rachischisis . . . . . . . . . .    congenital fissure of the vertebral col-
    (ra-KIS-kis-is)                      umn (also called *spina bifida* (Figure
                                         14-5)

26. scoliosis . . . . . . . . . . . .   abnormal (lateral) curve of the spine
    (*skō*-lē-Ō-sis)                     (Figure 13-8, B)

27. spondylarthritis . . . . . . .      inflammation of the vertebral joints
    (*spon*-dil-ar-THRĪ-tis)

28. synoviosarcoma . . . . . . .        a malignant tumor of the synovial mem-
    (si-nō-vē-ō-sar-KŌ-ma)               brane

29. tendinitis . . . . . . . . . . .    inflammation of a tendon
    (*ten*-di-NĪ-tis)

30. tenodynia . . . . . . . . . . .     pain in a tendon
    (*ten*-ō-DĪN-ē-a)

31. tenosynovitis . . . . . . . .    inflammation of the tendon and synovial
    (ten-ō-sin-ō-VĪ-tis)            membrane
    (NOTE: The "i" in synovi is
    dropped because the suffix be-
    gins with an "i")

Practice saying each of these terms aloud. To assist you in pronunciation, obtain the audiotape designed for use with this text. Learn the definitions and spellings of the diagnostic terms by completing the following exercises.

## EXERCISE 19

Analyze and define the following diagnostic terms.

1. osteitis _____

2. osteomyelitis _____

3. osteopetrosis _____

4. osteomalacia _____

5. osteocarcinoma _____

6. osteochondritis _____

7. osteofibroma _____

8. arthritis _____

9. arthrochondritis _____

10. myeloma _____

11. tendinitis _____

12. tenodynia _____

13. carpoptosis _____

14. bursitis _____

15. spondylarthritis _____

16. ankylosis _____

17. kyphosis _____

18. scoliosis _____

19. cranioschisis _____

20. maxillitis _____

21. meniscitis _____

22. rachischisis _____

23. bursolith _____

24. myasthenia _____

25. osteosarcoma _____

26. chondromalacia _____

27. synoviosarcoma _____

28. tenosynovitis _____

29. polymyositis _____

30. diskitis _____

31. lordosis _____

## EXERCISE 20

Build diagnostic terms for the following definitions by using the word parts you have learned.

1. cancerous tumor of the bone

  _____ / _____ / _____ / _____
   WR      CV      WR       S

2. inflammation of the bone and cartilage

  _____ / _____ / _____ / _____
   WR      CV      WR       S

3. tumor of the bone and fibrous tissue

  _____ / _____ / _____ / _____
   WR      CV      WR       S

4. inflammation of a joint

  _____ / _____
         WR             S

5. inflammation of joint cartilage

  _____ / _____ / _____ / _____
   WR      CV      WR       S

6. tumor of the bone marrow

  _____ / _____
         WR             S

7. inflammation of a tendon    _____
                                        WR    /    S

8. pain in a tendon    _____
                               WR    /    S

9. drooping wrist (wrist-drop)    _____
                                      WR   /   CV   /   S

10. inflammation of the bursa    _____
                                        WR    /    S

11. inflammation of the vertebral joints    _____
                                               WR   /   WR   /   S

12. abnormal condition of stiffness    _____
                                              WR    /    S

13. abnormal hump (of the thoracic spine)    _____
                                                    WR    /    S

14. abnormal (lateral) curve of the spine    _____
                                                    WR    /    S

15. fissure of the skull    _____
                               WR   /   CV   /   S

16. inflammation of the maxilla    _____
                                          WR    /    S

17. inflammation of the meniscus    _____
                                           WR    /    S

18. fissure of the vertebral column

                           WR    S

19. stone in the bursa

                     WR   CV   S

20. muscle weakness

                          WR   S

21. inflammation of the bone

                        WR   S

22. inflammation of the bone and bone marrow

          WR   CV   WR   S

23. abnormal condition of stone (marblelike bones)

          WR   CV   WR   S

24. softening of bones

            WR   CV   S

25. inflammation of the tendon and synovial membrane

          WR   CV   WR   S

26. malignant tumor of the synovial membrane

            WR   CV   S

27. malignant tumor of the bone

            WR   CV   S

28. softening of cartilage

            WR   CV   S

29. inflammation of an intervertebral disk

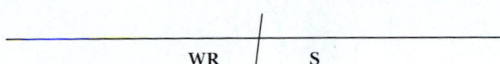

WR        S

30. inflammation of many
muscles

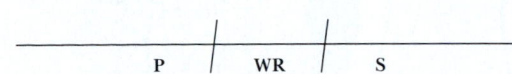

P        WR        S

31. abnormal condition of
bending forward

WR        S

## EXERCISE 21

Spell each of the diagnostic terms. Have someone dictate the terms on pp. 492 to 495 to you or say the words into a tape recorder; then spell the words from your recording as often as necessary. Think about the word parts before attempting to write the word. Study any you have spelled incorrectly.

1. _____          17. _____
2. _____          18. _____
3. _____          19. _____
4. _____          20. _____
5. _____          21. _____
6. _____          22. _____
7. _____          23. _____
8. _____          24. _____
9. _____          25. _____
10. _____         26. _____
11. _____         27. _____
12. _____         28. _____
13. _____         29. _____
14. _____         30. _____
15. _____         31. _____
16. _____

Place a check mark (√) in the box to indicate that you have completed Objective 3.

☐ **BUILD, ANALYZE, DEFINE, PRONOUNCE, AND SPELL THE DIAGNOSTIC TERMS RELATING TO THE MUSCULOSKELETAL SYSTEM.**

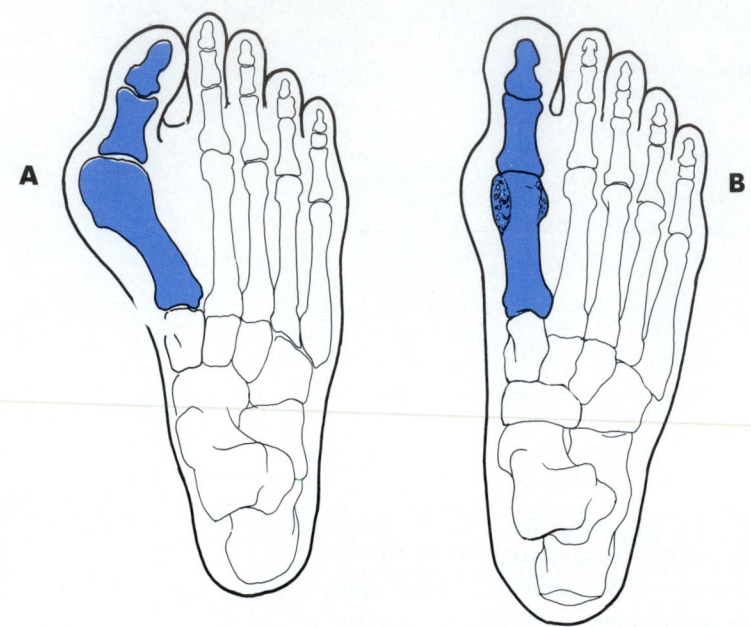

Figure 13-9

**A,** Bunion. **B,** Bunionectomy.

# Objective 4   DEFINE, PRONOUNCE, AND SPELL OTHER DIAGNOSTIC TERMS RELATED TO THE MUSCULOSKELETAL SYSTEM.

## Other Diagnostic Terms

| TERM | DEFINITION |
|---|---|
| 1. **ankylosing spondylitis** (an-kil-Ō-sing) (*spon*-di-LĪ-tis) | form of arthritis that first affects the spine and adjacent structures, and which, as it progresses, causes a forward bend of the spine. Also called *Strümpell-Marie arthritis* or disease, and *rheumatoid spondylitis*. |
| 2. **bunion** (BUN-yun) | abnormal enlargement of the joint at the base of the great toe, commonly caused by poorly fitted shoes (Figure 13-9, A) |
| 3. **carpal tunnel syndrome** | a common painful disorder of the wrist caused by compression of a nerve |
| 4. **exostosis** (*ex*-sos-TŌ-sis) | abnormal benign growth on the surface of a bone |
| 5. **fracture** (FRAK-chūr) | broken bone (Figure 13-10) |
| 6. **gout** (gowt) | disease in which an excessive amount of uric acid in the blood causes sodium urate crystals (*tophi*) to be deposited in the joints, especially that of the great toe (Figure 13-11) |

> Ernest Adolf Gustav Gottfried Strümpell (1853–1925) described **ankylosing spondylitis** in 1884; thus it became known as **Strümpell-Marie disease.**

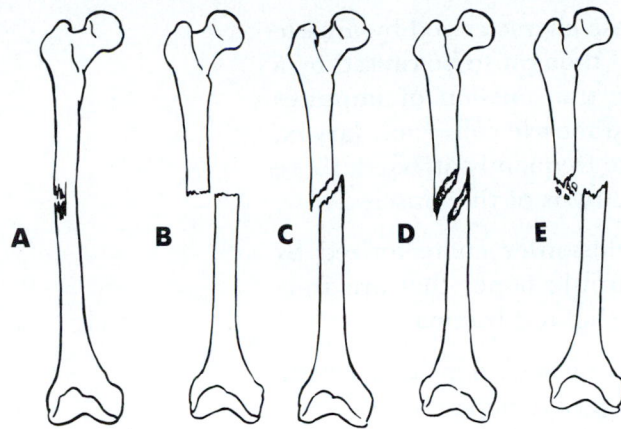

## Figure 13-10

Types of fractures. **A,** Greenstick, **B,** Transverse, **C,** Oblique, **D,** Spiral, **E,** Comminuted.

From Phipps WJ, Long BC, and Woods NF: *Shafer's medical-surgical nursing*, ed 7, St. Louis, 1980, Mosby.

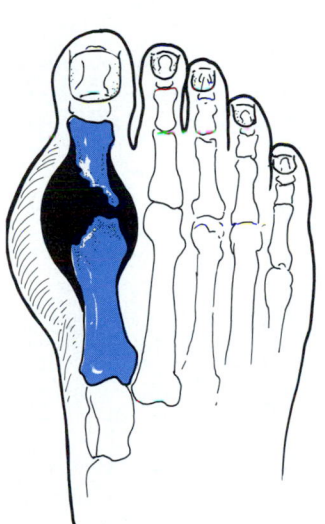

## Figure 13-11

Gout.

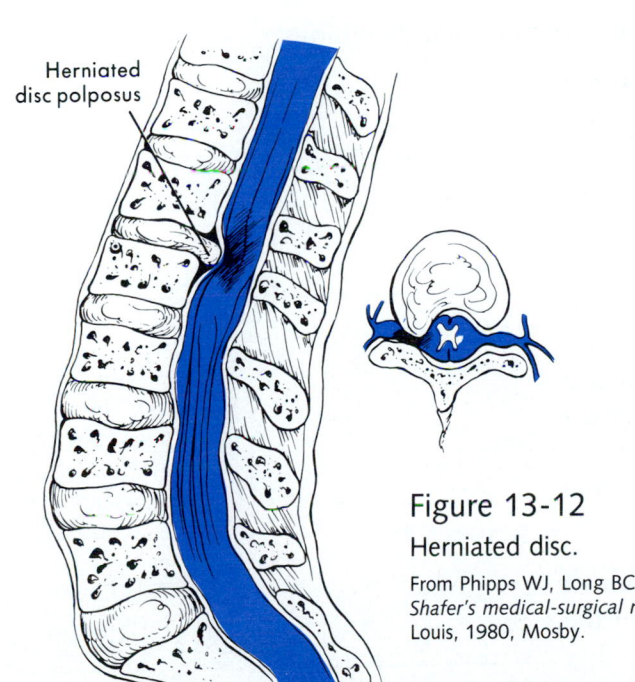

Herniated disc polposus

## Figure 13-12

Herniated disc.

From Phipps WJ, Long BC, and Woods NF: *Shafer's medical-surgical nursing*, ed 7, St. Louis, 1980, Mosby.

7. **herniated disc** . . . . . . . .
(HER-nē-āt-ed)

rupture of the intervertebral disc cartilage, which allows the contents to protrude through it, putting pressure on the spinal nerve roots (also called *slipped disc* or *ruptured disc*) (Figure 13-12)

8. **muscular dystrophy** . . . .
(DIS-trō-fē)

group of hereditary diseases characterized by degeneration of muscle and weakness

9.  myasthenia gravis...... chronic disease characterized by muscle
    (*mī*-as-THĔ-nē-a) (GRA-vis)    weakness and thought to be caused by a
    defect in the transmission of impulses
    from nerve to muscle cell. Face, larynx,
    and throat are frequently affected; there
    is no true paralysis of the muscles.

10. osteogenesis imperfecta . a hereditary disorder characterized by
    (os-tē-ō-JEN-e-sis) (im-per-    abnormally brittle bones that are frac-
    FEK-ta)                         tured by the slightest trauma

11. osteoporosis .......... abnormal loss of bone density occuring
    (*os*-tē-ō-po-RŌ-sis)           frequently in postmenopausal females

Practice saying each of these terms aloud. To assist you in pronunciation,
obtain the audiotape designed for use with this text. Learn the definitions
and spellings of the other diagnostic terms by completing the following
exercises.

## EXERCISE 22

Write the term for each of the following definitions.

1.  abnormal benign growth
    on the surface of a bone    _____

2.  group of hereditary dis-
    eases characterized by de-
    generation of muscle and
    weakness                    _____

3.  chronic disease character-
    ized by muscle weakness
    and thought to be caused
    by a defect in the trans-
    mission of impulses from
    nerve to muscle cell        _____

4.  abnormal enlargement of
    the joint at the base of the
    great toe                   _____

5.  form of arthritis that first
    affects the spine and adja-
    cent structures             _____

6.  disease in which an exces-
    sive amount of uric acid
    in the blood causes so-
    dium urate crystals (tophi)
    to be deposited in the
    joints                      _____

7. rupture of the intervertebral disc cartilage, which
   allows the contents to protrude through it, putting
   pressure on the spinal
   nerve roots

   a. _____

   b. _____

   c. _____

8. broken bone             _____

9. abnormal loss of bone
   density                 _____

10. a hereditary disorder
    characterized by abnor-
    mally brittle bones that
    are fractured by the
    slightest trauma        _____

11. a disorder of the wrist
    caused by compression of
    a nerve                 _____

## EXERCISE 23

Write the definitions of the following terms.

1. exostosis _____

2. muscular dystrophy _____

3. myasthenia gravis _____

4. bunion _____

5. ankylosing spondylitis _____

6. osteoporosis _____

7. gout _____

8. herniated disc, slipped disc, ruptured disc _____

9. fracture _____

10. carpal tunnel syndrome _____

11. osteogenesis imperfecta _____

## EXERCISE 24

Spell each of the other diagnostic terms. Have someone dictate the terms on pp. 500 to 502 to you or say the words into a tape recorder; then spell the words from your recording as often as necessary. Study any you have spelled incorrectly.

1. _____
2. _____
3. _____
4. _____
5. _____
6. _____

7. _____
8. _____
9. _____
10. _____
11. _____

Place a check mark (√) in the box to indicate that you have completed Objective 4.

☐ **DEFINE, PRONOUNCE, AND SPELL OTHER DIAGNOSTIC TERMS RELATED TO THE MUSCULOSKELETAL SYSTEM.**

# Objective 5    BUILD, ANALYZE, DEFINE, PRONOUNCE, AND SPELL THE SURGICAL TERMS RELATED TO THE MUSCULOSKELETAL SYSTEM.

## Surgical Terms

| TERM | DEFINITION |
|------|------------|
| 1. aponeurorrhaphy<br>(ap-ō-nū-RŌR-a-fē) | suture of an aponeurosis |
| 2. arthroclasia<br>(ar-thrō-KLĀ-zhē-a) | surgical breaking of a (stiff) joint |
| 3. arthrodesis<br>(ar-thrō-DĒ-sis) | surgical fixation of a joint |
| 4. arthroplasty<br>(AR-thrō-plas-tē) | surgical repair of a joint |
| 5. arthrotomy<br>(ar-THROT-ō-mē) | incision of a joint |
| 6. bursectomy<br>(bur-SEK-tō-mē) | excision of a bursa |
| 7. bursotomy<br>(bur-SOT-ō-mē) | incision of a bursa |
| 8. carpectomy<br>(kar-PEK-tō-mē) | excision of a carpal bone |
| 9. chondrectomy<br>(kon-DREK-tō-mē) | excision of a cartilage |
| 10. chondroplasty<br>(KON-drō-plas-tē) | surgical repair of a cartilage |

11. costectomy . . . . . . . . . .     excision of a rib
    (kos-TEK-tō-mē)

12. cranioplasty . . . . . . . . . .     surgical repair of the skull
    (KRĀ-nē-ō-plas-tē)

13. craniotomy . . . . . . . . . .     incision into the skull (as for surgery of
    (krā-nē-OT-ō-mē)                   the brain)

14. diskectomy . . . . . . . . . .     excision of an intervertebral disk
    (dis-KEK-tō-mē)

15. laminectomy . . . . . . . . .     excision of the lamina (often done to re-
    (lam-i-NEK-tō-mē)               lieve the symptoms of a ruptured disc)

16. maxillectomy . . . . . . . .     excision of the maxilla
    (mak-si-LEK-tō-mē)

17. meniscectomy . . . . . . . .     excision of the meniscus (performed for
    (men-i-SEK-tō-mē)              a torn cartilage)

18. myoplasty . . . . . . . . . . .     surgical repair of a muscle
    (MĪ-ō-plas-tē)

19. myorrhaphy . . . . . . . . . .     suture of a muscle
    (mī-OR-a-fē)

20. ostectomy . . . . . . . . . . .     excision of bone
    (os-TEK-tō-mē)
    (NOTE: One e is dropped.)

21. osteoclasis . . . . . . . . . . .     surgical breaking of a bone (to correct a
    (os-tē-OK-la-sis)                deformity)

22. osteoplasty . . . . . . . . . .     surgical repair of the bone
    (OS-tē-ō-plas-tē)

23. osteotome . . . . . . . . . . .     instrument used for cutting the bone
    (OS-tē-ō-tōm)

24. osteotomy . . . . . . . . . . .     incision of the bone
    (os-tē-OT-ō-mē)

25. patellectomy . . . . . . . . . .     excision of the patella
    (pat-e-LEK-tō-mē)

26. phalangectomy . . . . . . . .     excision of a finger or toe bone
    (fal-an-JEK-tō-mē)

27. rachiotomy . . . . . . . . . . .     incision into the vertebral column
    (ra-kē-OT-ō-mē)

28. spondylosyndesis . . . . . .     fusing together of the spine (spinal fu-
    (spon-di-lō-SIN-dē-sis)         sion)
    (NOTE: The prefix syn- appears
    in the middle of the term.)

29. synovectomy . . . . . . . . .     excision of the synovial membrane (of a
    (sin-ō-VEK-tō-mē)             joint)
    (NOTE: The "i" in synovi is
    dropped because the suffix be-
    gins with a vowel.)

30. tarsectomy . . . . . . . . . . .     excision of one or more tarsal bones
    (tar-SEK-tō-mē)

31.  tenomyoplasty . . . . . . .     surgical repair of the tendon and mus-
     (ten-ō-MI-ō-plas-tē)            cle

32.  tenorrhaphy . . . . . . . . .     suture of a tendon
     (ten-ŌR-a-fē)

33.  tenotomy . . . . . . . . . .     incision of the tendon
     (ten-OT-ō-mē)

Practice saying each of the surgical terms aloud. To assist you in pronunciation, obtain the audiotape designed for use with this text. Learn the
definitions and spellings of the surgical terms by completing the following exercises.

## EXERCISE 25

Analyze and define the following surgical terms.

1.  osteoclasis _____

2.  ostectomy _____

3.  osteoplasty _____

4.  osteotomy _____

5.  osteotome _____

6.  arthroclasia _____

7.  arthrodesis _____

8.  arthroplasty _____

9.  arthrotomy _____

10.  chondrectomy _____

11.  chrondroplasty _____

12.  myoplasty _____

13.  myorrhaphy _____

14.  tenomyoplasty _____

15.  tenotomy _____

16.  tenorrhaphy _____

17.  costectomy _____

18.  patellectomy _____

19.  aponeurorrhaphy _____

20.  carpectomy _____

21.  phalangectomy _____

22. meniscectomy _____

23. spondylosyndesis _____

24. laminectomy _____

25. bursectomy _____

26. bursotomy _____

27. craniotomy _____

28. cranioplasty _____

29. maxillectomy _____

30. rachiotomy _____

31. tarsectomy _____

32. synovectomy _____

33. diskectomy _____

## EXERCISE 26

Build surgical terms for the following definitions by using the word parts you have learned.

1. surgical breaking of a bone (to correct a deformity)

   _____
   WR ┃ CV ┃ S

2. excision of bone

   _____
   WR ┃ S

3. surgical repair of the bone

   _____
   WR ┃ CV ┃ S

4. incision of the bone

   _____
   WR ┃ S

5. instrument used for cutting the bone

   _____
   WR ┃ CV ┃ S

6. surgical breaking of a (stiff) joint

   _____
   WR ┃ CV ┃ S

7. surgical fixation of a
   joint

   _____ / _____ / _____
   WR     CV     S

8. surgical repair of a joint

   _____ / _____ / _____
   WR     CV     S

9. incision of a joint

   _____ / _____
   WR     S

10. excision of a cartilage

    _____ / _____
    WR     S

11. surgical repair of a carti-
    lage

    _____ / _____ / _____
    WR     CV     S

12. surgical repair of a mus-
    cle

    _____ / _____ / _____
    WR     CV     S

13. suture of a muscle

    _____ / _____
    WR     S

14. surgical repair of a ten-
    don and muscle

    _____ / _____ / _____ / _____ / _____
    WR     CV     WR     CV     S

15. incision into the tendon

    _____ / _____
    WR     S

16. suture of a tendon

    _____ / _____
    WR     S

17. excision of a rib

    _____ / _____
    WR     S

18. excision of the patella

    _____ / _____
    WR     S

19. suture of an aponeurosis

    _____ / _____
    WR     S

20. excision of a carpal bone

    WR / S

21. excision of a finger or
    toe bone

    WR / S

22. excision of the meniscus

    WR / S

23. fusing together of the
    spine

    WR / CV / P / S

24. excision of the lamina

    WR / S

25. excision of a bursa

    WR / S

26. incision of a bursa

    WR / S

27. incision into the skull

    WR / S

28. surgical repair of the
    skull

    WR / CV / S

29. excision of the maxilla

    WR / S

30. incision into the verte-
    bral column

    WR / S

31. excision of one or more
    tarsal bones

    WR / S

32. excision of the synovial
    membrane

    _____/_____
                            WR        S

33. excision of an interverte-
    bral disk

    _____/_____
                            WR        S

## EXERCISE 27

Spell each of the surgical terms. Have someone dictate the terms on pp.
504 to 506 to you or say the words into a tape recorder; then spell the
words from your recording as often as necessary. Think about the word
parts before attempting to write the word. Study any you have spelled
incorrectly.

1. _____        18. _____
2. _____        19. _____
3. _____        20. _____
4. _____        21. _____
5. _____        22. _____
6. _____        23. _____
7. _____        24. _____
8. _____        25. _____
9. _____        26. _____
10. _____       27. _____
11. _____       28. _____
12. _____       29. _____
13. _____       30. _____
14. _____       31. _____
15. _____       32. _____
16. _____       33. _____
17. _____

Place a check mark (√) in the box to indicate that you have completed Objective 5.

☐ BUILD, ANALYZE, DEFINE, PRONOUNCE, AND SPELL THE SURGICAL TERMS RELATED TO THE
MUSCULOSKELETAL SYSTEM.

# Objective 6    BUILD, ANALYZE, DEFINE, PRONOUNCE, AND SPELL THE DIAGNOSTIC PROCEDURAL TERMS RELATED TO THE MUSCULOSKELETAL SYSTEM.

## Diagnostic Procedural Terms

| TERM<br>(built from word parts) | DEFINITION |
| --- | --- |
| 1. arthrocentesis<br>(ar-thrō-sen-TĒ-sis) | surgical puncture of a joint to aspirate fluid |
| 2. arthrogram<br>(AR-thrō-gram) | x-ray film of a joint |
| 3. arthroscopy<br>(ar-THROS-kō-pē) | visual examination inside a joint (Figure 13-13) |

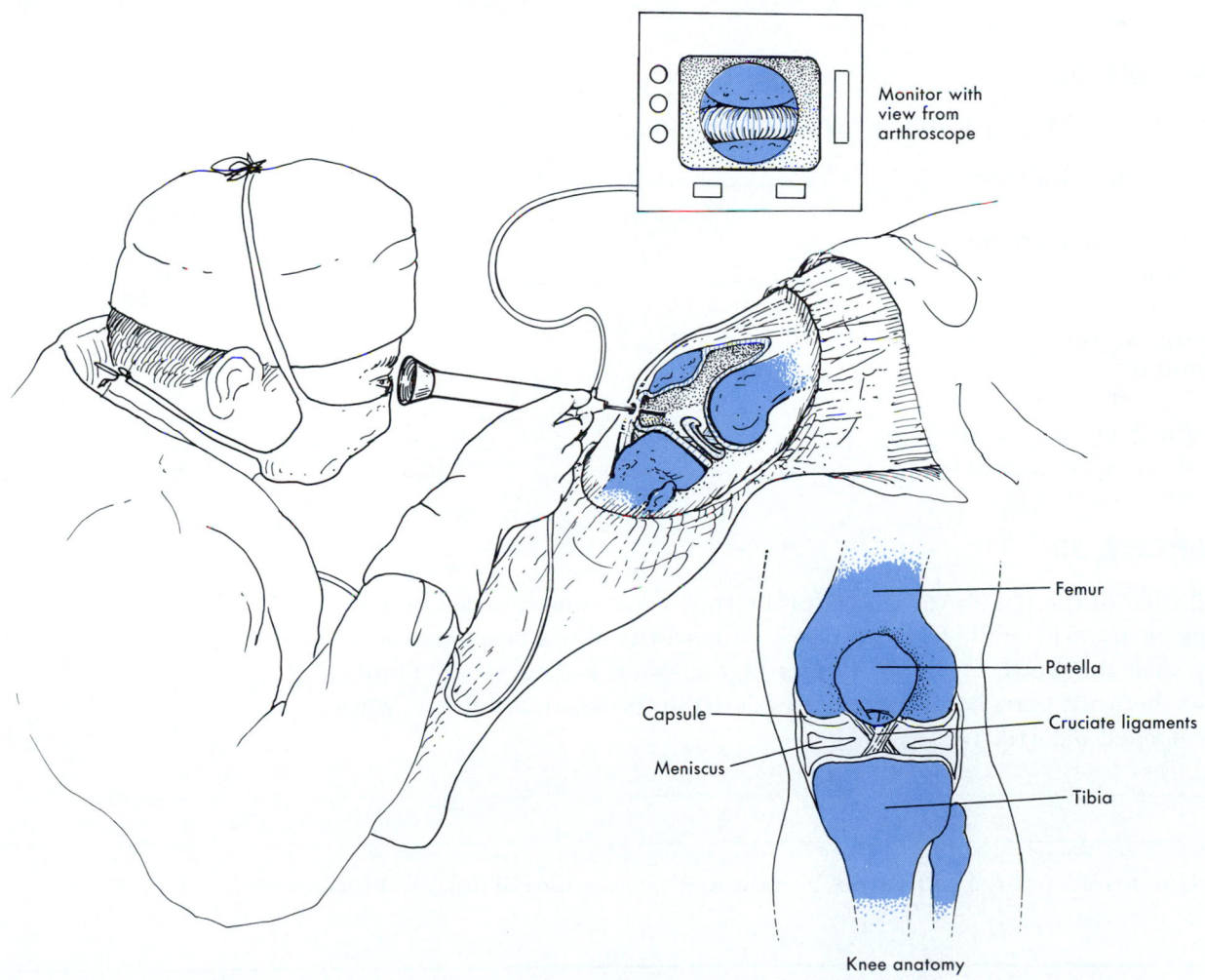

Monitor with view from arthroscope

Femur

Patella

Capsule

Cruciate ligaments

Meniscus

Tibia

Knee anatomy

**Figure 13-13**
Arthroscopy of the knee, performed for diagnostic purposes or for surgical repair of ligaments or the meniscus.

4. electromyogram . . . . . . . .    record of the (intrinsic) electric activity
    (ē-*lek*-trō-MĪ-ō-gram)     in a (skeletal) muscle

Practice saying each of these terms aloud. To assist you in pronunciation, obtain the audiotape designed for use with this text. Learn the definitions and spellings of the diagnostic procedural terms by completing the following exercises.

## EXERCISE 28

Analyze and define the following diagnostic procedural terms.

1. electromyogram _____

2. arthrogram _____

3. arthroscopy _____

4. arthrocentesis _____

## EXERCISE 29

Write the term for each of the following definitions.

1. x-ray film of a joint _____

2. visual examination inside a joint _____

3. surgical puncture of a joint to aspirate fluid _____

4. record of the electrical activity of a muscle _____

## EXERCISE 30

Spell each of the diagnostic procedural terms. Have someone dictate the terms on pp. 511 and 512 to you or say the words into a tape recorder; then spell the words from your recording as often as necessary. Think about the word parts before attempting to write the word. Study any you have spelled incorrectly.

1. _____     3. _____

2. _____     4. _____

Place a check mark (√) in the box to indicate that you have completed Objective 6.

☐ BUILD, ANALYZE, DEFINE, PRONOUNCE, AND SPELL THE DIAGNOSTIC PROCEDURAL TERMS RELATED TO THE MUSCULOSKELETAL SYSTEM.

# Objective 7

**BUILD, ANALYZE, DEFINE, PRONOUNCE, AND SPELL ADDITIONAL TERMS RELATED TO THE MUSCULOSKELETAL SYSTEM.**

## Additional Terms

| TERM (built from word parts) | DEFINITION |
|---|---|
| 1. **arthralgia** (ar-THRAL-jē-a) | pain in the joint |
| 2. **bradykinesia** (brād-ē-kin-Ē-zhē-a) | slow movement |
| 3. **carpal** (KAR-pal) | pertaining to the wrist |
| 4. **dyskinesia** (dis-ki-NĒ-zhē-a) | difficult movement |
| 5. **femoral** (FEM-ō-ral) | pertaining to the femur |
| 6. **humeral** (HŪ-mer-al) | pertaining to the humerus |
| 7. **hyperkinesia** (hī-per-kin-Ē-zhē-a) | excessive movement (overactive) |
| 8. **iliofemoral** (il-ē-ō-FEM-ō-ral) | pertaining to the ilium and femur |
| 9. **intervertebral** (in-ter-VER-te-bral) | pertaining to between the vertebrae |
| 10. **intracranial** (in-tra-KRĀ-nē-al) | pertaining to within the cranium |
| 11. **ischiofibular** (is-kē-ō-FIB-ū-lar) | pertaining to the ischium and fibula |
| 12. **ischiopubic** (is-kē-ō-PŪ-bik) | pertaining to the ischium and pubis |
| 13. **osteoblast** (OS-tē-ō-blast) | developing bone cell |
| 14. **osteocyte** (OS-tē-ō-sīt) | bone cell |
| 15. **osteonecrosis** (os-tē-ō-ne-KRŌ-sis) | (abnormal) death of bone tissues |
| 16. **pubofemoral** (pū-bō-FEM-ō-ral) | pertaining to the pubis and femur |
| 17. **sternoclavicular** (ster-nō-kla-VIK-ū-lar) | pertaining to the sternum and clavicle |
| 18. **sternoid** (STER-noyd) | resembling the sternum |
| 19. **subcostal** (sub-KOS-tal) | pertaining to below the rib |

20. submandibular........     pertaining to below the mandible
    (*sub*-man-DIB-ū-lar)

21. submaxillary.........     pertaining to below the maxilla
    (sub-MAK-si-lăr-ē)

22. subscapular .........     pertaining to below the scapula
    (sub-SKAP-ū-lar)

23. suprascapular........     pertaining to above the scapula
    (*sū*-pra-SKAP-ū-lar)

24. symphysis...........     growing together
    (SIM-fi-sis)

25. vertebrocostal........     pertaining to the vertebrae and ribs
    (*ver*-te-brō-KOS-tal)

Practice saying each of the additional terms aloud. To assist you in pronunciation, obtain the audiotape designed for use with this text. Learn the definitions and spellings of the additional terms by completing the following exercises.

## EXERCISE 31

Analyze and define the following additional terms.

1. symphysis _____

2. femoral _____

3. humeral _____

4. intervertebral _____

5. hyperkinesia _____

6. dyskinesia _____

7. bradykinesia _____

8. intracranial _____

9. sternoclavicular _____

10. iliofemoral _____

11. ischiofibular _____

12. submaxillary _____

13. ischiopubic _____

14. submandibular _____

15. pubofemoral _____

16. suprascapular _____

17. subcostal _____

18. vertebrocostal _____

19. subscapular _____

20. osteoblast _____

21. osteocyte _____

22. osteonecrosis _____

23. sternoid _____

24. arthralgia _____

25. carpal _____

## EXERCISE 32

Build terms for the following definitions by using the word parts you have learned.

1. growing together

    P | S(WR)

2. pertaining to the femur

    WR | S

3. pertaining to the humerus

    WR | S

4. pertaining to between the vertebrae

    P | WR | S

5. excessive movement (overactivity)

    P | WR | S

6. difficult movement

    P | WR | S

7. slow movement

    P | WR | S

8. pertaining to within the cranium

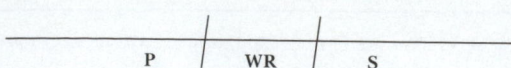

_____|_____|_____
      P     WR     S

9. pertaining to the sternum and clavicle

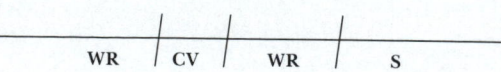

_____|_____|_____|_____
  WR   CV   WR    S

10. pertaining to the ilium and femur

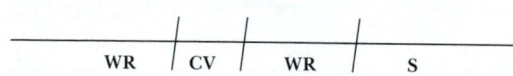

_____|_____|_____|_____
  WR   CV   WR    S

11. pertaining to the ischium and fibula

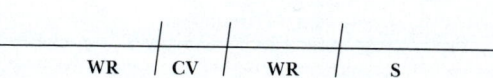

_____|_____|_____|_____
  WR   CV   WR    S

12. pertaining to below the maxilla

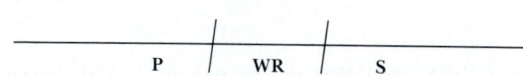

_____|_____|_____
      P     WR     S

13. pertaining to the ischium and pubis

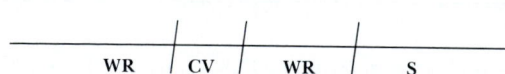

_____|_____|_____|_____
  WR   CV   WR    S

14. pertaining to below the mandible

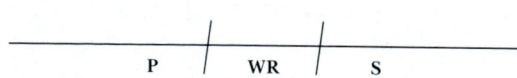

_____|_____|_____
      P     WR     S

15. pertaining to the pubis and femur

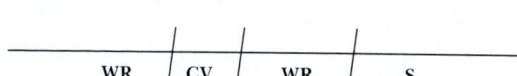

_____|_____|_____|_____
  WR   CV   WR    S

16. pertaining to above the scapula

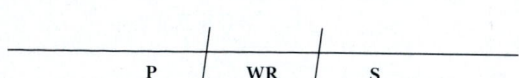

_____|_____|_____
      P     WR     S

17. pertaining to below the rib

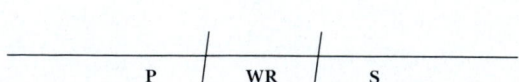

_____|_____|_____
      P     WR     S

18. pertaining to the vertebrae and ribs

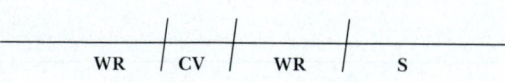

_____|_____|_____|_____
  WR   CV   WR    S

19. pertaining to below the scapula

<u>       /     /     </u>
       P    WR    S

20. developing bone cell

<u>       /     /     </u>
    WR   CV   WR

21. bone cell

<u>       /     /     </u>
    WR   CV   S

22. (abnormal) death of bone (tissues)

<u>       /     /     /     </u>
   WR   CV   WR   S

23. resembling the sternum

<u>       /     </u>
    WR   S

24. pain in the joint

<u>       /     </u>
    WR   S

25. pertaining to the wrist

<u>       /     </u>
    WR   S

## EXERCISE 33

Spell each of the additional terms. Have someone dictate the terms on pp. 513 and 514 to you or say the words into a tape recorder; then spell the words from your recording as often as necessary. Think about the word parts before attempting to write the word. Study any you have spelled incorrectly.

1. _____
2. _____
3. _____
4. _____
5. _____
6. _____
7. _____
8. _____
9. _____
10. _____
11. _____
12. _____
13. _____

14. _____
15. _____
16. _____
17. _____
18. _____
19. _____
20. _____
21. _____
22. _____
23. _____
24. _____
25. _____

Place a check mark (√) in the box to indicate that you have completed Objective 7.

☐ **BUILD, ANALYZE, DEFINE, PRONOUNCE, AND SPELL ADDITIONAL TERMS RELATED TO THE MUSCULOSKELETAL SYSTEM.**

## Objective 8   DEFINE, PRONOUNCE, AND SPELL THE OTHER ADDITIONAL TERMS RELATED TO THE MUSCULOSKELETAL SYSTEM.

## Other Additional Terms

| TERM | DEFINITION |
|---|---|
| 1. chiropodist (ki-ROP-ō-dist) OR podiatrist (pō-DĪ-a-trist) | specialist in treating and diagnosing foot disease and disorders such as corns and ingrown toenails. |
| 2. chiropractic (kī-rō-PRAK-tik) | system of therapy that consists of manipulation of the vertebral column |
| 3. chiropractor (KĪ-rō-prak-tor) | specialist in chiropractic |
| 4. orthopedics (or-thō-PĒ-diks) | branch of medicine dealing with the study and treatment of diseases and abnormalities of the musculoskeletal system |
| 5. orthopedist (or-thō-PĒ-dist) | physician who specializes in orthopedics |
| 6. orthotics (or-THOT-iks) | making and fitting of orthopedic appliances, such as arch supports, used to support, align, prevent, or correct deformities |
| 7. orthotist (ŌR-thō-tist) | one who is skilled in orthotics |
| 8. osteopathy (os-tē-OP-ath-ē) | system of medicine that utilizes usual forms of diagnosis and treatment but places greater emphasis on the role of the relationship between the body organs and the musculoskeletal system; manipulation may be used in addition to other treatment |
| 9. osteopath (OS-tē-ō-path) | physician who specializes in osteopathy |
| 10. prosthesis (pros-THĒ-sis) | an artificial substitute for a missing body part such as a leg or eye |

**Chiropodist** is made up of the Greek word roots **chir**, meaning **hand**, and **pod**, meaning **foot**, plus **ist**, meaning **one who practices.** The term was probably applied to mean persons who manually, or by using their hands, treat disorders of the feet.

**Chiropractic** is composed of the Greek **chir** and the English **practice.** Chiropractic was discovered in 1895 by D.D. Palmer, and the school was later founded by his son, B.J. Palmer. The degree Doctor of Chiropractic, or D.C., is awarded for completion of 2 years of premedical study followed by 4 years of training in an approved school.

A French physician, Dr. Nicolas Andry, devised the word **orthopedic** in 1741 from the Greek **orthos**, meaning **straight** and **ped**, meaning **child.** The word implies **to straighten a child.** During this time rickets, osteomyelitis, poliomyelitis, and tuberculosis were the main causes of orthopedic problems. All left their victims with severe deformities.

Practice saying these terms aloud. To assist you in pronunciation, obtain the audiotape designed for use with this text. Learn the definitions and spellings of the terms by completing the following exercises.

## EXERCISE 34

Match the definitions in the first column with the correct terms in the second column. The terms in the second column may be used more than once.

_c_ 1. specialist in manipulation of the vertebral column

_f_ 2. branch of medicine dealing with treatment of diseases of the musculoskeletal system

_d,g_ 3. physician

_a,h_ 4. foot specialist

_j_ 5. substitute for a body part

_b_ 6. system of therapy

_e_ 7. system of medicine

_i_ 8. making of orthopedic appliances

_k_ 9. skilled in orthotics

a. chiropodist
b. chiropractic
c. chiropractor
d. osteopath
e. osteopathy
f. orthopedics
g. orthopedist
h. podiatrist
i. orthotics
j. prosthesis
k. orthotist

Dr. Andrew Taylor Still, an American physician, founded osteopathy in 1874. It was the first system to treat disease by adjustment. Still believed that bones, ligaments, and muscles that are out of adjustment cause disease. He named the system **osteopathy,** from the word parts **oste,** meaning **bone,** and **path,** meaning **disease.** The practice of osteopathy is currently similar to conventional medical practice.

## EXERCISE 35

Write the definitions of the following.

1. chiropractor _____

2. chiropractic _____

3. orthopedics _____

4. orthopedist _____

5. chiropodist _____

6. podiatrist _____

7. osteopath _____

8. osteopathy _____

9. orthotics _____

10. prosthesis _____

11. orthotist _____

## EXERCISE 36

Spell each of the other additional terms. Have someone dictate the terms on p. 518 to you or say the words into a tape recorder; then spell the words from your recording as often as necessary. Study any you have spelled incorrectly.

1. _____   7. _____
2. _____   8. _____
3. _____   9. _____
4. _____   10. _____
5. _____   11. _____
6. _____

Place a check mark (√) in the box to indicate that you have completed Objective 8.

☐ **BUILD, ANALYZE, DEFINE, PRONOUNCE, AND SPELL THE OTHER ADDITIONAL TERMS RELATED TO THE MUSCULOSKELETAL SYSTEM.**

**Case History:** This 37-year-old married African-American male is admitted to the orthopedic service of the hospital. He complains of pain when walking and golfing. He says that his knees have "been painful" for many years since he quit playing semiprofessional football, but the pain has become very severe in the last six months. He is scheduled for arthroscopy. His preoperative diagnosis is degenerative arthritis, left knee, with possible tear, medial meniscus.

**Operative Report:** After induction of spinal anesthetic, patient was positioned on the operating table and a tourniquet applied over the upper left thigh. Following positioning of the leg in a circumferential holder, the end of the table was flexed to allow the leg to hang freely. The patient's left leg was prepped and draped in the usual manner. Following exsanguination of the leg with an Esmarch bandage, the tourniquet was inflated to 300 mm Hg. The knee was inspected using anterolateral and anteromedial parapatellar port holes.

**Findings:** The synovium in the suprapatellar pouch showed moderate to severe inflammatory changes with villi formation and hyperemia. The undersurface of the patella showed loss of normal articular cartilage on the lateral patellar facet with exposed bone in that area and moderate to severe chondromalacia of the medial facet. Similar changes were noted in the intercondylar groove. In the medial compartment, the patient had smooth articular cartilage on the femur and moderate chondromalacia of the tibial plateau. The lateral meniscus appeared normal with no evidence of tears and a smooth articular surface on the femoral condyle. The examination and probing were repeated with no additional pathology being identified. The tourniquet was then released and the knee flushed with Ringer's Lactate until the bleeding was slowed. The wounds were Steri-stripped closed, a sterile bandage with an external Ace wrap applied, and the patient returned to the postoperative recovery area in stable condition.

## EXERCISE 37

To test your understanding of the terms introduced in this chapter, circle the words that correctly complete the sentences. The italicized words refer to the correct answer.

1. The medical term for *hunchback* is (kyphosis, ankylosis, scoliosis).
2. Surgical treatment for a degenerative, painful hip joint may be *surgical repair of the joint,* or (arthroplasty, arthrodesis, arthroclasia).
3. The medical term for *excision of a cartilage* is (carpectomy, chondrectomy, costectomy).
4. *Difficult movement* is (hyperkinesia, bradykinesia, dyskinesia).
5. Vitamin D deficiency in adults may cause *osteomalacia,* or (muscle weakness, marblelike bones, softening of bones).
6. The *surgical breaking of a bone* to correct a deformity is called (osteoclasis, arthroclasia, osteoplasty).
7. The medical term that means *pertaining to below the rib* is (subscapular, subcostal, submandibular).
8. The medical term for *growing together* is (diaphysis, epiphysis, symphysis).
9. A(n) (orthopedist, podiatrist, chiropractor) is *competent to treat* a person with a *fractured femur.*
10. (Osteoporosis, osteopetrosis, osteomyelitis) is the *abnormal loss of bone density.*
11. A common *disorder of the wrist caused by compression of a nerve* is called (lordosis, carpal tunnel syndrome, osteogenesis imperfecta).

## EXERCISE 38

Unscramble the following mixed-up terms. The word on the left indicates the prefix in each of the following.

1. within

     / / / / / a / / / / / a / /
     r   a   n   l   a   i   n   a   c   t   r   i

2. above

     / / / / / a / / / a / / / / /
     r   a   c   p   u   l   s   a   r   s   u   p   a

3. together

     / / / / / / y / / / /
     m   i   s   s   s   y   p   y   h

4. below

     / / / / / o / / / /
     b   a   c   t   u   s   o   s   l

5. many

     / / / / / m / / / / / / / /
     m   p   i   s   i   y   o   y   l   o   s   t

## EXERCISE 39

The terms listed below are made up of word parts you have studied in this chapter, but the complete words have not been presented. Find their definitions by translating the word parts literally.

1. **craniorachischisis** _____
   (*krā*-nē-ō-ra-KIS-ki-sis)

2. **humeroradial** _____
   (*hu*-mer-ō-RĀ-dē-al)

3. **interpubic** _____
   (*in*-ter-PŪ-bik)

4. **intrasternal** _____
   (*in*-tra-STERN-al)

5. **myokinesis** _____
   (*mī*-ō-ki-NĒ-sis)

6. **osteoarthropathy** _____
   (*os*-tē-ō-ar-THROP-a-thē)

7. **osteolysis** _____
   (os-tē-OL-i-sis)

8. **osteoma** _____
   (os-tē-Ō-ma)

9. **osteometry** _____
   (*os*-tē-OM-e-trē)

10. **osteosclerosis** _____
    (os-tē-ō-skle-RŌ-sis)

11. **polyarthritis** _____
    (*pol*-ē-ar-THRĪ-tis)

12. **spondylodynia** _____
    (*spon*-di-lō-DĪN-ē-a)

13. **tenalgia** _____
    (ten-AL-jē-a)

14. **vertebrosternal** _____
    (*ver*-te-brō-STERN-al)

## COMBINING FORMS CROSSWORD PUZZLE

### ACROSS CLUES

1. cartilage
2. ulna
6. scapula
9. tendon
10. developing cell
12. bursa
14. clavicle
16. maxilla
18. vertebra, spinal column
19. ischia
22. tibia
26. stone
28. aponeurosis
29. crooked
31. fibula
32. tarsus
37. spinal (vertebral) column
38. joint

### DOWN CLUES

1. skull
3. movement, motion
4. mandible
5. pubis
7. finger or toe bone
8. hump
11. rib
13. kneecap
15. meniscus
17. ilium
20. wrist bone
21. bone marrow
23. spinal column
24. sternum
25. radius
27. bone
30. lamina
33. abbreviation for alarm reaction
34. abbreviation for rheumatoid arthritis
35. abbreviation for science
36. abbreviation for occupational history

# Summary

*Can you build, analyze, define, spell, and pronounce the following terms built from word parts?* yes □ no □

| DIAGNOSTIC | SURGICAL | PROCEDURAL | ADDITIONAL |
|---|---|---|---|
| ankylosis<br>(an-kil-Ō-sis) | aponeurorrhaphy<br>(*ap*-ō-nū-RŌR-a-fē) | arthrocentesis<br>(*ar*-thrō-sen-TĒ-sis) | arthralgia<br>(ar-THRAL-jē-a) |
| arthritis<br>(ar-THRĪ-tis) | arthroclasia<br>(*ar*-thrō-KLĀ-zhē-a) | arthrogram<br>(AR-thrō-gram) | bradykinesia<br>(*brād*-ē-kin-Ē-zhē-a) |
| arthrochondritis<br>(*ar*-thrō-kon-DRĪ-tis) | arthrodesis<br>(*ar*-thrō-DĒ-sis) | arthroscopy<br>(ar-THROS-kō-pē) | carpal<br>(KAR-pal) |
| bursitis<br>(bur-SĪ-tis) | arthroplasty<br>(AR-thrō-plas-tē) | electromyogram<br>(ē-*lek*-trō-MĪ-ō-gram) | dyskinesia<br>(dis-ki-NĒ-zhē-a) |
| bursolith<br>(BER-sō-lith) | arthrotomy<br>(ar-THROT-ō-mē) | | femoral<br>(FEM-ō-ral) |
| carpoptosis<br>(*kar*-pōp-TŌ-sis) | bursectomy<br>(bur-SEK-tō-mē) | | humeral<br>(HŪ-mer-al) |
| chondromalacia<br>(kon-drō-ma-LĀ-shē-a) | bursotomy<br>(bur-SOT-ō-mē) | | hyperkinesia<br>(*hī*-per-kin-Ē-zhē-a) |
| cranioschisis<br>(*krā*-nē-OS-ki-sis) | carpectomy<br>(kar-PEK-tō-mē) | | iliofemoral<br>(*il*-ē-ō-FEM-ō-ral) |
| diskitis<br>(dis-KĪ-tis) | chondrectomy<br>(kon-DREK-tō-mē) | | intervertebral<br>(*in*-ter-VER-te-bral) |
| kyphosis<br>(kī-FŌ-sis) | chondroplasty<br>(KON-drō-plas-tē) | | intracranial<br>(*in*-tra-KRĀ-nē-al) |
| lordosis<br>(lōr-DŌ-sis) | costectomy<br>(kos-TEK-tō-mē) | | ischiofibular<br>(*is*-kē-ō-FIB-ū-lar) |
| maxillitis<br>(*mak*-si-LĪ-tis) | cranioplasty<br>(KRĀ-nē-ō-plas-tē) | | ischiopubic<br>(*is*-kē-ō-PŪ-bik) |
| meniscitis<br>(*men*-i-SĪ-tis) | craniotomy<br>(*krā*-nē-OT-ō-mē) | | osteoblast<br>(OS-tē-ō-blast) |
| myasthenia<br>(*mī*-as-THĒ-nē-a) | diskectomy<br>(dis-KEK-tō-mē) | | osteocyte<br>(OS-tē-ō-sīt) |
| myeloma<br>(*mī*-e-LŌ-ma) | laminectomy<br>(*lam*-i-NEK-tō-mē) | | osteonecrosis<br>(*os*-tē-ō-ne-KRŌ-sis) |
| osteitis<br>(*os*-tē-Ī-tis) | maxillectomy<br>(*mak*-si-LEK-tō-mē) | | pubofemoral<br>(*pū*-bō-FEM-ō-ral) |
| osteocarcinoma<br>(*os*-tē-ō-*kar*-si-NŌ-ma) | meniscectomy<br>(*men*-i-SEK-tō-mē) | | sternoclavicular<br>(*ster*-nō-kla-VIK-ū-lar) |
| osteochondritis<br>(*os*-tē-ō-kon-DRĪ-tis) | myoplasty<br>(MĪ-ō-plas-tē) | | sternoid<br>(STER-noyd) |

## DIAGNOSTIC—cont'd

osteofibroma
(*os*-tē-ō-fĭ-BRŌ-ma)

osteomalacia
(*os*-tē-ō-ma-LĀ-shē-a)

osteomyelitis
(*os*-tē-ō-*mĭ*-e-LĪ-tis)

osteopetrosis
(*os*-tē-ō-pe-TRŌ-sis)

osteosarcoma
(os-tē-ō-sar-KŌ-ma)

polymyositis
(pol-ē-mī-ō-SĪ-tis)

rachischisis
(ra-KIS-kis-is)

scoliosis
(*skō*-lē-Ō-sis)

spondylarthritis
(*spon*-dĭl-ar-THRĪ-tis)

synoviosarcoma
(si-nō-vē-ō-sar-KŌ-ma)

tendinitis
(*ten*-di-NĪ-tis)

tenodynia
(*ten*-ō-DĬN-ē-a)

tenosynovitis
(ten-ō-sin-ō-VĪ-tis)

## SURGICAL—cont'd

myorrhaphy
(mī-OR-a-fē)

ostectomy
(os-TEK-tŏ-mē)

osteoclasis
(*os*-tē-OK-la-sis)

osteoplasty
(OS-tē-ō-plas-tē)

osteotome
(OS-tē-ō-tōm)

osteotomy
(*os*-tē-OT-ŏ-mē)

patellectomy
(*pat*-e-LEK-tō-mē)

phalangectomy
(*fal*-an-JEK-tō-mē)

rachiotomy
(*ra*-kē-OT-ō-mē)

spondylosyndesis
(*spon*-di-lō-SIN-dē-sis)

synovectomy
(sin-ō-VEK-tō-mē)

tarsectomy
(tar-SEK-tō-mē)

tenomyoplasty
(*ten*-ō-MĪ-ō-plas-tē)

tenorrhaphy
(ten-ŌR-a-fē)

tenotomy
(ten-OT-ŏ-mē)

## ADDITIONAL—cont'd

subcostal
(sub-KOS-tal)

submandibular
(*sub*-man-DIB-ū-lar)

submaxillary
(sub-MAK-si-lăr-ē)

subscapular
(sub-SKAP-ū-lar)

suprascapular
(*sū*-pra-SKAP-ū-lar)

symphysis
(SIM-fi-sis)

vertebrocostal
(*ver*-te-brō-KOS-tal)

# Summary

Can you define, pronounce, and spell the following terms *not built from word parts?* yes ☐ no ☐

**DIAGNOSTIC**

ankylosing spondylitis
(an-kil-Ō-sing)(*spon*-di-LĪ-tis)

bunion
(BUN-yun)

carpal tunnel syndrome

exostosis
(*ex*-sos-TŌ-sis)

fracture
(FRAK-chūr)

gout
(gowt)

herniated disc
(HER-nē-āt-ed)

muscular dystrophy
(DIS-trō-fē)

myasthenia gravis
(*mī*-as-THḖ-nē-a (GRA-vis))

osteogenesis imperfecta
(os-tē-ō-JEN-e-sis)

osteoporosis
(*os*-tē-ō-po-RŌ-sis)

**ADDITIONAL**

chiropodist
(ki-ROP-ō-dist)

podiatrist
(pō-DĪ-a-trist)

chiropractic
(*kī*-rō-PRAK-tik)

chiropractor
(KĪ-rō-prak-tor)

orthopedics
(*or*-thō-PḖ-diks)

orthopedist
(*or*-thō-PḖ-dist)

orthotics
(or-THOT-iks)

orthotist
(ŌR-thō-tist)

osteopathy
(*os*-tē-OP-ath-ē)

osteopath
(OS-tē-ō-path)

prosthesis
(pros-THḖ-sis)

# Answers

## Exercise 1

1. d   3. h   5. f   7. b
2. c   4. a   6. g

## Exercise 2

1. scapula
2. sternum
3. mandible
4. clavicle
5. humerus
6. a. ulna
   b. radius
7. tarsals
8. phalanges
9. metatarsals
10. metacarpals
11. femur
12. fibula, tibia
13. patella
14. cervical vertebrae
15. lumbar
16. pubis
17. sacrum
18. ischium
19. coccyx
20. ilium
21. carpals

## Exercise 3

1. m   4. a   7. h   10. b
2. c   5. l   8. i   11. f
3. e   6. d   9. k   12. g

## Exercise 4

**Figure 13-2**
Mandible: mandibul/o
Cranium: crani/o
Clavicle: clavic/o, clavicul/o
Ribs: cost/o
Femur: femor/o
Fibula: fibul/o
**Figure 13-5**
Humerus: humer/o
Carpals: carp/o
Ilium: ili/o
Ischium: ischi/o

## Exercise 5

1. clavicle
2. rib
3. skull, cranium
4. femur
5. clavicle
6. humerus
7. ilium
8. ischium
9. carpals
10. fibula
11. mandible

## Exercise 6

1. a. clavicul/o
   b. clavic/o
2. cost/o
3. crani/o
4. femor/o
5. humer/o
6. carp/o
7. ischi/o
8. fibul/o
9. ili/o
10. mandibul/o

## Exercise 7

**Figure 13-2**
Sternum: stern/o
Patella: patell/o
Tarsals: tars/o
Phalanges: phalang/o
Maxilla: maxill/o
Tibia: tibi/o

**Figure 13-5**
Vertebral column:
  vertebr/o, rachi/o,
  spondyl/o
Scapula: scapul/o
Ulna: uln/o
Radius: radi/o
Pubis: pub/o

## Exercise 8

1. vertebra
2. patella
3. vertebra
4. maxilla
5. phalanges
6. ulna
7. radius
8. tibia
9. pubis
10. tarsals
11. scapula
12. sternum
13. vertebra

## Exercise 9

1. maxill/o
2. uln/o
3. radi/o
4. tibi/o
5. pub/o
6. tars/o
7. a. vertebr/o
   b. spondyl/o
   c. rachi/o
8. stern/o
9. scapul/o
10. patell/o
11. phalang/o

## Exercise 10

**Figure 13-3**
Intervertebral disk: disk/o
**Figure 13-6**
Synovial membrane:
  synovi/o
Joint: arthr/o
Meniscus: menisc/o
Tendon: ten/o, tend/o,
  tendin/o
Cartilage: chondr/o
Bursa: burs/o

## Exercise 11

1. joint
2. aponeurosis
3. meniscus
4. tendon
5. cartilage
6. tendon
7. bursa
8. tendon
9. synovia, synovial membrane
10. intervertebral disk

## Exercise 12

1. menisc/o
2. aponeur/o
3. arthr/o
4. chrondr/o
5. a. tendin/o
   b. ten/o
   c. tend/o
6. burs/o
7. synovi/o
8. disk/o

## Exercise 13

1. muscle
2. stone
3. movement, motion
4. bone
5. lamina
6. bone marrow
7. hump
8. crooked, stiff, bent
9. crooked, curved
10. bone marrow
11. muscle
12. bent forward

## Exercise 14

1. my/o, myos/o
2. petr/o
3. kinesi/o
4. oste/o
5. lamin/o
6. a. myel/o
   b. myelon/o
7. kyph/o
8. ankyl/o
9. scoli/o
10. lord/o

## Exercise 15

1. above   2. together, joined   3. between

## Exercise 16

1. syn-, sym-   2. inter-   3. supra-

## Exercise 17

1. growth
2. break
3. fusion, surgical fixation
4. break
5. fissure, split
6. break
7. weakness

## Exercise 18

1. -physis
2. -asthenia
3. a. -clasis
   b. -clast
   c. -clasia
4. -desis
5. -schisis

## Exercise 19

1. oste/itis (WR S) — inflammation of the bone
2. oste/ o /myel/itis (WR CV WR S, CF) — inflammation of the bone and bone marrow
3. oste/ o /petr/osis (WR CV WR S, CF) — abnormal condition of stone (marblelike bones)
4. oste/ o /malacia (WR CV S, CF) — softening of bones
5. oste/ o /carcin/oma (WR CV WR S, CF) — cancerous tumor of the bone
6. oste/ o /chondr/itis (WR CV WR S, CF) — inflammation of the bone and cartilage
7. oste/ o /fibr/oma (WR CV WR S, CF) — tumor of the bone and fibrous tissue
8. arthr/itis (WR S) — inflammation of a joint
9. arthr/ o /chondr/itis (WR CV WR S, CF) — inflammation of the joint cartilages
10. myel/oma (WR S) — tumor in the bone marrow
11. tendin/itis (WR S) — inflammation of a tendon
12. ten/odynia (WR S) — pain in a tendon
13. carp/ o /ptosis (WR CV S, CF) — drooping wrist (wrist drop)
14. burs/itis (WR S) — inflammation of the bursa
15. spondyl/arthr/itis (WR WR S) — inflammation of the vertebral joints
16. ankyl/osis (WR S) — abnormal condition of stiffness
17. kyph/osis (WR S) — abnormal hump of the thoracic spine (also called *hunchback*)
18. scoli/osis (WR S) — abnormal (lateral) curve of the spine
19. crani/ o /schisis (WR CV S, CF) — fissure of the skull
20. maxill/itis (WR S) — inflammation of maxilla
21. menisc/itis (WR S) — inflammation of the meniscus
22. rachi/schisis (WR S) — fissure of the vertebral column
23. burs/ o /lith (WR CV WR, CF) — stone in the bursa
24. my/asthenia (WR S) — muscle weakness
25. oste/ o /sarcoma (WR CV S, CF) — malignant tumor of the bone
26. chondr/ o /malacia (WR CV S, CF) — softening of cartilage
27. synovi/ o /sarcoma (WR CV S, CF) — a malignant tumor of the synovial membrane
28. ten/ o /synov/itis (WR CV WR S, CF) — inflammation of the tendon and synovial membrane

P    WR   S
29. poly/myos/itis          inflammation of many
                            muscles

WR   S
30. disk/itis               inflammation of an inter-
                            vertebral disk

WR   S
31. lord/osis               abnormal condition of
                            bending forward.

## Exercise 20

1. oste/o/carcin/oma
2. oste/o/chondr/itis
3. oste/o/fibr/oma
4. arthr/itis
5. arthr/o/chondr/itis
6. myel/oma
7. tendin/itis
8. ten/odynia
9. carp/o/ptosis
10. burs/itis
11. spondyl/arthr/itis
12. ankyl/osis
13. kyph/osis
14. scoli/osis
15. crani/o/schisis
16. maxill/itis
17. menisc/itis
18. rachi/schisis
19. burs/o/lith
20. my/asthenia
21. oste/itis
22. oste/o/myel/itis
23. oste/o/petr/osis
24. oste/o/malacia
25. ten/o/synov/itis
26. synovi/o/sarcoma
27. oste/o/sarcoma
28. chondr/o/malacia
29. disk/itis
30. poly/myos/itis
31. lord/osis

## Exercise 21

Spelling exercise; *see* text, p. 499.

## Exercise 22

1. exostosis
2. muscular dystrophy
3. myasthenia gravis
4. bunion
5. ankylosing spondylitis
6. gout
7. a. herniated disc
   b. slipped disc
   c. ruptured disc
8. fracture
9. osteoporosis
10. osteogenesis imper-
    fecta
11. carpal tunnel syn-
    drome

## Exercise 23

1. abnormal benign growth on the surface of a bone
2. group of hereditary diseases characterized by degeneration of muscle and weakness
3. chronic disease characterized by muscle weakness and thought to be caused by a defect in the transmission of impulses from nerve to muscle cell
4. abnormal enlargement of the joint at the base of the great toe
5. form of arthritis that first affects the spine and adjacent structures
6. abnormal loss of bone density
7. disease in which an excessive amount of uric acid in the blood causes sodium urate crystals (tophi) to be deposited in the joints
8. rupture of the intervertebral disc cartilage, which allows the contents to protrude through it, putting pressure on the spinal nerve roots
9. broken bone
10. a hereditary disorder characterised by abnormally brittle bones that are fractured by the slightest trauma
11. a disorder of the wrist caused by compression of the nerve

## Exercise 24

Spelling exercise; *see* txt, p. 504.

## Exercise 25

WR  CV   S
1. oste/ o /clasis          surgical breaking of a
      CF                    bone

WR     S
2. ost/ectomy               excision of bone

WR  CV   S
3. oste/ o /plasty          surgical repair of the
      CF                    bone

WR     S
4. oste/otomy               incision of the bone

WR  CV   S
5. oste/ o /tome            instrument used for cut-
      CF                    ting the bone

WR  CV   S
6. arthr/ o /clasia         surgical breaking of a
      CF                    (stiff) joint

WR  CV   S
7. arthr/ o /desis          surgical fixation of a joint
      CF

WR  CV   S
8. arthr/ o /plasty         surgical repair of a joint
      CF

WR     S
9. arthr/otomy              incision of a joint

WR     S
10. chondr/ectomy           excision of a cartilage

WR   CV   S
11. chondr/ o /plasty       surgical repair of a carti-
       CF                   lage

WR  CV   S
12. my/ o /plasty           surgical repair of a mus-
      CF                    cle

WR     S
13. my/orrhaphy             suture of a muscle

14. 
```
WR CV WR CV   S
ten/ o /my/ o /plasty
   CF    CF
```
surgical repair of the tendon and muscle

15. 
```
WR    S
ten/otomy
```
incision of the tendon

16. 
```
WR    S
ten/orrhaphy
```
suture of a tendon

17. 
```
WR    S
cost/ectomy
```
excision of a rib

18. 
```
WR    S
patell/ectomy
```
excision of the patella

19. 
```
WR    S
aponeur/orrhaphy
```
suture of an aponeurosis

20. 
```
WR    S
carp/ectomy
```
excision of a carpal bone

21. 
```
WR    S
phalang/ectomy
```
excision of a finger or toe bone

22. 
```
WR    S
menisc/ectomy
```
excision of the meniscus

23. 
```
WR  CV  P   S
spondyl/ o /syn/desis
    CF
```
fusing together of the spine

24. 
```
WR    S
lamin/ectomy
```
excision of the lamina

25. 
```
WR    S
burs/ectomy
```
excision of a bursa

26. 
```
WR    S
burs/otomy
```
incision of a bursa

27. 
```
WR    S
crani/otomy
```
incision into the skull

28. 
```
WR  CV  S
crani/ o /plasty
   CF
```
surgical repair of the skull

29. 
```
WR    S
maxill/ectomy
```
excision of the maxilla

30. 
```
WR    S
rachi/otomy
```
incision into the vertebral column

31. 
```
WR    S
tars/ectomy
```
excision of one or more tarsal bones

32. 
```
WR    S
synov/ectomy
```
excision of the synovial membrane

33. 
```
WR    S
disk/ectomy
```
excision of an intervertebral disk

## Exercise 26

1. oste/o/clasis
2. ost/ectomy
3. oste/o/plasty
4. oste/otomy
5. oste/o/tome
6. arthr/o/clasia
7. arthr/o/desis
8. arthr/o/plasty
9. arthr/otomy
10. chondr/ectomy
11. chondr/o/plasty
12. my/o/plasty
13. my/orrhaphy
14. ten/o/my/o/plasty
15. ten/otomy
16. ten/orrhaphy
17. cost/ectomy
18. patell/ectomy
19. aponeur/orrhaphy
20. carp/ectomy
21. phalang/ectomy
22. menisc/ectomy
23. spondyl/o/syn/desis
24. lamin/ectomy
25. burs/ectomy
26. burs/otomy
27. crani/otomy
28. crani/o/plasty
29. maxill/ectomy
30. rachi/otomy
31. tars/ectomy
32. synov/ectomy
33. disk/ectomy

## Exercise 27

Spelling exercise; *see* text, p. 510.

## Exercise 28

1. 
```
WR  CV WR CV   S
electr/ o /my/ o /gram
     CF    CF
```
record of the electrical activity in a muscle

2. 
```
WR CV   S
arthr/ o /gram
     CF
```
x-ray film of a joint

3. 
```
WR  CV   S
arthr/ o /scopy
     CF
```
visual examination inside a joint

4. 
```
WR  CV   S
arthr/ o /centesis
     CF
```
surgical puncture of a joint to aspirate fluid

## Exercise 29

1. arthrogram    3. arthrocentesis
2. arthroscopy    4. electromyogram

## Exercise 30

Spelling exercise; *see* text, p. 512.

## Exercise 31

1. 
```
  P   S(WR)
sym/physis
```
growing together

2. 
```
WR    S
femor/al
```
pertaining to the femur

|   | | |
|---|---|---|
| WR S | | |
| 3. humer/al | pertaining to the hu-merus | |
| P WR S | | |
| 4. inter/vertebr/al | pertaining to between the vertebrae | |
| P WR S | | |
| 5. hyper/kinesi/a | excessive movement (overactivity) | |
| P WR S | | |
| 6. dys/kinesi/a | difficult movement | |
| P WR S | | |
| 7. brady/kinesi/a | slow movement | |
| P WR S | | |
| 8. intra/crani/al | pertaining to within the cranium | |
| WR CV WR S | | |
| 9. stern/ o /clavicul/ar | pertaining to the sternum and clavicle | |
| CF | | |
| WR CV WR S | | |
| 10. ili / o /femor/al | pertaining to the ilium and femur | |
| CF | | |
| WR CV WR S | | |
| 11. ischi/ o /fibul/ar | pertaining to the ischium and fibula | |
| CF | | |
| P WR S | | |
| 12. sub/maxill/ary | pertaining to below the maxilla | |
| WR CV WR S | | |
| 13. ischi/ o /pub/ic | pertaining to the ischium and pubis | |
| CF | | |
| P WR S | | |
| 14. sub/mandibul/ar | pertaining to below the mandible | |
| WR CV WR S | | |
| 15. pub/ o /femor/al | pertaining to the pubis and femur | |
| CF | | |
| P WR S | | |
| 16. supra/scapul/ar | pertaining to above the scapula | |
| P WR S | | |
| 17. sub/cost/al | pertaining to below the rib | |
| WR CV WR S | | |
| 18. vertebr/ o /cost/ar | pertaining to the verte-brae and ribs | |
| CF | | |
| P WR S | | |
| 19. sub/scapul/ar | pertaining to below the scapula | |
| WR CV WR | | |
| 20. oste/ o /blast | developing bone cell | |
| CF | | |
| WR CV S | | |
| 21. oste/ o /cyte | bone cell | |
| CF | | |

WR CV WR S
22. oste/ o /necr/osis    (abnormal) death of bone
    CF                     tissues

WR S
23. stern/oid    resembling the sternum

WR S
24. arthr/algia    pain in the joint

WR S
25. carp/al    pertaining to the wrist

## Exercise 32

| 1. sym/physis | 14. sub/mandibul/ar |
|---|---|
| 2. femor/al | 15. pub/o/femor/al |
| 3. humer/al | 16. supra/scapul/ar |
| 4. inter/vertebr/al | 17. sub/cost/al |
| 5. hyper/kinesi/a | 18. vertebr/o/cost/al |
| 6. dys/kinesi/a | 19. sub/scapul/ar |
| 7. brady/kinesi/a | 20. oste/o/blast |
| 8. intra/crani/al | 21. oste/o/cyte |
| 9. stern/o/clavicul/ar | 22. oste/o/necr/osis |
| 10. ili/o/femor/al | 23. stern/oid |
| 11. ischi/o/fibul/ar | 24. arthr/algia |
| 12. sub/maxill/ary | 25. carp/al |
| 13. ischi/o/pub/ic | |

## Exercise 33

Spelling exercise; *see* text, p. 517.

## Exercise 34

| 1. c | 3. d, g | 5. j | 7. e | 9. k |
|---|---|---|---|---|
| 2. f | 4. a, h | 6. b | 8. i | |

## Exercise 35

1. specialist in chiropractic
2. system of therapy that consists of manipulation of the vertebral column
3. branch of medicine dealing with the study and treatment of diseases and abnormalities of the musculoskeletal system
4. physician who specializes in orthopedics
5. specialist in treating and diagnosing foot diseases and disorders
6. specialist in treating and diagnosing foot diseases and disorders
7. physician who specializes in osteopathy
8. system of medicine in which emphasis is on the relationship between body organs and the musculoskeletal system
9. making and fitting of orthopedic appliances
10. an artificial substitute for a missing body part
11. one who is skilled in orthotics

## Exercise 36

Spelling exercise; *see* text, p. 520.

## Exercise 37

1. kyphosis
2. arthroplasty
3. chondrectomy
4. dyskinesia
5. softening of the bones
6. osteoclasis
7. subcostal
8. symphysis
9. orthopedist
10. osteoporosis
11. carpal tunnel syndrome

## Exercise 38

1. intracranial
2. suprascapular
3. symphysis
4. subcostal
5. polymyositis

## Exercise 39

1. (congenital) fissure of the skull and vertebral column
2. pertaining to the humerus and radius
3. between the pubic bones
4. pertaining to within the sternum
5. muscular movement
6. any disease of the joints and bones
7. dissolution of bone
8. tumor composed of bone
9. measurement of bone

10. hardening of bone
11. inflammation of many joints
12. pain in the vertebra
13. pain in the tendon
14. pertaining to the vertebrae and sternum

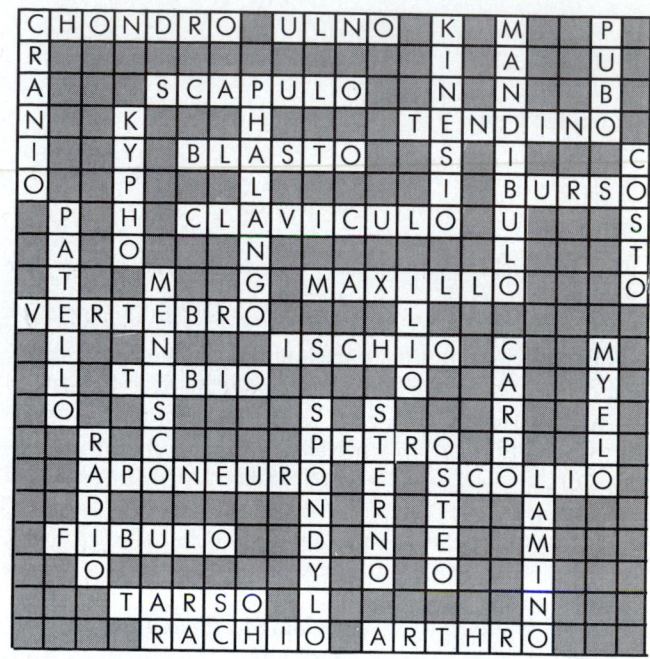

# 14

# Nervous System

## Objectives

Upon completion of this chapter you will be able to:

1. Define the anatomical terms of the nervous system.

2. Write the definitions of the word parts included in this chapter.

3. Build, analyze, define, pronounce, and spell the diagnostic terms related to the nervous system.

4. Define, pronounce, and spell other diagnostic terms related to the nervous system.

5. Build, analyze, define, pronounce, and spell the surgical terms related to the nervous system.

6. Build, analyze, define, pronounce, and spell the diagnostic procedural terms related to the nervous system.

7. Define, pronounce, and spell other diagnostic procedural terms related to the nervous system.

8. Build, analyze, define, pronounce, and spell additional terms related to the nervous system.

9. Define, pronounce, and spell the other additional terms related to the nervous system.

## Objective 1 DEFINE THE ANATOMICAL TERMS RELATED TO THE NERVOUS SYSTEM.

## Anatomical Terms

The nervous system and the endocrine system cooperate in regulating and controlling the activities of the other body systems.

The nervous system may be separated into two divisions: the *central nervous system* (CNS) and the *peripheral nervous system* (PNS). The central nervous system consists of the brain and the spinal cord. The peripheral nervous system is made up of *cranial nerves*, which carry impulses between the brain and neck and head, and *spinal nerves*, which carry messages between the spinal cord and abdomen, limbs, and chest.

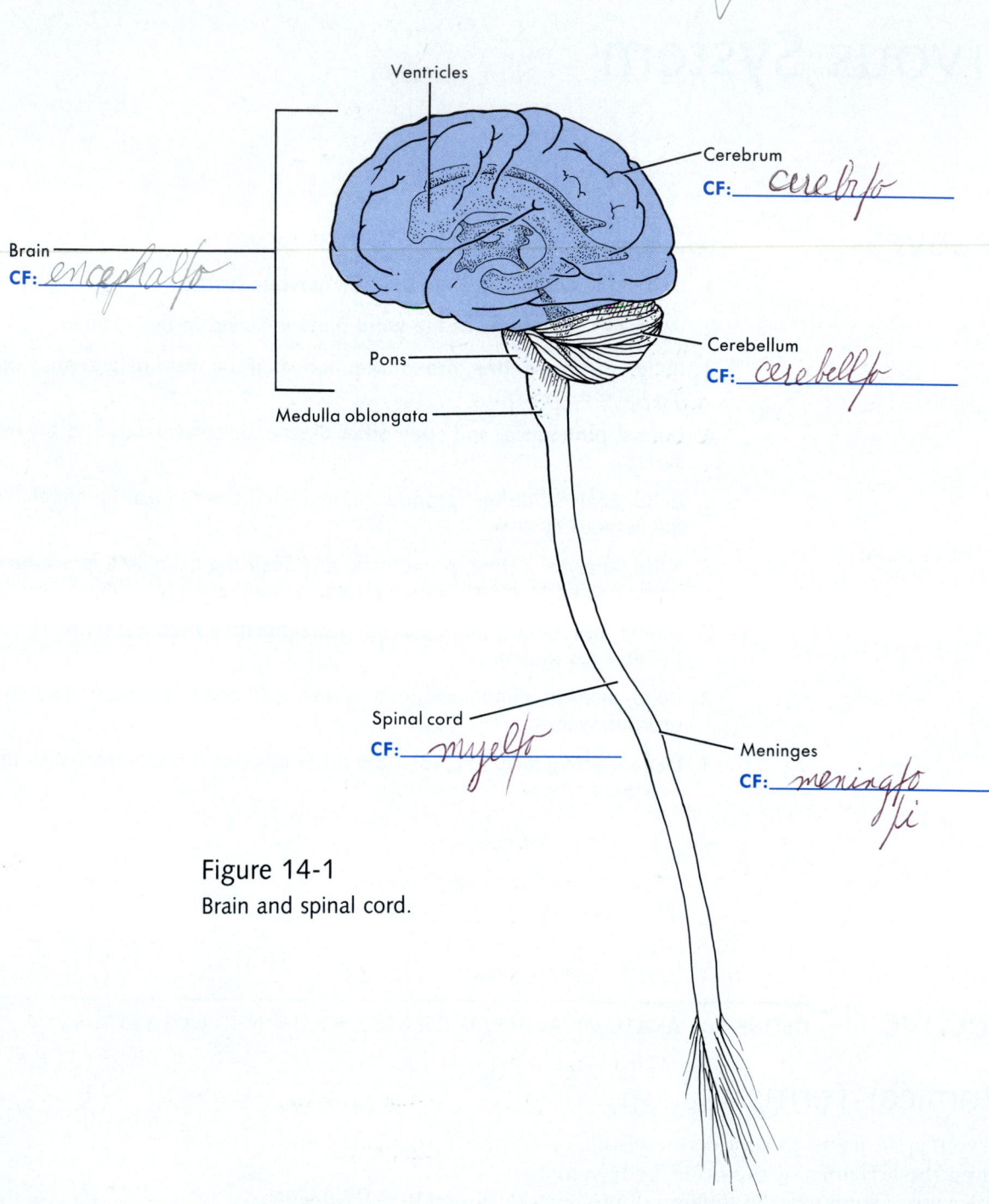

Ventricles

Cerebrum
CF: _cerebro_

Brain
CF: _encephalo_

Pons

Cerebellum
CF: _cerebello_

Medulla oblongata

Spinal cord
CF: _myelo_

Meninges
CF: _meningo_
_i_

Figure 14-1
Brain and spinal cord.

# ORGANS OF THE CENTRAL NERVOUS SYSTEM

1. brain . . . . . . . . . . . . . . . Major portion of the central nervous system (Figure 14-1).

    a. cerebrum . . . . . . . . . Largest portion of the brain, divided into left and right hemispheres. The cerebrum controls the skeletal muscles, interprets general senses (such as temperature, pain, and touch), and contains centers for sight and hearing. Intellect, memory, and emotional reactions also take place in the cerebrum.

       (1) ventricles . . . . . . Spaces within the cerebrum that contain a fluid called *cerebrospinal fluid*. The cerebrospinal fluid flows through the subarachnoid space around the brain and spinal cord.

    b. cerebellum . . . . . . . . Sometimes referred to as the *hindbrain*. It is located under the posterior portion of the cerebrum. Its function is to assist in the coordination of skeletal muscles and to maintain balance.

    c. brain stem . . . . . . . . Stemlike portion of the brain, which connects with the spinal cord.

       (1) pons . . . . . . . . . Literally means *bridge*. It connects the cerebrum with the cerebellum and brain stem.

       (2) medulla oblongata . . . . . . . . . Located between the pons and spinal cord. It contains centers that control respiration, heart rate, and the muscles in the blood vessel walls, which assist in determining blood pressure.

2. spinal cord . . . . . . . . . . . Passes through the vertebral canal extending from the medulla oblongata to the level of the second lumbar vertebra. The spinal cord conducts nerve impulses to and from the brain and initiates reflex action to sensory information without input from the brain.

3. meninges . . . . . . . . . . . . Three layers of membrane that cover the brain and spinal cord (Figure 14-2).

    a. dura mater . . . . . . . . Tough outer layer of the meninges.

    b. arachnoid . . . . . . . . . Delicate middle layer of the meninges. The arachnoid membrane is loosely attached to the pia mater by weblike fibers, which allow for the *subarachnoid space*.

    c. pia mater . . . . . . . . . Thin inner layer of the meninges.

---

Erasistratus, in the third century BC, named both the cerebrum and cerebellum. **Cerebellum** literally means **little brain** and is the diminutive of **cerebrum,** meaning **brain.** Although it was named long ago, its function was not understood until the nineteenth century.

---

The meninges were first named by a Persian physician in the tenth century. When translated into Latin they became **dura mater,** meaning **hard mother** (because it is a tough membrane), and **pia mater,** meaning **soft mother** (because it is a delicate membrane). **Mater** was used because the Arabians believed that the meninges were the mother of all other body membranes.

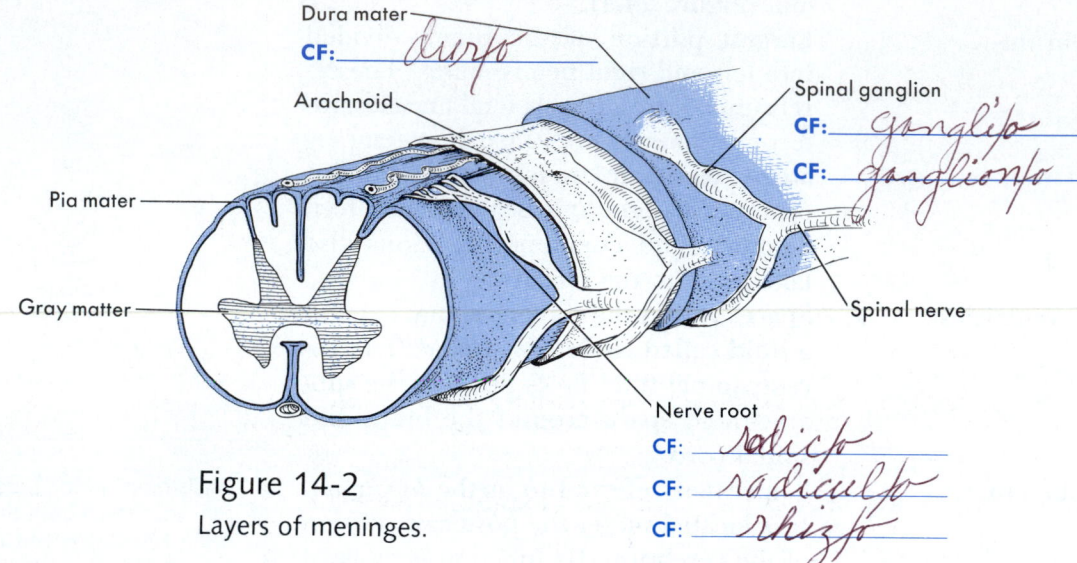

Dura mater

CF: _dur/o_

Arachnoid

Spinal ganglion

CF: _gangli/o_

CF: _ganglion/o_

Pia mater

Gray matter

Spinal nerve

Nerve root

CF: _radic/o_

CF: _radicul/o_

CF: _rhiz/o_

Figure 14-2
Layers of meninges.

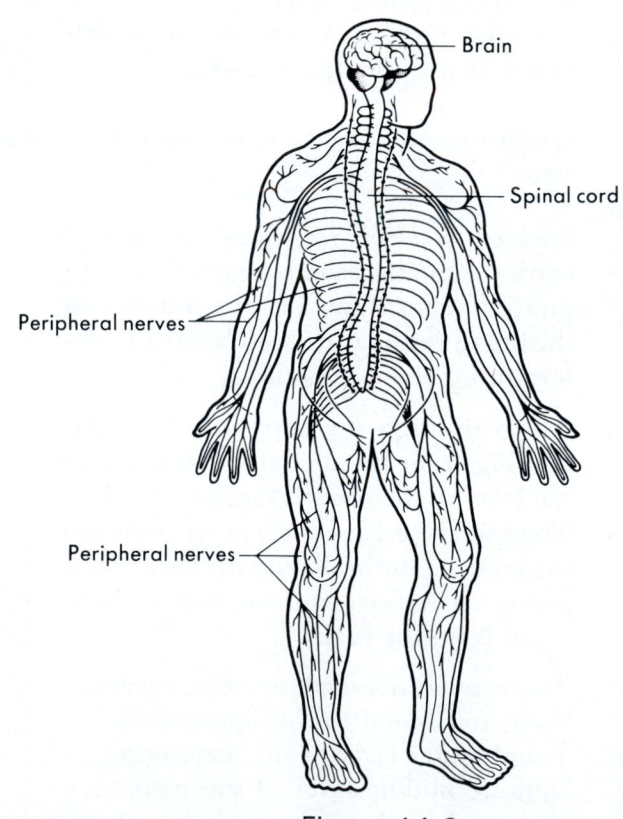

Brain

Spinal cord

Peripheral nerves

Peripheral nerves

Figure 14-3
Nervous system.

## ORGANS OF THE PERIPHERAL NERVOUS SYSTEM

1. nerve . . . . . . . . . . . . . . .    Cordlike structure that carries impulses from one part of the body to another. There are 12 pairs of cranial nerves and 31 pairs of spinal nerves (Figure 14-3).

2. ganglion (*pl*, ganglia) . . . .    Group of nerve cells located outside the central nervous system.

Learn the anatomical terms by completing the following exercises.

## EXERCISE 1

Fill in the blanks with the correct terms.
The layer of membrane that covers the brain and spinal cord is called

the (1) *meninges* It is composed of three layers called

(2) *dura mater*, (3) *arachnoid*, and (4) *pia*

*mater*. Below the middle layer is a space called the (5) *subarachnoid* ~~ventricles~~

*space* through which (6) *cerebrospinal fluid*

flows around the brain and spinal cord.

## EXERCISE 2

Match the definitions in the first column with the correct terms in the second column.

*d*   1. maintains balance

*f*   2. connects the cerebrum with the cerebellum and brain stem

*g*   3. spaces within the cerebrum

*e*   4. contains the control center for respiration

*a*   5. carries impulses from one part of the body to another

*h*   6. conducts impulses to and from the brain

*b*   7. group of nerve cells outside the CNS

a. nerve

b. ganglion

c. pia mater

d. cerebellum

e. medulla oblongata

f. pons

g. ventricles

h. spinal cord

Place a check mark (√) in the box to indicate that you have completed Objective 1.

☐ DEFINE THE ANATOMICAL TERMS OF THE NERVOUS SYSTEM.

# Objective 2   WRITE THE DEFINITIONS OF THE WORD PARTS INCLUDED IN THIS CHAPTER.

## Nervous System Word Parts

Study the word parts and their definitions listed as follows. Learning will be made easier by completing the exercises that follow.

| COMBINING FORM | DEFINITION |
|---|---|
| 1. cerebell/o . . . . . . . . . . . . | cerebellum |
| 2. cerebr/o . . . . . . . . . . . . . | cerebrum, brain |
| 3. dur/o . . . . . . . . . . . . . . | hard, dura mater |
| 4. encephal/o . . . . . . . . . . . | brain |
| 5. gangli/o, ganglion/o . . . . . | ganglion |
| 6. mening/i, mening/o . . . . . | meninges |

(NOTE: Both *i* and *o* are used as combining vowels with *mening*.)

| | |
|---|---|
| 7. myel/o . . . . . . . . . . . . . . | spinal cord |

(NOTE: *Myel/o* also means *bone marrow;* see Chapter 13.)

| | |
|---|---|
| 8. neur/o. . . . . . . . . . . . . . | nerve |

(NOTE: *Neur/o* was introduced in Chapter 2.)

| | |
|---|---|
| 9. radic/o, radicul/o, rhiz/o . | nerve root |

Learn the anatomical locations and definitions of the combining forms by completing the following exercises.

## EXERCISE 3

Write the combining forms in the spaces provided on the diagrams in Figures 14-1 and 14-2, pp. 534 and 536.

## EXERCISE 4

Write the definitions of the following combining forms.

1. cerebell/o _____ *cerebellum* _____
2. neur/o _____ *nerve* _____
3. myel/o _____ *spinal cord* _____
4. mening/o, mening/i _____ *meninges* _____
5. encephal/o _____ *brain* _____
6. cerebr/o _____ *cerebrum* _____
7. radicul/o _____ *nerve root* _____

8. gangli/o _____ *ganglion*

9. radic/o _____ *nerve root*

10. dur/o _____ *hard, dura mater*

11. ganglion/o _____ *ganglion*

12. rhiz/o _____ *nerve root*

## EXERCISE 5

Write the combining form for each of the following.

1. cerebellum _____ *cerebell/o*

2. nerve _____ *neur/o*

3. spinal cord _____ *myel/o*

4. meninges   a. _____ *mening/o*

             b. _____ *meningi/o*

5. brain _____ *encephal/o*

6. cerebrum _____ *cerebr/o*

7. nerve root   a. _____ *radic/o*

             b. _____ *radicul/o*

             c. _____ *rhiz/o*

8. hard, dura mater _____ *dur/o*

9. ganglion   a. _____ *gangli/o*

             b. _____ *ganglion/o*

# Other Word Parts

| COMBINING FORM | DEFINITION |
| --- | --- |
| 1. esthesi/o . . . . . . . . . . . . | sensation, sensitivity, feeling |
| 2. mon/o . . . . . . . . . . . . . . | one |
| 3. phas/o . . . . . . . . . . . . . . | speech |
| 4. poli/o . . . . . . . . . . . . . . | gray matter |
| 5. psych/o<br>   ment/o<br>   phren/o . . . . . . . . . . . . . . | mind |

6. quadr/i . . . . . . . . . . . . . .    four
   (NOTE: An *i* is the combining
   vowel in *quadr/i.*)

Learn the other combining forms by completing the following exercises.

## EXERCISE 6

Write the definitions of the following combining forms.

1. mon/o _____ *one*

2. psych/o _____ *mind*

3. quadr/i _____ *four*

4. ment/o _____ *mind*

5. phas/o _____ *speech*

6. esthesi/o _____ *sensation, sensitivity, feeling*

7. phren/o _____ *mind*

8. poli/o _____ *gray matter*

## EXERCISE 7

Write the combining form for each of the following.

1. four _____ *quadri*

2. one _____ *mono*

3. mind      a. _____ *mento*
             b. _____ *phreno*
             c. _____ *psycho*

4. speech _____ *phaso*

5. gray matter _____ *olio*

6. sensation, sensitivity, feeling _____ *esthesio*

## Prefixes

| PREFIX | DEFINITION |
|---|---|
| 1. hemi- . . . . . . . . . . . . . . . | half |
| 2. pre-. . . . . . . . . . . . . . . . | before |
| 3. tetra-. . . . . . . . . . . . . . . | four |

Learn the prefixes by completing the following exercises.

## EXERCISE 8

Write the definitions of the following prefixes.

1. tetra- _*four*_
2. hemi- _*half*_
3. pre- _*before*_

## EXERCISE 9

Write the prefix for each of the following definitions.

1. half _*hemi*_
2. four _*tetra*_
3. before _*pre*_

# Suffixes

| SUFFIX | DEFINITION |
|---|---|
| 1. -iatry | physician, treatment |
| 2. -ictal | seizure, attack |
| 3. -paresis | slight paralysis |

Learn the suffixes by completing the following exercises.

## EXERCISE 10

Write the definitions for the following suffixes.

1. -paresis _*slight paralysis*_
2. -iatry _*physician, treatment*_
3. -ictal _*seizure, attack*_

## EXERCISE 11

Write the suffix for each of the following definitions.

1. slight paralysis _*paresis*_
2. physician, treatment _*iatry*_
3. seizure _*ictal*_

Place a check mark (√) in the box to indicate that you have completed Objective 2.

☐ **WRITE THE DEFINITION OF THE WORD PARTS INCLUDED IN THIS CHAPTER.**

## Medical Terms

The terms you need to learn to complete this chapter are listed as follows. Now that you know the meaning of the word parts, the exercises found at the end of the list will assist you to learn the definition and the spelling of each word.

## Objective 3    BUILD, ANALYZE, DEFINE, PRONOUNCE, AND SPELL THE DIAGNOSTIC TERMS RELATED TO THE NERVOUS SYSTEM.

## Diagnostic Terms

| TERM (built from word parts) | DEFINITION |
|---|---|
| 1. cerebellitis<br>(sãr-e-bel-Ī-tis) | inflammation of the cerebellum |
| 2. cerebral thrombosis<br>(ser-Ē-bral) (throm-BŌ-sis) | condition of a blood clot in the cerebrum (Figure 14-4) |
| 3. duritis<br>(du-RĪ-tis) | inflammation of the dura mater |
| 4. encephalitis<br>(en-sef-a-LĪ-tis) | inflammation of the brain |

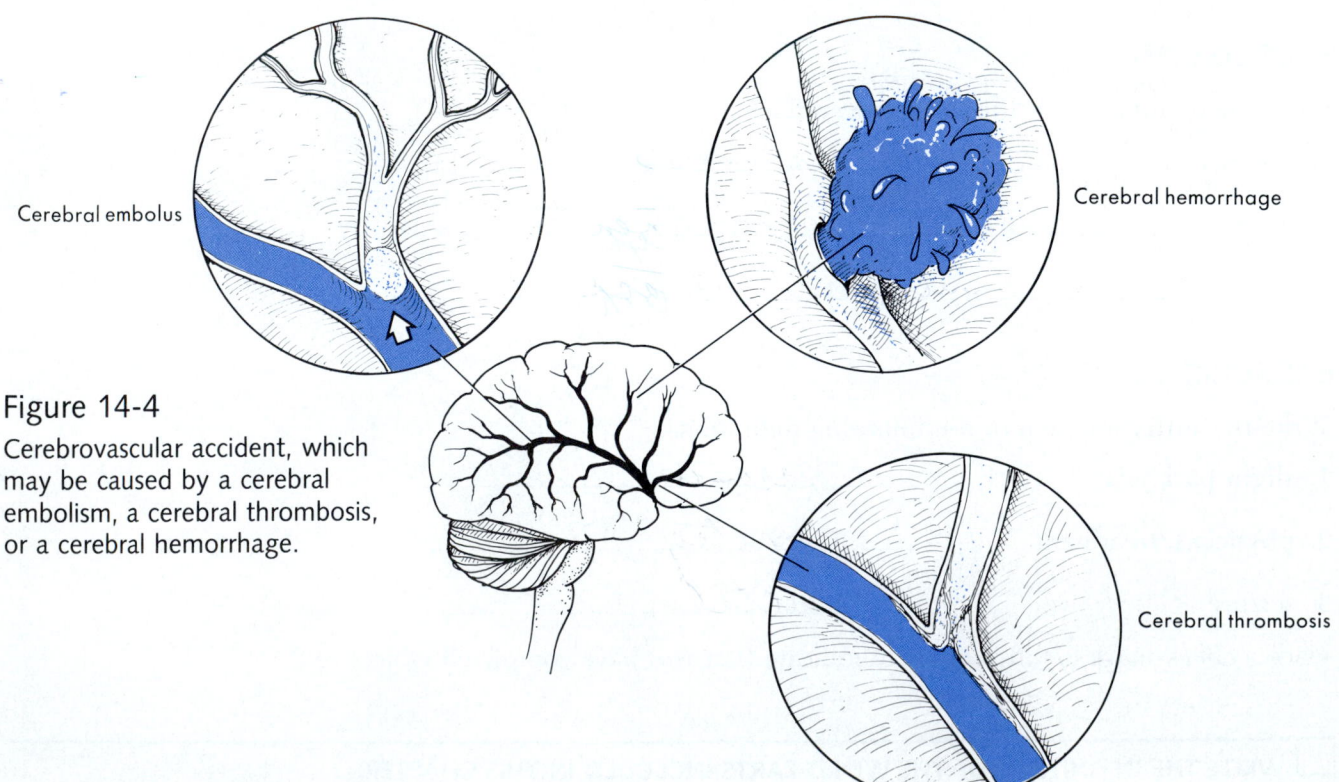

Cerebral embolus

Cerebral hemorrhage

Cerebral thrombosis

Figure 14-4
Cerebrovascular accident, which may be caused by a cerebral embolism, a cerebral thrombosis, or a cerebral hemorrhage.

5.  encephalomalacia......    softening of the brain
    (en-*sef*-a-lō-ma-LĀ-shē-a)

6.  encephalomyeloradiculi-
    tis .................    inflammation of the brain, spinal cord,
    (en-*sef*-a-lō-*mī*-e-lō-ra-*dik*-ū-    and nerve roots
    LĪ-tis)

7.  gangliitis ...........    inflammation of the ganglion
    (*gang*-glē-Ī-tis)

8.  meningitis ...........    inflammation of the meninges
    (*men*-in-JĪ-tis)

9.  meningocele..........    protrusion of the meninges (through a
    (me-NING-gō-sēl)    defect in the skull or vertebral column)

10. meningomyelocele.....    protrusion of the meninges and spinal
    (me-*ning*-gō-MĪ-e-lō-*sēl*)    cord (through the vertebral column)
                                     (Figure 14-5)

11. neuralgia ............    pain in a nerve
    (nū-RAL-jē-a)

12. neuroarthropathy......    disease of nerves and joints
    (*nūr*-ō-ar-THROP-a-thē)

13. neurasthenia ........    nerve weakness (nervous exhaustion, fa-
    (*nū*-ras-THĒ-nē-a)    tigue, and weakness)

14. neuritis..............    inflammation of the nerve
    (nū-RI-tis)

15. neuroblast ..........    developing nerve cell
    (NŪ-rō-blast)

## Figure 14-5
Spina bifida and meningomyelocele.

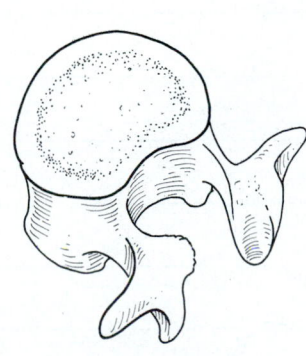

Spina bifida

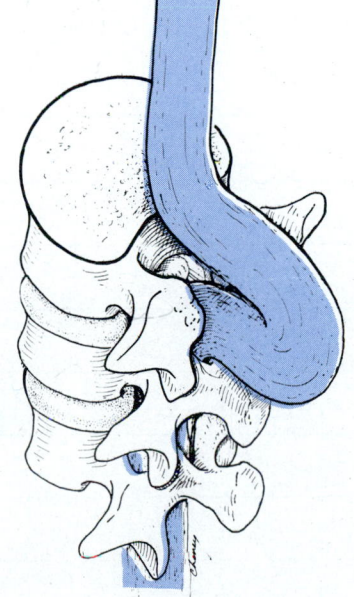

Meningomyelocele

16. neuroma . . . . . . . . . . . .     tumor made up of nerve cells
    (nū-RŌ-ma)

17. poliomyelitis . . . . . . . . .     inflammation of the gray matter of the
    (pō-lē-ō-mī-e-LĪ-tis)               spinal cord. This infectious disease,
                                        commonly referred to as polio, is caused
                                        by one of three polio viruses

18. polyneuritis . . . . . . . . .     inflammation of many nerves
    (pol-ē-nū-RĪ-tis)

19. radiculitis . . . . . . . . . . .   inflammation of the (spinal) nerve roots
    (ra-dik-ū-LĪ-tis)

20. rhizomeningomyelitis . .           inflammation of the nerve root, menin-
    (rī-zō-men-ning-gō-mī-e-           ges, and spinal cord
    LĪ-tis)

21. subdural hematoma . . . .          blood tumor below the dura (*hematoma*,
    (sub-DŪ-ral) (hĕm-a-TŌ-ma)         literally translated, means *blood tumor*;
                                        however, a hematoma is a tumorlike
                                        mass produced by the collection of blood
                                        in a tissue or cavity)

Practice saying each of these terms aloud. To assist you in pronunciation, obtain the audiotape designed for use with this text. Learn the definitions and spellings of the diagnostic terms by completing the following exercises.

## EXERCISE 12

Analyze and define the following diagnostic terms.

1. neuritis _____

2. neuroma _____

3. neuralgia _____

4. neuroarthropathy _____

5. neuroblast _____

6. neurasthenia _____

7. encephalomalacia _____

8. encephalitis _____

9. encephalomyeloradiculitis _____

10. meningitis _____

11. meningocele _____

12. meningomyelocele _____

13. radiculitis _____

14. cerebellitis _____

15. gangliitis _____

16. duritis _____

17. polyneuritis _____

18. poliomyelitis _____

19. cerebral thrombosis _____

20. subdural hematoma _____

21. rhizomeningomyelitis _____

## EXERCISE 13

Build diagnostic terms for the following definitions by using the word parts you have learned.

1. inflammation of the
   nerve
   _____ / _____
   WR            S

2. tumor made up of nerve
   cells
   _____ / _____
   WR            S

3. pain in a nerve
   _____ / _____
   WR            S

4. disease of nerves and
   joints
   _____ / ___ / _____ / ___ / _____
   WR    CV    WR    CV    S

5. developing nerve cell
   _____ / ___ / _____
   WR    CV    WR

6. nerve weakness (nervous
   exhaustion, fatigue, and
   weakness)
   _____ / _____
   WR            S

7. softening of the brain
   _____ / ___ / _____
   WR    CV    S

8. inflammation of the brain

$$\underline{\hspace{3cm}}\ \underset{\text{WR}}{\Big|}\ \underset{\text{S}}{}\underline{\hspace{3cm}}$$

9. inflammation of the brain, spinal cord, and nerve roots

$$\underline{\hspace{1cm}}\ \underset{\text{WR}}{\Big|}\ \underset{\text{CV}}{\Big|}\ \underset{\text{WR}}{\Big|}\ \underset{\text{CV}}{\Big|}\ \underset{\text{WR}}{\Big|}\ \underset{\text{S}}{}$$

10. inflammation of the meninges

$$\underline{\hspace{3cm}}\ \underset{\text{WR}}{\Big|}\ \underset{\text{S}}{}\underline{\hspace{3cm}}$$

11. protrusion of the meninges (through a defect in the skull or vertebral column)

$$\underline{\hspace{2cm}}\ \underset{\text{WR}}{\Big|}\ \underset{\text{CV}}{\Big|}\ \underset{\text{S}}{}\underline{\hspace{2cm}}$$

12. protrusion of the meninges and spinal cord (through the vertebral column)

$$\underline{\hspace{1cm}}\ \underset{\text{WR}}{\Big|}\ \underset{\text{CV}}{\Big|}\ \underset{\text{WR}}{\Big|}\ \underset{\text{CV}}{\Big|}\ \underset{\text{S}}{}$$

13. inflammation of the (spinal) nerve roots

$$\underline{\hspace{3cm}}\ \underset{\text{WR}}{\Big|}\ \underset{\text{S}}{}\underline{\hspace{3cm}}$$

14. inflammation of the cerebellum

$$\underline{\hspace{3cm}}\ \underset{\text{WR}}{\Big|}\ \underset{\text{S}}{}\underline{\hspace{3cm}}$$

15. inflammation of the ganglion

$$\underline{\hspace{3cm}}\ \underset{\text{WR}}{\Big|}\ \underset{\text{S}}{}\underline{\hspace{3cm}}$$

16. inflammation of the dura mater

$$\underline{\hspace{3cm}}\ \underset{\text{WR}}{\Big|}\ \underset{\text{S}}{}\underline{\hspace{3cm}}$$

17. inflammation of many nerves

$$\underline{\hspace{2cm}}\ \underset{\text{P}}{\Big|}\ \underset{\text{WR}}{\Big|}\ \underset{\text{S}}{}\underline{\hspace{2cm}}$$

18. inflammation of the gray matter of the spinal cord

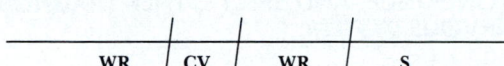

WR / CV / WR / S

19. condition of a blood clot in a blood vessel of the cerebrum

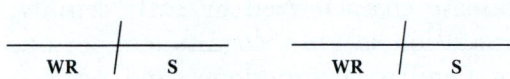

WR / S        WR / S

20. blood tumor below the dura

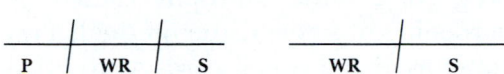

P / WR / S        WR / S

21. inflammation of the nerve root, meninges, and spinal cord

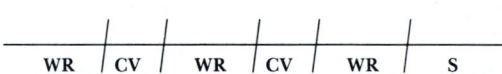

WR / CV / WR / CV / WR / S

## EXERCISE 14

Spell each of the diagnostic terms. Have someone dictate the terms on pp. 542 to 544 to you or say the words into a tape recorder; then spell the words from your recording as often as necessary. Think about the word parts before attempting to write the word. Study any you have spelled incorrectly.

1. _____    12. _____
2. _____    13. _____
3. _____    14. _____
4. _____    15. _____
5. _____    16. _____
6. _____    17. _____
7. _____    18. _____
8. _____    19. _____
9. _____    20. _____
10. _____   21. _____
11. _____

Place a check mark (√) in the box to indicate that you have completed Objective 3.

☐ **BUILD, ANALYZE, DEFINE, PRONOUNCE, AND SPELL THE DIAGNOSTIC TERMS RELATED TO THE NERVOUS SYSTEM.**

# Objective 4 DEFINE, PRONOUNCE, AND SPELL OTHER DIAGNOSTIC TERMS RELATED TO THE NERVOUS SYSTEM.

## Other Diagnostic Terms

| TERM | DEFINITION |
|---|---|
| 1. Alzheimer's disease . . . . (AHLTS-hī-merz) | disease characterized by early senility, confusion, loss of recognition of persons or familiar surroundings, and restlessness |
| 2. amyotrophic lateral sclerosis (ALS) . . . . . . . . . . (a-mī-ō-TROF-ik) (LAT-er-al) (skle-RŌ-sis) | progressive muscle atrophy caused by hardening of nerve tissue on the lateral columns of the spinal cord. Also called *Lou Gehrig's disease.* |
| 3. cerebral aneurysm . . . . . (se-RĒ-bral) (AN-ū-rizm) | aneurysm in the cerebrum (see aneurysm p. 320) |
| 4. cerebral palsy (CP). . . . . (se-RĒ-bral) (PAWL-zē) | condition characterized by lack of muscle control and partial paralysis, caused by a brain defect or lesion present at birth or shortly after |
| 5. cerebrovascular accident (CVA) . . . . . . . . . . . . . . . (se-rē-brō-VAS-kū-lar) | interruption of blood supply to the brain caused by a cerebral thrombosis, cerebral embolism, or cerebral hemorrhage. The patient may experience mild to severe paralysis. Also called a *stroke*, or *apoplexy.* (Figure 14-4) |
| 6. epilepsy . . . . . . . . . . . . (EP-i-lep-sē) | disorder in which the main symptom is recurring seizures |
| 7. hydrocephalus . . . . . . . . (hī-drō-SEF-a-lus) | increased amount of cerebral spinal fluid in the ventricles of the brain, which causes enlargement of the cranium |
| 8. multiple sclerosis (MS). . (skle-RŌ-sis) | degenerative disease characterized by sclerotic patches along the brain and spinal cord |
| 9. neurosis . . . . . . . . . . . . (nū-RŌ-sis) | emotional disorder that involves an ineffective way of coping with anxiety or inner conflict |
| 10. Parkinson's disease. . . . . | chronic degenerative disease of the central nervous system. Symptoms include muscular tremors, rigidity, expressionless face, and shuffling gait. It usually occurs after the age of 50. |
| 11. psychosis . . . . . . . . . . . (sī-KŌ-sis) | major mental disorder characterized by extreme derangement, often with delusions and hallucinations |

Cerebrovascular accident is the most common disease of the nervous system. It is the third-highest cause of death in the United States, claiming 200,000 lives every year.

Hippocrates, in 400 BC, wrote of epilepsy in a book entitled **Sacred Disease.** It was believed at one time that epilepsy was a punishment for offending the gods. The Greek **epilepsia** meant **seizure** and is derived from **epi,** meaning **upon,** and **lambaneia,** meaning **to seize.** The term literally means **seized upon** (by the gods).

Hydrocephalus literally means **water in the head** and is made of the word parts **hydro,** meaning **water** and **cephal,** meaning **head.** The condition was first described in approximately AD 30 in the book **De Medicina.**

Parkinson's disease is also called **parkinsonism, paralysis agitans,** and **shaking palsy.** Since Dr. James Parkinson, an English professor, described the disease in 1817 in his **Essay on the Shaking Palsy,** it has often been referred to as Parkinson's disease.

12. **Reye's syndrome** . . . . . .
    (RĪZ)

    disease of the brain and other organs such as the liver. Affects children and adolescents. The cause is unknown, but typically follows a viral infection.

13. **sciatica** . . . . . . . . . . . . .
    (sī-AT-i-ka)

    inflammation of the sciatic nerve, causing pain that travels from thigh through leg to foot and toes

14. **shingles** . . . . . . . . . . . .

    viral disease that affects the peripheral nerves and causes blisters on the skin that follow the course of the affected nerves. Also called *herpes zoster*.

15. **transient ischemic attack**
    **(TIA)** . . . . . . . . . . . . . .
    (is-KĒM-ik)

    sudden deficient supply of blood to the brain lasting a short time. (see coronary ischemia, pg. 315)

Practice saying each of these terms. To assist you in pronunciation, obtain the audiotape designed for use with this text. Learn the definitions and spellings of the other diagnostic terms by completing the following exercises.

## EXERCISE 15

Many of the other diagnostic terms include word parts you have studied in this or previous chapters. To help you become familiar with the terms write the definition of the italicized word part in each of the following.

1. *cerebro*vascular accident _____

2. *psych*osis _____

3. *epi*lepsy _____

4. multiple *sclerosis* _____

5. hydro*cephalus* _____

6. *neur*osis _____

7. *cerebral* palsy _____

## EXERCISE 16

Match the diseases listed in the first column with the corresponding symptoms in the second column.

*b* 1. psychosis

*a* 2. sciatica

*n* 3. transient ischemic attack

*j* 4. Parkinson's disease

a. causes pain from thigh to toes

b. derangement, possibly including delusions and hallucinations

c. enlargement of the cranium

d. hardened patches scattered along the brain and spinal cord

___l___ 5. cerebral palsy

___c___ 6. hydrocephalus

___e___ 7. neurosis

___g___ 8. cerebrovascular accident

___i___ 9. Alzheimer's disease

___m___ 10. Reye's syndrome

___f___ 11. epilepsy

___k___ 12. multiple sclerosis

___h___ 13. shingles

___o___ 14. amyotrophic lateral sclerosis

e.  inability to cope with anxiety or inner conflict

f.  recurring seizures

g.  mild to severe paralysis

h.  blisters on the skin

i.  early senility

j.  muscle tremors and rigidity

k.  inflammation of spinal cord

l.  lack of muscle control

m.  affects children and adolescents, typically following viral infection

n.  deficient supply of blood to the brain

o.  also called Lou Gehrig's disease

## EXERCISE 17

Spell each of the other diagnostic terms. Have someone dictate the terms on pp. 548 and 549 to you or say the words into a tape recorder; then spell the words from your recording as often as necessary. Study any you have spelled incorrectly.

1. _____      9. _____

2. _____     10. _____

3. _____     11. _____

4. _____     12. _____

5. _____     13. _____

6. _____     14. _____

7. _____     15. _____

8. _____

Place a check mark (√) in the box to indicate that you have completed Objective 4.

☐ DEFINE, PRONOUNCE, AND SPELL THE OTHER DIAGNOSTIC TERMS RELATED TO THE NERVOUS SYSTEM.

# Objective 5   BUILD, ANALYZE, DEFINE, PRONOUNCE, AND SPELL THE SURGICAL TERMS RELATED TO THE NERVOUS SYSTEM.

## Surgical Terms

| TERM (built from word parts) | DEFINITION |
|---|---|
| 1. ganglionectomy . . . . . . . . (gang-glē-on-EK-tō-mē) | excision of a ganglion (also called *gangliectomy*) |

2. **neurectomy** . . . . . . . . . . .    excision of a nerve
   (nū-REK-tō-mē)

3. **neurolysis** . . . . . . . . . . . .    separating a nerve (from adhesions)
   (nū-ROL-i-sis)

4. **neuroplasty** . . . . . . . . . .    surgical repair of a nerve
   (NŪ-rŏ-plas-tē)

5. **neurorrhaphy** . . . . . . . . .    suture of a nerve
   (nū-RŌR-a-fē)

6. **neurotomy** . . . . . . . . . . .    incision into the nerves
   (nū-ROT-ō-mē)

7. **radicotomy** . . . . . . . . . . .
   (*rad*-i-KOT-ō-mē)
   } incision into a nerve root (Figure 14-6)

8. **rhizotomy** . . . . . . . . . . .
   (rī-ZOT-ō-mē)

Practice saying each of these terms aloud. To assist you in pronunciation, obtain the audiotape designed for use with this text. Learn the definitions and spellings of the surgical terms by completing the following exercises.

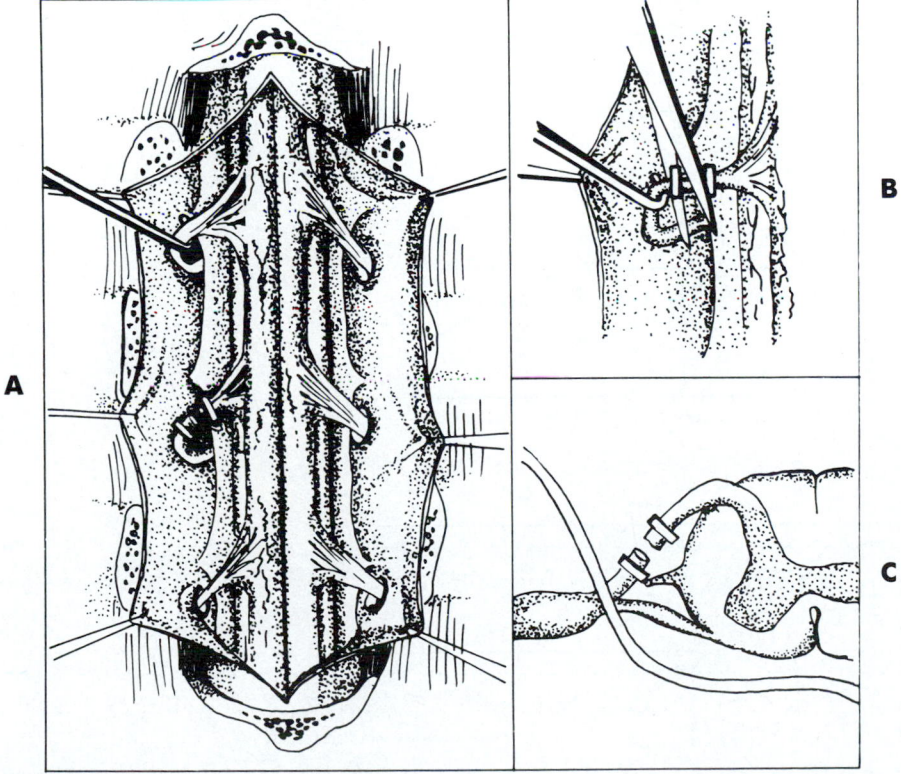

Figure 14-6

Rhizotomy after laminectomy. **A,** Spinal cord and roots exposed. **B,** Posterior root indentified. **C,** Diagram showing cross-section of spinal cord and divided posterior root.

From Carini E and Owens G: *Neurological and neurosurgical nursing,* ed 6, St. Louis, 1974, Mosby.

## EXERCISE 18

Analyze and define the following surgical terms.

1. radicotomy _____

2. neurectomy _____

3. neurorrhaphy _____

4. ganglionectomy _____

5. neurotomy _____

6. neurolysis _____

7. neuroplasty _____

8. rhizotomy _____

## EXERCISE 19

Build terms for the following definitions by using the word parts you have learned.

1. incision into a nerve
   root

   a. _____ / _____
                        WR         S

   b. _____ / _____
                        WR         S

2. excision of a nerve

   _____ / _____
                    WR         S

3. suture of a nerve

   _____ / _____
                    WR         S

4. excision of a ganglion

   _____ / _____
                    WR         S

5. incision into the nerves

   _____ / _____
                    WR         S

6. separating a nerve (from
   adhesions)

   _____ / _____ / _____
              WR       CV       S

7. surgical repair of a nerve

   _____ / _____ / _____
              WR       CV       S

**EXERCISE 20**

Spell each of the surgical terms. Have someone dictate the terms on pp. 550 and 551 to you or say the words into a tape recorder; then spell the words from your recording as often as necessary. Think of the word parts before attempting to write the word. Study any you have spelled incorrectly.

1. _____    5. _____

2. _____    6. _____

3. _____    7. _____

4. _____    8. _____

Place a check mark (√) in the box to indicate that you have completed Objective 5.

☐ BUILD, ANALYZE, DEFINE, PRONOUNCE, AND SPELL THE SURGICAL TERMS RELATED TO THE NERVOUS SYSTEM.

# Objective 6    BUILD, ANALYZE, DEFINE, PRONOUNCE, AND SPELL THE DIAGNOSTIC PROCEDURAL TERMS RELATED TO THE NERVOUS SYSTEM.

## Diagnostic Procedural Terms

| TERM (built from word parts) | DEFINITION |
|---|---|
| 1. cerebral angiography .... (sē-RĒ-bral) (an-jē-OG-ra-fē) | process of x-ray filming of the blood vessels in the brain (after an injection of contrast medium) |
| 2. echoencephalography ... (ek-ō-en-*sef*-a-LOG-ra-fē) | process of recording brain structures by use of sound (also called *ultrasonography*) |
| 3. electroencephalogram (EEG) ................ (e-*lek*-trō-en-SEF-a-lō-gram) | record of the electrical impulse of the brain |
| 4. electroencephalograph... (e-*lek*-trō-en-SEF-a-lō-graf) | instrument used for recording the electrical impulses of the brain |
| 5. electroencephalography.. (e-*lek*-trō-en-*sef*-a-LOG-ra-fē) | process of recording the electrical impulses of the brain |
| 6. myelogram ............ (MĪ-e-lō-gram) | x-ray film of the spinal cord (after injection of dye into the spinal fluid that surrounds the spinal cord) (Figure 14-7) |

Practice saying each of these above words aloud. To assist you in pronunciation, obtain the audiotape designed for use with this text. Learn the definitions and spellings of the diagnostic procedural terms by completing the following exercises.

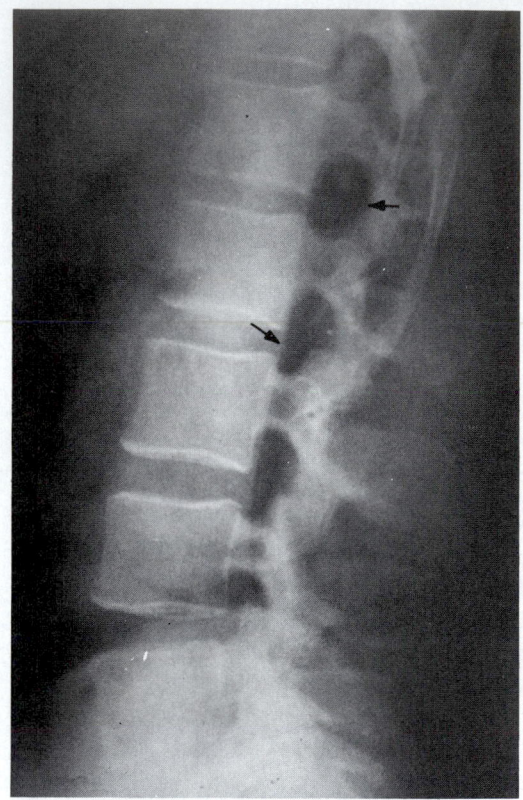

**Figure 14-7**

Lateral myelogram showing gas in spinal canal *(arrows)*.

From Ballinger PW: *Merrill's atlas of radiographic positions and radiologic procedures,* ed 7, St. Louis, 1991, Mosby.

## EXERCISE 21

Analyze and define the following diagnostic procedural terms.

1. electroencephalogram _____

2. electroencephalograph _____

3. electroencephalography _____

4. echoencephalography _____

5. myelogram _____

6. cerebral angiography _____

## EXERCISE 22

Write the term for each of the following definitions.

1. process of recording brain
(structures) by use of
sound

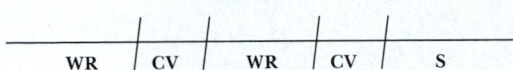

     WR   CV   WR   CV   S

2. record of the electrical
impulses of the brain

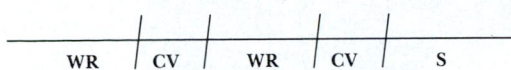

     WR   CV   WR   CV   S

3. instrument used for recording the electrical impulses of the brain

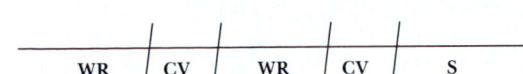

     WR   CV   WR   CV   S

4. process of recording the
electrical impulses of the
brain

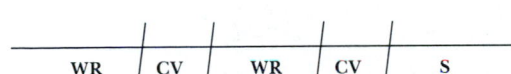

     WR   CV   WR   CV   S

5. x-ray film of the spinal
cord

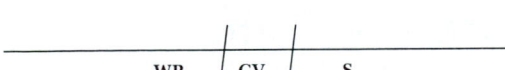

         WR   CV   S

6. process of x-ray filming of
the blood vessels in the
brain

     WR   S        WR   CV   S

## EXERCISE 23

Spell each of the diagnostic procedural terms. Have someone dictate the terms on p. 553 to you. Think about the word parts before attempting to write the word or say the words into a tape recorder; then spell the words from your recording as often as necessary. Study any you have spelled incorrectly.

1. _____    4. _____

2. _____    5. _____

3. _____    6. _____

Place a check mark (√) in the box to indicate that you have completed Objective 6.

☐ **BUILD, ANALYZE, DEFINE, PRONOUNCE, AND SPELL THE DIAGNOSTIC PROCEDURAL TERMS RELATED TO THE NERVOUS SYSTEM.**

**Figure 14-8**
**A,** CT scanner capable of examining the head only. **B,** CT scanner capable of examining any part of the body.

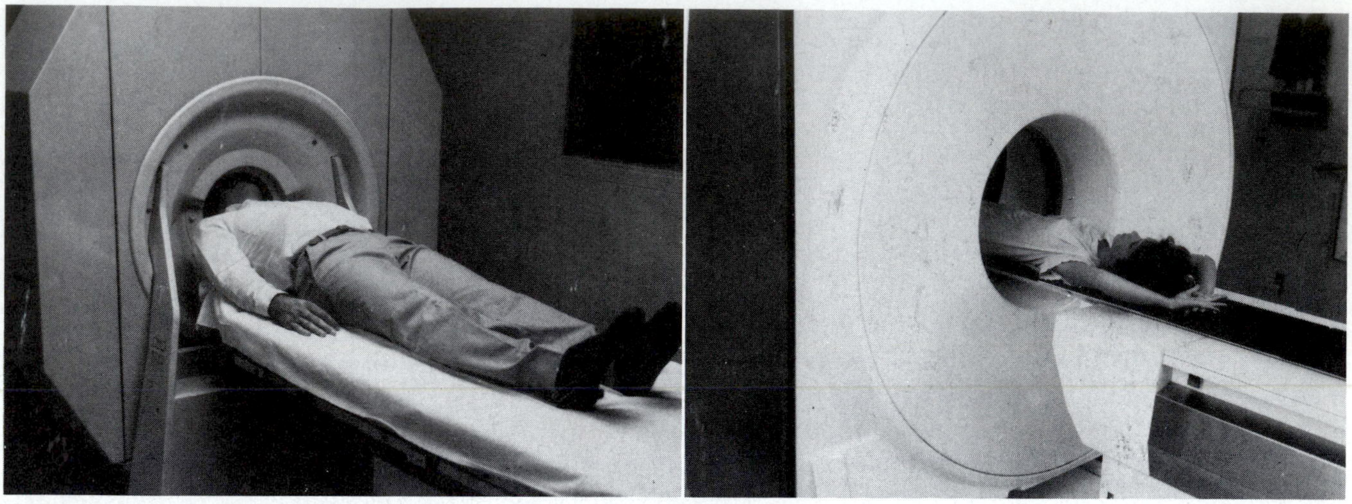

From Ballinger PW: *Merrill's atlas of radiographic positions and radiologic procedures,* ed 5, St. Louis, 1982, Mosby.

# Objective 7   DEFINE, PRONOUNCE, AND SPELL OTHER DIAGNOSTIC PROCEDURAL TERMS RELATED TO THE NERVOUS SYSTEM.

## Other Diagnostic Procedural Terms

| TERM | DEFINITION |
|---|---|
| 1. computed tomography of the brain . . . . . . . . . . . . (tō-MOG-ra-fē) | process that includes the use of a computer to produce a series of images of the tissues of the brain at any desired depth. The procedure is noninvasive, painless, and particularly useful in diagnosing brain tumors. Also referred to as a *CT scan* or *CAT scan* for *computed axial tomography* (Figures 14-8 and 14-9). |
| 2. lumbar puncture (LP) . . . (LUM-bar) | insertion of a needle into the subarachnoid space between the third and fourth lumbar vertebrae. It is performed for many reasons, including the removal of cerebrospinal fluid for diagnostic purposes (Figure 14-10). |
| 3. magnetic resonance imaging of the head (MRI) . . . (mag-NET-ik) (re-zo-NANCE) (IM-a-jing) | a noninvasive technique that produces cross-sectional and vertical images of cranial structures by use of magnetic waves. Unlike CT scan, MRI produces images without use of radiation or contrast medium. (Figure 14-11). |

> The first full-scale CT unit for head scanning was installed in a hospital in Wimbledon, United Kingdom in 1971. Its ability to provide neurological diagnostic information gained rapid recognition. The first units in the United States were used in 1973. The first scanner for visualizing sections of the body other than the brain was developed in 1974 by Dr. Robert Ledly at Georgetown University Medical Center.

> Magnetic resonance imaging scanner was first used in the United States in 1981. The scanner was developed in England and installed there in 1975.

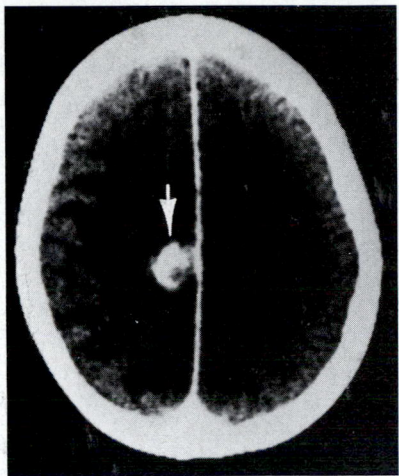

**Figure 14-9**

CT scan showing metastatic brain tumor *(arrow)*.

From Ballinger PW: *Merrill's atlas of radiographic positions and radiologic procedures,* ed 5, St. Louis, 1982, Mosby.

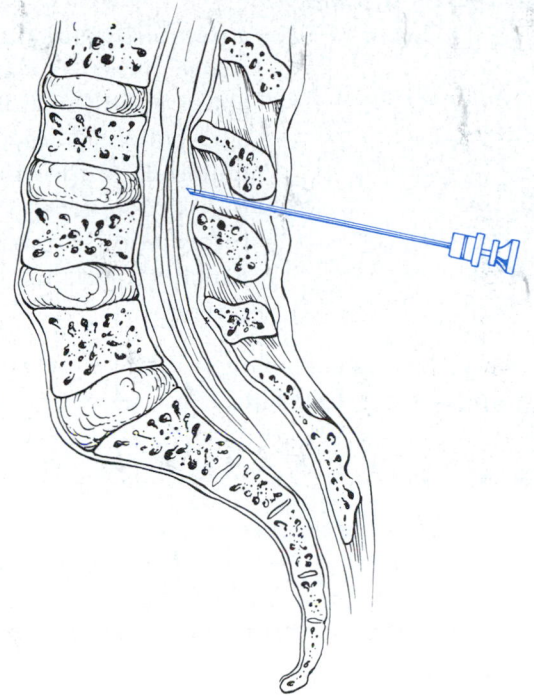

**Figure 14-10**

Lumbar puncture with needle in place.

From Phipps WJ, Long BC, and Woods NF: *Medical-surgical nursing,* ed 4, St. Louis, 1991, Mosby.

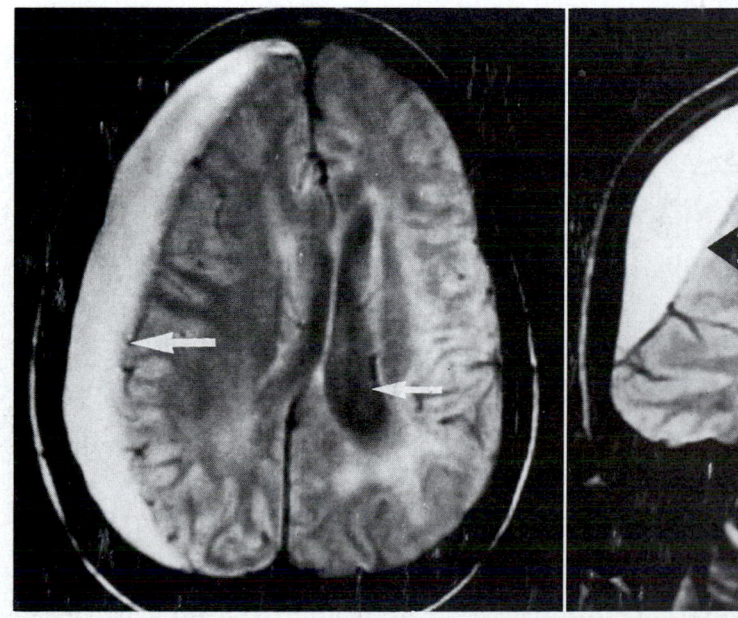

**Figure 14-11**

**A** and **B,** Magnetic resonance images show left subdural hematoma *(large arrow)* produces midline shift with enlargement of the left lateral ventricle *(small arrow).* **A,** Axial image. **B,** Coronal image.

From Stark DD and Bradley WG: *Magnetic resonance imaging,* ed 2, St. Louis, 1991, Mosby.

4. positron emission tomography of the brain (PET scan)............... (POS-i-tron) (e-MI-shun) (tō-MOG-ra-fē)     a new technique that permits viewing of a slice of the brain and gives information about brain function such as blood flow. The patient is injected with radioactive material. A special camera records the radioactive decay within the brain. The information is transmitted to a computer which projects images onto a television screen.

Learn the definitions and spellings of the other diagnostic procedural terms by completing the following exercises.

## EXERCISE 24

Fill in the blanks with the correct terms.

1. A computer is used to produce images during _computed_ _tomography_ .

2. A needle is inserted into the subarachnoid space during a _lumbar_ _puncture_ .

3. Produces images reflecting brain function _positron_ _emission_ _tomography_ .

4. Uses magnetic waves to produce images _____ _____ _____ .

## EXERCISE 25

Write the definitions of the following terms.

1. lumbar puncture _____

2. computer tomography of the brain _____

3. magnetic resonance imaging of the head _____

4. positron emission tomography of the brain _____

_____

## EXERCISE 26

Spell each of the other diagnostic procedural terms. Have someone dictate the terms on pp. 556 and 558 to you or say the words into a tape recorder; then spell the words from your recording as often as necessary. Study any you have spelled incorrectly.

1. _____    3. _____

2. _____    4. _____

Place a check mark (√) in the box to indicate that you have completed Objective 7.

☐ **DEFINE, PRONOUNCE, AND SPELL OTHER DIAGNOSTIC PROCEDURAL TERMS RELATED TO THE NERVOUS SYSTEM.**

# Objective 8
### BUILD, ANALYZE, DEFINE, PRONOUNCE, AND SPELL ADDITIONAL TERMS RELATED TO THE NERVOUS SYSTEM.

## Additional Terms

**TERM**
(built from word parts)

**DEFINITION**

1. **anesthesia**............ loss of feeling or sensation
   (*an*-es-THĒ-zē-a)

2. **aphasia**............. condition of loss or impairment of the ability to speak
   (a-FĀ-zē-a)

3. **cephalalgia**........... pain in the head, headache
   (*sef*-el-AL-jē-a)

4. **cerebral**............ pertaining to the cerebrum
   (se-RĒ-bral)

5. **craniocerebral**....... pertaining to the cranium and cerebrum
   (*krā*-nē-ō-sar-Ē-bral)

6. **dysphasia**........... condition of difficulty in speaking
   (dis-FĀ-zē-a)

7. **encephalosclerosis**..... hardening of the brain
   (en-*sef*-a-lō-skle-RŌ-sis)

8. **hemiparesis**.......... slight paralysis of half (right or left side of the body)
   (*hem*-i-pār-Ē-sis)

9. **hemiplegia**........... paralysis of half (right or left side) of the body; cerebrovascular accident is the most common cause of hemiplegia (Figure 14-12, *A*)
   (*hem*-i-PLĒ-jē-a)

10. **hyperesthesia**........ condition of excessive sensitivity (to stimuli)
    (*hī*-per-es-THĒ-zē-a)

11. **interictal**............ occurring between seizures or attacks
    (in-ter-IK-tal)

12. **monoparesis**.......... slight paralysis of one (limb)
    (mon-ō-pa-RĒ-sis)

13. **monoplegia**.......... paralysis of one (limb)
    (*mon*-ō-PLĒ-jē-a)

14. **myelomalacia**........ softening of the spinal cord
    (*mī*-e-lō-ma-LĀ-shē-a)

15. **neuroid**.............. resembling a nerve
    (NŪ-royd)

16. **neurologist**........... physician who specializes in neurology
    (nū-ROL-ō-jist)

17. **neurology**............ branch of medicine dealing with the nervous system's function and disorders
    (nū-ROL-ō-jē)

18. **panplegia**........... total paralysis (also spelled pamplegia)
    (pan-PLĒ-jē-a)

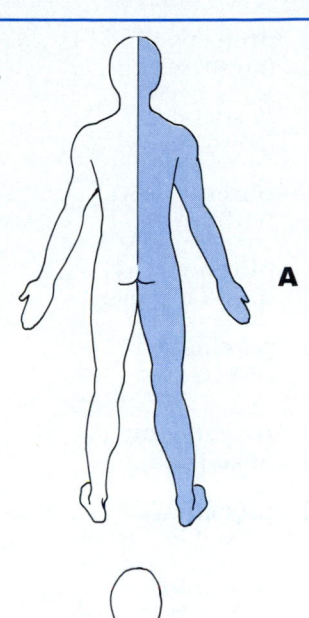

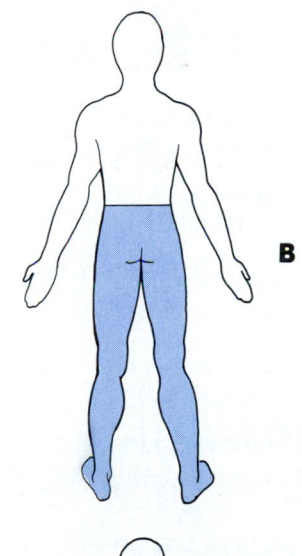

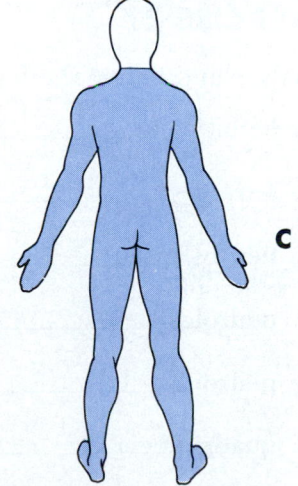

**Figure 14-12**

Types of paralysis. **A**, Hemiplegia. **B**, Paraplegia, **C**, Quadriplegia, or tetraplegia.

19. preictal . . . . . . . . . . . . . occurring before a seizure or attack
    (prē-IK-tal)

20. postictal . . . . . . . . . . . occurring after a seizure or attack
    (pōst-IK-tal)

21. phrenic . . . . . . . . . . . . pertaining to the mind
    (FREN-ik)

22. phrenopathy . . . . . . . . . mental disease
    (fre-NOP-a-thē)

23. psychiatry . . . . . . . . . . . branch of medicine that deals with the
    (sī-KĪ-a-trē)                   treatment of mental disorders

24. psychogenic . . . . . . . . . originating within the mind
    (sī-kō-JEN-ik)

25. psychologist . . . . . . . . . specialist in the study of psychology
    (sī-KOL-ō-jist)

26. psychology . . . . . . . . . . study of the mind (mental processes and
    (sī-KOL-ō-jē)                  behavior)

27. psychopathy . . . . . . . . . (any) disease of the mind
    (sī-KOP-a-thē)

28. psychosomatic . . . . . . . pertaining to the interrelations of body
    (sī-ko-sō-MAT-ik)              and mind

29. quadriplegia . . . . . . . . . paralysis of four (limbs) (Figure 14-12,
    (kwod-ri-PLĒ-jē-a)             C)

30. subdural . . . . . . . . . . . . pertaining to below the dura mater
    (sub-DŪ-ral)

31. tetraplegia . . . . . . . . . . paralysis of four (limbs) (synonymous
    (te-tra-PLĒ-jē-a)              with *quadriplegia*) (Figure 14-12, *C*)

## EXERCISE 27

Analyze and define the following additional terms.

1. hemiplegia _____

2. tetraplegia _____

3. neurologist _____

4. neurology _____

5. neuroid _____

6. quadriplegia _____

7. cerebral _____

8. monoplegia _____

9. aphasia _____

10. dysphasia _____

11. hemiparesis _____

12. anesthesia _____

13. hyperesthesia _____

14. subdural _____

15. cephalalgia _____

16. psychosomatic _____

17. psychopathy _____

18. psychology _____

19. psychiatry _____

20. psychologist _____

21. psychogenic _____

22. phrenic _____

23. phrenopathy _____

24. craniocerebral _____

25. myelomalacia _____

26. encephalosclerosis _____

27. postictal _____

28. panplegia _____

29. interictal _____

30. monoparesia _____

31. preictal _____

## EXERCISE 28

Build terms for the following definitions by using the word parts you have learned.

1. slight paralysis of half (right or left side of the body)

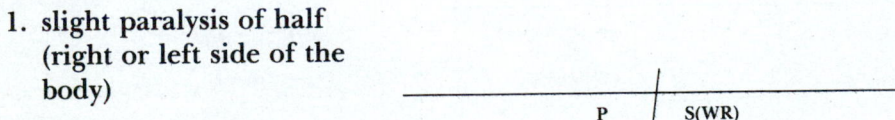

P / S(WR)

2. loss of feeling or sensation

         P   /   WR   /   S

3. excessive sensitivity (to stimuli)

         P   /   WR   /   S

4. below the dura mater

         P   /   WR   /   S

5. pain in the head, headache

         WR   /   S

6. pertaining to the interrelations of body and mind

         WR   /   CV   /   WR   /   S

7. (any) disease of the mind

         WR   /   CV   /   S

8. study of the mind

         WR   /   S

9. branch of medicine that deals with the treatment of mental disorders

         WR   /   S

10. specialist in the study of psychology

         WR   /   S

11. originating within the mind

         WR   /   CV   /   S

12. pertaining to the mind

         WR   /   S

13. mental disease

         WR   /   CV   /   S

14. pertaining to the cranium and cerebrum

_____ / _____ / _____ / _____
WR      CV      WR      S

15. softening of the spinal cord

_____ / _____ / _____
WR      CV      S

16. hardening of the brain

_____ / _____ / _____
WR      CV      S

17. paralysis of half (left or right side) of the body

_____ / _____
P      S(WR)

18. paralysis of four (limbs)

_____ / _____
P      S(WR)

19. physician who specializes in neurology

_____ / _____
WR      S

20. branch of medicine dealing with the nervous system's function and disorders

_____ / _____
WR      S

21. resembling a nerve

_____ / _____
WR      S

22. paralysis of four (limbs)

_____ / _____ / _____
WR      CV      S

23. pertaining to the cerebrum

_____ / _____
WR      S

24. paralysis of one (limb)

_____ / _____ / _____
WR      CV      S

25. condition of loss or impairment of the ability to speak

_____
P | WR | S

26. condition of difficulty in speaking

_____
P | WR | S

27. occurring before a seizure or attack

_____
P | S(WR)

28. slight paralysis of one (limb)

_____
WR | CV | S

29. occurring after a seizure

_____
P | S(WR)

30. total paralysis

_____
P | S(WR)

31. occurring between seizures or attacks

_____
P | S(WR)

## EXERCISE 29

Spell each of the additional terms. Have someone dictate the terms on pp. 559 and 560 to you or say the words into a tape recorder; then spell the words from your recording as often as necessary. Think about the word parts before attempting to write the word. Study any you have spelled incorrectly.

1. _____     9. _____

2. _____     10. _____

3. _____     11. _____

4. _____     12. _____

5. _____     13. _____

6. _____     14. _____

7. _____     15. _____

8. _____     16. _____

17. _____          25. _____

18. _____          26. _____

19. _____          27. _____

20. _____          28. _____

21. _____          29. _____

22. _____          30. _____

23. _____          31. _____

24. _____

Place a check mark (√) in the box to indicate that you have completed Objective 8.

☐ **BUILD, ANALYZE, DEFINE, PRONOUNCE, AND SPELL ADDITIONAL TERMS RELATED TO THE NERVOUS SYSTEM.**

## Objective 9 DEFINE, PRONOUNCE, AND SPELL THE OTHER ADDITIONAL TERMS RELATED TO THE NERVOUS SYSTEM.

## Other Additional Terms

| TERM | DEFINITION |
|---|---|
| 1. ataxia . . . . . . . . . . . . . .<br>(a-TAK-sē-a) | lack of muscle coordination |
| 2. coma. . . . . . . . . . . . . . .<br>(KŌ-ma) | state of profound unconsciousness |
| 3. concussion . . . . . . . . . . .<br>(kon-KUSH-un) | violent jarring or shaking that results in an injury. Brain concussions are caused by slight or severe head injury; symptoms include vertigo and loss of consciousness. |
| 4. conscious . . . . . . . . . . . .<br>(KON-shus) | awake, alert, aware of one's surroundings |
| 5. convulsion . . . . . . . . . . .<br>(kun-VUL-zhun) | sudden, involuntary contraction of a group of muscles |
| 6. dementia . . . . . . . . . . . .<br>(de-MEN-shē-a) | mental decline |
| 7. gait. . . . . . . . . . . . . . . .<br>(gāt) | a manner or style of walking |
| 8. paraplegia . . . . . . . . . . .<br>(păr-a-PLĒ-jē-ā) | paralysis from the waist down caused by damage to the lower level of the spinal cord (Figure 14-12, *B*) |
| 9. seizure . . . . . . . . . . . . .<br>(SĒ-zher) | sudden attack |

**Paraplegia** is composed of the Greek **para**, meaning **beside**, and **plegia**, meaning **paralysis.** It has been used since Hippocrates' times and at first meant paralysis of any limb or side of the body. Since the nineteenth century it has been used to mean paralysis from the waist down.

10. shunt . . . . . . . . . . . . . .     tube implanted in the body to redirect the flow of a fluid

11. syncope. . . . . . . . . . . . .     fainting or sudden loss of consciousness caused by lack of blood supply to the ce-
    (SIN-cō-pē)                          rebrum

12. unconsciousness . . . . . . .     state of being unaware of surroundings and incapable of responding to stimuli
    (un-KON-shus-nes)                   as a result of injury, shock, or illness

Practice saying each of these terms aloud. To assist you in pronunciation, obtain the audiotape designed for use with this text. Learn the definitions and spellings of the other additional terms by completing the following exercises.

## EXERCISE 30

Write the term for each of the following definitions.

1. violent jarring or shaking that results in an injury     _____Concussion_____

2. state of being unaware of surroundings and incapable of responding to stimuli as a result of injury, shock, or illness     _____unconscious_____

3. awake, alert, aware of one's surroundings     _____conscious_____

4. sudden attack     _____seizure_____

5. sudden, involuntary contraction of a group of muscles     _____Convulsion_____

6. tube implanted in the body to redirect the flow of a fluid     _____shunt_____

7. paralysis from the waist down caused by damage to the lower level of the spinal cord     _____paraplegia_____

8. state of profound unconsciousness     _____Coma_____

9. fainting     _____syncope_____

10. lack of muscle coordination     _ataxia_

11. a manner or style of walking     _gait_

12. mental decline     _dementia_

## EXERCISE 31

Write the definitions for the following terms.

1. shunt _____

2. paraplegia _____

3. coma _____

4. concussion _____

5. unconsciousness _____

6. conscious _____

7. seizure _____

8. convulsion _____

9. syncope _____

10. ataxia _____

11. dementia _____

12. gait _____

## EXERCISE 32

Spell each of the other additional terms. Have someone dictate the terms on pp. 565 and 566 to you or say the words into a tape recorder; then spell the words from your recording as often as necessary. Study any you have spelled incorrectly.

1. _____     7. _____
2. _____     8. _____
3. _____     9. _____
4. _____     10. _____
5. _____     11. _____
6. _____     12. _____

Place a check mark (√) in the box to indicate that you have completed Objective 9.

☐ DEFINE, PRONOUNCE, AND SPELL THE OTHER ADDITIONAL TERMS RELATED TO THE NERVOUS SYSTEM.

**Case History:** This 30-year-old white male was initially injured in a train accident approximately 1 year ago when he jumped from a moving boxcar. X-ray showed a forced flexion injury to the cervical spine compressing C-6 and C-7 vertebral bodies, C-6 vertebra dislocated forward on C-7. Compression of spinal cord was evident with subsequent quadriplegia. His condition was first treated and stabilized in an acute care facility. He was transferred to this facility for rehabilitation. He has been referred to Collaborative Care for discharge planning.

**Collaborative Care Conference: Nurse Practitioner**—This patient continues to have a chronic sacral decubitus, stage 2, which has not resolved with Duoderm or with wet to dry dressings. He has a urinary tract infection that has been resolved with a negative urine culture 1 week ago. His bladder spasms are well controlled at this time with Baclofen, Valium, and Talwin. **Occupational Therapy**—His treatment regimen consists of activities encouraging functional range of motion and ADL tid. A tenodesis splint has been ordered for left upper extremity. Short-term goal: OT for increased functional use of left hand when patient's tenodesis splint is completed. **Physical Therapy**—In addition to treatment regimen in OT, PT tid is given to increase vital capacity, which appears to have peaked at 60% to 67% of the expected norm. Patient is independent in getting on and off the bus. **Medical Social Service**—Patient will be discharged to home in 1 week with mother as primary caretaker. Home supportive services will be instated when he is discharged. He is on state disability and has been cleared for Independent Living Centers. He knows how to contact these resources.

## EXERCISE 33

To test your understanding of the terms introduced in this chapter, circle the words that correctly complete the sentences. The italicized words refer to the correct answer.

1. *Tetraplegia* is synonymous with (paraplegia, monoplegia, hemiplegia, quadriplegia).
2. *The inability to speak* or (aphagia, aphasia, dysphasia, dysphagia) may be an aftereffect of cerebrovascular accident.
3. A symptom of brain concussion is *vertigo,* or dizziness, and may cause a patient to be *unaware of his or her surroundings* and *unable to respond to stimuli,* that is, to be (subconscious, unconscious, convulsive).
4. The newborn had *meninges protruding through a defect in his skull,* or a (meningocele, myelomeningocele, myelomalacia).
5. *The branch of medicine that deals with the treatment of mental disorders* is (neurology, psychology, psychiatry).
6. *Multiple sclerosis* is a common disease of the nervous system and generally occurs in young adults. It is characterized by (seizures, hardened patches along the brain and spinal cord, muscular tremors).
7. *The recording of electrical impulses of the brain,* or (echoencephalogram, electroencephalogram, electroencephalograph, electroencephalography), is used to study brain function and is valuable for diagnosing epilepsy, tumors, and other brain diseases.
8. Cerebral *thrombosis,* or (blood clot, infection, hardened patches), may cause a stroke.

9. The patient was admitted to the neurology unit of the hospital with a diagnosis of cerebrovascular accident. The physician ordered *a diagnostic procedure that would give information on brain function* or (computed tomography, positron emission tomography, magnetic resonance).

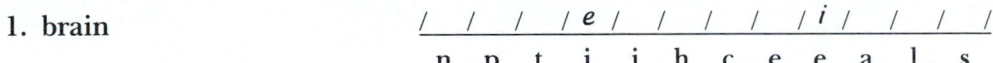

## EXERCISE 34

Unscramble the following mixed-up terms. The word on the left indicates the organs affected by the disease process named by the scrambled word.

1. brain

   /  /  /  / *e* /  /  /  / *i* /  /  /
   n  p  t  i  i  h  c  e  e  a  l   s

2. meninges

   /  /  /  /  /  / *i* /  /  /
   s  i  t  g  i  n  m  e  i   n

3. cranium

   /  /  /  / *o* /  /  /  / *a* /  /  /
   y  o  c  d  e  l  h  a  p  u  s   h  r

4. nerve

   /  /  /  /  /  /  / *i* /  /
   a  l  a  n  u  r  e  g   i

5. nerve roots
   meninges
   spinal cord

   /  /  /  /  / *m* /  /  /  /  /  /  /  /  / *i* /  /  /
   l  n  i  n  i  t  i  s  i  y  m  e  m  h  r  z  o  g   o

## EXERCISE 35

The following definitions are of medical terms that did not appear in this or the previous chapters; but they are made up of word parts you have studied. Test your knowledge by building the term to match the definition.

1. paralysis of one muscle    _____

2. many pregnancies (the word has an *is* suffix)    _____

3. inflammation of many cartilages of the body    _____

4. disease of the gray matter of the spinal cord    _____

5. surgical removal of      _____
   the colon and rectum

6. suture of the muscle    _____

7. excision of half of     _____
   the colon

8. excision of the ova-    _____
   ries and uterus

## COMBINING FORMS CROSSWORD PUZZLE

### Across Clues

2. mind
4. cerebellum
6. abbreviation for diabetes insipidus
7. abbreviation for undetermined origin
8. brain
13. nerve root
14. mind
15. ganglion
16. speech

### Down Clues

1. four
2. spinal cord
3. gray matter
5. sensation
6. dura mater
9. cerebrum
10. meninges
11. one
12. mind

# Summary

Can you build, analyze, define, spell, and pronounce the following terms *built from word parts?*   yes □   no □

## DIAGNOSTIC

cerebellitis
(sār-e-bel-Ī-tis)

cerebral thrombosis
(ser-Ē-bral) (throm-BŌ-sis)

duritis
(du-RĪ-tis)

encephalitis
(*en*-sef-a-LĪ-tis)

encephalomalacia
(en-*sef*-a-lō-ma-LĀ-shē-a)

encephalomyeloradicu-
litis
(en-*sef*-a-lō-*mī*-e-lō-ra-*dik*-ū-
LĪ-tis)

gangliitis
(*gang*-glē-Ī-tis)

meningitis
(*men*-in-JĪ-tis)

meningocele
(me-NING-gō-sēl)

meningomyelocele
(me-*ning*-gō-MĪ-e-lō-*sēl*)

neuralgia
(nū-RAL-jē-a)

neuroarthropathy
(*nŭr*-ō-ar-THROP-a-thē)

neurasthenia
(*nū*-ras-THĒ-nē-a)

neuritis
(nū-RĪ-tis)

neuroblast
(NŪ-rō-blast)

neuroma
(nū-RŌ-ma)

poliomyelitis
(*pō*-lē-ō-*mī*-e-LĪ-tis)

polyneuritis
(*pol*-ē-nū-RĪ-tis)

## SURGICAL

ganglionectomy
(*gang*-glē-on-EK-tō-mē)

neurectomy
(nū-REK-tō-mē)

neurolysis
(nū-ROL-i-sis)

neuroplasty
(NŪ-rō-plas-tē)

neurorrhaphy
(nū-RŌR-a-fē)

neurotomy
(nū-ROT-ō-mē)

radicotomy
(*rad*-i-KOT-ō-mē)

rhizotomy
(rī-ZOT-ō-mē)

## PROCEDURAL

cerebral angiography
(se-RĒ-bral)
(an-jē-OG-ra-fē)

echoencephalography
(*ek*-o-en-*sef*-a-LOG-ra-fē)

electroencephalogram
(e-*lek*-trō-en-SEF-a-lō-gram)

electroencephalograph
(e-*lek*-trō-en-SEF-a-lō-graf )

electroencephalography
(e-*lek*-trō-en-*sef*-a-LOG-ra-fē)

myelogram
(MĪ-e-lō-gram)

## ADDITIONAL

anesthesia
(*an*-es-THĒ-zē-a)

aphasia
(a-FĀ-zē-a)

cephalalgia
(*sef*-el-AL-jē-a)

cerebral
(se-RĒ-bral)

craniocerebral
(*krā*-nē-ō-sār-Ē-bral)

dysphasia
(dis-FĀ-zē-a)

encephalosclerosis
(en-*sef*-a-lo-skle-RŌ-sis)

hemiparesis
(*hem*-i-pār-Ē-sis)

hemiplegia
(*hem*-i-PLĒ-jē-a)

hyperesthesia
(*hī*-per-es-THĒ-zē-a)

interictal
(in-ter-IK-tal)

monoparesis
(mon-ō-pa-RĒ-sis)

monoplegia
(*mon*-ō-PLĒ-jē-a)

myelomalacia
(*mī*-e-lō-ma-LĀ-shē-a)

neuroid
(NŪ-royd)

neurologist
(nū-ROL-ō-jist)

neurology
(nū-ROL-ō-jē)

panplegia
(pan-PLĒ-jē-a)

preictal
(prē-IK-tal)

## DIAGNOSTIC—CONT'D

radiculitis
(ra-*dik*-ū-LĪ-tis)

rhizomeningomyelitis
(rī-zō-men-ning-gō-mī-e-LĪ-tis)

subdural hematoma
(sub-DŪ-ral)
(*hēm*-a-TŌ-ma)

## ADDITIONAL—CONT'D

postictal
(pōst-IK-tal)

phrenic
(FREN-ik)

phrenopathy
(fre-NOP-a-thē)

psychiatry
(sī-KĪ-a-trē)

psychogenic
(*sī*-kō-JEN-ik)

psychologist
(sī-KOL-ō-jist)

psychology
(sī-KOL-ō-jē)

psychopathy
(sī-KOP-a-thē)

psychosomatic
(*sī*-ko-sō-MAT-ik)

quadriplegia
(*kwod*-ri-PLĒ-jē-a)

subdural
(sub-DŪ-ral)

tetraplegia
(*te*-tra-PLĒ-jē-a)

# Summary

Can you define, pronounce, and spell the following terms *not built from word parts?*   yes □   no □

## DIAGNOSTIC

Alzheimer's disease
(AHLTS-hī-merz)

amyotrophic lateral
   sclerosis
(a-mī-ō-TROF-ik)
(LAT-er-al) (skle-RŌ-sis)

cerebral aneurysm
(se-RĒ-bral) (AN-ū-rizm)

cerebral palsy
(se-RĒ-bral) (PAWL-zē)

cerebrovascular
   accident
(se-re-brō-VAS-ku-lar)

## PROCEDURAL

computed tomography
   of the brain
(tō-MOG-ra-fē)

lumbar puncture
(LUM-bar)

magnetic resonance
   imaging
(mag-NET-ik)
(re-zo-NANCE) (IM-a-jing)

positron emission
   tomography of the
   brain
(POS-i-tron) (e-MI-shun
(tō-MOG-ra-fē)

## ADDITIONAL

ataxia
(a-TAK-sē-a)

coma
(KŌ-ma)

concussion
(kon-KUSH-un)

conscious
(KON-shus)

convulsion
(kun-VUL-zhun)

dementia
(de-MEN-she-a)

## DIAGNOSTIC—CONT'D

epilepsy
(EP-i-lep-sē)

hydrocephalus
(hī-drō-SEF-a-lus)

multiple sclerosis
(skle-RŌ-sis)

neurosis
(nū-RŌ-sis)

Parkinson's disease

psychosis
(sī-KŌ-sis)

Reye's syndrome
(RĪZ)

sciatica
(sī-AT-i-ka)

shingles

transient ischemic
    attack
(is-KĒM-ik)

## ADDITIONAL—CONT'D

gait
(gāt)

paraplegia
(*pār*-a-PLĒ-jē-ā)

seizure
(SĒ-zher)

shunt

syncope
(SIN-cō-pē)

unconsciousness
(un-KON-shus-nes)

# Answers

### Exercise 1
1. meninges     3. arachnoid     5. subarachnoid space
2. dura mater   4. pia mater     6. cerebrospinal fluid

### Exercise 2
1. d     3. g     5. a     7. b
2. f     4. e     6. h

### Exercise 3
**Figure 14-1**

| | |
|---|---|
| Brain: encephal/o | Cerebellum: cerebell/o |
| Spinal cord: myel/o | Meninges: mening/i, |
| Cerebrum: cerebr/o |     mening/o |

**Figure 14-2**

| | |
|---|---|
| Dura mater: dur/o | Nerve root: radic/o, |
| Spinal ganglion: gangli/o, |     radicul/o, rhiz/o |
|     ganglion/o | |

### Exercise 4
1. cerebellum     5. brain      9. nerve root
2. nerve          6. cerebrum   10. hard, dura mater
3. spinal cord    7. nerve root 11. ganglion
4. meninges       8. ganglion   12. nerve root

### Exercise 5
1. cerebell/o            6. cerebr/o
2. neur/o                7. radicul/o, radic/o,
3. myel/o                    rhiz/o
4. mening/o, mening/i    8. dur/o
5. encephal/o            9. gangli/o, ganglion/o

### Exercise 6
1. one     5. speech
2. mind    6. sensation, sensitivity,
3. four        feeling
4. mind    7. mind
           8. gray matter

### Exercise 7
1. quadr/i     4. phas/o
2. mon/o       5. poli/o
3. a. phren/o  6. esthesi/o
   b. psych/o
   c. ment/o

### Exercise 8
1. four     2. half     3. before

## Exercise 9

1. hemi-   2. tetra-   3. pre-

## Exercise 10

1. slight paralysis          3. seizure, attack
2. physician, treatment

## Exercise 11

1. -paresis   2. -iatry   3. -ictal

## Exercise 12

WR  S
1. neur/itis                     inflammation of
                                 the nerve

WR   S
2. neur/oma                      tumor made up of
                                 nerve cells

WR   S
3. neur/algia                    pain in a nerve

WR CV  WR CV  S
4. neur/ o /arthr/ o /pathy      disease of nerves
   CF        CF                  and joints

WR CV  WR
5. neur/ o /blast                developing nerve
   CF                            cell

WR     S
6. neur/asthenia                 nerve weakness
                                 (nervous ex-
                                 haustion, fa-
                                 tigue, and weak-
                                 ness)

WR    CV   S
7. encephal/ o /malacia          softening of the
   CF                            brain

WR     S
8. encephal/itis                 inflammation of
                                 the brain

WR    CV  WR CV  WR   S
9. encephal/ o /myel/ o /radicul/itis   inflammation of
   CF         CF                        the brain, spinal
                                        cord, and nerve
                                        roots

WR    S
10. mening/itis                  inflammation of
                                 the meninges

WR    CV  S
11. mening/ o /cele              protrusion of the
    CF                           meninges

WR    CV  WR CV  S
12. mening/ o /myel/ o /cele     protrusion of the
    CF        CF                 meninges and
                                 spinal cord

WR     S
13. radicul/itis                 inflammation of
                                 the spinal nerve
                                 roots

WR     S
14. cerebell/itis                inflammation of
                                 the cerebellum

WR   S
15. gangli/itis                  inflammation of
                                 the ganglion

WR  S
16. dur/itis                     inflammation of
                                 the dura mater

P   WR  S
17. poly/neur/itis               inflammation of
                                 many nerves

WR CV  WR  S
18. poli/ o /myel/itis           inflammation of
    CF                           the gray matter
                                 of the spinal
                                 cord

WR   S  WR    S
19. cerebr/al thromb/osis        condition of a
                                 blood clot in a
                                 blood vessel of
                                 the cerebrum

P   WR S  WR    S
20. sub/dur/al hemat/oma         blood tumor below
                                 the dura

WR CV   WR   CV  WR  S
21. rhiz/ o /mening/ o /myel/itis   inflammation of
    CF          CF                  the nerve root,
                                    meninges, and
                                    spinal cord

## Exercise 13

1. neur/itis
2. neur/oma
3. neur/algia
4. neur/o/arthr/o/pathy
5. neur/o/blast
6. neur/asthenia
7. encephal/o/malacia
8. encephal/itis
9. encephal/o/myel/o/radicul/itis
10. mening/itis
11. mening/o/cele
12. mening/o/myel/o/cele
13. radicul/itis
14. cerebell/itis
15. gangli/itis
16. dur/itis
17. poly/neur/itis
18. poli/o/myel/itis
19. cerebr/al thromb/osis
20. sub/dur/al hemat/oma
21. rhiz/o/mening/o/myel/itis

## Exercise 14

Spelling exercise; *see* text, p. 547.

## Exercise 15

1. cerebrum (brain)  5. head
2. mind             6. nerve
3. upon             7. cerebrum (brain)
4. hardening

## Exercise 16

| | | | | |
|---|---|---|---|---|
| 1. b | 4. j | 7. e | 10. m | 13. h |
| 2. a | 5. l | 8. g | 11. f | 14. o |
| 3. n | 6. c | 9. i | 12. d | |

## Exercise 17

Spelling exercise; *see* text, p. 550.

## Exercise 18

1. radic/otomy  (WR  S)          incision into a nerve root
2. neur/ectomy  (WR  S)          excision of a nerve
3. neur/orrhaphy  (WR  S)        suture of a nerve
4. ganglion/ectomy  (WR  S)      excision of a ganglion
5. neur/otomy  (WR  S)           incision into the nerves
6. neur/ o /lysis  (WR  CV  S / CF)   separating a nerve (from adhesions)
7. neur/ o /plasty  (WR  CV  S / CF)   plastic repair of a nerve
8. rhiz/otomy  (WR  S)           incision into a nerve root

## Exercise 19

1. a. radic/otomy       5. neur/otomy
   b. rhiz/otomy        6. neur/o/lysis
2. neur/ectomy          7. neur/o/plasty
3. neur/orrhaphy
4. ganglion/ectomy

## Exercise 20

Spelling exercise; *see* text, p. 553.

## Exercise 21

1. electr/ o /encephal/ o /gram  (WR  CV  WR  CV  S / CF  CF)
   record of the electrical impulses of the brain

2. electr/ o /encephal/ o /graph  (WR  CV  WR  CV  S / CF  CF)
   instrument used for recording the electrical impulses of the brain

3. electr/ o /encephal/ o /graphy  (WR  CV  WR  CV  S / CF  CF)
   process of recording the electrical impulses of the brain

4. ech/ o /encephal/ o /graphy  (WR  CV  WR  CV  S / CF  CF)
   process of recording brain (structures) by use of sound

5. myel/ o /gram  (WR  CV  S / CF)
   x-ray film of the spinal cord

6. cerebr/al angi/ o /graphy  (WR  S  WR  CV  S / CF)
   process of x-ray filming of the blood vessels in the brain

## Exercise 22

1. ech/o/encephal/o/graphy
2. electr/o/encephal/o/gram
3. electr/o/encephal/o/graph
4. electr/o/encephal/o/graphy
5. myel/o/gram
6. cerebr/al angi/o/graphy

## Exercise 23

Spelling exercise; *see* text, p. 553.

## Exercise 24

1. computer tomography
2. lumbar puncture
3. positron emission tomography of the brain
4. magnetic resonance imaging of the head

## Exercise 25

1. insertion of a needle into the subarachnoid space
2. process that includes the use of a computer to produce a series of images of the brain tissues at any desired depth
3. produces cross-sectional images of cranial structure by use of magnetic waves
4. a technique that gives information about brain function

## Exercise 26

Spelling exercise; *see* text, pp. 556 and 558.

## Exercise 27

      P  S(WR)
1. hemi/plegia — paralysis of half (left or right side of the body)

      P  S(WR)
2. tetra/plegia — paralysis of four (limbs)

     WR    S
3. neur/ologist — physician who specializes in neurology

     WR    S
4. neur/ology — branch of medicine dealing with the nervous system's function and disorders

     WR    S
5. neur/oid — resembling a nerve

    WR  CV   S
6. quadr/ i /plegia — paralysis of four (limbs)
       CF

     WR    S
7. cerebr/al — pertaining to the cerebrum

    WR CV   S
8. mon/ o /plegia — paralysis of one (limb)
      CF

    P  WR  S
9. a/phas/ia — condition of loss or impairment of the ability to speak

    P  WR  S
10. dys/phas/ia — condition of difficulty in speaking

     P  S(WR)
11. hemi/paresis — slight paralysis of half (right or left side of the body)

    P   WR  S
12. an/esthesi/a — loss of feeling or sensation

    P    WR  S
13. hyper/esthesi/a — condition of excessive sensitivity (to stimuli)

    P  WR  S
14. sub/dur/al — pertaining to below the dura mater

     WR    S
15. cephal/algia — pain in the head, headache

    WR  CV  WR  S
16. psych/ o /somat/ic — pertaining to the body and mind
       CF

    WR  CV   S
17. psych/ o /pathy — any disease of the mind
       CF

    WR    S
18. psych/ology — study of the mind (mental processes and behavior)

    WR    S
19. psych/iatry — branch of medicine that deals with the treatment of mental disorders

    WR    S
20. psych/ologist — specialist in the study of psychology

    WR CV   S
21. psych/ o /genic — originating within the mind
      CF

    WR    S
22. phren/ic — pertaining to the mind

    WR CV   S
23. phren/ o /pathy — mental disease
      CF

    WR CV  WR  S
24. crani/ o /cerebr/al — pertaining to the cranium and cerebrum
      CF

    WR CV   S
25. myel/ o /malacia — softening of the spinal cord
      CF

    WR   CV   S
26. encephal/ o /sclerosis — hardening of the brain
      CF

    P  S(WR)
27. post/ ictal — occurring after a seizure or attack

    P  S(WR)
28. pan/plegia — total paralysis

    P  S(WR)
29. inter/ ictal — occurring between seizures, or attacks

    WR CV   S
30. mon/ o /paresis — slight paralysis of one (limb)
      CF

    P  S(WR)
31. pre/ ictal — occurring before a seizure or attack

## Exercise 28

1. hemi/paresis
2. an/esthesi/a
3. hyper/esthesi/a
4. sub/dur/al
5. cephal/algia
6. psych/o/somat/ic
7. psych/o/pathy
8. psych/ology
9. psych/iatry
10. psych/ologist
11. psych/o/genic
12. phren/ic
13. phren/o/pathy
14. crani/o/cerebr/al
15. myel/o/malacia
16. encephal/o/sclerosis
17. hemi/plegia
18. tetra/plegia
19. neur/ologist
20. neur/ology
21. neur/oid
22. quadr/i/plegia
23. cerebr/al
24. mon/o/plegia
25. a/phas/ia
26. dys/phas/ia
27. pre/ictal
28. mon/o/paresis
29. post/ictal
30. pan/plegia
31. inter/ictal

## Exercise 29

Spelling exercise; *see* text, p. 564.

## Exercise 30

| | | |
|---|---|---|
| 1. concussion | 5. convulsion | 9. syncope |
| 2. unconsciousness | 6. shunt | 10. ataxia |
| 3. conscious | 7. paraplegia | 11. gait |
| 4. seizure | 8. coma | 12. dementia |

## Exercise 31

1. tube implanted in the body to redirect the flow of a fluid
2. paralysis from the waist down caused by damage to the lower level of the spinal cord
3. state of profound unconsciousness
4. violent jarring or shaking that results in an injury
5. state of being unaware of surroundings and incapable of responding to stimuli as a result of injury, shock, or illness
6. awake, alert, aware of one's surroundings
7. sudden attack
8. sudden, involuntary contraction of a group of muscles
9. fainting, or sudden loss of consciousness
10. lack of muscle coordination
11. mental decline
12. a manner or style of walking

## Exercise 32

Spelling exercise; *see* text, p. 567.

## Exercise 33

| | |
|---|---|
| 1. quadriplegia | 6. hardened patches along brain and spinal cord |
| 2. aphasia | |
| 3. unconscious | |
| 4. meningocele | 7. electroencephalogram |
| 5. psychiatry | 8. blood clot |
| | 9. positron emission tomography |

## Exercise 34

| | |
|---|---|
| 1. encephalitis | 4. neuralgia |
| 2. meningitis | 5. rhizomeningomyelitis |
| 3. hydrocephalus | |

## Exercise 35

| | |
|---|---|
| 1. monomyoplegia | 5. coloproctectomy |
| 2. polycyesis | 6. myorrhaphy |
| 3. polychondritis | 7. hemicolectomy |
| 4. poliomyelopathy | 8. oophorohysterectomy |

# 15

# Endocrine System

## Objectives

**Upon completion of this chapter you will be able to:**

1. Define the anatomical terms of the endocrine system.

2. Write the definitions of the word parts included in this chapter.

3. Build, analyze, define, pronounce, and spell the diagnostic terms related to the endocrine system.

4. Define, pronounce, and spell other diagnostic terms related to the endocrine system.

5. Build, analyze, define, pronounce, and spell the surgical terms related to the endocrine system.

6. Build, analyze, define, pronounce, and spell additional terms related to the endocrine system.

7. Define, pronounce, and spell the other additional terms related to the endocrine system.

## Objective 1   DEFINE THE ANATOMICAL TERMS OF THE ENDOCRINE SYSTEM.

## Anatomical Terms

The endocrine system is composed of a series of glands located in various parts of the body. These glands are called *ductless glands,* because they have no ducts or tubes to carry the secretions they produce to other body parts. Their secretions, called *hormones,* are secreted directly into the blood. Only those terms related to the major endocrine glands—pituitary, thyroid, parathyroid, adrenals, and the islets of Langerhans in the pancreas—are studied in this chapter. The thymus and the male and female sex glands were discussed in previous chapters.

### ENDOCRINE GLANDS

1. pituitary gland, or hypophysis . . . . . . . . . . . . .    Sometimes referred to as the "master gland," since its hormones stimulate the function of other endocrine glands. It is approximately the size of a pea and is located at the base of the brain. The pituitary is divided into two lobes (Figure 15-1).

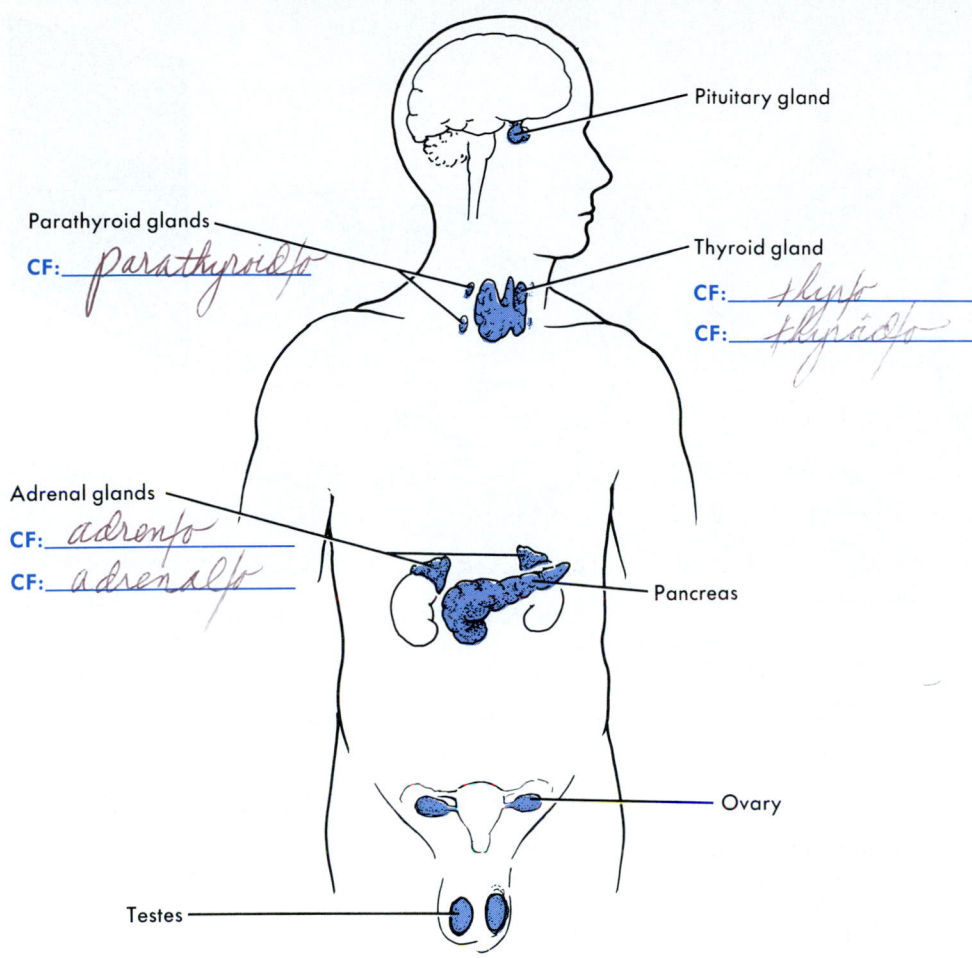

**Pituitary gland**

**Parathyroid glands**
CF: _parathyroid/o_

**Thyroid gland**
CF: _thyr/o_
CF: _thyroid/o_

**Adrenal glands**
CF: _adren/o_
CF: _adrenal/o_

**Pancreas**

**Ovary**

**Testes**

Figure 15-1

Diagram of endocrine glands in
the human body.

a.  anterior lobe, or ade-
    nohypophysis. . . . . . .    Produces and secretes the following
                                 hormones:

    (1)  growth hormone
         (GH). . . . . . . . .   Regulates the growth of the body.
    (2)  adrenocortico-
         tropic hormone
         (ACTH),. . . . . . .    Stimulates the adrenal cortex.
    (3)  thyroid-stimu-
         lating hormone
         (TSH). . . . . . . .    Stimulates the thyroid gland.
    (4)  other hormones .        Affect the male and female reproduc-
                                 tive system.

b.  posterior lobe or
    neurohypophysis . . . .      Stores and releases the following hor-
                                 mones:

    (1)  antidiuretic hor-
         mone (ADH) . . .        Stimulates the kidney to reabsorb wa-
                                 ter.

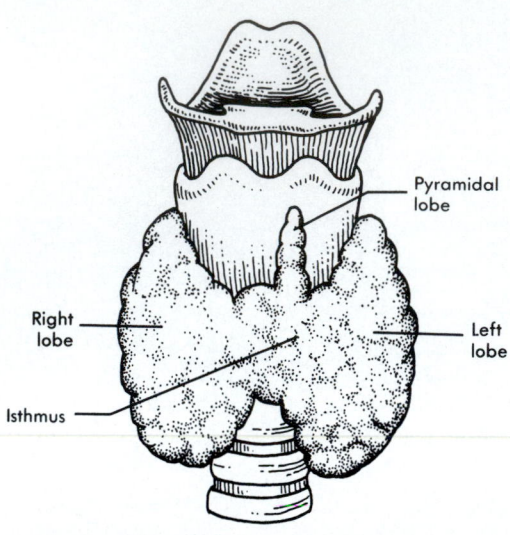

**Figure 15-2**

Structure of thyroid gland showing lobes and isthmus.

From Urdang L: *Mosby's medical and nursing dictionary,*
St. Louis, 1983, Mosby.

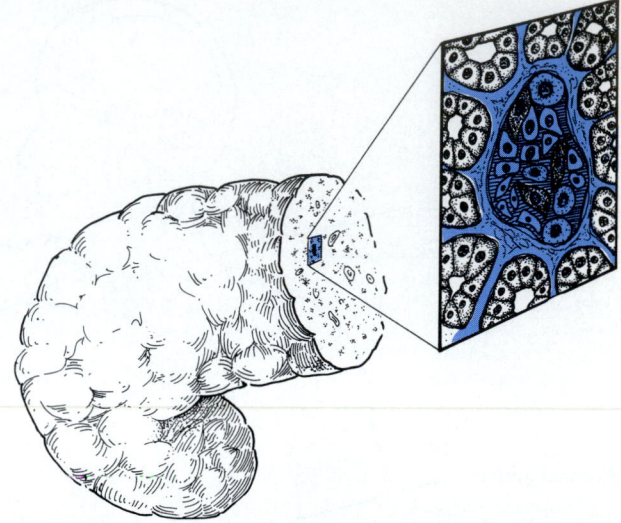

**Figure 15-3**

Pancreas, with islets of Langerhans.

| | |
|---|---|
| (2)  oxytocin . . . . . . . | Stimulates uterine contractions during labor and postpartum. |
| 2. thyroid gland . . . . . . . . . | Largest endocrine gland. It is located in the neck in the area of the larynx and is comprised of bilateral lobes connected by an isthmus (Figure 15-2). The thyroid gland secretes the hormone *thyroxine*, which requires iodine for its production. Thyroxine is necessary for body cell metabolism. |
| 3. parathyroid glands . . . . . . | Four small bodies lying directly behind the thyroid. *Parathormone*, the hormone produced by the glands, helps to maintain the level of calcium in the blood. |
| 4. islets of Langerhans. . . . . | Cellular clusters found throughout the pancreas that secrete the insulin necessary to control carbohydrate metabolism. Different cells found throughout the pancreas perform nonendocrine functions such as digestion (Figure 15-3). |
| 5. adrenal glands, or suprarenals . . . . . . . . . . . . | Located one above each kidney. The outer portion is called the *cortex,* and the inner portion is called the *medulla* |

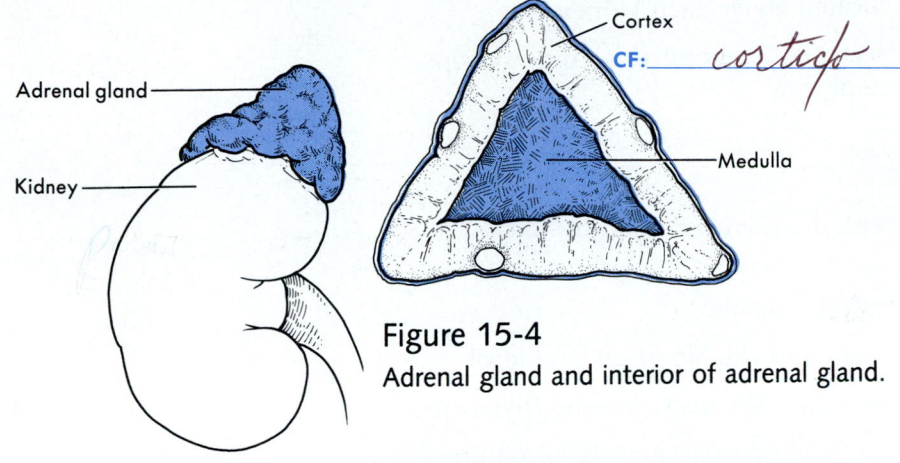

Adrenal gland

Kidney

Cortex

CF: _cortico_

Medulla

**Figure 15-4**
Adrenal gland and interior of adrenal gland.

(Figure 15-4). The following hormones are secreted by the adrenal glands:

a.  cortisol . . . . . . . . . . . Secreted by the cortex. It aids the body during stress and in the metabolism of food.

b.  aldosterone . . . . . . . Secreted by the cortex. Electrolytes (mineral salts) that are necessary for normal body function are regulated by this hormone.

c.  epinephrine (adrenaline), and norepinephrine . . . . . . . . . Secreted by the medulla. These hormones assist the body to deal with stress by increasing the blood pressure, heart beat, and respirations.

The following exercises will help you to learn the anatomical terms of the endocrine system.

## EXERCISE 1A

Match the terms in the first column with the correct definitions in the second column.

_b_ 1. adrenal cortex

_g_ 2. adrenal glands

_d_ 3. adrenaline

_h_ 4. adrenal medulla

_a_ 5. adrenocorticotropic hormone

_c_ 6. adenohypophysis

_e_ 7. aldosterone

a.  stimulates the adrenal cortex

b.  secretes cortisol and aldosterone

c.  anterior lobe of pituitary that secretes growth hormone and thyroid-stimulating hormone

d.  another name for epinephrine

e.  assists in regulating body electrolytes

f.  another name for norepinephrine

g. located above each kidney

h. secretes epinephrine and norepi-nephrine

## EXERCISE 1B

Match the terms in the first column with the correct definitions in the second column.

_d_ 1. antidiuretic hormone    a. secretes insulin

_a_ 2. islets of Langerhans    b. maintains the blood calcium level

_e_ 3. neurohypophysis    c. located in the neck, secretes thyroxine

_b_ 4. parathyroid gland    d. secreted by posterior lobe of pituitary

_g_ 5. pituitary gland    e. stores and releases antidiuretic hormone and oxytocin

_c_ 6. thyroid gland

f. another name for the anterior lobe of the pituitary

g. master gland

Place a check mark (√) in the box to indicate that you have completed Objective 1.

☐ **DEFINE THE ANATOMICAL TERMS OF THE ENDOCRINE SYSTEM.**

# Objective 2   WRITE THE DEFINITIONS OF THE WORD PARTS INCLUDED IN THIS CHAPTER.

## Endocrine System Word Parts

Study the word parts and their definitions listed as follows. Learning will be made easier by completing the exercises that follow.

| COMBINING FORM | DEFINITION |
|---|---|
| 1. adren/o, adrenal/o | adrenal glands |
| 2. cortic/o | cortex (the outer layer of a body organ) |
| 3. endocrin/o | endocrine |
| 4. parathyroid/o | parathyroid glands |
| 5. thyroid/o, thyr/o | thyroid gland |

Learn the anatomical locations and definitions of the combining forms by completing the following exercises.

## EXERCISE 2

Write the combining forms in the spaces marked CF on the diagrams in Figures 15-1 and 15-4, pp. 579 and 581.

## EXERCISE 3

Write the definitions of the following combining forms.

1. cortic/o _____ *cortex* _____
2. adren/o _____ *adrenal glands* _____
3. parathyroid/o _____ *parathyroid glands* _____
4. thyroid/o _____ *thyroid glands* _____
5. adrenal/o _____ *adrenal glands* _____
6. thyr/o _____ *thyroid glands* _____
7. endocrin/o _____ *endocrine* _____

## EXERCISE 4

Write the combining form for each of the following.

1. adrenal      a. _____ *adrenal/o* _____

               b. _____ *adren/o* _____

2. thyroid      a. _____ *thyr/o* _____

               b. _____ *thyroid/o* _____

3. endocrine      _____ *endocrin/o* _____

4. cortex      _____ *cortic/o* _____

5. parathyroid      _____ *parathyroid/o* _____

# Related Word Parts

| COMBINING FORM | DEFINITION |
| --- | --- |
| 1. acr/o . . . . . . . . . . . . . . . | extremities, height |
| 2. calc/i . . . . . . . . . . . . . . . <br> (NOTE: The combining vowel is *i*.) | calcium |
| 3. dips/o . . . . . . . . . . . . . . | thirst |
| 4. kal/i . . . . . . . . . . . . . . . <br> (NOTE: The combining vowel is *i*.) | potassium |
| 5. toxic/o . . . . . . . . . . . . . | poison |

Learn the related combining forms by completing the following exercises.

## EXERCISE 5

Write the definitions of the following combining forms.

1. dips/o ___*thirst*___

2. toxic/o ___*poison*___

3. kal/i ___*potassium*___

4. calc/i ___*calcium*___

5. acr/o ___*extremities, height*___

## EXERCISE 6

Write the combining form for each of the following.

1. poison ___*toxic/o*___

2. extremities, height ___*acr/o*___

3. calcium ___*calc/i*___

4. thirst ___*dips/o*___

5. potassium ___*kal/i*___

# Prefix and Suffix

| PREFIX | DEFINITION |
|---|---|
| ex-, exo- . . . . . . . . . . . . . . . . | outside, outward |

| SUFFIX | DEFINITION |
|---|---|
| -drome . . . . . . . . . . . . . . . . | run, running |

Learn the prefix and suffix by completing the following exercises.

## EXERCISE 7

Write the definitions of the following word parts.

1. ex-, exo- ___*outside, outward*___

2. -drome ___*run, running*___

## EXERCISE 8

Write the prefix and suffix in the following:

1. run, running ___*-drome*___

2. outside, outward   a. ___*ex-*___

   b. ___*exo-*___

Place a check mark (√) in the box to indicate that you have completed Objective 2.

☐ **WRITE THE DEFINITIONS OF THE WORD PARTS INCLUDED IN THIS CHAPTER.**

# Medical Terms

The terms you need to learn to complete this chapter are listed as follows. Now that you know the meaning of the word parts, the exercises found at the end of the list will assist you to learn the definition and the spelling of each word.

## Objective 3 BUILD, ANALYZE, DEFINE, PRONOUNCE, AND SPELL THE DIAGNOSTIC TERMS RELATED TO THE ENDOCRINE SYSTEM.

# Diagnostic Terms

| TERM<br>(built from word parts) | DEFINITION |
|---|---|
| 1. acromegaly<br>(ak-rō-MEG-a-lē) | enlargement of the extremities (and bones of the face caused by excessive production of the growth hormone) (Figure 15-5) |
| 2. adrenalitis<br>(ad-*rēn*-al-Ī-tis) | inflammation of an adrenal gland |
| 3. adrenomegaly<br>(ad-*rēn*-o-MEG-a-lē) | enlargement (of one or both) of the adrenal glands |
| 4. hypercalcemia<br>(*hī*-per-kal-SĒ-mē-a) | excessive calcium in the blood |
| 5. hyperglycemia<br>(*hī*-per-glī-SĒ-mē-a) | excessive sugar in the blood |
| 6. hyperkalemia<br>(*hī*-per-ka-LĒ-mē-a) | excessive potassium in the blood |
| 7. hyperthyroidism<br>(*hī*-per-THĪ-royd-izm) | state of excessive production of the thyroid hormone |
| 8. hypocalcemia<br>(*hī*-pō-kal-SĒ-mē-a) | deficient level of calcium in the blood |
| 9. hypoglycemia<br>(*hī*-pō-glī-SĒ-mē-a) | deficient level of sugar in the blood |
| 10. hypokalemia<br>(*hī*-pō-ka-LĒ-mē-a) | deficient level of potassium in the blood |
| 11. hypothyroidism<br>(*hī*-pō-THĪ-royd-izm) | state of deficient thyroid gland activity |

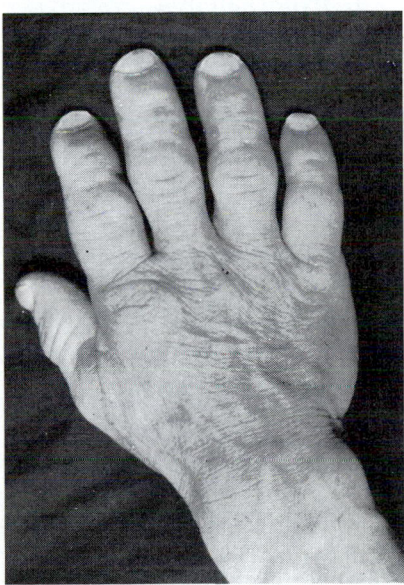

**Figure 15-5**

Hand with characteristics of acromegaly.

From Schottelius BA and Schottelius DD: *Textbook of physiology*, ed 18, St. Louis, 1978, Mosby.

12. parathyroidoma . . . . . . .    tumor of the parathyroid gland
    (pār-a-THĪ-roy-dō-ma)

13. thyrotoxicosis . . . . . . . .    abnormal condition of poisoning caused
    (thī-rō-tok-si-KŌ-sis)          by excessive thyroid gland activity (also
                                     called hyperthyroidism)

Practice saying each of these terms aloud. To assist you in pronunciation, obtain th audiotape designed for use with this text. Learn the definitions and spellings of the diagnostic terms by completing the following exercises.

## EXERCISE 9

Analyze and define the following diagnostic terms.

1. adrenalitis _____

2. hypocalcemia _____

3. hyperthyroidism _____

4. hyperkalemia _____

5. thyrotoxicosis _____

6. hyperglycemia _____

7. adrenomegaly _____

8. hypothyroidism _____

9. hypokalemia _____

10. parathyroidoma _____

11. acromegaly _____

12. hypoglycemia _____

13. hypercalcemia _____

## EXERCISE 10

Build diagnostic terms for the following definitions by using the word parts you have learned.

1. enlargement of the adrenal gland
   
   _____ / ____ / _____
        WR      CV      S

2. state of deficient thyroid
   gland activity
   
   _____ / ____ / _____
        P       WR       S

3. enlargement of extremities

    ———————————————————
    WR    CV    S

4. deficient level of sugar in the blood

    ———————————————————
    P    WR    S

5. excessive potassium in the blood

    ———————————————————
    P    WR    S

6. deficient level of calcium in the blood

    ———————————————————
    P    WR    S

7. state of excessive production of the thyroid hormone

    ———————————————————
    P    WR    S

8. excessive calcium in the blood

    ———————————————————
    P    WR    S

9. abnormal condition of poisoning caused by excessive thyroid gland activity

    ———————————————————
    WR    CV    WR    S

10. tumor of the parathyroid

    ———————————————————
    WR    S

11. excessive sugar in the blood

    ———————————————————
    P    WR    S

12. deficient level of potassium in the blood

    ———————————————————
    P    WR    S

13. inflammation of the adrenal gland

    ———————————————————
    WR    S

## EXERCISE 11

Spell each of the diagnostic terms. Have someone dictate the terms on pp. 585 and 586 to you or say the words into a tape recorder; then spell the words from your recording as often as necessary. Think about the word parts before attempting to write the word. Study any you have spelled incorrectly.

1. _____    8. _____

2. _____    9. _____

3. _____   10. _____

4. _____   11. _____

5. _____   12. _____

6. _____   13. _____

7. _____

Place a check mark (√) in the box to indicate that you have completed Objective 3.

☐ **BUILD, ANALYZE, DEFINE, PRONOUNCE, AND SPELL THE DIAGNOSTIC TERMS RELATED TO THE ENDOCRINE SYSTEM.**

# Objective 4 — DEFINE, PRONOUNCE, AND SPELL OTHER DIAGNOSTIC TERMS RELATED TO THE ENDOCRINE SYSTEM.

# Other Diagnostic Terms

| TERM | DEFINITION |
|---|---|
| 1. acidosis . . . . . . . . . . . . . (*as*-i-DŌ-sis) | condition brought about by an abnormal accumulation of acid products of metabolism, seen frequently in uncontrolled diabetes mellitus (see below for a discussion of diabetes mellitus) |
| 2. Addison's disease . . . . . . | chronic syndrome resulting from a deficiency in the hormonal secretion of the adrenal cortex. Symptoms may include weakness, darkening of skin, loss of appetite, depression, and other emotional problems. |
| 3. cretinism . . . . . . . . . . . (KRÉ-tin-izm) | condition caused by congenital absence or atrophy (wasting away) of the thyroid gland, resulting in hypothyroidism. The disease is characterized by puffy features, mental deficiency, large tongue, and dwarfism. |

**Addison's disease** was named in 1855 for Thomas Addison, an English physician and pathologist. He described the disease as a "morbid state with feeble heart action, anemia, irritability of the stomach, and a peculiar change in the color of the skin."

4.  Cushing's syndrome . . . .     group of symptoms that are attributed to the excessive production of cortisol by the adrenal cortices (*pl.* of cortex). This syndrome may be the result of a pituitary tumor. Symptoms include abnormally pigmented skin, "moonface," pads of fat on chest and abdomen, and wasting away of muscle.

> **Cushing's syndrome** was named for an American neurosurgeon, Harvey William Cushing (1869-1939), after he described adrenal cortical hyperfunction.

5.  diabetes insipidus . . . . . .
    (dī-a-BĒ-tēz) (in-SIP-i-dus)     result of decreased activity of the antidiuretic hormone of the posterior lobe of the pituitary gland. Patients complain of excessive thirst *(polydipsia)* and pass large amounts of urine *(polyuria)*.

6.  diabetes mellitus . . . . . .
    (dī-a-BĒ-tēz) (mel-LĪ-tus)     chronic disease involving a disorder of carbohydrate metabolism. Diabetes mellitus is caused by underactivity of the islets of Langerhans in the pancreas, which results in too little production of insulin. When the disease is not controlled or is untreated, the patient may develop ketosis (see below), acidosis, and finally coma.

7.  gigantism . . . . . . . . . . .
    (jī-GAN-tizm)     condition brought about by overproduction of the pituitary growth hormone

8.  goiter . . . . . . . . . . . . . .
    (GOY-ter)     enlargement of the thyroid gland

9.  ketosis . . . . . . . . . . . . . .
    (kē-TŌ-sis)     condition resulting from uncontrolled diabetes mellitus, in which the body has an abnormal concentration of ketone bodies (compounds that are a normal product of fat metabolism)

10. myxedema . . . . . . . . . . .
    (mik-se-DĒ-ma)     condition resulting from a deficiency of the thyroid hormone, thyroxine

11. tetany . . . . . . . . . . . . . .
    (TET-a-nē)     condition resulting in spasms of the nerves and muscles, which result from low amounts of calcium in the blood caused by a deficiency of the parathyroid hormone

Practice saying each of these terms aloud. To assist you in pronunciation, obtain the audiotape designed for use with this text. Learn the definitions and spellings of the other diagnostic terms by completing the following exercises.

## EXERCISE 12

Match the terms in the first column with the correct definitions in the second column.

_d_ 1. acidosis

_a_ 2. Addison's disease

_j_ 3. cretinism

_b_ 4. Cushing's disease

_h_ 5. diabetes insipidus

_c_ 6. diabetes mellitus

_l_ 7. gigantism

_e_ 8. goiter

_k_ 9. ketosis

_i_ 10. myxedema

_f_ 11. tetany

a. results from a deficiency in the hormonal secretion of the adrenal cortex

b. attributed to the excessive production of cortisol

c. caused by underactivity of the islets of Langerhans

d. abnormal accumulation of acid products of metabolism

e. enlargement of the thyroid gland

f. results from low blood calcium

g. caused by an excessive amount of parathormone

h. result of a decreased activity of antidiuretic hormone

i. caused by deficiency of the thyroid hormone

j. caused by a wasting away of the thyroid gland

k. abnormal concentration of compounds resulting from fat metabolism

l. caused by overproduction of the pituitary growth hormone

## EXERCISE 13

Write the name of the endocrine gland responsible for each of the following conditions.

1. myxedema _____

2. tetany _____

3. ketosis _____

4. gigantism _____

5. goiter _____

6. Addison's disease _____

7. diabetes mellitus _____

8. cretinism _____

9. acidosis  _____

10. Cushing's syndrome  _____

11. diabetes insipidus  _____

## EXERCISE 14

Spell each of the other diagnostic terms. Have someone dictate the terms on pp. 588 and 589 to you or say the words into a tape recorder; then spell the words from your recording as often as necessary. Study any you have spelled incorrectly.

1. _____  7. _____

2. _____  8. _____

3. _____  9. _____

4. _____  10. _____

5. _____  11. _____

6. _____

Place a check mark (√) in the box to indicate that you have completed Objective 4.

☐ DEFINE, PRONOUNCE, AND SPELL OTHER DIAGNOSTIC TERMS RELATED TO THE ENDOCRINE SYSTEM.

# Objective 5  BUILD, ANALYZE, DEFINE, PRONOUNCE, AND SPELL THE SURGICAL TERMS RELATED TO THE ENDOCRINE SYSTEM.

## Surgical Terms

**TERM**
(built from word parts)

**DEFINITION**

1. adrenalectomy . . . . . . . . . excision of an adrenal gland
   (ad-rē-nal-EK-tō-mē)

2. parathyroidectomy . . . . . . excision of a parathyroid gland
   (pār-a-thī-royd-EK-tō-mē)

3. thyroidectomy . . . . . . . . excision of the thyroid gland
   (thī-royd-EK-tō-mē)

4. thyroidotomy . . . . . . . . . incision into the thyroid gland
   (thī-royd-OT-ō-mē)

5. thyroparathyroidectomy . . excision of the thyroid and parathyroid
   (thī-rō-pār-a-thī-royd-EK-tō-  glands
   mē)

Practice saying each of these words aloud. To assist you in pronunciation, obtain the audiotape designed for use with this text. Learn the definitions and spellings of the terms by completing the following exercises.

## EXERCISE 15

Analyze and define the following surgical terms.

1. thyroidotomy _____

2. adrenalectomy _____

3. thyroparathyroidectomy _____

4. thyroidectomy _____

5. parathyroidectomy _____

## EXERCISE 16

Build surgical terms for the following definitions by using the word parts you have learned.

1. excision of the thyroid
   gland

   _____ / _____
          WR        S

2. excision of the thyroid
   and parathyroid glands

   _____ / _____ / _____ / _____
      WR    CV    WR    S

3. excision of the adrenal
   gland

   _____ / _____
          WR        S

4. excision of the parathyroid gland

   _____ / _____
          WR        S

5. incision into the thyroid
   gland

   _____ / _____
          WR        S

## EXERCISE 17

Spell each of the surgical terms. Have someone dictate the terms on p. 591 to you or say the words into a tape recorder; then spell the words from your recording as often as necessary. Think about the word parts before attempting to write the word. Study any you have spelled incorrectly.

1. _____    4. _____

2. _____    5. _____

3. _____

Place a check mark (√) in the box to indicate that you have completed Objective 5.

☐ BUILD, ANALYZE, DEFINE, PRONOUNCE, AND SPELL THE SURGICAL TERMS RELATED TO THE ENDOCRINE SYSTEM.

## Objective 6  BUILD, ANALYZE, DEFINE, PRONOUNCE, AND SPELL ADDITIONAL TERMS RELATED TO THE ENDOCRINE SYSTEM.

## Additional Terms

| TERM (built from word parts) | DEFINITION |
|---|---|
| 1. adrenocorticohyperplasia.................<br>(a-*drē*-nō-*kōr*-ti-kō-*hī*-per-PLĀ-zhē-a)<br>(NOTE: *Hyper*, a prefix, appears within this word.) | excessive development of the adrenal cortex |
| 2. adrenopathy.........<br>(*ad*-rēn-OP-a-thē) | disease of the adrenal gland |
| 3. calcipenia...........<br>(kal-si-PĒ-nē-a) | deficiency of calcium |
| 4. cortical.............<br>(KŌR-ti-kal) | pertaining to the cortex |
| 5. corticoid............<br>(KŌR-ti-koyd) | resembling the cortex |
| 6. endocrinologist ......<br>(en-dō-kri-NOL-ō-jist) | a physician who specializes in endocrinology |
| 7. endocrinology ........<br>(en-dō-kri-NOL-ō-jē) | the study of endocrine glands |
| 8. endocrinopathy ......<br>(en-dō-kri-NOP-a-thē) | any disease of the endocrine system |
| 9. euthyroid ...........<br>(ū-THĪ-royd) | resembling a normal thyroid |
| 10. exophthalmic........<br>(*ek*-sof-THAL-mik) | pertaining to eyes (bulging) outward (abnormal protrusion of the eyeball) (Figure 15-6) |
| 11. polydipsia...........<br>(*pol*-ē-DIP-sē-a) | abnormal state of much thirst |
| 12. syndrome...........<br>(SIN-drōm) | set of symptoms that run (occur) together |

> **Exophthalmic** is derived from the Greek **ex,** meaning **outward,** and **ophthalmos,** meaning **eye.** Protrusion of the eyeball is sometimes a symptom of hyperthyroidism, which was first described by Dr. Robert Graves in 1835 and is frequently called **Graves' disease.**

Practice saying each of these terms aloud. To assist you in pronunciation, obtain the audiotape designed for use with this text. Learn the definitions and spellings of the additional terms by completing the following exercises.

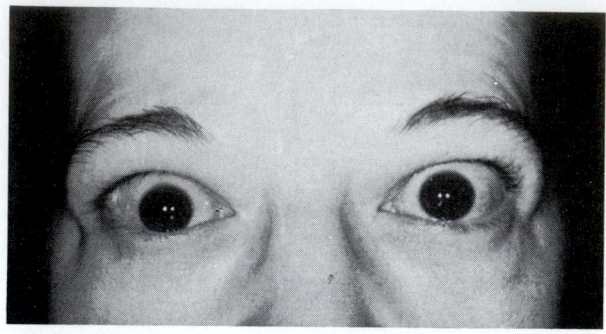

Figure 15-6
Protrusion of eyes, a characteristic of exophthalmic thyroid disease.

From Saunders WH and others: *Nursing care in eye, ear, nose,
and throat disorders,* ed 4, St. Louis, 1979, Mosby.

## EXERCISE 18

Analyze and define the following additional terms.

1. corticoid _____

2. exophthalmic _____

3. syndrome _____

4. adrenopathy _____

5. endocrinologist _____

6. polydipsia _____

7. calcipenia _____

8. endocrinopathy _____

9. adrenocorticohyperplasia _____

10. euthyroid _____

11. cortical _____

12. endocrinology _____

## EXERCISE 19

Build additional terms for the following definitions by using the word
parts you have learned.

1. pertaining to eyes bulg-
   ing out            _____ / _____ / _____
                          P          WR          S

2. any disease of the endocrine system

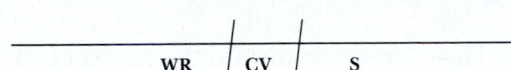

WR | CV | S

3. resembling the cortex

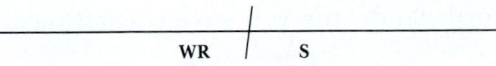

WR | S

4. set of symptoms that run
   (occur) together

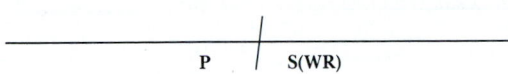

P | S(WR)

5. excessive development of
   the adrenal cortex

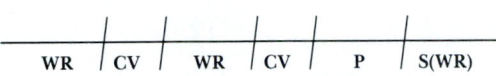

WR | CV | WR | CV | P | S(WR)

6. the study of endocrine
   glands

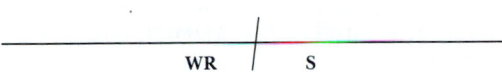

WR | S

7. abnormal state of much
   thirst

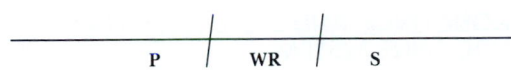

P | WR | S

8. disease of the adrenal
   gland

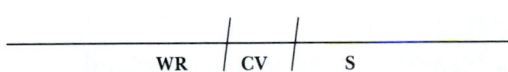

WR | CV | S

9. deficiency of calcium

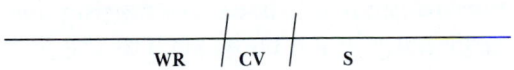

WR | CV | S

10. resembling normal thy-
    roid

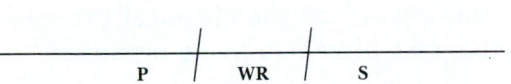

P | WR | S

11. pertaining to the cortex

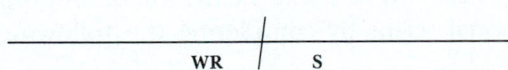

WR | S

12. a physician who special-
    izes in endocrinology

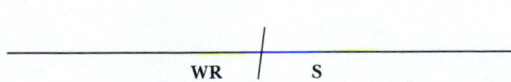

WR | S

## EXERCISE 20

Spell each of the additional terms. Have someone dictate the terms on p. 593 to you or say the words into a tape recorder; then spell the words from your recording as often as necessary. Think about the word parts before attempting to write the word. Study any you have spelled incorrectly.

1. _____      7. _____
2. _____      8. _____
3. _____      9. _____
4. _____      10. _____
5. _____      11. _____
6. _____      12. _____

Place a check mark (√) in the box to indicate that you have completed Objective 6.

☐ **BUILD, ANALYZE, DEFINE, PRONOUNCE, AND SPELL ADDITIONAL TERMS RELATED TO THE ENDOCRINE SYSTEM.**

## Objective 7    DEFINE, PRONOUNCE, AND SPELL THE OTHER ADDITIONAL TERMS RELATED TO THE ENDOCRINE SYSTEM.

## Other Additional Terms

| TERM | DEFINITION |
|---|---|
| 1. hormone............<br>(HOR-mōn) | a secretion of an endocrine gland |
| 2. isthmus.............<br>(IS-mus) | narrow strip of tissue connecting two large parts in the body, such as the isthmus that connects the two lobes of the thyroid gland (Figure 15-2). |
| 3. metabolism...........<br>(me-TAB-ō-lizm) | sum total of all the chemical processes that take place in a living organism |

Practice saying each of these terms aloud. To assist you in pronunciation, obtain the audiotape designed for use with this text. Learn the definitions and spellings of the other additional terms by completing the following exercises.

## EXERCISE 21

Fill in the blanks with the correct terms.

1. The total of all the chemical processes that take place in a living organism is called its _____ .

2. The secretion from an endocrine gland is called a

_____ .

3. A narrow strip of tissue connecting large parts in the body is called a(n)

_____ .

## EXERCISE 22

Write the definitions of the following terms.

1. isthmus _____

2. metabolism _____

3. hormone _____

## EXERCISE 23

Spell each of the other additional terms. Have someone dictate the terms on p. 596 to you or say the words into a tape recorder; then spell the words from your recording as often as necessary. Study any you have spelled incorrectly.

1. _____     3. _____

2. _____

Place a check mark (√) in the box to indicate that you have completed Objective 7.

☐ **DEFINE, PRONOUNCE, AND SPELL THE OTHER ADDITONAL TERMS RELATED TO THE ENDOCRINE SYSTEM.**

---

**Case History:** This 53-year-old female Mexican-American executive secretary presents to the clinic with complaints of excessive urination and thirst for the last month. She has also lost about ten pounds.

---

**History and Physical: Chief Complaint: Polyuria, polydipsia**

History of Present Illness: This patient presented to emergency room following an episode of syncope at work. She was oriented × 3, but responses to questions were sluggish. Routine lab work was ordered. Blood sugar was discovered to be over 600. Urinalysis showed moderate ketonuria. For the past four weeks she had been experiencing polyuria and polydipsia, drinking 3-4 quarts of water daily for the past ten days. This has also resulted in nocturia. She denies anorexia, nausea, vomiting, or any abdominal pain.

Past Medical History: No allergies; no previous hospitalizations. Does not smoke or drink. She has had no recent illnesses.

*Continued.*

**History and Physical:**Chief Complaint: Polyuria, polydipsia—cont'd

Family History; Social History: Mother died of a cerebrovascular accident at age 78. Father is still living at the age of 85, but has had diabetes mellitus for twenty years. She has two brothers, no sisters. She has no children and has never been married.

Review of Systems: Essentially unremarkable, except for occasional headaches and blurred vision. No chest pain, no awareness of cardiac palpitations or irregularities. Denies nausea, vomiting, hematochezia, or hematemesis, although has lost ten pounds in the past month.

Admission Physical Examination: A 53-year-old female in no acute distress. BP 120/84, respiratory rate of 22, pulse rate of 76.
**HEENT:** Clear, nonicteric sclerae. Pupils equal, round, reactive to light; funduscopic examination is benign.
**CHEST:** Clear to auscultation and percussion.
**HEART:** JVD is flat; PMI fifth left intercostal space, left midclavicular line; S1 and S2 are appreciated, no S3 or S4. No murmurs, no lifts, heaves, or thrills. Sinus rhythm.
**EXTREMITIES:** Negative for clubbing, cyanosis, or edema. Pulses intact.
**ABDOMEN:** Soft, nontender, bowel sounds normal, without evidence of organomegaly.
**RECTAL:** Unremarkable, guaiac negative.
**NEUROLOGIC:** Alert, oriented to time, person, and place; cranial nerves II through XII are grossly within normal limits.

**ASSESSMENT:** Diabetic ketoacidosis, cause needs to be ascertained. Most likely adult onset diabetes mellitus.

# EXERCISE 24

To test your understanding of the terms introduced in this chapter, circle the words that successfully complete the sentences. The italicized words refer to the correct answer.

1. A patient who has an *enlargement of the thyroid gland* has (myxedema, tetany, goiter).
2. A condition that results from *uncontrolled diabetes mellitus* is (calcipenia, ketosis, tetany).
3. *Addison's disease* is caused by an *underfunctioning* of the (adrenal, pituitary, thyroid) gland.
4. *Decreased activity* of the (thyroid, antidiuretic hormone, adrenals) may cause *diabetes insipidus*.
5. *Cushing's syndrome* is caused by (overactivity, underactivity) of the *adrenal cortices*.
6. A *wasting away of the thyroid gland* may result in (cretinism, myxedema, tetany).

# EXERCISE 25

Unscramble the following mixed-up terms. The word on the left hints at the condition named by the scrambled term.

1. thyroid       / / / / / /
                r  o  i  g  e  t

2. potassium    / / / /e/ / / /e/ / /
p a y m e h r l a i e k

3. thirst    / / / / / /i/ / / /
y o p p l i d i a s

4. adrenal    / / / /e/ / / /e/ / / /
o n g e m a a y l e r d

5. calcium    / / / /o/ / / / /e/ / /
l o a m p e c a y h i c

## EXERCISE 26

The following words did not appear in this chapter but are composed of word parts studied in this or the previous chapters. Find their definitions by translating the word parts literally.

1. **acrodermatitis** _____
   (*ak*-rō-der-ma-TĪ-tis)

2. **calciuria** _____
   (*kal*-sē-Ū-rē-a)

3. **interalveolar** _____
   (*in*-ter-al-VĒ-ō-lar)

4. **kalemia** _____
   (ka-LĒ-mē-a)

5. **neurotripsy** _____
   (NŪ-rō-trip-sē)

6. **ophthalmomalacia** _____
   (of-*thal*-mō-ma-LĀ-she-a)

7. **pancreatography** _____
   (*pan*-krē-a-TOG-ra-fē)

8. **phlebosclerosis** _____
   (*fleb*-ō-skle-RŌ-sis)

9. **pneumomelanosis** _____
   (*nū*-mō-mel-a-NŌ-sis)

10. **rectoscope** _____
    (REK-tō-skōp)

# Summary

Can you build, analyze, define, spell, and pronounce the following terms built from word parts?   yes ☐   no ☐

| DIAGNOSTIC | SURGICAL | ADDITIONAL |
|---|---|---|
| acromegaly<br>(*ak*-rō-MĔG-a-lē) | adrenalectomy<br>(ad-*rē*-nal-EK-tō-mē) | adrenocorticohyperplasia<br>(a-*drē*-nō-*kōr*-ti-kō-*hī*-per-PLĀ-zhē-a) |
| adrenalitis<br>(ad-*rēn*-al-Ī-tis) | parathyroidectomy<br>(*pār*-a-*thī*-royd-EK-tō-mē) | adrenopathy<br>(*ad*-rēn-ŎP-a-thē) |
| adrenomegaly<br>(ad-*rēn*-ō-MĔG-a-lē) | thyroidectomy<br>(*thī*-royd-EK-tō-mē) | calcipenia<br>(kal-si-PĒ-nē-a) |
| hypercalcemia<br>(*hī*-per-kal-SĒ-mē-a) | thyroidotomy<br>(*thī*-royd-OT-ō-me) | cortical<br>(KŌR-ti-kal) |
| hyperglycemia<br>(*hī*-per-glī-SĒ-mē-a) | thyroparathyroidectomy<br>(*thī*-rō-pār-a-*thī*-royd-EK-tō-mē) | corticoid<br>(KŌR-ti-koyd) |
| hyperkalemia<br>(*hī*-per-ka-LĒ-mē-a) | | endocrinologist<br>(en-dō-kri-NOL-ō-jist) |
| hyperthyroidism<br>(*hī*-per-THĪ-royd-izm) | | endocrinology<br>(en-dō-kri-NOL-ō-jē) |
| hypocalcemia<br>(*hī*-pō-kal-SĒ-mē-a) | | endocrinopathy<br>(en-dō-kri-NOP-a-thē) |
| hypoglycemia<br>(*hī*-pō-glī-SĒ-me-a) | | euthyroid<br>(ū-THĪ-royd) |
| hypokalemia<br>(*hī*-pō-ka-LĒ-mē-a) | | exophthalmic<br>(*ek*-sof-THAL-mik) |
| hypothyroidism<br>(*hī*-pō-THĪ-royd-izm) | | polydipsia<br>(*pol*-ē-DIP-sē-a) |
| parathyroidoma<br>(*pār*-a-THĪ-roy-*dō*-ma) | | syndrome<br>(SIN-drōm) |
| thyrotoxicosis<br>(*thī*-rō-*tok*-si-KŌ-sis) | | |

# Summary

Can you define, pronounce, and spell the following terms *not built from word parts?*  yes □  no □

## DIAGNOSTIC

acidosis
(*as*-i-DŌ-sis)

Addison's disease

cretinism
(KRĒ-tin-izm)

Cushing's syndrome

diabetes insipidus
(*dī*-a-BĒ-tēz) (in-SIP-i-dūs)

diabetes mellitus
(*dī*-a-BĒ-tēz) (mel-LĪ-tus)

gigantism
(jī-GAN-tizm)

goiter
(GOY-ter)

ketosis
(kē-TŌ-sis)

myxedema
(*mik*-se-DĒ-ma)

tetany
(TET-a-nē)

## ADDITIONAL

hormone
(HOR-mōn)

isthmus
(IS-mus)

metabolism
(me-TAB-ō-lizm)

# Answers

### Exercise 1A

1. b    3. d    5. a    7. e
2. g    4. h    6. c

### Exercise 1B

1. d    3. e    5. g
2. a    4. b    6. c

### Exercise 2

**Figure 15-1**
Parathyroid glands:
   parathyroid/o
Adrenal glands: adren/o,
   adrenal/o
Thyroid gland: thyroid/o,
   thyr/o
**Figure 15-4**
Cortex: cortic/o

### Exercise 3

1. cortex        5. adrenal
2. adrenal       6. thyroid
3. parathyroid   7. endocrine
4. thyroid

### Exercise 4

1. a. adren/o     2. a. thyroid/o    3. endocrin/o
   b. adrenal/o       b. thyr/o          4. cortic/o
                                5. parathyroid/o

### Exercise 5

1. thirst    3. potassium    5. extremities, height
2. poison    4. calcium

### Exercise 6

1. toxic/o    3. calc/i    5. kal/i
2. acr/o      4. dips/o

## Exercise 7

1. outside, outward    2. run, running

## Exercise 8

1. -drome    2. a. ex-
                    b. exo-

## Exercise 9

|  |  |
|---|---|
| WR  S<br>1. adrenal/itis | inflammation of an adrenal gland |
| P  WR  S<br>2. hypo/calc/emia | deficient level of calcium in the blood |
| P    WR    S<br>3. hyper/thyroid/ism | state of excessive production of thyroid hormone |
| P  WR  S<br>4. hyper/kal/emia | excessive potassium in the blood |
| WR CV WR  S<br>5. thyr/ o /toxic/osis<br>   CF | abnormal condition of poisoning caused by excessive thyroid gland activity |
| P  WR  S<br>6. hyper/glyc/emia | excessive sugar in the blood |
| WR CV  S<br>7. adren/ o /megaly<br>   CF | enlargement of the adrenal gland |
| P   WR   S<br>8. hypo/thyroid/ism | state of deficient thyroid gland activity |
| P  WR  S<br>9. hypo/kal/emia | deficient level of potassium in the blood |
| WR    S<br>10. parathyroid/oma | tumor of the parathyroid gland |
| WR CV  S<br>11. acr/ o /megaly<br>   CF | enlargement of the extremities (and facial bones) |
| P  WR  S<br>12. hypo/glyc/emia | deficient level of sugar in the blood |
| P  WR  S<br>13. hyper/calc/emia | excessive calcium in the blood |

## Exercise 10

1. adren/o/megaly
2. hypo/thyroid/ism
3. acr/o/megaly
4. hypo/glyc/emia
5. hyper/kal/emia
6. hypo/calc/emia
7. hyper/thyroid/ism
8. hyper/calc/emia
9. thyr/o/toxic/osis
10. parathyroid/oma
11. hyper/glyc/emia
12. hypo/kal/emia
13. adrenal/itis

## Exercise 11

Spelling exercise: *see* text, p. 588.

## Exercise 12

1. d    4. b    7. l    10. i
2. a    5. h    8. e    11. f
3. j    6. c    9. k

## Exercise 13

1. thyroid
2. parathyroid
3. islets of Langerhans (pancreas)
4. pituitary
5. thyroid
6. adrenal
7. islets of Langerhans (pancreas)
8. thyroid
9. islets of Langerhans (pancreas)
10. adrenal
11. pituitary

## Exercise 14

Spelling exercise; *see* text, p. 591.

## Exercise 15

|  |  |
|---|---|
| WR    S<br>1. thyroid/otomy | incision into the thyroid gland |
| WR    S<br>2. adrenal/ectomy | excision of the adrenal gland |
| WR CV    WR     S<br>3. thyr/ o /parathyroid/ectomy<br>   CF | excision of the thyroid and parathyroid glands |
| WR    S<br>4. thyroid/ectomy | excision of the thyroid gland |
| WR     S<br>5. parathyroid/ectomy | excision of the parathyroid gland |

## Exercise 16

1. thyroid/ectomy
2. thyr/o/parathyroid/ ectomy
3. adrenal/ectomy
4. parathyroid/ectomy
5. thyroid/otomy

## Exercise 17

Spelling exercise; *see* text, p. 591.

## Exercise 18

1.
```
 WR   S
```
cortic/oid — resembling the cortex

2.
```
 P    WR    S
```
ex/ophthalm/ic — pertaining to eyes bulging outward

3.
```
 P   S(WR)
```
syn/drome — set of symptoms that run together

4.
```
 WR  CV   S
```
adren/ o /pathy — disease of the adrenal gland
```
    CF
```

5.
```
 WR       S
```
endocrin/ologist — a physician who specializes in endocrinology

6.
```
 P   WR S
```
poly/dips/ia — abnormal state of much thirst

7.
```
 WR CV   S
```
calc/ i /penia — deficiency of calcium
```
   CF
```

8.
```
 WR    CV   S
```
endocrin/ o /pathy — any disease of the endocrine system
```
    CF
```

9.
```
 WR  CV  WR  CV   P   S(WR)
```
adren/ o /cortic/ o /hyper/plasia — excessive development of the adrenal cortex
```
    CF      CF
```

10.
```
 P   WR  S
```
eu/thyr/oid — resembling normal thyroid

11.
```
 WR   S
```
cortic/al — pertaining to the cortex

12.
```
 WR      S
```
endocrin/ology — the study of endocrine glands

## Exercise 19

1. ex/ophthalm/ic
2. endocrin/o/pathy
3. cortic/oid
4. syn/drome
5. adren/o/cortic/o/ hyper/plasia
6. endocrin/ology
7. poly/dips/ia
8. adren/o/pathy
9. calc/i/penia
10. eu/thyr/oid
11. cortic/al
12. endocrin/ologist

## Exercise 20

Spelling exercise; *see* text, p. 596.

## Exercise 21

1. metabolism   2. hormone   3. isthmus

## Exercise 22

1. narrow strip of tissue connecting large parts in the body
2. total of all the chemical processes that take place in living organisms
3. a secretion of an endocrine gland

## Exercise 23

Spelling exercise; *see* text, p. 597.

## Exercise 24

1. goiter
2. ketosis
3. adrenal
4. antidiuretic hormone
5. overactivity
6. cretinism

## Exercise 25

1. goiter
2. hyperkalemia
3. polydipsia
4. adrenomegaly
5. hypocalcemia

## Exercise 26

1. inflammation of the skin of the extremities
2. calcium in the urine
3. pertaining to between the alveoli
4. potassium in the blood
5. surgical crushing of a nerve
6. softening of the eye
7. process of x-ray filming the pancreas
8. hardening of a vein
9. abnormal condition of a black lung
10. instrument to examine the rectum

# 16

# Directional Terms, Anatomical Planes and Regions, and Additional Terms

## Objectives

**Upon completion of this chapter you will be able to:**

1. Define, pronounce, and spell the terms used to describe the body directions.

2. Define, pronounce, and spell the terms used to describe the anatomical planes.

3. Define, pronounce, and spell the terms used to describe the anatomical abdominal regions.

4. Define, pronounce, and spell additional terms related to the body.

In the description of body directions and planes a position of reference is used. In the anatomical position, as it is called, the body is viewed as erect, arms at the side with the palms of the hands facing forward and feet placed side by side. Whether the patient is standing or lying down face up, the directional terms are the same.

## Objective 1
**DEFINE, PRONOUNCE, AND SPELL THE TERMS USED TO DESCRIBE THE BODY DIRECTIONS (SEE FIGURE 16-1).**

## Body Directional Terms

| TERM | DEFINITION |
|---|---|
| 1. a. cephalic (head). . . . . . <br> (se-FAL-ik) | toward the top of the body |
| b. superior (above) <br> (su-PĒR-ē-or) | |
| 2. a. caudal (tail) . . . . . . . . <br> (CAW-dal) | toward the lower end of the body |
| b. inferior (below) <br> (in-FĒR-ē-or) | |

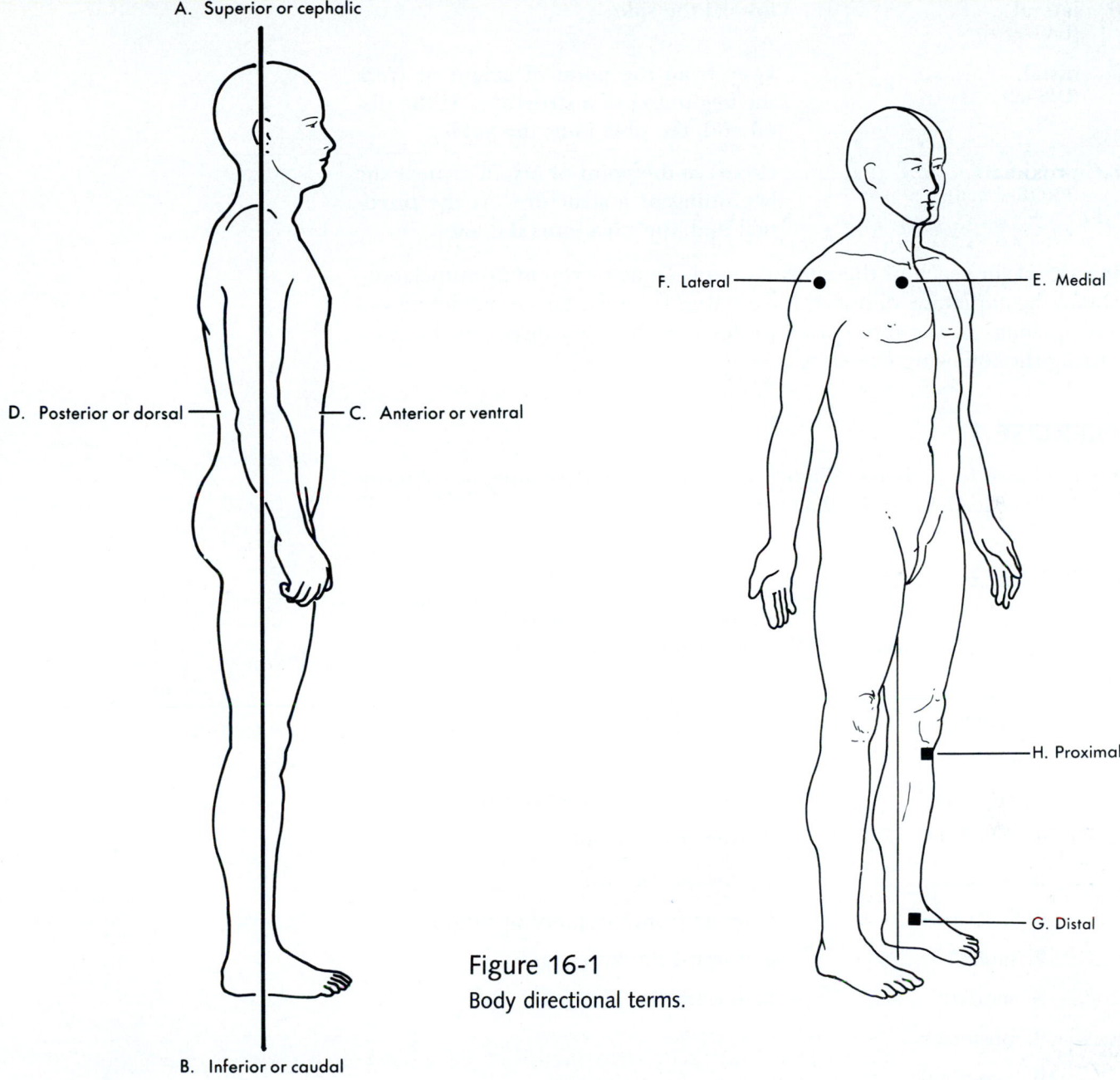

A. Superior or cephalic

D. Posterior or dorsal — — C. Anterior or ventral

B. Inferior or caudal

F. Lateral — E. Medial

H. Proximal

G. Distal

Figure 16-1
Body directional terms.

3. a. **anterior** . . . . . . . . . . .    toward the front of the body
    (an-TĒR-ē-or)
   b. **ventral**
    (VEN-tral)

4. a. **posterior**. . . . . . . . . .    toward the back of the body
    (pos-TĒR-ē-or)
   b. **dorsal**
    (DŌR-sal)

5. **medial** . . . . . . . . . . . . . .    toward the midline or middle
   (MĒ-dē-al)

6. lateral . . . . . . . . . . . . . . . . . toward the side
   (LAT-er-al)

7. distal . . . . . . . . . . . . . . . away from the point of origin or from the beginning of a structure. At the distal end, the tibia joins the ankle.
   (DIS-tal)

8. proximal . . . . . . . . . . . . . closest to the point of origin or near the beginning of a structure. At the proximal end, the tibia joins the knee.
   (PROK-si-mal)

Practice saying each of these terms aloud. To assist you in pronunciation, obtain the audiotape designed for use with this text. Learn the definitions and spellings of the terms used to describe the body directions by completing the following exercises.

## EXERCISE 1

Study Figure 16-1; then on Figure 16-2 write the correct directional terms on the lines leading to the diagram.

## EXERCISE 2

Match the terms in the first column with the correct definitions in the second column. The answers in the second column may be used more than once.

_d_ 1. anterior          a. toward the top
_g_ 2. caudal            b. toward the side
_a_ 3. cephalic          c. closest to the point of origin
_f_ 4. distal            d. toward the front
_e_ 5. dorsal            e. toward the back
_g_ 6. inferior          f. away from the point of origin
_b_ 7. lateral           g. toward the lower end
_h_ 8. medial            h. toward the middle
_e_ 9. posterior
_c_ 10. proximal
_a_ 11. superior
_d_ 12. ventral

## EXERCISE 3

Fill in the blanks with the correct terms. The italicized words refer to the correct answer.

1. _Cephalic,_ or _____Superior_____, means ____toward the top____.

2. _____Posterior_____, or _____dorsal_____, means _toward the back of the body._

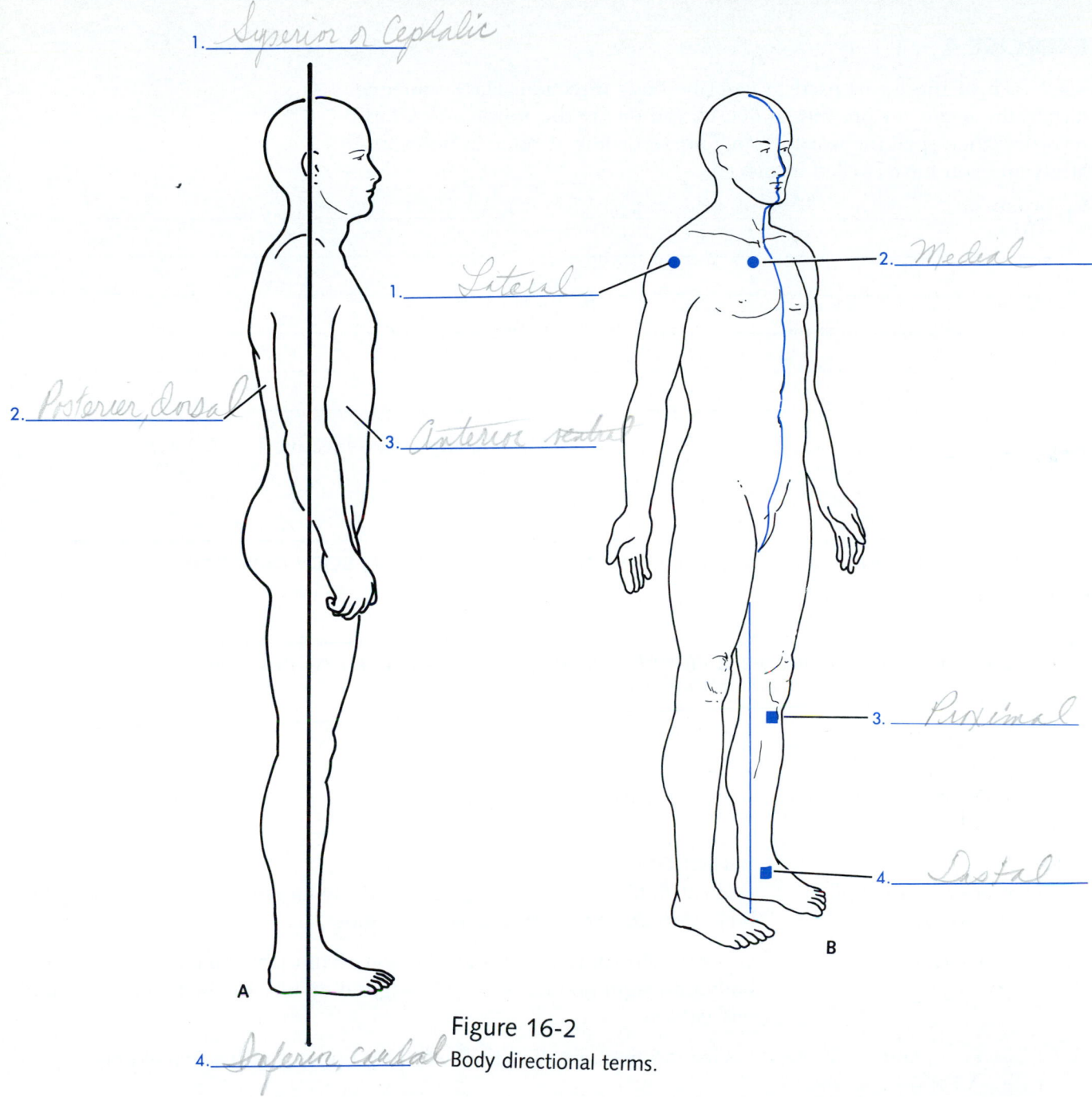

1. _Superior or Cephalic_

1. _Lateral_

2. _Medial_

2. _Posterior, dorsal_

3. _Anterior ventral_

3. _Proximal_

4. _Distal_

A

B

4. _Inferior, caudal_

**Figure 16-2**
Body directional terms.

3. _Anterior,_ or _____ventral_____, means _towards the front._
4. _____Inferior_____, or _____caudal_____, means _toward the lower end of the body._
5. _Medial_ means _____toward the middle_____
6. _____Proximal_____ means _closest to the point of origin._
7. _Distal_ means _away from point of origin_

## EXERCISE 4

Spell each of the terms used to describe body direction. Have someone dictate the terms on pp. 604 to 606 to you or say the words into a tape recorder; then spell the words from your recording as often as necessary. Study any you have spelled incorrectly.

1. _____     7. _____

2. _____     8. _____

3. _____     9. _____

4. _____     10. _____

5. _____     11. _____

6. _____     12. _____

Place a check mark (√) in the box to indicate that you have completed Objective 1.

☐ DEFINE, PRONOUNCE, AND SPELL THE TERMS USED TO DESCRIBE THE BODY DIRECTIONS.

## Objective 2   DEFINE, PRONOUNCE, AND SPELL THE TERMS USED TO DESCRIBE THE ANATOMICAL PLANES.

## Anatomical Planes

Planes are imaginary flat fields used as points of reference to identify the position of parts of the body (Figure 16-3).

| TERM | DEFINITION |
| --- | --- |
| 1. frontal or coronal plane . (KOR-ō-nal) | vertical field passing through the body from side to side, dividing the body into anterior and posterior portions |
| 2. sagittal plane . . . . . . . . . . (SAJ-i-tal) | vertical field running through the body from front to back, dividing the body into right and left sides. Midsagittal divides the body into right and left halves. |
| 3. transverse plane . . . . . . . . (trans-VERS) | horizontal field dividing the body into upper and lower portions |

Learn the definitions and spellings of the terms used to describe the anatomical planes by completing the following exercises.

## EXERCISE 5

Write the terms used to describe anatomical planes in the spaces provided on the diagram in Figure 16-4.

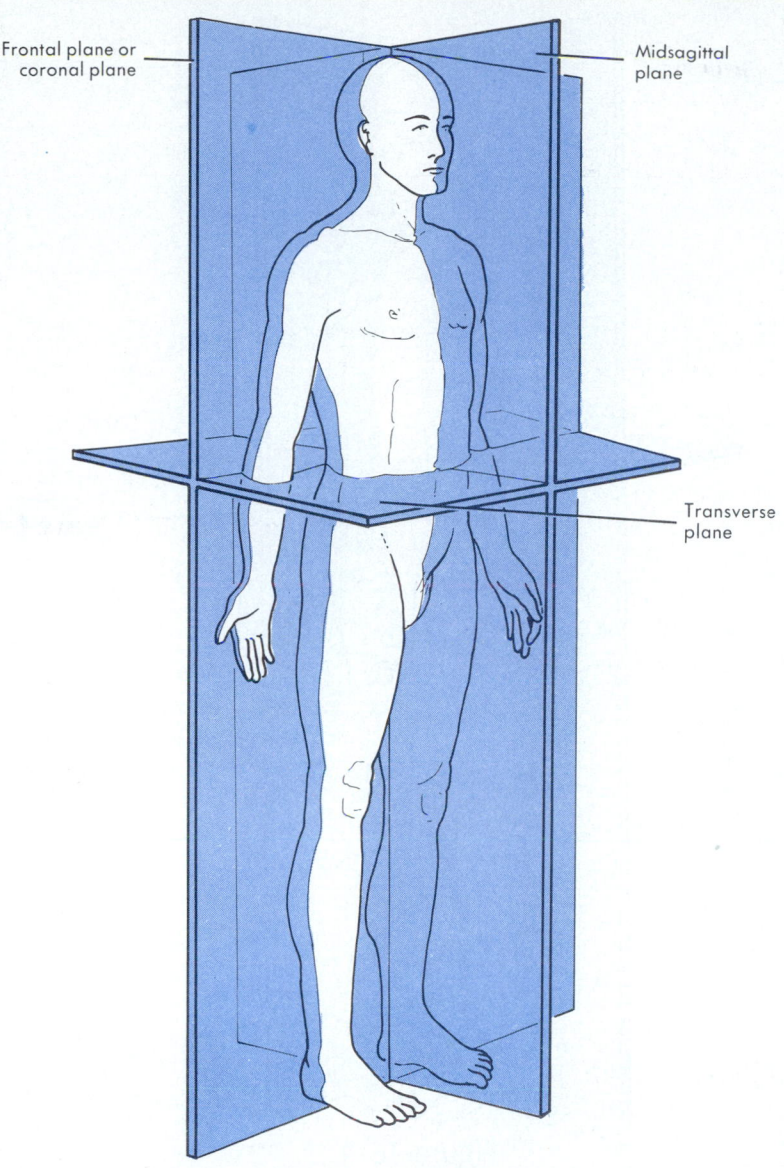

Frontal plane or
coronal plane

Midsagittal
plane

Transverse
plane

Figure 16-3
Anatomical planes.

## EXERCISE 6

Fill in the blanks with the correct terms.

1. The plane that divides the body into superior and inferior portions is the _____ plane.

2. The plane that divides the body into right and left halves is the _____ plane.

3. The plane that divides the body into anterior and posterior portions is the _____ plane.

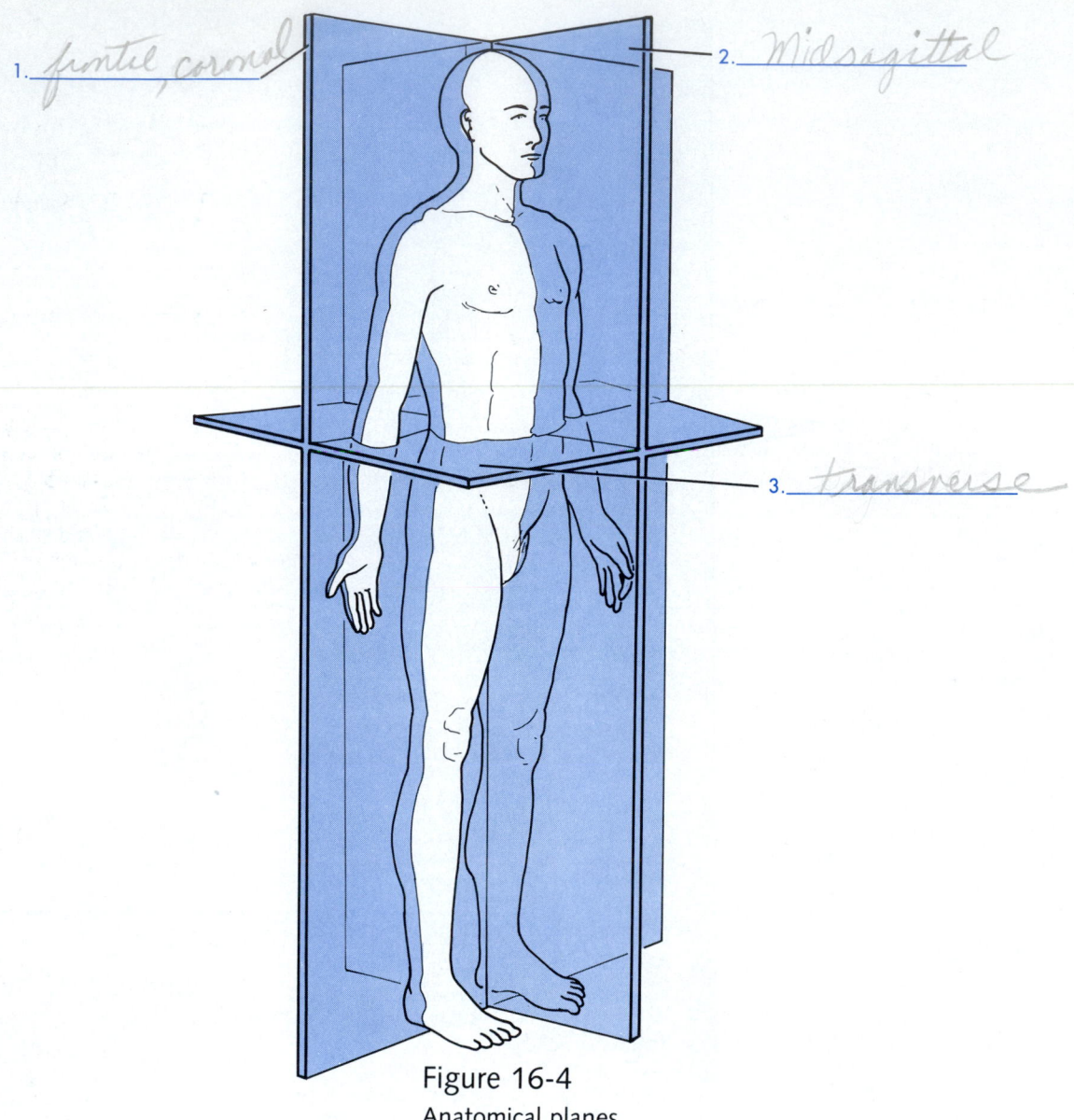

1. *frontal, coronal*    2. *Midsagittal*

3. *transverse*

**Figure 16-4**
Anatomical planes.

## EXERCISE 7

Spell each of the terms used to describe the anatomical planes. Have someone dictate the terms on p. 608 to you or say the words into a tape recorder; then spell the words from your recording as often as necessary. Study any you have spelled incorrectly.

1. *frontal coronal*    3. *midsagittal*

2. *transverse*    4. _____

Place a check mark (√) in the box to indicate that you have completed Objective 2.

☐ **DEFINE, PRONOUNCE, AND SPELL THE TERMS USED TO DESCRIBE THE ANATOMICAL PLANES.**

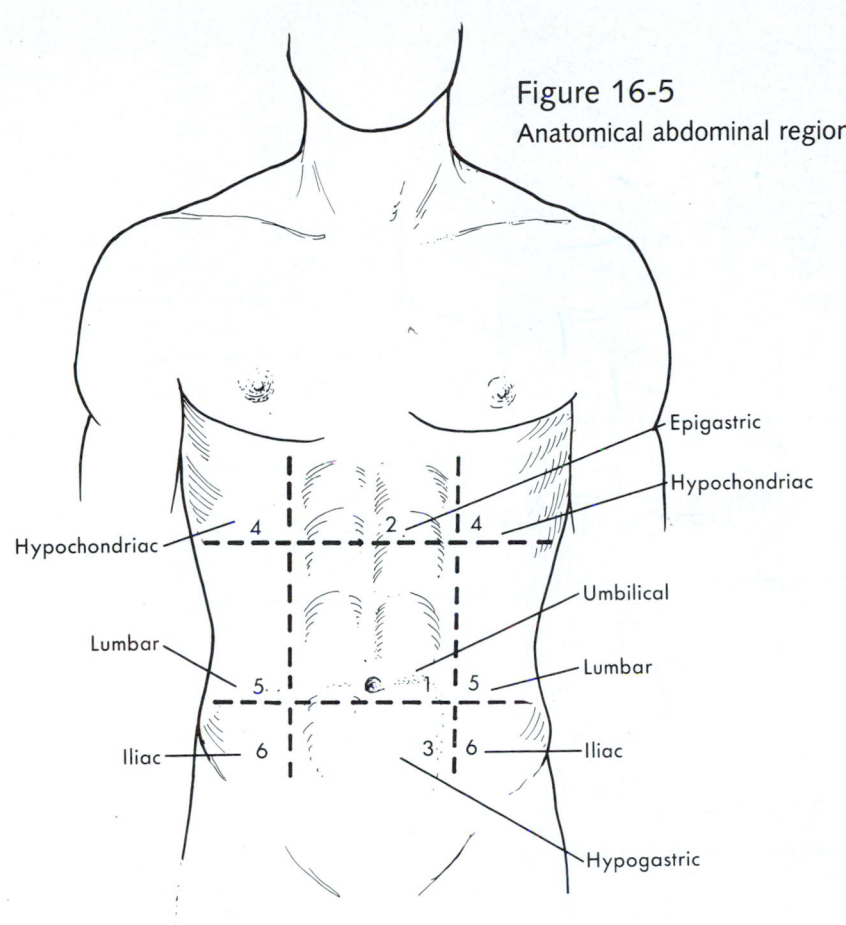

Figure 16-5
Anatomical abdominal regions.

Epigastric

Hypochondriac

Hypochondriac

Umbilical

Lumbar

Lumbar

Iliac

Iliac

Hypogastric

The term **umbilicus** is derived from the Latin **umbo,** which denoted the boss, or protuberant part, of a shield. Around the first century the term was used to designate either a raised or a depressed spot in the middle of anything.

The term **epigastric** is composed of the Greek **epi,** meaning **upon,** and **gaster,** meaning **belly.** In the first century the term referred to the area between the breast and the umbilicus. The term now designates only the upper middle portion of the abdomen.

## Objective 3    DEFINE, PRONOUNCE, AND SPELL THE TERMS USED TO DESCRIBE THE ANATOMICAL ABDOMINAL REGIONS.

## Anatomical Abdominal Regions

To assist medical personnel to locate medical problems with greater accuracy and for identification purposes, the abdomen is divided into regions (Figure 16-5).

**Hypogastric** is composed of the Greek **hypo,** meaning **under,** and **gaster,** meaning **belly.** It literally means **beneath or under the belly.**

| TERM | DEFINITION |
|---|---|
| 1. umbilical region. . . . . . . (um-BIL-i-kal) | around the navel (umbilicus) |
| 2. epigastric region . . . . . . . (*ep*-i-GAS-trik) | directly above the umbilical region |
| 3. hypogastric region . . . . . . (*hī*-pō-GAS-trik) | directly below the umbilical region |
| 4. hypochondriac regions . . (*hī*-pō-KON-drē-ak) | to the right and left of the epigastric region |
| 5. lumbar regions. . . . . . . . . (LUM-bar) | to the right and left of the umbilical region |
| 6. iliac regions . . . . . . . . . . . (IL-ē-ak) | to the right and left of the hypogastric region |

**Hypochondriac** is derived from the Greek **hypo,** meaning **under,** and **chondros,** meaning **cartilage.** This ancient term was used by Hippocrates to refer to the region just below the cartilages of the ribs. In 1765 the term was first used to refer to people who experienced discomfort or painful sensations in this area but had no organic findings. Now, a person who has an imaginary illness is referred to as a **hypochondriac.**

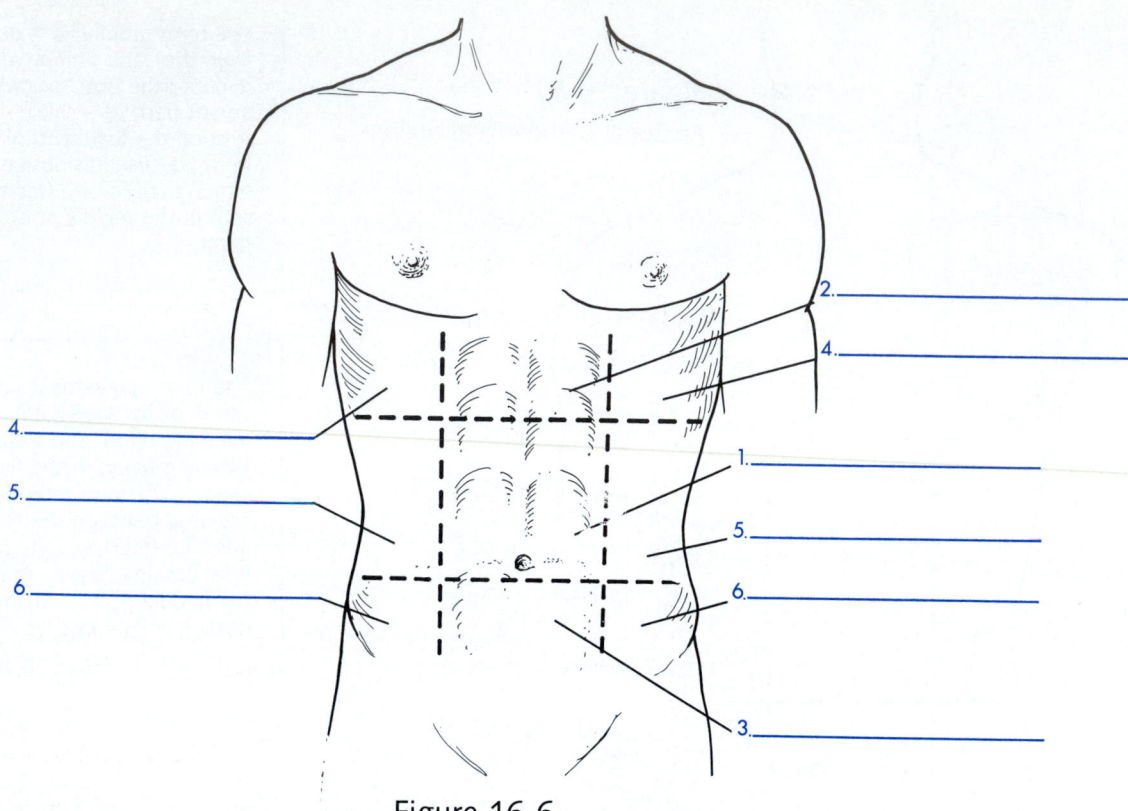

**Figure 16-6**
Anatomical abdominal regions.

Practice saying each of these words aloud. To assist you in pronunciation, obtain the audiotape designed for use with this text. Learn the definitions and spellings of the terms used to describe the anatomical abdominal regions by completing the following exercises.

## EXERCISE 8

Name the anatomical abdominal regions in the spaces provided on the diagram in Figure 16-6 above.

## EXERCISE 9

Fill in the blanks with the correct terms.

1. The regions to the right and left of the hypogastric region are the _____ regions.

2. The _____ region is directly above the umbilical region.

3. Inferior to the umbilical region is the _____ region.

4. The _____ are the regions to the right and left of the epigastric region.

5. Superior to the hypogastric region is the _____ region.

6. To the right and the left of the umbilical region are the _____ regions.

## EXERCISE 10

Match the terms in the first column with the correct definitions in the second column.

_____ 1. epigastric

_____ 2. hypochondriac

_____ 3. hypogastric

_____ 4. iliac

_____ 5. lumbar

_____ 6. umbilical

a. inferior to the navel

b. superior to the navel

c. right and left of the umbilical region

d. right and left of the epigastric region

e. right and left of the hypogastric region

f. below the hypogastric region

g. inferior to the epigastric region

## EXERCISE 11

Spell each of the terms used to describe the anatomical abdominal regions. Have someone dictate the terms on p. 611 to you or say the words into a tape recorder; then spell the words from your recording as often as necessary. Study any you have spelled incorrectly.

1. _____

2. _____

3. _____

4. _____

5. _____

6. _____

Place a check mark (√) in the box to indicate that you have completed Objective 3.

☐ DEFINE, PRONOUNCE, AND SPELL THE TERMS USED TO DESCRIBE THE ANATOMICAL ABDOMINAL REGIONS.

## Objective 4  DEFINE, PRONOUNCE, AND SPELL ADDITIONAL TERMS RELATED TO THE BODY.

## Additional Terms

| TERM | DEFINITION |
|------|------------|
| 1. extension (ek-STEN-shun) | movement in which a limb is placed in a straight position |
| 2. flexion (FLEK-shun) | movement in which a limb is bent |
| 3. afferent (AF-er-ent) | conveying toward a center (for example, afferent nerves carry impulses to the central nervous system) |
| 4. efferent (EF-er-ent) | conveying away from the center (for example, efferent nerves carry information away from the central nervous system to muscles and glands) |

5. **plantar** . . . . . . . . . . . . .    pertaining to the sole of the foot
   (PLAN-tar)

6. **palmar** . . . . . . . . . . . . .    pertaining to the palm of the hand
   (PAL-mar)

7. **prone** . . . . . . . . . . . . . . .    lying straight on one's front; facedown
   (prōn)

8. **supine** . . . . . . . . . . . . . .    lying straight on one's back; faceup
   (sū-PĪN)

9. **deep** . . . . . . . . . . . . . . . .    situated far below the surface
   (dēp)

10. **superficial** . . . . . . . . . . .    situated near the surface
    (sū-per-FISH-al)

11. **adduction** . . . . . . . . . . .    state of drawing toward the middle
    (ad-DUK-shun)

12. **abduction** . . . . . . . . . . .    state of drawing away from the middle
    (ab-DUK-shun)

13. **eversion** . . . . . . . . . . . .    state of turning outward
    (ē-VER-zhun)

14. **inversion** . . . . . . . . . . .    state of turning inward
    (in-VER-zhun)

15. **bilateral** . . . . . . . . . . . .    pertaining to both sides
    (bī-LAT-er-al)

16. **unilateral** . . . . . . . . . . .    pertaining to one side only
    (ū-ni-LAT-er-al)

Practice saying each of these terms aloud. To assit you in pronunciation, obtain the audiotape designed for use with this text. Learn the definitions and spellings of the additional terms by completing the following exercises.

## EXERCISE 12

Write the definitions of the following terms.

1. abduction _____

2. unilateral _____

3. superficial _____

4. plantar _____

5. prone _____

6. efferent _____

7. extension _____

8. eversion _____

9. palmar _____

10. adduction _____

11. bilateral _____

12. deep _____

13. supine _____

14. afferent _____

15. flexion _____

16. inversion _____

## EXERCISE 13

Match the terms in the first column with the correct definitions in the second column.

_____  1. abduction

_____  2. adduction

_____  3. afferent

_____  4. bilateral

_____  5. deep

_____  6. efferent

_____  7. eversion

_____  8. extension

_____  9. flexion

_____ 10. inversion

_____ 11. palmar

_____ 12. plantar

_____ 13. prone

_____ 14. superficial

_____ 15. supine

_____ 16. unilateral

a.  movement in which the limb is placed in a straight position

b.  pertaining to the palm of the hand

c.  lying straight on one's front; face-down

d.  state of turning outward

e.  conveying away from center

f.  situated near the surface

g.  pertaining to both sides

h.  state of drawing toward the middle

i.  pertaining to the sole of the foot

j.  conveying toward the center

k.  lying straight on one's back; faceup

l.  situated far below the surface

m.  state of turning inward

n.  pertaining to one side only

o.  movement in which the limb is bent

p.  about the navel

q.  state of drawing away from the middle

## EXERCISE 14

Spell each of the additional terms. Have someone dictate the terms on pp. 613 and 614 to you or say the words into a tape recorder; then spell the words from your recording as often as necessary. Study any you have spelled incorrectly.

1. _____    9. _____

2. _____    10. _____

3. _____    11. _____

4. _____    12. _____

5. _____    13. _____

6. _____    14. _____

7. _____    15. _____

8. _____    16. _____

## EXERCISE 15

Fill in the blanks with the correct terms. The italicized words refer to the correct answer.

While examining the patient the physician did the following:

1. Brought the arm *toward the middle of the body, or* _____ the arm.

2. Examined the patient's eyes and found _____ cataracts, or cataracts *in both* eyes.

3. Tested the reflexes *on the sole,* or _____ side, of the foot.

4. Placed the patient on the examining table in a *faceup,* or _____ , position.

5. Noticed small hemorrhages *situated near the surface* of the skin and noted on the chart that the hemorrhages were _____ .

6. _____ , or *bent,* the patient's knee.

7. Turned the patient over in a *facedown,* or _____ , position.

Place a check mark (√) in the box to indicate that you have completed Objective 4.

☐ DEFINE, PRONOUNCE, AND SPELL ADDITIONAL TERMS RELATED TO THE BODY.

## EXERCISE 16

The following words did not appear in this chapter but are made up of word parts studied in this or the previous chapters. Find their definitions by translating the word parts literally.

1. adenochondroma _____
   (*ad*-e-nō-kon-DRŌ-ma)

2.  **cardiodiaphragmatic** _____
    (*kar*-dē-ō-*dī*-a-frag-MAT-ik)

3.  **chromatometer** _____
    (*kro*-ma-TOM-e-ter)

4.  **dacryosinusitis** _____
    (*dak*-rē-ō-*sī*-nus-Ī-tis)

5.  **endogastric** _____
    (*en*-dō-GAS-trik)

6.  **enterocele** _____
    (EN-ter-ō-sēl)

7.  **esophagodynia** _____
    (e-*sof*-a-go-DĪN-ē-a)

8.  **gastropulmonary** _____
    (*gas*-trō-PUL-mo-nār-ē)

9.  **intracephalic** _____
    (*in*-tra-se-FAL-ik)

10. **myelopathic** _____
    (*mī*-e-lō-PATH-ik)

11. **neurotripsy** _____
    (NŪ-rō-trip-sē)

12. **parasplenic** _____
    (*pār*-a-SPLEN-ik)

13. **peritonsillar** _____
    (*per*-i-TON-si-lar)

14. **pylorotomy** _____
    (*pī*-lōr-OT-ō-mē)

15. **pyogenic** _____
    (*pī*-ō-JEN-ik)

16. **splenolymphatic** _____
    (*splen*-ō-lim-FAT-ik)

17. **suprascapular** _____
    (*sū*-pra-SKAP-ū-lar)

18. **vesicoabdominal** _____
    (*ves*-i-kō-ab-DOM-i-nal)

## TERMS CROSSWORD PUZZLE

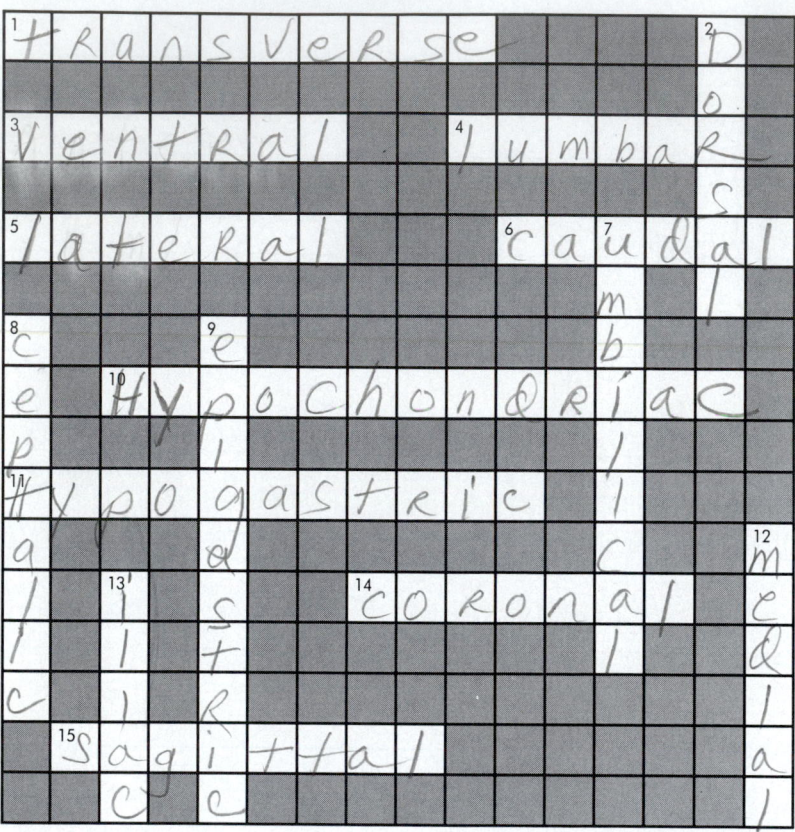

### Across Clues

1. plane that divides the body into upper and lower portions
3. toward the front of the body
4. regions to the right and left of the umbilical region
5. toward the side
6. toward the lower end of the body
10. regions to the right and left of the epigastric region
11. region directly below the umbilical region
14. plane dividing the body into anterior and posterior portions
15. plane dividing the body into right and left sides

### Down Clues

2. toward the back of the body
7. region around the navel
8. toward the top of the body
9. region directly above the umbilical region
12. toward the midline or middle
13. regions to the right and left of the hypogastric region

## MORE TERMS CROSSWORD PUZZLE

### Across Clues

1. drawing toward the middle
2. situated far below the surface
4. pertaining to one side only
5. conveying toward a center
8. straight positioning of a limb
9. turning inward
11. lying facedown
13. situated near the surface
14. lying faceup

### Down Clues

1. drawing away from the middle
3. pertaining to both sides
6. turning outward
7. bending of a limb
10. conveying away from a center
11. pertaining to the palm of the hand
12. pertaining to the sole of the foot

# Summary

Can you define, pronounce and spell the following terms?   yes ☐   no ☐

| BODY DIRECTIONAL TERMS | ANATOMICAL PLANES | ANATOMICAL ABDOMINAL REGIONS | ADDITIONAL TERMS |
|---|---|---|---|
| cephalic<br>(se-FAL-ik) | frontal or coronal<br>   plane<br>(KOR-ō-nal) | umbilical region<br>(um-BIL-i-kal) | extension<br>(ek-STEN-shun) |
| superior<br>(su-PĒR-ē-or) | sagittal plane<br>(SĂJ-i-tal) | epigastric region<br>(*ep*-i-GAS-trik) | flexion<br>(FLEK-shun) |
| caudal<br>(CAW-dal) | transverse plane<br>(trans-VERS) | hypogastric region<br>(*hī*-pō-GAS-trik) | afferent<br>(AF-er-ent) |
| inferior<br>(in-FĒR-ē-or) | | hypochondriac regions<br>(*hī*-pō-KON-drē-ak) | efferent<br>(EF-er-ent) |
| anterior<br>(an-TĒR-ē-or) | | lumbar regions<br>(LUM-bar) | plantar<br>(PLAN-tar) |
| ventral<br>(VEN-tral) | | iliac region<br>(IL-ē-ak) | palmar<br>(PAL-mar) |
| posterior<br>(pos-TĒR-ē-or) | | | prone<br>(prōn) |
| dorsal<br>(DŌR-sal) | | | supine<br>(sū-PĪN) |
| medial<br>(MĒ-dē-al) | | | deep<br>(dēp) |
| lateral<br>(LAT-er-al) | | | superficial<br>(sū-per-FISH-al) |
| distal<br>(DIS-tal) | | | adduction<br>(ad-DUK-shun) |
| proximal<br>(PROK-si-mal) | | | abduction<br>(ab-DUK-shun) |
| | | | eversion<br>(ē-VER-zhun) |
| | | | inversion<br>(in-VER-zhun) |
| | | | bilateral<br>(bī-LAT-er-al) |
| | | | unilateral<br>(ū-ni-LAT-er-al) |

# Answers

## Exercise 1

**Figure 16-2, A**
1. Superior or cephalic    3. Anterior or ventral
2. Posterior or dorsal    4. Inferior or caudal

**Figure 16-2, B**
1. Lateral    3. Proximal
2. Medial    4. Distal

## Exercise 2

1. d    4. f    7. b    10. c
2. g    5. e    8. h    11. a
3. a    6. g    9. e    12. d

## Exercise 3

1. superior; toward the top of the body
2. dorsal; posterior
3. ventral; toward the front of the body
4. inferior; caudal
5. toward the midline or middle
6. proximal
7. away from the point of origin

## Exercise 4

Spelling exercise; *see* text, p. 608.

## Exercise 5

**Figure 16-4**
1. coronal or frontal plane    3. transverse plane
2. midsagittal plane

## Exercise 6

1. transverse    3. coronal, or frontal
2. midsagittal

## Exercise 7

Spelling exercise; *see* text, p. 610.

## Exercise 8

**Figure 16-6**
1. umbilical    4. hypochondriac
2. epigastric    5. lumbar
3. hypogastric    6. iliac

## Exercise 9

1. iliac    3. hypogastric    5. umbilical
2. epigastric    4. hypochondriac    6. lumbar

## Exercise 10

1. b    3. a    5. c
2. d    4. e    6. g

## Exercise 11

Spelling exercise; *see* text p. 613.

## Exercise 12

1. state of drawing away from the middle
2. pertaining to one side only
3. situated near the surface
4. pertaining to the sole of the foot
5. lying straight on one's front; facedown
6. conveying away from the center
7. movement in which a limb is placed in a straight position
8. state of turning outward
9. pertaining to the palm of the hand
10. state of drawing toward the middle
11. pertaining to both sides
12. situated far below the surface
13. lying straight on one's back; faceup
14. conveying to a center
15. movement in which a limb is bent
16. state of turning inward

## Exercise 13

1. q    5. l    9. o    13. c
2. h    6. e    10. m    14. f
3. j    7. d    11. b    15. k
4. g    8. a    12. i    16. n

## Exercise 14

Spelling exercise; *see* text, pp. 613 and 614.

## Exercise 15

1. adducted    4. supine    7. prone
2. bilateral    5. superficial
3. plantar    6. flexed

## Exercise 16

1. tumor of gland and cartilage
2. pertaining to the heart and diaphragm
3. instrument for measuring color
4. inflammation of the tear duct and sinuses
5. inside the stomach
6. hernia of the intestine
7. pain in the esophagus
8. pertaining to the stomach and lungs
9. pertaining to within the head

10. pertaining to disease of the spinal cord
11. surgical crushing of a nerve
12. pertaining to beside the spleen
13. pertaining to around the tonsils
14. surgical incision of the pylorus
15. pertaining to formation of pus
16. pertaining to the spleen and lymph glands
17. above the shoulder blade
18. pertaining to the bladder and abdomen

Crossword 1:

Row 1: T R A N S V E R S E   D
Row 2: (O)
Row 3: V E N T R A L   L U M B A R   R
Row 4: S
Row 5: L A T E R A L   C A U D A L
Row 6: M   L
Row 7: C   E   B
Row 8: E   H Y P O C H O N D R I A C
Row 9: P   I   L
Row 10: H Y P O G A S T R I C   I
Row 11: A   A   C   M
Row 12: L   I   S   C O R O N A L   E
Row 13: I   L   T   L   D
Row 14: C   I   R   I
Row 15: S A G I T T A L   A
Row 16: C   C   L

Crossword 2:

Row 1: A D D U C T I O N   D E E P
Row 2: B
Row 3: D   B
Row 4: U N I L A T E R A L
Row 5: C   L
Row 6: T   A F F E R E N T   F
Row 7: I   T   V   L
Row 8: O   E X T E N S I O N   E
Row 9: N   R   R   X
Row 10: A   S   I
Row 11: L   I N V E R S I O N
Row 12: O   F   N
Row 13: P R O N E   F   P
Row 14: A   E   L
Row 15: L   S U P E R F I C I A L
Row 16: M   E   N
Row 17: A   S U P I N E   T
Row 18: R   T   A
Row 19: R

# Appendix A

## Combining Forms, Prefixes, and Suffixes Alphabetized According to Word Part

| COMBINING FORM | DEFINITION | CHAPTER |
|---|---|---|
| abdomin/o | abdomen | 10 |
| acou/o | hearing | 12 |
| acr/o | extremities, height | 15 |
| adenoid/o | adenoids | 4 |
| aden/o | gland | 3 |
| adrenal/o | adrenal gland | 15 |
| adren/o | adrenal gland | 15 |
| albumin/o | albumin | 5 |
| alveol/o | alveolus | 4 |
| amni/o | amnion | 8 |
| amnion/o | amnion | 8 |
| andr/o | male | 6 |
| angi/o | vessel | 9 |
| ankyl/o | crooked, stiff, bent | 13 |
| antr/o | antrum | 10 |
| an/o | anus | 10 |
| aort/o | aorta | 9 |
| aponeur/o | aponeurosis | 13 |
| appendic/o | appendix | 10 |
| arche/o | first, beginning | 7 |
| arteri/o | artery | 9 |
| arthr/o | joint | 13 |
| atel/o | imperfect, incomplete | 4 |
| ather/o | yellowish, fatty plaque | 9 |
| atri/o | atrium | 9 |

| COMBINING FORM | DEFINITION | CHAPTER |
|---|---|---|
| aur/i | ear | 12 |
| aur/o | ear | 12 |
| aut/o | self | 3 |
| azot/o | urea, nitrogen | 5 |
| bacteri/o | bacteria | 9 |
| balan/o | glans penis | 6 |
| bi/o | life | 3 |
| blast/o | developing cell | 5 |
| blephar/o | eyelid | 11 |
| bronch/i | bronchus | 4 |
| bronchiol/o | bronchiole | 4 |
| bronch/o | bronchus | 4 |
| burs/o | bursa (cavity) | 13 |
| calc/i | calcium | 15 |
| cancer/o | cancer | 2 |
| carcin/o | cancer | 2 |
| cardi/o | heart | 9 |
| carp/o | carpals (wrist bones) | 13 |
| cec/o | cecum | 10 |
| celi/o | abdomen (abdominal cavity) | 10 |
| cephal/o | head | 8 |
| cerebell/o | cerebellum | 14 |
| cerebr/o | cerebrum, brain | 14 |
| cervic/o | cervix | 7 |
| cheil/o | lip | 10 |
| cholangi/o | bile duct | 10 |
| chol/e | gall, bile | 10 |
| choledoch/o | common bile duct | 10 |
| chondr/o | cartilage | 13 |
| chori/o | chorion | 8 |
| chrom/o | color | 2 |
| clavic/o | clavicle (collarbone) | 13 |

| COMBINING FORM | DEFINITION | CHAPTER |
|---|---|---|
| clavicul/o | clavicle (collarbone) | 13 |
| col/o | colon | 10 |
| colp/o | vagina | 7 |
| coni/o | dust | 3 |
| conjunctiv/o | conjunctiva | 11 |
| core/o | pupil | 11 |
| corne/o | cornea | 11 |
| coron/o | heart | 9 |
| cortic/o | cortex (outer layer of body organ) | 15 |
| cor/o | pupil | 11 |
| cost/o | rib | 13 |
| crani/o | cranium (skull) | 13 |
| cry/o | cold | 11 |
| crypt/o | hidden | 3 |
| culd/o | cul-de-sac | 7 |
| cutane/o | skin | 3 |
| cyan/o | blue | 2 |
| cyes/i | pregnancy | 8 |
| cyes/o | pregnancy | 8 |
| cyst/o | bladder, sac | 5 |
| cyt/o | cell | 2 |
| dacry/o | tear, tear duct | 11 |
| dermat/o | skin | 3 |
| derm/o | skin | 3 |
| diaphragmat/o | diaphragm | 4 |
| dipl/o | two, double | 11 |
| dips/o | thirst | 15 |
| disk/o | intervertebral disk | 13 |
| diverticul/o | diverticulum | 10 |
| duoden/o | duodenum | 10 |
| dur/o | hard, dura mater | 14 |
| ech/o | sound | 9 |
| electr/o | electricity, electrical activity | 9 |

| COMBINING FORM | DEFINITION | CHAPTER |
|---|---|---|
| embry/o | embryo, to be full | 8 |
| encephal/o | brain | 14 |
| endocrin/o | endocrine | 15 |
| enter/o | intestines | 10 |
| epididym/o | epididymis | 6 |
| epiglott/o | epiglottis | 4 |
| episi/o | vulva | 7 |
| epitheli/o | epithelium | 2 |
| erythr/o | red | 2 |
| esophag/o | esophagus | 8, 10 |
| esthesi/o | sensation, sensitivity, feeling | 14 |
| eti/o | cause (of disease) | 2 |
| femor/o | femur (upper leg bone) | 13 |
| fet/i | fetus, unborn child | 8 |
| fet/o | fetus, unborn child | 8 |
| fibr/o | fibrous tissue, fibers | 3 |
| fibul/o | fibula (lower leg bone) | 13 |
| gangli/o | ganglion | 14 |
| ganglion/o | ganglion | 14 |
| gastr/o | stomach | 10 |
| gingiv/o | gum | 10 |
| glomerul/o | glomerulus | 5 |
| gloss/o | tongue | 10 |
| glyc/o | sugar | 5 |
| glycos/o | sugar | 5 |
| gnos/o | knowledge | 2 |
| gravid/o | pregnancy | 8 |
| gynec/o | woman | 7 |
| gyn/o | woman | 7 |
| hem/o | blood | 4 |
| hemat/o | blood | 4 |
| hepat/o | liver | 10 |
| herni/o | hernia | 10 |

| COMBINING FORM | DEFINITION | CHAPTER |
|---|---|---|
| heter/o | other | 3 |
| hidr/o | sweat | 3 |
| hist/o | tissue | 2 |
| humer/o | humerus (upper arm bone) | 13 |
| hydr/o | water | 5 |
| hymen/o | hymen | 7 |
| hyster/o | uterus | 7 |
| iatr/o | medicine, physician | 2 |
| ile/o | ileum | 10 |
| ili/o | ilium | 13 |
| irid/o | iris | 11 |
| iri/o | iris | 11 |
| ischi/o | ischium | 13 |
| isch/o | deficiency, blockage | 9 |
| jejun/o | jejunum | 10 |
| kal/i | potassium | 15 |
| kary/o | nucleus | 2 |
| kerat/o | cornea | 11 |
| kerat/o | horny tissue, hard | 3 |
| kinesi/o | movement, motion | 13 |
| kyph/o | hump | 13 |
| labyrinth/o | labyrinth | 12 |
| lacrim/o | tear duct, tear | 11 |
| lact/o | milk | 8 |
| lamin/o | lamina (thin, flat plate or layer) | 13 |
| lapar/o | abdomen | 10 |
| laryng/o | larynx | 4 |
| lei/o | smooth | 2 |
| leuk/o | white | 2 |
| lingu/o | tongue | 10 |
| lip/o | fat | 2 |
| lith/o | stone, calculus | 5 |
| lob/o | lobe | 4 |

| COMBINING FORM | DEFINITION | CHAPTER |
|---|---|---|
| lord/o | bent forward | 13 |
| lymph/o | lymph | 9 |
| mamm/o | breast | 7 |
| mandibul/o | mandible (lower jawbone) | 13 |
| mast/o | breast | 7 |
| mastoid/o | mastoid | 12 |
| maxill/o | maxilla (upper jawbone) | 13 |
| meat/o | meatus (opening) | 5 |
| melan/o | black | 2 |
| mening/i | meninges | 14 |
| mening/o | meninges | 14 |
| menisc/o | meniscus (crescent) | 13 |
| men/o | menstruation | 7 |
| ment/o | mind | 14 |
| metr/i | uterus | 7 |
| metr/o | uterus | 7 |
| mon/o | one | 14 |
| muc/o | mucus | 4 |
| myc/o | fungus | 3 |
| myel/o | bone marrow | 13 |
| myel/o | spinal cord | 14 |
| myelon/o | bone marrow | 13 |
| myos/o | muscle | 13 |
| myring/o | eardrum | 12 |
| my/o | muscle | 2, 13 |
| nas/o | nose | 4 |
| nat/o | birth | 8 |
| necr/o | death (cells, body) | 3 |
| nephr/o | kidney | 5 |
| neur/o | nerve | 2, 14 |
| noct/i | night | 5 |
| ocul/o | eye | 11 |
| olig/o | scanty, few | 5 |
| omphal/o | umbilicus, navel | 8 |

| COMBINING FORM | DEFINITION | CHAPTER |
|---|---|---|
| onc/o | tumor | 2 |
| onych/o | nail | 3 |
| oophor/o | ovary | 7 |
| ophthalm/o | eye | 11 |
| opt/o | vision | 11 |
| orchid/o | testis, testicle | 6 |
| orchi/o | testis, testicle | 6 |
| orch/o | testis, testicle | 6 |
| organ/o | organ | 2 |
| or/o | mouth | 10 |
| orth/o | straight | 4 |
| oste/o | bone | 13 |
| ot/o | ear | 12 |
| ox/i | oxygen | 4 |
| ox/o | oxygen | 4 |
| pachy/o | thick | 3 |
| palat/o | palate | 10 |
| pancreat/o | pancreas | 10 |
| parathyroid/o | parathyroid gland | 15 |
| par/o | bear, give birth to, labor | 8 |
| patell/o | patella (kneecap) | 13 |
| path/o | disease | 2 |
| part/o | bear, give birth to, labor | 8 |
| pelv/i | pelvis, pelvic bone | 8 |
| pelv/o | pelvis, pelvic bone | 8 |
| perine/o | perineum | 7 |
| peritone/o | peritoneum | 10 |
| petr/o | stone | 13 |
| phalang/o | phalanx (finger or toe bone) | 13 |
| pharyng/o | pharynx | 4 |
| phas/o | speech | 14 |
| phleb/o | vein | 9 |
| phot/o | light | 11 |

| COMBINING FORM | DEFINITION | CHAPTER |
|---|---|---|
| phren/o | mind | 14 |
| plasm/o | plasma | 9 |
| pleur/o | pleura | 4 |
| pneumat/o | lung, air | 4 |
| pneum/o | lung, air | 4 |
| pneumon/o | lung, air | 4 |
| poli/o | gray matter | 14 |
| polyp/o | polyp, small growth | 10 |
| prim/i | first | 8 |
| proct/o | rectum | 10 |
| prostat/o | prostate gland | 6 |
| pseud/o | false | 8 |
| psych/o | mind | 14 |
| pub/o | pubis | 13 |
| puerper/o | childbirth | 8 |
| pulmon/o | lung | 4 |
| pupill/o | pupil | 11 |
| pyel/o | renal pelvis | 5 |
| pylor/o | pylorus (pyloric sphincter) | 8, 10 |
| py/o | pus | 4 |
| quadr/i | four | 14 |
| rachi/o | vertebra, spinal or vertebral column | 13 |
| radic/o | nerve root | 14 |
| radicul/o | nerve root | 14 |
| radi/o | radius (lower arm bone) | 13 |
| rect/o | rectum | 10 |
| ren/o | kidney | 5 |
| retin/o | retina | 11 |
| rhabd/o | rod-shaped, striated | 2 |
| rhin/o | nose | 4 |
| rhytid/o | wrinkles | 3 |
| rhiz/o | nerve root | 14 |
| salping/o | fallopian (uterine) tube | 7 |

| COMBINING FORM | DEFINITION | CHAPTER |
|---|---|---|
| sarc/o | flesh, connective tissue | 2 |
| scapul/o | scapula (shoulder bone) | 13 |
| scler/o | sclera | 11 |
| scoli/o | crooked, curved | 13 |
| seb/o | sebum (oil) | 3 |
| sept/o | septum | 4 |
| sial/o | saliva | 10 |
| sigmoid/o | sigmoid | 10 |
| sinus/o | sinus | 4 |
| somat/o | body | 2 |
| son/o | sound | 5 |
| spermat/o | spermatozoan, sperm | 6 |
| sperm/o | spermatozoan, sperm | 6 |
| sphygm/o | pulse | 9 |
| spir/o | breathe, breathing | 4 |
| splen/o | spleen | 9 |
| spondyl/o | vertebra, spinal or vertebral column | 13 |
| staped/o | stapes (middle ear bone) | 12 |
| staphyl/o | grapelike clusters | 3 |
| stern/o | sternum (breastbone) | 13 |
| steth/o | chest | 9 |
| stomat/o | mouth | 10 |
| strept/o | twisted chains | 3 |
| synovi/o | synovia, synovial membrane | 13 |
| system/o | system | 2 |
| tars/o | tarsals (ankle bones) | 13 |
| tendin/o | tendon | 13 |
| tend/o | tendon | 13 |
| ten/o | tendon | 13 |
| test/o | testis, testicle | 6 |
| therm/o | heat | 9 |
| thorac/o | thorax (chest) | 4 |

| COMBINING FORM | DEFINITION | CHAPTER |
|---|---|---|
| thromb/o | clot | 9 |
| thym/o | thymus gland | 9 |
| thyroid/o | thyroid gland | 15 |
| thyr/o | thyroid gland | 15 |
| tibi/o | tibia (lower leg bone) | 13 |
| tom/o | cut, section | 5 |
| ton/o | tension, pressure | 11 |
| tonsill/o | tonsils | 4 |
| toxic/o | poison | 15 |
| trachel/o | neck, necklike | 5 |
| trache/o | trachea | 4 |
| trich/o | hair | 3 |
| tympan/o | eardrum, middle ear | 12 |
| uln/o | ulna (lower arm bone) | 13 |
| ungu/o | nail | 3 |
| ureter/o | ureter | 5 |
| urethr/o | urethra | 5 |
| urin/o | urine, urinary tract | 5 |
| ur/o | urine, urinary tract | 5 |
| uter/o | uterus | 7 |
| uvul/o | uvula | 10 |
| vagin/o | vagina | 7 |
| valv/o | valve | 9 |
| valvul/o | valve | 9 |
| vas/o | vessel, duct | 6 |
| ven/o | vein | 5 |
| ventricul/o | ventricle | 9 |
| vertebr/o | vertebra, spinal or vertebral column | 13 |
| vesic/o | bladder, sac | 5 |
| vesicul/o | seminal vesicles | 6 |
| viscer/o | internal organs | 2 |
| vulv/o | vulva | 7 |
| xanth/o | yellow | 2 |
| xer/o | dry | 3 |

| PREFIX | DEFINITION | CHAPTER |
|--------|-----------|---------|
| a- | without or absence of | 4 |
| an- | without or absence of | 4 |
| ante- | before | 8 |
| bi- | two | 11 |
| bin- | two | 11 |
| brady- | slow | 9 |
| dia- | through, complete | 2 |
| dys- | difficult, labored, painful, abnormal | 2 |
| endo- | within | 4 |
| epi- | on, upon, over | 3 |
| eu- | normal, good | 4 |
| ex- | outside, outward | 15 |
| exo- | outside, outward | 15 |
| hemi- | half | 13 |
| hyper- | above, excessive | 2 |
| hypo- | below, incomplete, deficient | 2 |
| inter- | between | 13 |
| intra- | within | 3 |
| meta- | after, beyond, change | 2 |
| micro- | small | 8 |
| multi- | many | 8 |
| neo- | new | 2 |
| nulli- | none | 8 |
| pan- | all, total | 4 |
| para- | beside, beyond, around | 3 |
| per- | through | 3 |
| peri- | surrounding (outer) | 7 |
| poly- | many, much | 5 |
| post- | after | 8 |
| pre- | before | 14 |
| pro- | before | 2 |

| PREFIX | DEFINITION | CHAPTER |
|---|---|---|
| sub- | under, below | 3 |
| supra- | above | 13 |
| sym- | together, joined | 13 |
| syn- | together, joined | 13 |
| tachy- | fast, rapid | 9 |
| tetra- | four | 13 |
| trans- | through, across, beyond | 6 |

| SUFFIX | DEFINITION | CHAPTER |
|---|---|---|
| -ac | pertaining to | 9 |
| -al | pertaining to | 2 |
| -algia | pain | 4 |
| -apheresis | removal | 9 |
| -ar | pertaining to | 4 |
| -ary | pertaining to | 4 |
| -asthenia | weakness | 13 |
| -atresia | absence of a normal body opening, occlusion, closure | 7 |
| -capnia | carbon dioxide | 4 |
| -cele | hernia, protrusion | 4 |
| -centesis | surgical puncture to aspirate fluid | 4 |
| -clasia | break | 13 |
| -clasis | break | 13 |
| -clast | break | 13 |
| -coccus (*pl.* cocci) | berry-shaped (a form of bacterium) | 3 |
| -crit | to separate | 9 |
| -cyte | cell | 2 |
| -desis | surgical fixation, fusion | 13 |
| -drome | run, running | 15 |
| -eal | pertaining to | 4 |
| -ectasis | stretching out, dilatation, expansion | 4 |
| -ectomy | excision or surgical removal | 3 |

| SUFFIX | DEFINITION | CHAPTER |
|---|---|---|
| -emia | blood condition | 4 |
| -esis | condition | 5 |
| -gen | substance or agent that produces or causes | 2 |
| -genesis | origin, cause | 2 |
| -genic | producing, originating, causing | 2 |
| -gram | record, x-ray film | 4 |
| -graph | instrument used to record | 9 |
| -graphy | process of recording, x-ray filming | 4 |
| -ia | condition of diseased or abnormal state | 3 |
| -ial | pertaining to | 7 |
| -iasis | condition | 5 |
| -iatry | physician, treatment | 14 |
| -ic | pertaining to | 2 |
| -ician | one who | 11 |
| -ictal | seizure, attack | 14 |
| -ism | state of | 6 |
| -itis | inflammation | 3 |
| -lysis | loosening, dissolution, separating | 5 |
| -malacia | softening | 3 |
| -megaly | enlargement | 5 |
| -meter | instrument used to measure | 4 |
| -metry | measurement | 4 |
| -odynia | pain | 9 |
| -oid | resembling | 2 |
| -ologist | one who studies and practices (specialist) | 2 |
| -ology | study of | 2 |
| -oma | tumor, swelling | 2 |
| -opia | vision (condition) | 11 |
| -opsy | to view | 3 |

| SUFFIX | DEFINITION | CHAPTER |
|--------|-----------|---------|
| -orrhagia | rapid flow of blood | 4 |
| -orrhaphy | suturing, repairing | 5 |
| -orrhea | flow, excessive discharge | 3 |
| -orrhexis | rupture | 8 |
| -osis | abnormal condition (means increased when used with blood cell word roots) | 2 |
| -ostomy | creation of an artificial opening | 4 |
| -otomy | cut into or incision | 4 |
| -ous | pertaining to | 2 |
| -oxia | oxygen | 4 |
| -paresis | slight paralysis | 14 |
| -pathy | disease | 2 |
| -penia | abnormal reduction in number | 9 |
| -pepsia | digestion | 10 |
| -pexy | surgical fixation, suspension | 4 |
| -phagia | eating, swallowing | 3 |
| -phobia | abnormal fear of or aversion to specific objects or things | 11 |
| -phonia | sound or voice | 4 |
| -physis | growth | 13 |
| -plasia | formation, development, a growth | 2 |
| -plasm | growth, substance, formation | 2 |
| -plasty | plastic or surgical repair | 3 |
| -plegia | paralysis | 11 |
| -pnea | breathing | 4 |
| -poiesis | formation | 9 |
| -ptosis | dropping, sagging, prolapse | 5 |

| SUFFIX | DEFINITION | CHAPTER |
|---|---|---|
| -salpinx | fallopian tube | 6 |
| -sarcoma | malignant tumor | 2 |
| -schisis | split, fissure | 13 |
| -sclerosis | hardening | 9 |
| -scope | instrument used for visual examination | 4 |
| -scopy | visual examination | 4 |
| -scopic | visual examination | 4 |
| -sis | state of | 2 |
| -spasm | sudden involuntary muscle contraction | 4 |
| -stasis | control, stop | 2 |
| -stenosis | constriction, narrowing | 4 |
| -thorax | chest | 4 |
| -tocia | birth, labor | 8 |
| -tome | instrument used to cut | 3 |
| -tripsy | surgical crushing | 5 |
| -trophy | nourishment, development | 5 |
| -uria | urine, urination | 5 |

# Appendix B

## Combining Forms, Prefixes, and Suffixes Alphabetized According to the Meaning of the Word Part

| DEFINITION | COMBINING FORM | CHAPTER |
|---|---|---|
| abdomen | abdomin/o | 10 |
| abdomen | lapar/o | 10 |
| abdomen (abdominal cavity) | celi/o | 10 |
| adenoids | adenoid/o | 4 |
| adrenal gland | adren/o | 15 |
| adrenal gland | adrenal/o | 15 |
| albumin | albumin/o | 5 |
| alveolus | alveol/o | 4 |
| amnion | amni/o | 8 |
| amnion | amnion/o | 8 |
| antrum | antr/o | 10 |
| anus | an/o | 10 |
| aorta | aort/o | 9 |
| aponeurosis | aponeur/o | 13 |
| appendix | appendic/o | 10 |
| artery | arteri/o | 9 |
| atrium | atri/o | 9 |
| bacteria | bacteri/o | 9 |
| bear, give birth to, labor | part/o | 8 |
| bear, give birth to, labor | par/o | 8 |
| bent forward | lord/o | 13 |
| bile duct | cholangi/o | 10 |
| birth | nat/o | 8 |
| black | melan/o | 2 |

| DEFINITION | COMBINING FORM | CHAPTER |
|---|---|---|
| bladder, sac | cyst/o | 5 |
| bladder, sac | vesic/o | 5 |
| blood | hemat/o | 4 |
| blood | hem/o | 4 |
| blue | cyan/o | 2 |
| body | somat/o | 2 |
| bone | oste/o | 13 |
| bone marrow | myelon/o | 13 |
| bone marrow | myel/o | 13 |
| brain | encephal/o | 14 |
| breast | mamm/o | 7 |
| breast | mast/o | 7 |
| breathe, breathing | spir/o | 4 |
| bronchus | bronch/i, bronch/o | 4 |
| bronchiole | bronchiol/o | 4 |
| bursa (cavity) | burs/o | 13 |
| calcium | calc/i | 15 |
| cancer | cancer/o | 2 |
| cancer | carcin/o | 2 |
| carpus (wrist bone) | carp/o | 13 |
| cartilage | chondr/o | 13 |
| cause (of disease) | eti/o | 2 |
| cecum | cec/o | 10 |
| cell | cyt/o | 2 |
| cerebellum | cerebell/o | 14 |
| cerebrum, brain | cerebr/o | 14 |
| cervix | cervic/o | 7 |
| chest | steth/o | 9 |
| childbirth | puerper/o | 8 |
| chorion | chori/o | 8 |
| clavicle (collar bone) | clavic/o | 13 |
| clavicle (collar bone) | clavicul/o | 13 |
| clot | thromb/o | 9 |
| cold | cry/o | 11 |

| DEFINITION | COMBINING FORM | CHAPTER |
|---|---|---|
| colon | col/o | 10 |
| color | chrom/o | 2 |
| common bile duct | choledoch/o | 10 |
| conjunctiva | conjunctiv/o | 11 |
| cornea | corne/o | 11 |
| cornea | kerat/o | 11 |
| cortex | cortic/o | 15 |
| cranium, skull | crani/o | 13 |
| crooked, curved | scoli/o | 13 |
| crooked, stiff, bent | ankyl/o | 13 |
| cul-de-sac | culd/o | 7 |
| cut, section | tom/o | 5 |
| death (cells, body) | necr/o | 3 |
| deficiency, blockage | isch/o | 9 |
| developing cell | blast/o | 5 |
| diaphragm | diaphragmat/o | 4 |
| disease | path/o | 2 |
| diverticulum | diverticul/o | 10 |
| dry | xer/o | 3 |
| duodenum | duoden/o | 10 |
| dust | coni/o | 3 |
| ear | ot/o | 12 |
| ear | aur/i, aur/o | 12 |
| eardrum | myring/o | 12 |
| eardrum, middle ear | tympan/o | 12 |
| electricity, electrical activity | electr/o | 9 |
| embryo, to be full | embry/o | 8 |
| endocrine | endocrin/o | 16 |
| epididymis | epididym/o | 6 |
| epiglottis | epiglott/o | 4 |
| epithelium | epitheli/o | 2 |
| esophagus | esophag/o | 8, 10 |
| extremities, height | acr/o | 15 |
| eye | ophthalm/o | 11 |
| eye | ocul/o | 11 |

| DEFINITION | COMBINING FORM | CHAPTER |
|---|---|---|
| eyelid | blephar/o | 11 |
| fallopian tube | salping/o | 7 |
| false | pseud/o | 8 |
| fat | lip/o | 2 |
| femur (upper leg bone) | femor/o | 13 |
| fetus, unborn child | fet/o, fet/i | 8 |
| fibrous tissue, fibers | fibr/o | 3 |
| fibula (lower leg bone) | fibul/o | 13 |
| first | prim/i | 8 |
| first, beginning | arche/o | 7 |
| flesh, connective tissue | sarc/o | 2 |
| four | quadr/i | 14 |
| fungus | myc/o | 3 |
| gall, bile | chol/e | 10 |
| ganglion | gangli/o | 14 |
| ganglion | ganglion/o | 14 |
| gland | aden/o | 3 |
| glans penis | balan/o | 6 |
| glomerulus | glomerul/o | 5 |
| grape-like clusters | staphyl/o | 3 |
| gray matter | poli/o | 14 |
| gum | gingiv/o | 10 |
| hair | trich/o | 3 |
| hard, dura mater | dur/o | 14 |
| head | cephal/o | 8 |
| hearing | aud/i | 12 |
| hearing | acou/o | 12 |
| heart | cardi/o, coron/o | 9 |
| heat | therm/o | 9 |
| hernia | herni/o | 10 |
| hidden | crypt/o | 3 |
| horny tissue, hard | kerat/o | 3 |
| humerus (upper arm bone) | humer/o | 13 |
| hump | kyph/o | 13 |
| hymen | hymen/o | 7 |

| DEFINITION | COMBINING FORM | CHAPTER |
|---|---|---|
| ileum | ile/o | 10 |
| ilium | ili/o | 13 |
| imperfect, incomplete | atel/o | 4 |
| internal organs | viscer/o | 2 |
| intervertebral disk | disk/o | 13 |
| intestines | enter/o | 10 |
| iris | irid/o | 11 |
| iris | iri/o | 11 |
| ischium | ischi/o | 13 |
| jejunum | jejun/o | 10 |
| joint | arthr/o | 13 |
| kidney | nephr/o | 5 |
| kidney | ren/o | 5 |
| knowledge | gnos/o | 2 |
| labyrinth | labyrinth/o | 12 |
| lamina (thin flat plate or layer) | lamin/o | 13 |
| larynx | laryng/o | 4 |
| life | bi/o | 3 |
| light | phot/o | 11 |
| lip | cheil/o | 10 |
| liver | hepat/o | 10 |
| lobe | lob/o | 4 |
| lung | pulmon/o | 4 |
| lung, air | pneumat/o | 4 |
| lung, air | pneum/o | 4 |
| lung, air | pneumon/o | 4 |
| lymph | lymph/o | 9 |
| male | andr/o | 6 |
| mandible (upper jaw bone) | mandibul/o | 13 |
| mastoid | mastoid/o | 12 |
| maxilla (lower jaw bone) | maxill/o | 13 |
| meatus (opening) | meat/o | 5 |
| medicine | iatr/o | 2 |
| meninges | mening/o, mening/i | 14 |

| DEFINITION | COMBINING FORM | CHAPTER |
|---|---|---|
| meniscus (crescent) | menisc/o | 13 |
| menstruation | men/o | 7 |
| milk | lact/o | 8 |
| mind | ment/o | 14 |
| mind | psych/o | 14 |
| mind | phren/o | 14 |
| mouth | or/o | 10 |
| mouth | stomat/o | 10 |
| movement, motion | kinesi/o | 13 |
| mucus | muc/o | 4 |
| muscle | my/o | 2, 13 |
| muscle | myos/o | 13 |
| nail | ungu/o | 3 |
| nail | onych/o | 3 |
| neck, neck-like | trachel/o | 5 |
| nerve | neur/o | 2, 14 |
| nerve root | radicul/o | 14 |
| nerve root | radic/o | 14 |
| nerve root | rhiz/o | 14 |
| night | noct/i | 5 |
| nose | rhin/o | 4 |
| nose | nas/o | 4 |
| nucleus | kary/o | 2 |
| one | mon/o | 14 |
| organ | organ/o | 2 |
| other | heter/o | 3 |
| ovary | oophor/o | 7 |
| oxygen | ox/o, ox/i | 4 |
| palate | palat/o | 10 |
| pancreas | pancreat/o | 10 |
| parathyroid gland | parathyroid/o | 15 |
| patella (kneecap) | patell/o | 13 |
| pelvis, pelvic bone | pelv/i, pelv/o | 8 |
| perineum | perine/o | 7 |

| DEFINITION | COMBINING FORM | CHAPTER |
|---|---|---|
| peritoneum | peritone/o | 10 |
| phalanx, finger or toe bone | phalang/o | 13 |
| pharynx | pharyng/o | 4 |
| physician | iatr/o | 2 |
| plasma | plasm/o | 9 |
| pleura | pleur/o | 4 |
| poison | toxic/o | 15 |
| potassium | kal/i | 15 |
| pregnancy | cyes/o, cyes/i | 8 |
| pregnancy | gravid/o | 8 |
| prostate gland | prostat/o | 6 |
| pubis | pub/o | 13 |
| pulse | sphygm/o | 9 |
| pupil | core/o, cor/o | 11 |
| pupil | pupill/o | 11 |
| pus | py/o | 4 |
| pylorus, pyloric sphincter | pylor/o | 10, 8 |
| radius (lower arm bone) | radi/o | 13 |
| rectum | proct/o | 10 |
| rectum | rect/o | 10 |
| red | erythr/o | 2 |
| renal pelvis | pyel/o | 5 |
| retina | retin/o | 11 |
| rib | cost/o | 13 |
| rod shaped, striated | rhabd/o | 2 |
| saliva | sial/o | 10 |
| scanty, few | olig/o | 5 |
| scapula (shoulder bone) | scapul/o | 13 |
| sclera | scler/o | 11 |
| sebum (oil) | seb/o | 3 |
| self | aut/o | 3 |
| seminal vesicles | vesicul/o | 6 |
| sensation, sensitivity, feeling | esthesi/o | 14 |

| DEFINITION | COMBINING FORM | CHAPTER |
|---|---|---|
| septum | sept/o | 4 |
| sigmoid | sigmoid/o | 10 |
| sinus | sinus/o | 4 |
| skin | cutane/o | 3 |
| skin | dermat/o | 3 |
| skin | derm/o | 3 |
| small growth | polyp/o | 10 |
| smooth | lei/o | 2 |
| sound | son/o | 5 |
| sound | ech/o | 9 |
| speech | phas/o | 14 |
| spermatozoa, sperm | sperm/o | 6 |
| spermatozoa, sperm | spermat/o | 6 |
| spinal cord | myel/o | 14 |
| spleen | splen/o | 9 |
| stapes | staped/o | 12 |
| sternum (breast bone) | stern/o | 13 |
| stomach | gastr/o | 10 |
| stone | petr/o | 13 |
| stone, calculus | lith/o | 5 |
| straight | orth/o | 4 |
| sugar | glycos/o | 5 |
| sugar | glyc/o | 5 |
| sweat | hidr/o | 3 |
| synovia, synovial membrane | synovi/o | 13 |
| system | system/o | 2 |
| tarsus (ankle bone) | tars/o | 13 |
| tear duct, tear | lacrim/o | 11 |
| tear, tear duct | dacry/o | 11 |
| tendon | ten/o | 13 |
| tendon | tendin/o | 13 |
| tendon | tend/o | 13 |
| tension, pressure | ton/o | 11 |

| DEFINITION | COMBINING FORM | CHAPTER |
|---|---|---|
| testis, testicle | orch/o | 6 |
| testis, testicle | test/o | 6 |
| testis, testicle | orchi/o | 6 |
| testis, testicle | orchid/o | 6 |
| thick | pachy/o | 3 |
| thorax (chest) | thorac/o | 4 |
| thirst | dips/o | 15 |
| thymus gland | thym/o | 9 |
| thyroid gland | thyroid/o | 15 |
| thyroid gland | thyr/o | 15 |
| tibia (lower leg bone) | tibi/o | 13 |
| tissue | hist/o | 2 |
| tongue | lingu/o | 10 |
| tongue | gloss/o | 10 |
| tonsils | tonsill/o | 4 |
| trachea | trache/o | 4 |
| tumor | onc/o | 2 |
| twisted chains | strept/o | 3 |
| two, double | dipl/o | 11 |
| ulna (lower arm bone) | uln/o | 13 |
| umbilicus, navel | omphal/o | 8 |
| urea, nitrogen | azot/o | 5 |
| ureter | ureter/o | 5 |
| urethra | urethr/o | 5 |
| urinary bladder | vesic/o | 5 |
| urine, urinary tract | urin/o | 5 |
| urine, urinary tract | ur/o | 5 |
| uterus | uter/o | 7 |
| uterus | metr/o, metr/i | 7 |
| uterus | hyster/o | 7 |
| uvula | uvul/o | 10 |
| vagina | vagin/o | 7 |
| vagina | colp/o | 7 |
| valve | valv/o | 9 |

| DEFINITION | COMBINING FORM | CHAPTER |
|---|---|---|
| valve | valvul/o | 9 |
| vein | phleb/o | 9 |
| vein | ven/o | 5 |
| ventricle | ventricul/o | 9 |
| vertebra, spinal column, vertebral column | vertebr/o | 13 |
| vertebra, spinal column, vertebral column | spondyl/o | 13 |
| vertebra, spinal or vertebral column | rachi/o | 13 |
| vessel | angi/o | 9 |
| vessel, duct | vas/o | 6 |
| vision | opt/o | 11 |
| vulva | vulv/o | 7 |
| vulva | episi/o | 7 |
| water | hydr/o | 5 |
| white | leuk/o | 2 |
| woman | gyn/o | 7 |
| woman | gynec/o | 7 |
| wrinkles | rhytid/o | 3 |
| yellow | xanth/o | 2 |
| yellowish, fatty plaque | ather/o | 9 |

| DEFINITION | PREFIX | CHAPTER |
|---|---|---|
| above | supra- | 13 |
| above, excessive | hyper- | 2 |
| after | post- | 8 |
| after, beyond, change | meta- | 2 |
| all, total | pan- | 4 |
| before | ante- | 8 |
| before | pro- | 2 |
| below, incomplete, deficient | hypo- | 2 |
| beside, beyond, around | para- | 3 |
| between | inter- | 13 |
| difficult, labored, painful, abnormal | dys- | 2 |

| DEFINITION | PREFIX | CHAPTER |
|---|---|---|
| fast, rapid | tachy- | 9 |
| four | tetra- | 13 |
| half | hemi- | 13 |
| many | multi- | 8 |
| many, much | poly- | 5 |
| new | neo- | 2 |
| none | nulli- | 8 |
| normal | eu- | 4 |
| on, upon, over | epi- | 3 |
| outside, outward | ex, exo- | 13 |
| slow | brady- | 9 |
| small | micro- | 8 |
| surrounding (outer) | peri- | 7 |
| through, complete | per- | 3 |
| through | dia- | 2 |
| through, across, beyond | trans- | 6 |
| together, joined | sym- | 13 |
| together, joined | syn- | 13 |
| two | bin- | 13 |
| two | bi- | 13 |
| under, below | sub- | 3 |
| within | intra- | 3 |
| within | endo- | 4 |
| without or absence of | a, an- | 4 |

| DEFINITION | SUFFIX | CHAPTER |
|---|---|---|
| abnormal fear of or aversion to specific objects or things | -phobia | 11 |
| abnormal condition (means increased when used with blood cell word roots) | -osis | 2 |
| abnormal reduction in number | -penia | 9 |
| absence of a normal opening, occlusion, closure | -atresia | 7 |

| DEFINITION | SUFFIX | CHAPTER |
|---|---|---|
| berry-shaped (a form of bacterium) | -coccus (cocci, pl.) | 3 |
| birth, labor | -tocia | 8 |
| blood condition | -emia | 4 |
| break | -clasis | 13 |
| break | -clasia | 13 |
| break | -clast | 13 |
| breathing | -pnea | 4 |
| carbon dioxide | -capnia | 4 |
| cell | -cyte | 2 |
| chest | -thorax | 4 |
| condition | -iasis | 5 |
| condition | -esis | 5 |
| constriction, narrowing | -stenosis | 5 |
| control, stop | -stasis | 2 |
| constricted or narrowing | -stenosis | 4 |
| creation of an artificial opening | -ostomy | 4 |
| cut into or incision | -otomy | 4 |
| digestion | -pepsia | 10 |
| disease | -pathy | 2 |
| diseased or abnormal state | -ia | 3 |
| drooping, sagging, prolapse | -ptosis | 5 |
| eating, swallowing | -phagia | 3 |
| enlargement | -megaly | 5 |
| excision or surgical removal | -ectomy | 3 |
| fallopian tube | -salpinx | 6 |
| flow, excessive discharge | -orrhea | 3 |
| formation | -poiesis | 9 |
| formation, development, a growth | -plasia | 2 |
| growth | -physis | 13 |
| growth, substance, (formation) | -plasm | 2 |
| hardening | -sclerosis | 9 |
| hernia, protrusion | -cele | 4 |

| DEFINITION | SUFFIX | CHAPTER |
|---|---|---|
| inflammation | -itis | 3 |
| instrument for visual examination | -scope | 4 |
| instrument to measure | -meter | 4 |
| instrument used to cut | -tome | 3 |
| instrument used to record | -graph | 9 |
| loosening, dissolution, separating | -lysis | 5 |
| malignant tumor | -sarcoma | 2 |
| measurement | -metry | 4 |
| nourishment, development | -trophy | 5 |
| one who | -ician | 11 |
| one who studies and practices (specialist) | -ologist | 2 |
| origin, cause | -genesis | 2 |
| oxygen | -oxia | 4 |
| pain | -odynia | 9 |
| pain | -algia | 4 |
| paralysis | -plegia | 11 |
| pertaining to | -ac | 9 |
| pertaining to | -ous | 5 |
| pertaining to | -ar | 4 |
| pertaining to | -ic | 2 |
| pertaining to | -ial | 7 |
| pertaining to | -eal | 4 |
| pertaining to | -ary | 4 |
| pertaining to | -al | 2 |
| pertaining to | -ous | 2 |
| pertaining to sound or voice | -phonia | 4 |
| physician, treatment | -iatry | 14 |
| plastic or surgical repair | -plasty | 3 |
| process of recording, x-ray filming | -graphy | 4 |

| DEFINITION | SUFFIX | CHAPTER |
|---|---|---|
| producing, originating, causing | -genic,-genesis | 2 |
| rapid flow of blood | -orrhagia | 4 |
| record, x-ray | -gram | 4 |
| removal | -apheresis | 9 |
| resembling | -oid | 2 |
| run, running | -drome | 15 |
| rupture | -orrhexis | 8 |
| seizure, attack | -ictal | 14 |
| slight paralysis | -paresis | 14 |
| softening | -malacia | 3 |
| split, fissure | -schisis | 13 |
| state | -ism | 6 |
| state of | -sis | 2 |
| stretch out, dilatation, expansion | -ectasis | 4 |
| study of | -ology | 2 |
| substance or agent that produces or causes | -gen | 2 |
| sudden involuntary muscle contraction | -spasm | 4 |
| surgical crushing | -tripsy | 5 |
| surgical fixation, fusion | -desis | 13 |
| surgical fixation, suspension | -pexy | 4 |
| surgical puncture to aspirate fluid | -centesis | 4 |
| suturing, repairing | -orrhaphy | 5 |
| to separate | -crit | 9 |
| to view | -opsy | 3 |
| tumor, swelling | -oma | 2 |
| urine, urination | -uria | 5 |
| vision (condition) | -opia | 11 |
| visual examination | -scopic | 4 |
| visual examination | -scopy | 4 |
| weakness | -asthenia | 13 |

# Appendix C

## Additional Combining Forms, Prefixes, and Suffixes

The following word parts were not included in the text. They are listed here for your easy reference.

| COMBINING FORM | DEFINITION |
| --- | --- |
| acanth/o | thorny, spiny |
| acetabul/o | acetabulum (hip socket) |
| actin/o | ray, radius |
| aer/o | air, gas |
| algesi/o | pain |
| ambly/o | dull, dim |
| amyl/o | starch |
| anis/o | unequal, dissimilar |
| arteriol/o | arteriole (small artery) |
| articul/o | joint |
| axill/o | armpit |
| bil/i | bile |
| brachi/o | arm |
| bucc/o | cheek |
| caud/o | tail, toward the lower part of the body |
| cerumin/o | cerumen (earwax) |
| chir/o | hand |
| dactyl/o | fingers or toes |
| dent/i | tooth |
| dextr/o | right |
| diaphor/o | sweat |
| dors/i | back (of the body) |
| dors/o | back (of the body) |
| dynam/o | power or strength |

| COMBINING FORM | DEFINITION |
|---|---|
| ectop/o | located away from usual place |
| emmetr/o | a normal measure |
| faci/o | face |
| ger/o | old age, aged |
| geront/o | old age, aged |
| gluc/o | sweetness, sugar |
| gnath/o | jaw |
| gon/o | seed |
| home/o | sameness, unchanging |
| hom/o | same |
| hypn/o | sleep |
| ichthy/o | fish |
| immun/o | immune |
| is/o | equal, same |
| kin/e | movement |
| labi/o | lips |
| later/o | side |
| macr/o | abnormal largeness |
| morph/o | form, shape |
| narc/o | stupor |
| nyct/o | night |
| nyctal/o | night |
| oo/o | egg, ovum |
| ov/i | egg |
| ov/o | egg |
| papill/o | nipple |
| pector/o | chest |
| ped/o | child, foot |
| phac/o | lens of the eye |
| phag/o | eat, swallow |
| phak/o | lens of the eye |
| physi/o | nature |
| pod/o | foot |
| poikil/o | varied, irregular |

| COMBINING FORM | DEFINITION |
|---|---|
| poster/o | back (of body) |
| pyr/o | fever, heat |
| somn/i | sleep |
| tars/o | edge of eyelid, tarsal (instep of foot) |
| top/o | place |

| PREFIX | DEFINITION |
|---|---|
| ab- | from, away from |
| ad- | to, toward |
| ana- | up, again, backward |
| anti- | against |
| apo- | upon |
| cata- | down |
| con- | together |
| contra- | against |
| de- | from, down from, lack of |
| dis- | to undo. free from |
| ecto- | outside, outer |
| eso- | inward |
| extra- | outside of, beyond |
| in- | in, into, not |
| infra- | under, below |
| mal- | bad |
| meso- | middle |
| pre- | in front of, before |
| re- | back |
| retro- | back, behind |
| semi- | half |
| super- | over, above |
| tri- | three |
| ultra- | beyond, excess |
| uni- | one |

| SUFFIX | DEFINITION |
|---|---|
| -agra | excessive pain |
| -ase | enzyme |
| -cidal | killing |
| -clysis | irrigating, washing |
| -crine | separate, secrete |
| -ectopia | displacement |
| -emesis | vomiting |
| -er | one who |
| -lepsy | seizure |
| -lytic | destroy, reduce |
| -mania | madness, insane desire |
| -morph | form, shape |
| -odia | smell |
| -opia | vision |
| -philia | love |
| -phily | love |
| -phoria | feeling |
| -porosis | passage |
| -prandial | meal |
| -praxia | in front of, before |
| -ptysis | spitting |
| -sepsis | infection |
| -stalsis | contraction |
| -ule | little |

# Appendix D

## Abbreviations

These abbreviations are written as they appear most commonly in physician's orders and on patient charts. Some may also appear in both capital and small letters and with or without periods.

| COMMON MEDICAL ABBREVIATIONS | DEFINITION |
| --- | --- |
| @ | at |
| $\overline{\overline{aa}}$ | of each |
| AA | Alcoholics Anonymous |
| ab | abortion |
| abd | abdomen |
| ABG | arterial blood gas |
| ac | before meals |
| ACTH | adrenocorticotropic hormone |
| ADL | activities of daily living |
| ad lib | as desired |
| adm | admission |
| ADT | admission, discharge, transfer |
| AFB | acid-fast bacillus |
| AgNO$_3$ | silver nitrate |
| alb | albumin |
| alka phos | alkaline phosphatase |
| alt dieb | alternate days (every other day) |
| alt hor | alternate hours |
| alt noct | alternate nights |
| ALS | amyotrophic lateral sclerosis |

| COMMON MEDICAL ABBREVIATIONS | DEFINITION |
|---|---|
| AM | between midnight and noon |
| AMA | against medical advice |
| amb | ambulate, ambulatory |
| amp | ampule |
| amt | amount |
| ant | anterior |
| AP | anterior-posterior |
| A&P | auscultation and percussion |
| aq | aqueous |
| ARDS | adult respiratory disease syndrome |
| ARM | artificial rupture of membranes |
| ASA | aspirin |
| ASAP | as soon as possible |
| as tol | as tolerated |
| AV | arteriovenous |
| ax | axillary |
| BE | barium enema |
| bid | twice a day |
| BK | below knee |
| BM | bowel movement |
| BP | blood pressure |
| BR | bedrest |
| BRP | bathroom privileges |
| BS | blood sugar, bowel sounds, breath sounds |
| c̄ | with |
| C | Celsius |
| Ca | calcium |
| CABG | coronary artery bypass graft |

| COMMON MEDICAL ABBREVIATIONS | DEFINITION |
|---|---|
| cal | calorie |
| cap | capsule |
| CAPD | continuous ambulatory peritoneal dialysis |
| CAT | computed axial tomography |
| cath | catheter, catheterize |
| CBC | complete blood count |
| CBR | complete bed rest |
| CC | chief complaint |
| CC | colony count |
| CCU | coronary care unit |
| CEA | carcinoma embryonic antigen |
| CHO | carbohydrate |
| chol | cholesterol |
| CIP | computerized impedance plethysmography |
| circ | circumcision |
| cl | clinic |
| Cl | chloride |
| cl liq | clear liquid |
| cm | centimeter |
| CMV | cytomegalovirus |
| CNS | central nervous system |
| c/o | complains of |
| CO | carbon monoxide |
| $CO_2$ | carbon dioxide |
| comp | compound |
| cond | condition |
| CPK | creatine phosphokinase |
| CPR | cardiopulmonary resuscitation |
| CRNA | certified registered nurse-anesthetist |
| C&S | culture and sensitivity |

**COMMON**
**MEDICAL**
**ABBREVIATIONS**     **DEFINITION**

| | |
|---|---|
| CSF | cerebrospinal fluid |
| CSR | central service room |
| CT | computed tomography |
| Cu | copper |
| CVA | cerebrovascular accident |
| CVP | central venous pressure |
| cx | cervix |
| CXR | chest x-ray film |
| DAT | diet as tolerated |
| DC | discontinued |
| del | delivery |
| diff | differential (part of complete blood count) |
| disch | discharge |
| DOA | dead on arrival |
| dr | dram |
| DRG | diagnosis-related groupings |
| D/S | dextrose in saline |
| DVT | deep-vein thrombosis |
| DW | distilled water |
| D/W | dextrose in water |
| Dx | diagnosis |
| E | enema |
| EBL | estimated blood loss |
| ECG | electrocardiogram |
| ECT | electroconvulsive therapy |
| EDC | expected date of confinement |
| EEG | electroencephalogram |
| EENT | eye, ear, nose, and throat |
| EGD | esophagogastroduodenoscopy |
| EKG | electrocardiogram |
| elix | elixir |
| EMG | electromyogram |

**COMMON**
**MEDICAL**
**ABBREVIATIONS**          **DEFINITION**

ENG . . . . . . . .   electronystagmography

ENT . . . . . . . .   ear, nose, and throat

ER. . . . . . . . . .   emergency room

ESR. . . . . . . . .   erythrocyte sedimentation rate

ESWL . . . . . . . .   extracorporeal shock-wave
                          lithotripsy

etiol . . . . . . . .   etiology

exam . . . . . . . .   examination

ext. . . . . . . . . .   extract

ext. . . . . . . . . .   external

F . . . . . . . . . . .   Fahrenheit

FBS. . . . . . . . .   fasting blood sugar

Fe . . . . . . . . . .   iron

FHT . . . . . . . .   fetal heart tones

Fr . . . . . . . . . .   French (catheter size)

FSH . . . . . . . .   follicle-stimulating hormone

FTT . . . . . . . .   failure to thrive

Fx . . . . . . . . . .   fracture

g . . . . . . . . . . .   gram

GB . . . . . . . . .   gall bladder

GI . . . . . . . . . .   gastrointestinal

gtt . . . . . . . . . .   drop

GTT . . . . . . . .   glucose tolerance test

GU . . . . . . . . .   genitourinary

Gyn. . . . . . . . .   gynecology

h . . . . . . . . . . .   hour

H . . . . . . . . . .   hypodermic

H&H. . . . . . . .   hemoglobin and hematocrit

HCl. . . . . . . . .   hydrochloric acid

$HCO_3$ . . . . . . .   bicarbonate

Hct . . . . . . . . .   hematocrit

Hg . . . . . . . . .   mercury

hgb . . . . . . . . .   hemoglobin

**COMMON
MEDICAL
ABBREVIATIONS**    **DEFINITION**

| | |
|---|---|
| $H_2O$ | water |
| $H_2O_2$ | hydrogen peroxide (hydrogen dioxide) |
| HOB | head of bed |
| H&P | history and physical |
| hs | hour of sleep (bedtime) |
| ht | height |
| Hx | history |
| hypo | hypodermic |
| IBS | irritable bowel syndrome |
| ICU | intensive care unit |
| IM | intramuscular |
| I&O | intake and output |
| IPPB | intermittent positive pressure breathing |
| irrig | irrigation |
| isol | isolation |
| IUD | intrauterine device |
| IV | intravenous |
| IVC | intravenous cholangiogram |
| IVP | intravenous pyelogram |
| K | potassium |
| KCl | potassium chloride |
| kg | kilogram |
| KO | keep open |
| KUB | kidneys, ureters, bladder |
| KVO | keep vein open |
| L | liter |
| lab | laboratory |
| lac | laceration |
| lap | laparotomy |
| lat | lateral |
| L&D | labor and delivery |

| COMMON MEDICAL ABBREVIATIONS | DEFINITION |
|---|---|
| LDH | lactic dehydrogenase |
| lg | large |
| LLL | left lower lobe |
| LLQ | left lower quadrant |
| LMP | last menstrual period |
| LP | lumbar puncture |
| LPN | licensed practical nurse |
| LR | lactated Ringer's (IV solution) |
| lt | left |
| LUL | left upper lobe |
| LUQ | left upper quadrant |
| μg | microgram |
| MCH | mean corpuscular hemoglobin |
| MCV | mean corpuscular volume |
| mEq | millequivalent |
| mg | milligram |
| mL | milliliter |
| mm | millimeter |
| MOM | milk of magnesia |
| MRI | magnetic resonance imaging |
| MS | morphine sulfate |
| MS | multiple sclerosis |
| Na | sodium |
| NA | nursing assistant |
| NaCl | sodium chloride (salt) |
| NAS | no added salt |
| NB | newborn |
| neg | negative |
| neuro | neurology |
| NG | nasogastric |
| NICU | neurological intensive care unit, neonatal intensive care unit |

| COMMON MEDICAL ABBREVIATIONS | DEFINITION |
|---|---|
| noc | night |
| noct. | night |
| NPO | nothing by mouth |
| NS. | normal saline |
| NSR | normal sinus rhythm |
| N&V | nausea and vomiting |
| NVS | neuro vital signs |
| $O_2$ | oxygen |
| OB | obstetrics |
| OD | right eye |
| OD | overdose |
| oint | ointment |
| OOB | out of bed |
| OP | outpatient |
| Ophth | ophthalmic |
| OR | operating room |
| Ortho | orthopedic |
| OS. | left eye |
| OSA | obstructive sleep apnea |
| OT | occupational therapy |
| OU | both eyes |
| oz | ounce |
| p̄ | after |
| P | phosphorus |
| PA. | physician's assistant |
| PA. | posterior-anterior |
| pc | after meals |
| PCP. | pneumocystis carinii pneumonia |
| PCU | progressive care unit |
| PCV | packed cell volume |
| PDR | *Physician's Desk Reference* |
| Peds | pediatrics |

| COMMON MEDICAL ABBREVIATIONS | DEFINITION |
|---|---|
| PEEP | positive end expiratory pressure |
| per | by |
| PERLA | pupils equal, reactive to light and accommodation |
| PET | positron emission tomography |
| PICU | pediatric intensive care unit |
| PKU | phenylketonuria |
| PM | between noon and midnight |
| PNS | peripheral nervous system |
| PO | orally |
| PO | postoperative |
| PO | phone order |
| post-op | postoperatively |
| PP | postpartum |
| PP | postprandial (after meals) |
| PPD | purified protein derivative |
| PRBC | packed red blood cells |
| PRN | whenever necessary |
| pro time | prothrombin time |
| pt | patient |
| pt | pint |
| PT | physical therapy |
| PTCA | percutaneous transluminal coronary angioplasty |
| PTT | partial thromboplastin time |
| PUL | percutaneous ultrasound lithotripsy |
| q | every |
| qd | every day |
| q—h | every [number] hour (example: q2h) |
| qid | four times a day |
| qn | every night |

| COMMON MEDICAL ABBREVIATIONS | DEFINITION |
|---|---|
| qod | every other day |
| qoh | every other hour |
| qt | quart |
| R | rectal |
| RBC | red blood count |
| reg | regular |
| REM | rapid eye movement |
| resp. | respirations |
| RLL | right lower lobe |
| RLQ | right lower quadrant |
| RN | registered nurse |
| R/O | rule out |
| ROM | range of motion |
| RR | recovery room |
| rt. | right |
| rt. | routine |
| RT | respiratory therapy |
| RUL | right upper lobe |
| Rx | prescription |
| s̄ | without |
| sc. | subcutaneous |
| SICU | surgical intensive care unit |
| SLE | systemic lupus erythematosus |
| SMAC | sequential multiple analysis computer |
| ss | one-half |
| SSE | soap suds enema |
| stat | immediately |
| subq | subcutaneous |
| supp | suppository |
| surg. | surgical |
| SVN | small volume nebulizer |
| tab. | tablet |

| COMMON MEDICAL ABBREVIATIONS | DEFINITION |
|---|---|
| TAT | tetanus antitoxin |
| TCDB | turn, cough, deep breathe |
| TCT | thrombin clotting time |
| temp | temperature |
| TIA | transient ischemic attack |
| tid | three times a day |
| tinct | tincture |
| TLC | tender loving care |
| TO | telephone order |
| TPN | total parenteral nutrition |
| tr | tincture |
| trach | tracheostomy |
| TWE | tap water enema |
| Tx | traction |
| U | unit |
| UGI | upper gastrointestinal |
| Ung | ointment |
| UTI | urinary tract infection |
| vag | vaginal |
| VDRL | Venereal Disease Research Laboratory |
| VS | vital signs |
| WA | while awake |
| WBC | white blood count |
| W/C | wheelchair |
| wt | weight |

| ABBREVIATION OF DIAGNOSIS OR SURGICAL PROCEDURE | DEFINITION |
|---|---|
| ABE | acute bacterial endocarditis |
| AFIB | atrial fibrillation |
| AHD | arteriosclerotic heart disease |
| AI | aortic insufficiency |

| ABBREVIATION OF DIAGNOSIS OR SURGICAL PROCEDURE | DEFINITION |
|---|---|
| AIDS | acquired immune deficiency syndrome |
| AKA | above-knee amputation |
| ALL | acute lymphocytic leukemia |
| ALS | amyotrophic lateral sclerosis |
| AMI | acute myocardial infarction |
| AML | acute myelocytic leukemia |
| AOD | adult-onset diabetes |
| AP | angina pectoris |
| ARDS | acute respiratory distress syndrome |
| ASCVD | arteriosclerotic cardiovascular disease |
| ASD | atrial septal defect |
| ASHD | arteriosclerotic heart disease |
| AUL | acute undifferentiated leukemia |
| AVR | aortic valve replacement |
| BA | bronchial asthma |
| BBB | bundle branch block |
| BKA | below-knee amputation |
| BOM | bilateral otitis media |
| BPH | benign prostatic hypertrophy |
| BSO | bilateral salpingo-oophorectomy |
| CA | cancer, carcinoma |
| CABG | coronary artery bypass graft |
| CAD | coronary artery disease |
| CBS | chronic brain syndrome |
| CDH | congenital dislocation of the hip |
| CF | cystic fibrosis |
| CHB | complete heart block |
| CHD | coronary heart disease |

| ABBREVIATION OF DIAGNOSIS OR SURGICAL PROCEDURE | DEFINITION |
|---|---|
| CHF . . . . . . . . | congestive heart failure |
| CI . . . . . . . . . | coronary insufficiency |
| CLD . . . . . . . . | chronic liver disease |
| CLL . . . . . . . . | chronic lymphocytic leukemia |
| CML . . . . . . . . | chronic myelogenous leukemia |
| COLD . . . . . . . | chronic obstructive lung disease |
| COPD . . . . . . . | chronic obstructive pulmonary disease |
| CP . . . . . . . . . | cerebral palsy |
| CPD . . . . . . . . | cephalopelvic disproportion |
| CPN . . . . . . . . | chronic pyelonephritis |
| CRD . . . . . . . . | chronic respiratory disease |
| C-section . . . . . . | cesarean section |
| CVA . . . . . . . . | cerebrovascular accident |
| D&C . . . . . . . . | dilatation and curettage |
| DIC . . . . . . . . | diffuse intravascular coagulation |
| DLE . . . . . . . . | discoid lupus erythematosus |
| DM . . . . . . . . . | diabetes mellitus |
| DT . . . . . . . . . | delirium tremens |
| DVT . . . . . . . . | deep vein thrombosis |
| EP . . . . . . . . . | ectopic pregnancy |
| ERCP . . . . . . . | endoscopic retrograde cholangiopancreatography |
| FUO . . . . . . . . | fever of undetermined origin |
| GC . . . . . . . . . | gonorrhea |
| GSW . . . . . . . . | gunshot wound |
| HB . . . . . . . . . | heart block |
| HCVD . . . . . . . | hypertensive cardiovascular disease |
| HMD . . . . . . . | hyaline membrane disease |
| HNP . . . . . . . . | herniated nucleus pulposus |

| ABBREVIATION OF DIAGNOSIS OR SURGICAL PROCEDURE | DEFINITION |
|---|---|
| IBS . . . . . . . . . | irritable bowel syndrome |
| IDDM . . . . . . . | insulin dependent diabetes mellitus |
| I&D . . . . . . . . . | incision and drainage |
| IHD . . . . . . . . | ischemic heart disease |
| LE . . . . . . . . . . | lupus erythematosus |
| LTB . . . . . . . . | laryngotracheobronchitis |
| MD . . . . . . . . . | muscular dystrophy |
| MI . . . . . . . . . . | myocardial infarction |
| MM . . . . . . . . . | multiple myeloma |
| MS . . . . . . . . . | multiple sclerosis |
| MVP . . . . . . . . | mitral valve prolapse |
| OD . . . . . . . . . | overdose |
| OSA . . . . . . . . | obstructive sleep apnea |
| PAC . . . . . . . . | premature atrial contractions |
| PAT . . . . . . . . | paroxysmal atrial tachycardia |
| PCP . . . . . . . . . | pneumocystis carinii pneumonia |
| PD . . . . . . . . . . | Parkinson's disease |
| PDA . . . . . . . . | patent ductus arteriosus |
| PID . . . . . . . . . | pelvic inflammatory disease |
| PKU . . . . . . . . | phenylketonuria |
| PTCA . . . . . . . . | percutaneous transluminal coronary angioplasty |
| PVC . . . . . . . . | premature ventricular contractions |
| PVD . . . . . . . . | peripheral vascular disease |
| RA . . . . . . . . . . | rheumatoid arthritis |
| RDS . . . . . . . . | respiratory distress syndrome |
| RHD . . . . . . . . | rheumatic heart disease |
| SBE . . . . . . . . . | subacute bacterial endocarditis |
| SIDS . . . . . . . . | sudden infant death syndrome |

| ABBREVIATION OF DIAGNOSIS OR SURGICAL PROCEDURE | DEFINITION |
|---|---|
| SLE | systemic lupus erythematosus |
| SMR | submucous resection |
| SO | salpingo-oophorectomy |
| STAPH | staphylococcus |
| STD | sexually transmitted disease |
| STREP | streptococcus |
| SVD | spontaneous vaginal delivery |
| T&A | tonsillectomy and adenoidectomy |
| TAH | total abdominal hysterectomy |
| TB | tuberculosis |
| TIA | transient ischemic attack |
| TUR | transurethral resection |
| TURP | transurethral resection of prostate gland |
| TVH | total vaginal hysterectomy |
| UGI | upper gastrointestinal |
| UPPP | uvulopalatopharyngoplasty |
| URI | upper respiratory disease |
| UTI | urinary tract infection |
| VD | venereal disease |

# Appendix E

## Common Plural Endings for Medical Terms

In the English language one often forms plurals by simply adding *s* or *es* to the word. Forming plurals in the language of medicine is not so simple. Use the table below to learn the standard plural formation of medical terms.

| SINGULAR ENDING | PLURAL ENDING | EXAMPLE SINGULAR | PLURAL |
|---|---|---|---|
| -a | -ae | vertebra | vertebrae |
| -ax | -aces | thorax | thoraces |
| -ex | -ices | apex | apices |
| -is | -es | pubis | pubes |
| -ix | -es | cervix | cervices |
| -ma | -mata | sarcoma | sarcomata |
| -on | -a | ganglion | ganglia |
| -um | -a | ovum | ova |
| -us | -i | alveolus | alveoli |
| -y | -ies | biopsy | biopsies |

# Bibliography

American Medical Association: *Family medical guide,* New York, 1982, Random House.

Anthony CP and Thibodeau GA: *Structure and function of the body,* ed 7, St. Louis, 1984, Mosby.

Austrin MG and Austrin HR: *Young's learning medical terminology,* ed 6, St. Louis, 1987, Mosby.

Ballinger PW: *Merrill's atlas of radiographic positions and radiologic procedures,* ed 7, St. Louis, 1991, Mosby.

Behea DC: *Introductory maternity nursing,* ed 3, New York, 1979, JB Lippincott.

Bevan J: *The Simon and Schuster handbook of anatomy and physiology,* New York, 1978, Simon & Schuster.

Bickerton J and Small JC: *Neurology for nurses,* Baltimore, 1982, University Park Press.

Borror DJ: *Dictionary of word roots and combining forms,* Mountain View, Calif, 1960, Mayfield Publishing.

Brooks SM and Paynton-Brooks N: *The human body: structure and function in health and disease,* ed 2, St. Louis, 1980, Mosby.

Brunner LS and Suddarth DS: *Textbook of medical-surgical nursing,* ed 4, Philadelphia, 1980, JB Lippincott.

Brunner TF and Berkowitz L: *The elements of scientific and specialized terminology,* Minneapolis, 1967, Burgess Publishing.

Butnarescu GF and Tillotson DM: *Maternity nursing: theory to practice,* New York, 1983, John Wiley & Sons.

Chabner D: *The language of medicine,* ed 4, Philadelphia, 1991, WB Saunders.

Clinical highlights irritable bowel syndrome, *Hospital Medicine,* p 41, June 1992.

*Dorland's illustrated medical dictionary,* ed 27, Philadelphia, 1988 WB Saunders.

Frenay MA: *Understanding medical terminology,* ed 3, St. Louis, 1964, The Catholic Hospital Association.

Gilroy J and Holliday PL: *Basic neurology,* New York, 1982, Macmillan Publishing.

Gylys BA and Wedding ME: *Medical terminology,* Philadelphia, 1983, FA Davis.

Hamilton WJ, editor: *Textbook of human anatomy,* ed 2, St. Louis, 1976, Mosby.

Jacobs SW and Francone CA: *Structure and function in man,* ed 2, Philadelphia, 1970, WB Saunders.

Jaeger EC: *A source book of medical terms,* Springfield, Ill, 1953, Charles C Thomas, Publisher.

Jensen M and others: *Maternity care: the nurse and the family,* ed 2, St. Louis, 1981, Mosby.

Juneau PS: *Maternal and child nursing,* New York, 1979, Macmillan Publishing.

Lewis C: *Medical Latin,* Francestown, NH, 1948, Marshall Jones.

Long BC and Phipps WJ: *Medical-surgical nursing,* ed 2, St. Louis, 1989, Mosby.

Luckman J and Sorensen KC: *Medical-surgical nursing: a psycho-physiological approach,* ed 3, Philadelphia, 1987, WB Saunders.

Meeker MH and Rothrock JC: *Alexander's care of the patient in surgery,* ed 9, St. Louis, 1991, Mosby.

*Melloni's illustrated medical dictionary,* Baltimore, 1979, The Williams & Wilkins Co.

Memmler RL and Wood DL: *Structure and function of the human body,* ed 2, Philadelphia, 1977, JB Lippincott.

Miller and Keane: *Encyclopedia and dictionary of medicine, nursing, and allied health*, Philadelphia, 1987, WB Saunders.

*Mosby's medical, nursing, & allied health dictionary*, ed 3, St. Louis, 1990, Mosby.

*Mosby medical encyclopedia*, New York, 1985, New American Library.

Phipps WJ, Long BC, and Woods NF: *Shafer's medical-surgical nursing*, ed 7, St. Louis, 1980, Mosby.

Phipps WJ and others: *Medical surgical nursing*, ed 4, St. Louis, 1991, Mosby.

Prendergast A: *Medical terminology: a text/workbook*, ed 2, Menlo Park, Calif, 1983, Addison-Wesley Publishing.

Roberts F: *Medical terms: their origin and construction*, ed 4, London, 1966, William Heinemann Medical Books.

Saunders WH and others: *Nursing care in eye, ear, nose, and throat disorders*, ed 4, St. Louis, 1979, Mosby.

Septowitz KA and others: Pneumocystis carinii pneumonia among patients without AIDS at a cancer hospital, JAMA 267:6, p 832, 1992.

Skydell B and Crowder AS: *Diagnostic procedures*, Boston, 1975, Little, Brown & Co.

Sloane SB: *A word book in oncology and hematology*, St. Louis, 1992, Mosby.

Sloane SB: *The medical word book*, ed 3, Philadelphia, 1991, WB Saunders.

Smith BC and Smith BE: *Medical terminology for the health professions*, Orlando, 1986, Academic Press.

Smith GL and Davis PE: *Medical terminology: a programmed text*, ed 4, New York, 1963, John Wiley & Sons.

Spearman CB, Sheldon RL, and Egan DF: *Egan's fundamentals of respiratory therapy*, ed 4, 1982, Mosby.

*Springhouse diagnostics nurse's reference library*, ed 2, Springhouse, Pa, 1986, Springhouse Corp.

*Springhouse diagnostic tests nurse's ready reference*, Springhouse, Pa, 1991, Springhouse Corp.

*Springhouse treatments nurse's reference library*, Springhouse, Pa, 1988, Springhouse Corp.

Stark DD and Bradley WG: *Magnetic resonance imaging*, ed 2, St. Louis, 1991, Mosby.

*Taber's cyclopedic medical dictionary*, ed 15, Philadelphia, 1985, FA Davis.

Tampinco-Golos I: Endoscopic thoracotomy, a new approach to thoracic surgery, *Assoc Operat Room Nurs J* 55:5, p 1167, 1992.

Taylor JW and Ballenger S: *Neurological dysfunctions and nursing intervention*, New York, 1980, McGraw-Hill Book.

Tilkian SM, Conover MB, and Tilkian AG: *Clinical implications of laboratory tests*, ed 3, St. Louis, 1983, Mosby.

*Urdang dictionary of current medical terms*, New York, 1981, John Wiley & Sons.

Wain H: *The story behind the words*, Springfield, Ill, 1958, Charles C Thomas, Publisher.

*Webster's medical desk dictionary*, Massachusetts, 1986, Merriam-Webster.

White DP: Obstructive sleep apnea, *Hosp Prac*, p 57, May 30, 1992.

White RA and Stanley RK: *Endoscopic surgery*, St. Louis, 1991, Mosby.

White WF: *Language of the health sciences*, New York, 1977, John Wiley & Sons.

Wroble MW: *Terminology for the health professions*, Philadelphia, 1982, JB Lippincott.

# Index

| | |
|---|---|
| **xanth/o**<br><br>COMBINING FORM | **leuk/o**<br><br>COMBINING FORM |
| **viscer/o**<br><br>COMBINING FORM | **eti/o**<br><br>COMBINING FORM |
| **somat/o**<br><br>COMBINING FORM | **cancer/o**<br><br>COMBINING FORM |
| **organ/o**<br><br>COMBINING FORM | **kary/o**<br><br>COMBINING FORM |
| **epitheli/o**<br><br>COMBINING FORM | **carcin/o**<br><br>COMBINING FORM |
| **erythr/o**<br><br>COMBINING FORM | **onc/o**<br><br>COMBINING FORM |
| **lei/o**<br><br>COMBINING FORM | **cyan/o**<br><br>COMBINING FORM |

white **leuk/o**

yellow **xanth/o**

cause (of disease)
**eti/o**

internal organs **viscer/o**

cancer **cancer/o**

body **somat/o**

nucleus **kary/o**

organ **organ/o**

cancer **carcin/o**

epithelium **epitheli/o**

tumor **onc/o**

red **erythr/o**

blue **cyan/o**

smooth **lei/o**

| | |
|---|---|
| **sarc/o**<br><br>COMBINING FORM | **lip/o**<br><br>COMBINING FORM |
| **system/o**<br><br>COMBINING FORM | **chrom/o**<br><br>COMBINING FORM |
| **cyt/o**<br><br>COMBINING FORM | **hist/o**<br><br>COMBINING FORM |
| **path/o**<br><br>COMBINING FORM | **neur/o**<br><br>COMBINING FORM |
| **my/o**<br><br>COMBINING FORM | **-oma**<br><br>SUFFIX |
| **melan/o**<br><br>COMBINING FORM | **-osis**<br><br>SUFFIX |
| **rhabd/o**<br><br>COMBINING FORM | **-ous**<br><br>SUFFIX |

fat **lip/o**

flesh, connective tissue **sarc/o**

color **chrom/o**

system **system/o**

tissue **hist/o**

cell **cyt/o**

nerve **neur/o**

disease **path/o**

tumor, swelling **-oma**

muscle **my/o**

abnormal condition (means increased when used with blood cell word roots) **-osis**

black **melan/o**

pertaining to **-ous**

rod shaped, striated **rhabd/o**

# gnos/o

# iatr/o

# sis

knowledge   **gnos/o**

medicine, physician
**iatr/o**

state of   **sis**

| | |
|---|---|
| **-pathy**<br><br>SUFFIX | **-genic**<br><br>SUFFIX |
| **-plasia**<br><br>SUFFIX | **-ic**<br><br>SUFFIX |
| **-sarcoma**<br><br>SUFFIX | **-oid**<br><br>SUFFIX |
| **-genesis**<br><br>SUFFIX | **-ologist**<br><br>SUFFIX |
| **-al**<br><br>SUFFIX | **-ology**<br><br>SUFFIX |
| **-cyte**<br><br>SUFFIX | **-stasis**<br><br>SUFFIX |
| **-gen**<br><br>SUFFIX | **-plasm**<br><br>SUFFIX |

producing, originating, causing
**-genic**

disease **-pathy**

pertaining to **-ic**

formation, development, a growth **-plasia**

resembling **-oid**

malignant tumor **-sarcoma**

one who studies and practices (specialist, physician) **-ologist**

origin, cause **-genesis**

study of **-ology**

pertaining to **-al**

control, stop **-stasis**

cell **-cyte**

wth, substance ation) **-plasm**

substance or agent that produces or causes **-gen**